Pathophysiology
Applied to Nursing Practice

Pathophysiology
Applied to Nursing Practice

ESTHER CHANG
JOHN DALY
DOUG ELLIOTT

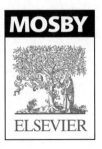

Sydney Edinburgh London New York Philadelphia St Louis Toronto

ELSEVIER

Mosby
is an imprint of Elsevier

Elsevier Australia
(a division of Reed International Books Australia Pty Ltd)
30–52 Smidmore Street, Marrickville, NSW 2204
ACN 001 002 357

This edition © 2006 Elsevier Australia

National Library of Australia Cataloguing-in-Publication Data

Pathophysiology applied to nursing practice.

  Includes index.
  For tertiary students.

  ISBN-13: 978-0-7295-3743-8
  ISBN-10: 0-7295-3743-9

1. Physiology, Pathological – Textbooks.   2. Nursing – Textbooks.
I. Chang, Esther May Lan.   II. Daly, John.
III. Elliott, Doug.   IV. Title.

616.07

Publishing Director: Vaughn Curtis
Developmental Editor: Suzanne Hall
Publishing Services Manager: Helena Klijn
Edited by Carolyn Beaumont
Proofread by Deborah McRitchie
Cover and internal design by Avril Makula
Illustrations by Lucia Diagraphics
Typeset by SNP Best-set Typesetter Ltd., Hong Kong
Indexed by Max McMaster
Printed in Australia by Ligare

Contents

Preface

One of the most challenging aspects of undergraduate nursing courses for students is the development of knowledge and understanding of pathophysiology, and the ability to apply this knowledge in practice. Sound nursing practice is based on careful clinical judgement. The capacity to engage in sound clinical judgement develops with experience, as long as this is supported by good skills in the application of relevant theory. Students need to master the theory in order to be able to apply it.

Many nursing texts that deal with pathophysiology are large, cumbersome and complex. This text has been designed to serve as a bridge to more complex theory for beginner nurses (years one to three), or for those embarking on a refresher course. The contributors have set out to make learning easier, applied and interesting. The book emphasises the clinical application of pathophysiological concepts in clinical practice, utilising relevant clinical case studies. Chapters in the book have been designed to facilitate access to concepts that need to be grasped in order to understand disease processes, and in order to facilitate holistic integration of concepts to develop understanding of rationales of nursing care. Concepts that are important in the treatment of a range of health breakdown problems are also included. The case studies build knowledge and understanding of pharmacology and the role of drug therapy in managing homeostatic irregularities.

We hope that you, as a student of nursing, find the book useful in your learning and development as a nurse. Remember good theory underpins good practice and has implications for the safety and quality of care of patients and clients.

Esther Chang
John Daly
Doug Elliott
Sydney June 2005

Contributors

Ms Vicki Baker RN, BN, Intensive Care Nursing Cert; Clinical Nurse; Shoalhaven District Memorial Hospital, Nowra, NSW

Dr Jennifer Blundell RN, CNN, BAppSc (Nursing), GradDipEd, PhD; Senior Lecturer; Faculty of Nursing and Midwifery, The University of Sydney, Sydney

Dr Ann Bonner RN, BAppSc (Nursing), MA, PhD, MRCNA; Senior Lecturer; School of Nursing, James Cook University, Townsville

Professor Sally Borbasi RN, BEd (Nursing), MA (Educ), PhD; School of Nursing and Midwifery, Griffith University, Adelaide

Ms Kate Cameron RN, MNSc; Department of Clinical Nursing, The University of Adelaide, Adelaide

Professor Esther Chang RN, CM, BAppSc (Adv Nursing), MEdAdmin, PhD, FCN (NSW); Director of Research; School of Nursing, Family and Community Health, University of Western Sydney, Sydney

Ms Kerry Chouzadjian RN, RM, BEd, MEd; Midwifery Educator; Women's and Children's Program, Monash Medical Centre, Melbourne

Dr Fiona Coyer RN, RM, ENB100, PGCEA, MSc (Nursing), PhD; Lecturer; School of Nursing, Queensland University of Technology, Brisbane

Professor Patrick Crookes PhD, BSc (Nursing), RGN (UK), RN (NSW), RNT, CertEd; Head of Department; Faculty of Health & Behavioural Science, University of Wollongong, Wollongong

Professor David Currow BMed, MPH, FRACP; Professor of Palliative & Supportive Services; School of Medicine, Flinders University of South Australia, Adelaide

Professor John Daly RN, BA, BHSc (Nursing), MEd (Hons), PhD, FCN (NSW), FINE, FRCNA; Foundation Head; School of Nursing, Family and Community Health, University of Western Sydney, Sydney

Associate Professor Patricia Davidson RN, BA, MEd, PhD; Clinical Nursing Research Unit (conjoint position); School of Nursing, Family and Community Health, University of Western Sydney and Sydney West Area Health Service, Sydney

Ms Kathleen Dixon RN, BA, MHAdmin; Lecturer; School of Nursing, Family and Community Health, University of Western Sydney, Sydney

Mr Malcolm Elliott DipHSc(Nursing), BN, MNurs, GradCert (Intensive Care), GradCert (Cardiac Nursing), GradCert (NursEd); Lecturer; Faculty of Health & Behavioural Science, University of Wollongong, Wollongong

Mr Scott Fanker Senior Nurse Manager; Area Mental Health, Sydney South West Area Health Service; and Senior Lecturer; University of Western Sydney, Sydney

Ms Janet Forber RN, BSci (BioChem), MSci; Clinical Nurse Consultant, Infection Control; Liverpool Health Service, Sydney

Dr Daniella Goldberg PhD, DipComm; Science Journalist; Gene Genie Media, Sydney

Dr Karen Hancock BSc (Psych) (Hons), PhD; Research Associate; School of Nursing, Family and Community Health, University of Western Sydney, Sydney

Ms Kathleen Harrison RN, BHSc; Area Director; Stream of Chronic & Complex Care, Lawson Community Health Centre, Lawson, NSW

Ms Deborah Hatcher RN, DipTeach (Phys.Ed), BHSc (Nursing), MHPEd; Lecturer; School of Nursing, Family and Community Health, University of Western Sydney, Sydney

Associate Professor Cecily Hengstberger–Sims RN, DipEd, CCU Cert, BSocSc, PhD, MHPEd; Head of Programs; School of Nursing, Family and Community Health, University of Western Sydney, Sydney

Professor Debra Jackson RN, PhD; Professorial Fellow; School of Nursing, Family and Community Health, University of Western Sydney, Sydney

Ms Amanda Johnson RN, DipTeach (Nursing), MHScEd; Lecturer; School of Nursing, Family and Community Health, University of Western Sydney, Sydney

Mr Robert Johnson RN, BHA, CertOnc; Executive Care Manager; Carlingford Centre for Aged Care, Baptist Community Services NSW & ACT, Sydney

Dr Linda Jones RN, CM, BAppSc (Nursing), GradDipEd (Nursing), MNA; Midwifery Programs Coordinator; Department of Nursing and Midwifery, Royal Melbourne Institute of Technology, Melbourne

Ms Kathleen Kilstoff RN, BA, DipEd, MA, FCN; Senior Lecturer; Faculty of Nursing, Midwifery and Health, University of Technology Sydney, Sydney

Ms Jane Koch RGN (UK), RN (NSW), RNT (UK), MA; Lecturer; School of Nursing, Family and Community Health, University of Western Sydney, Sydney

Dr Maria Cynthia Leigh RN, BSc, GradDipAppSc, PhD; Head of School; School of Nursing, Australian Catholic University, Sydney

Dr Dominic Leung MBBS, FRACP, PhD; Staff Cardiologist; Cardiology Department, Liverpool Hospital, Sydney South West Area Health Service, Sydney

Ms Julie Lewin MCogSc, BSc, RN, DipIntCareSc (Hons), MACE; formerly Lecturer; School of Arts and Science, NSW, Australian Catholic University, Sydney

Ms Megan Luhr-Taylor RN, DipAppSc, GradCert (Pall Care), GradCert (Onc Nursing); Clinical Nurse Consultant Palliative Care; Wentworth Area Health Service, Wentworth, NSW

Associate Professor Louise O'Brien RN, BA, PhD; School of Nursing, Family and Community Health, University of Western Sydney and Sydney West Area Health Service, Sydney

Professor Ian Olver MD, PhD, FRACP, MRACMA; Clinical Director; Royal Adelaide Hospital Cancer Centre, Adelaide

Ms Fran Owen RN, GradCert (PCN), GradCert (ON); Clinical Nurse Consultant; Cancer Care Services, Wollongong Hospital, Wollongong

Ms Joanne Ramsbotham RN, RM, GradCertAdultEd, MNursing (Child Health); Lecturer; School of Nursing, Queensland University of Technology, Brisbane

Dr Kathy Robinson BSc (Med) (Hons), PhD; Senior Lecturer; School of Arts and Sciences, Australian Catholic University, Sydney

Dr Yenna Salamonson RN, GradDipNsgEd, BSc, MA, PhD; Lecturer; School of Nursing, Family and Community Health, University of Western Sydney, Sydney

Dr John Sibbald BSc (Hons), PhD; Senior Lecturer; Faculty of Health & Behavioural Science, University of Wollongong, Wollongong

Dr Melissa Sinfield RN, BHSc (Nursing) (Hons), PhD; Lecturer (Aged Care Research); School of Nursing, Family and Community Health, University of Western Sydney and Our Lady of Consolation Aged Care Service, Sydney

Ms Ana Smith RN, CM, BA, MA (Education and Work); Director of Teaching and Learning, Senior Lecturer; School of Nursing, Family and Community Health, University of Western Sydney, Sydney

Ms Charlotte Thompson RN, BN; Clinician Nurse Educator; Emergency Department, Palmerston North Hospital, Palmerston North, NZ

Ms Yvonne White RN, RMN, RMCftN, RenalCert, BN, MN (Hons); Lecturer; Faculty of Health & Behavioural Science, University of Wollongong, Wollongong

Ms Kim van Wissen BN, BSc, MA; Lecturer; School of Health Sciences, Massey University, Wellington, NZ

About the Editors

Esther Chang RN, CM, BAppSc (Adv Nursing), MEdAdmin, PhD, FCN (NSW) is Professor of Nursing and Director of Research at the School of Nursing, Family and Community Health, University of Western Sydney. Esther has almost 25 years of clinical experience with an emphasis in aged care, and has held many senior leadership roles in the tertiary sector. She is also an active researcher and has published widely.

John Daly RN, BA, BHSc (Nursing), MEd (Hons), PhD, FCN (NSW), FINE, FRCNA is Professor of Nursing and Foundation Head of the School of Nursing, Family and Community Health at the University of Western Sydney. He has a clinical background in acute care nursing, and extensive experience as a leader and manager in nursing and higher education. John is also active in nursing research and has published extensively nationally and internationally.

Doug Elliott RN, PhD, MAppSc, BAppSc, IntCareCert, MCN has been a nursing academic for 20 years, most recently as a Clinical Professor at the University of Sydney. His clinical and research interests focus on critical care nursing. Doug publishes regularly in journals and has written 16 book chapters and has co-edited a nursing research text.

ACKNOWLEDGEMENTS

We would like to acknowledge a number of key people who contributed to and assisted us in the preparation of this book for publication. We extend our sincere thanks to the contributors for their scholarly, accessible, reality-based case studies. Our intention was to involve clinicians, academics and health professionals to produce a resource that is practical and useful for our readers. This book would not have been possible without them.

We are thankful for the assistance of Cheryl Bates, Patricia Corbett and Alison Sheppard at the University of Western Sydney who assisted us at various stages of development of the manuscript. We also extend our appreciation to Suzanne Hall and Vaughn Curtis and the rest of the team at Elsevier, who provided advice and support throughout the project.

Elsevier Australia and the editors would also like to thank Karen Scott, Moreton Institute of TAFE, and Jacinta Stewart, University of Tasmania, for their valuable feedback on the manuscript during the development of this edition.

1 | Health and Illness

AUTHORS

ESTHER CHANG

KAREN HANCOCK

ANA SMITH

LEARNING OBJECTIVES

When you have completed this chapter you will be able to explain
- The concepts of health and illness;
- The difference between illness and disease;
- How knowledge about the determinants of health and the aetiology of illness can assist in the prevention and treatment of disease and illness;
- How non-physical factors impact on health and illness and how this knowledge can increase a nurse's ability to provide appropriate care to a person who is ill;
- Various models of health and illness;
- The relationship between health, illness and individual attitudes toward health and health behaviours;
- Risk factors that predispose an individual to illness;
- Different ways individuals cope with illness;
- The role of the nurse in enabling health; and
- The role of the nurse in enhancing coping abilities in a person who is ill.

INTRODUCTION

Health and illness can be difficult concepts to define. Personal, cultural and social factors influence a person's ideas about the nature and meaning of health and illness so that definitions of health and illness vary from person to person. Cultural differences also affect how societies classify what is health and what is illness. Individual and cultural differences affect perceptions of how an illness is caused and treated. A person's perception of health and illness is socially constructed. For example, a person's social group may help that person recognise that they have a potential illness, and encourage them to seek health care. Long before there is a perception of illness, however, a person's family and cultural heritage will, among other things, have had a significant influence on the conduct and experience of various health issues: pregnancy and childbirth, the understanding of the role that food plays in the promotion of health, and the appropriate management of stressful situations[1]. What may be classed as an illness in one society may be viewed as quite normal in another society. For instance, until recent times, homosexuality was stigmatised by many people as a mental illness, requiring significant medical intervention[2]. Homosexuality is still considered unlawful in some societies[2].

In Australian Aboriginal and Torres Strait Island cultures, illness is a manifestation of spiritual, emotional and physical factors. Spiritual connections to the land and ancestors, as well as community relationships, particularly those with elders, have traditionally been central to health issues in Aboriginal and Torres Strait Islander peoples[3]. A recent qualitative study of health perceptions of an Aboriginal community in Australia confirmed that traditional Aboriginal beliefs regarding the concept of health and well-being still prevail[3]. The study found that well-being involved an interplay of identity, family and community kinship, culture and spirituality, and land. In 1999, the National Aboriginal Health Strategy defined Aboriginal people's perception of health in the following way:

> Health does not just mean the physical well-being of the individual but refers to the social, emotional, spiritual and cultural well-being of the whole community. This is a whole of life view and includes the cyclical concept of life-death-life[4].

It is argued that the fundamental cause of poor health among Aboriginal people is disempowerment, partly due to dispossession from land[3]. Thus, a multi-faceted approach to improving the health of Aboriginal people is needed that goes beyond treatment of physical symptoms of illness.

Similarly, the Māori people of New Zealand have poorer health compared with other New Zealanders[5]. The process of colonisation and the introduction of Western scientific medicine resulted in a suppression of traditional Māori medicine. The Māori philosophy towards health is based on a holistic approach, which encompasses spiritual, psychological, emotional, cultural, social, environmental, family aspects, and physical health. It has a long history and is characterised by oral transmission of knowledge, diversity of practice, and emphasis on the spiritual dimension of health[5]. For many Māori, the major deficiency in modern health services is *taha wairua* (spiritual dimension)[6]. Many Māori people are increasingly turning to their own traditional healers for health services, as they are more consistent with the way many Māori people view health and illness than is Western scientific medicine[5].

Educational differences, as well as class, gender and the structures within society, can influence an individual's perception of what constitutes illness and healthy behaviours[7]. In addition, personal perceptions can change over time: a child's definition of illness may alter by the time they reach adolescence, then again as an adult[8]. Health professionals may also have differing views of health and illness, with some regarding the concepts from a dualistic, biomedical perspective only (i.e., the mind and body are separate, with physical diseases located solely in the body)[9], while others take into account the social determinants of health and illness[10].

Although there are inherent difficulties in defining health and illness, it is important that nurses understand both these concepts because it influences their practice. For example, nurses need to be able to describe health and health problems when deciding if they can effectively manage an issue problem[8]. The practice of nursing is improved when nurses understand that their ideas of illness may differ from those of some of their clients. An appreciation of the reasons for a client's behaviour when ill allows nurses to appropriately accommodate the behaviour when implementing care[8]. A holistic understanding will better assist clients and their families in achieving optimal health. Enhancing wellness can improve quality of life, especially for those clients living with chronic illnesses or disabilities[8]. Being able to define illness also helps nurses to define our scope of practice and describe it to others[8]. Contemporary nursing practice involves provision of complex, holistic care in an environment where there is access to highly technological equipment and services. Consequently, it is important for the profession to develop and articulate its own perception of the meaning of health and illness[11,12].

This chapter, therefore, will also review concepts that are central to the meaning of health and illness:

- health as a holistic concept;
- the distinction between disease and illness;
- acute and chronic illnesses;
- disease categories;
- models of health and illness;
- coping with illness;
- illness behaviour;
- the impact of illness on the individual and the family; and
- how nurses enhance coping abilities in people who are ill.

Case studies with learning exercises are used to apply theory to practice.

WHAT IS HEALTH?

A number of concepts of health co-exist within current Western society and inform quite different approaches in the provision of health care. Early theories about health and illness proposed that the mind and body were connected. However, Descartes challenged this theory with the notion of dualism, where health was thought to exist only in the absence of disease, or where there has been medical cure of illness[13]. This medical model of health has existed for some time, but as this perspective does not begin to address the health inequities that exist throughout the world, the World Health Organization has advocated a holistic, social model of health as an alternative[14]. This model defines health as a multidimensional concept that is individually and socially constructed by the connection that exists between people's health choices, their 'social world' and the environment[15]. It is described as a fundamental human right that can only exist 'for all' in a socially just society. Health is not only the absence of disease but rather is

> the extent to which an individual or group is able on the one hand, to realise aspirations and satisfy needs, and on the other, to cope with and adapt to the environment. Health is seen as a positive concept, emphasising social and personal resources as well as physical capacity[16] (p. 1).

With reference to these definitions of health, consider the following examples from Wass[15] and think through who, in the following list, could be regarded as healthy. Would it be a person who

- Is free from disease but experiencing long-term grief?
- Has a serious chronic illness but is happy and lives an active life?
- Is free from disease but engages in risky behaviours?
- Is free from disease but is culturally isolated and depressed?
- Is living in poverty?

Nurses who view health from a holistic perspective are more likely to work with clients in a collaborative way, encouraging active participation in decision-making about how best to promote their client's health. This is a care rather than cure focus that also necessitates the inclusion of a client's social and family network[14,17].

WHAT IS ILLNESS?

Put simply, illness may be defined as a state of bad health or sickness[18] or a condition marked by deviation from the normal healthy state[19]. However, one of the limitations of defining an illness as a state identified by measurable deviations from the norm, is that a person with an amputated leg would be an example of someone who deviates from the norm. However, this person may adapt successfully to having a prosthesis, and therefore not be regarded as ill or disabled. According to Besson[20], there are six circumstances in which a person's health status does not easily fall under the category of 'healthy' or 'ill':

1. The person who feels well, but is in the early stages of an illness that will eventually manifest symptoms;
2. The person who feels well, but is exposed to risk factors, such as smoking;
3. The person who is temporarily overwhelmed by life's problems;
4. The physically well person who prefers the sick role;
5. The physically unwell person who refuses the sick role; and
6. The person who cannot be determined to be either sick or well, because he or she never presents for examination.

A more complex definition that considers more than the physical component, is that of illness as a process in which the functioning of a person is diminished or impaired in one or more dimensions (physical, emotional, intellectual, social, developmental, spiritual), when compared with the person's previous condition[21]. Central to this interpretation of illness is the meaning the person and their significant others give to living and coping with impairment or disablement[7].

THE DISTINCTION BETWEEN DISEASE AND ILLNESS

Although most people not working in health care would use the terms disease and illness interchangeably, health care professionals distinguish between the two terms. Suchman[12] suggests that disease is the medical condition defined in terms of medical and physiological functioning, while illness is a social response defined in terms of social functioning. According to the wellness–illness model[22], disease is an objective process, viewed as a dysfunction or alteration in functioning. It is measured by laboratory tests and direct observation. Illness is the human experience of the disease, affected by intrapersonal (e.g., personality, past experiences), interpersonal (social support, relationships) and extrapersonal (sociocultural and economic) factors[21].

The distinction between disease and illness is made clearer when one considers that two individuals may have the same disease, but different degrees of illness. Another example demonstrating the difference between the two is that a person may feel ill but there may be no disease identifiable, while another person may have a disease without feeling ill.

Boorse[23] views disease as an illness only if it is serious enough to be incapacitating, with social evaluations attached to it. An illness may be viewed as a subclass of diseases: a reasonably serious disease with incapacitating effects that make it undesirable. A person with a spinal injury may not feel ill, but on a physiological level, he or she has a disease/dysfunction. Another social connotation to illness is that when a disease is called an illness, the person is viewed as deserving special treatment and diminished moral accountability[23]. In terms of a nursing definition of illness, Wu[24] suggests that illness is best described as 'an event or happening that offers content for scientific observation and study, i.e., an experience that evokes a certain class of behaviours' (p. 6).

Mental illnesses also highlight the individual differences in definitions of illness. Weitz[25] contrasts the medical and sociological models of mental illness, suggesting that in the former, mental illness is a psychological, biological condition that requires medical treatment, while in the latter, the illness is thought to be socially as well as psychologically or biologically determined and thus may or may not respond to medical treatment. Like nurses and other health care professionals, lay people attribute their own meanings to mental illness. For example, one person may view depression as having a physical basis, while someone else may see it as a character weakness.

In summary, illness is not synonymous with disease. Disease may be classed as a physical response, while illness is a subjective experience; only the person can tell you whether or not he or she feels ill. Illness may or may not be detectable in terms of a pathological process. Disease, on the other hand, is a pathological process with verifiable, observable signs and symptoms that can change over time as the body struggles to maintain its equilibrium[26]. Disease has the potential to cause illness.

Nurses working in hospitals tend to focus on illness, which may include disease as well as its effects on functioning and all dimensions of well-being.[21] It is important that nurses determine how the patient experiences their own health state (i.e., whether they view themselves as ill) when planning care.

Case study

Ms Tsang, 35, sustained an incomplete spinal cord injury following a car accident. She requires medication for her skeletal muscle spasms, and self-catheterises to empty her bladder. However, she has adapted well enough to walk unaided, and leads a full life.

● Case study

Mrs Andrews experiences ongoing headaches that prevent her from being able to hold down a job. However, no identifiable cause has been found.

LEARNING EXERCISES

1. In what way(s) would you say Ms Tsang has a disease?
2. Would you say Ms Tsang has an illness? Why/why not?
3. To what extent would you consider Ms Tsang and Mrs Andrews to be healthy?
4. What nursing care could you offer Mrs Andrews?

BENEFITS OF ILLNESS

Craven and Hirnle[27] conceptualise illness as

> the body's way of signalling that a person has exceeded the natural capacity to mediate between the internal and external environments. Illness can be an opportunity to discover meaning in life and to heal, identifying areas of disharmony and determining how best to move toward a natural state of harmony (p. 259).

For some people, a positive aspect of being ill is the increased attention one receives. For others, it can mean a break from usual roles and responsibilities.

A simple exercise to identify the needs being met through illness is to

1. List the five most important benefits you received from an illness in your life;
2. Consider the needs that were met by your illness: relief from stress, love and attention, opportunity to renew energy, and so forth; and
3. Identify the rules or beliefs that limit you from meeting each of these needs when you are well[28].

ACUTE AND CHRONIC ILLNESSES

The incidence (number of cases with onset during a specific time period) and prevalence (total number of cases at any given point in time) of chronic diseases have increased since the beginning of the twentieth century. The reason is that fewer persons are dying from acute diseases. Decreases in deaths due to infectious diseases are due to improved sanitation, vaccines, and antibiotics[29]. Decreases in deaths are also due to effective treatments for some cancers[29]. Worldwide, the major causes of ill health and death today are heart disease, stroke, cancers and accidents[29].

An acute illness is one caused by a disease that produces symptoms and signs soon after exposure to the cause, that runs a short course, and from which there is usually a full recovery or an abrupt termination in death[29]. The symptoms usually have a rapid onset, are intense, and often subside after a short time period. Influenza is an example of an acute illness. A chronic illness is one caused by a disease that produces symptoms and signs within a variable time period, that runs a long course, and from which there is only partial recovery. A chronic illness usually persists longer than six months. An example is bronchiectasis. Criteria that may be used to define chronic conditions are: 1) the conditions were first noticed 3 months or more before the date of the interview, or 2) they belong to a group of conditions (including heart disease and diabetes) that are considered chronic, regardless of when they began[29] (p. 72).

These criteria are in accordance with the definition of the Commission on Chronic Illness[30], which views chronic illness as an impairment that is characterised by one or more of the following. The illness

1. Is permanent;
2. Leaves residual disability;
3. Is caused by nonreversible pathologic alteration; or
4. Requires a long period of supervision, observation or care.

Chronic physical conditions may be placed into the following categories: 1) selected skin and musculoskeletal conditions, 2) impairments (visual, hearing, speech, paralysis, deformity, or orthopaedic impairment), 3) selected digestive conditions, 4) selected conditions of the genitourinary, nervous, endocrine, metabolic, and blood and blood-forming systems, 5) selected circulatory conditions, and 6) selected respiratory conditions[29] (p. 72).

Acute attacks in chronic illness can also occur. An example is asthma, where the person has a chronic condition, but under certain conditions (e.g., viral) an acute asthma attack can be precipitated. The person requires more intensive medical treatment at this time, while at other times they will take preventive medication to reduce the occurrences of acute attacks.

The needs of patients, in terms of treatments and nursing care, and patients' responses to treatment recommendations, can be very different in a patient with an acute illness compared with a patient with a chronic illness.

DISEASE CATEGORIES

Diseases can be caused by disruptions to the body's structure or function. Some diseases have no known cause, and are called idiopathic. Diseases can be caused by

1. *Microorganisms.* Types of microorganisms causing infectious diseases include bacteria, fungi, viruses and protozoa. Some of the diseases produced by bacteria include whooping cough, tuberculosis, and *Salmonella* infections. Some examples of viral-induced diseases include acquired immune deficiency syndrome (AIDS), severe acute respiratory syndrome (SARS), and common coughs and colds;

2. *Inflammation*. Some pathogenic microorganisms cause other infections that produce inflammation of, for example, body organs such as the bronchi (bronchitis). An inflammatory response can also be triggered by allergy, extremes of cold or heat, and chemicals and friction. It can be acute or chronic;

3. *Trauma*. Trauma causes many types of wounds involving tissue and/or organs, and may cause sprains, fractures or paralysis. Thus the person may be rendered ill either temporarily or permanently;

4. *Insects transmitting disease*. Insects such as fleas, lice, mosquitoes and ticks can transmit diseases to humans through the microorganisms they carry (e.g., dengue fever, malaria);

5. *Genetic and developmental changes*. These are diseases that are caused by abnormalities in the genetic makeup of the individual, or abnormalities due to changes during embryonic and fetal development. This broad range of abnormalities ranges from congenital deformities to biochemical changes caused by genes that are expressed later in life under the influence of the environment (e.g., diabetes mellitus)[31];

6. *Degenerative process*. Degenerative processes in the tissues can change their structure and function, leading to illness;

7. *Hyperplasias and neoplasms*. These are diseases that have increases in the numbers of cells. Hyperplasia is 'a proliferative reaction to a prolonged external stimulus and will usually regress when the stimulus is removed'[31] (p. 5). Neoplasia results from 'a genetic change producing a single population of new (neoplastic) cells, which can proliferate beyond the degree allowed by the mechanisms that normally govern cell proliferation'[31] (p. 5). There are two types of neoplasms, benign and malignant. Malignancy refers to cancerous or diseased cells that have the capacity to spread, invade and destroy tissue[32]. The cells may occur in epithelial tissue (carcinoma) or connective tissue (sarcoma). Benign neoplasms remain localised to their region of origin;

8. *Internal causes*. There are three large categories of internal causes of disease, including vascular (obstruction of blood supply to an organ or tissue, bleeding, or altered blood flow); immunologic (caused by immune deficiency or allergy); or metabolic (abnormal metabolism or deficiency of lipid, carbohydrate, protein, mineral, vitamins, or fluids). Some examples of these diseases may also fall into other categories (e.g., metabolic diseases can be genetic in origin); or

9. *Stress*. Stress may be 'both a cause of illness and a determinant of illness behavior'[24] (p. 146). Stress is described as a state of disruption to the body's equilibrium[29].

Although these are the major categories of diseases, sociocultural, economic, environmental and psychological factors also can predispose people to illness. The distinction between functional and structural diseases becomes blurred when one considers the case of mental illness. Once considered a functional disease (i.e., where no structural abnormality is found), there is growing evidence of a genetic and/or biochemical basis to many types of mental illness[31]. The above clinical issues are discussed more fully in the following chapters.

STRESS AND ILLNESS

Hans Seyle first described the stress response in the 1950s, and this provides a link through which psychological factors can influence physical illness; for example, susceptibility to infection, leading to ulcers. Seyle described the process by which the body responded to the disruption (caused by stressors) as the General Adaptation Syndrome[26]. This syndrome is comprised of three stages: a) alarm reaction (otherwise known as 'fight or flight'); b) resistance; and c) exhaustion:

a) In the alarm phase, physiological reactions include the activation of the sympathetic nervous system by the hypothalamus, leading to increased blood and glucose supply to muscles, increased heart and respiratory rates and blood pressure, release of adrenocorticotrophic and antidiuretic hormones.[26] This hormonal activity can influence the immune system as both T-cells and B-cells have receptors for glucocorticoids, noradrenaline and adrenaline[33];

b) The body moves into the adaptation, resistance stage if the stress continues. Physiological reactions include increased sodium and water retention as a result of secretion of cortisol and an anti-inflammatory response to the release of aldosterone. A prolonged stage of resistance leads to 'diseases of adaptation'[34] (p. 117); and

c) The exhaustion stage is reached when the body is no longer capable of resisting the stress and cannot use coping mechanisms to return to a state of equilibrium[34]. The exhaustion phase results in pathology and disease if there has been no relief from the stress during the alarm reaction and resistance stages[26].

Not everybody believes that it is possible to identify a causal link between stress and illness. As stressed people may report more illnesses because they expect to be ill, the experience of illness may be worse under stress, or stress may cause illness-inducing behavioural changes rather than the illness itself (e.g., sleep deprivation, poor diet)[34].

As discussed above, there is now increasing evidence for the link between emotional factors such as stress and disease[35,36]. It is important to use this knowledge because preventing and treating illnesses effectively occurs only if the aetiology is understood. If a nurse understands how other variables influence illness, apart from physical factors, this can improve the care they provide to a person who is ill.

MODELS OF HEALTH AND ILLNESS

Models of health and illness can be used to understand the complex relationship between health, illness and a client's attitudes toward health and health behaviours[21]. Nurses use models of health and illness to understand the relationships between the concepts of health, wellness, and illness. Nurses can then promote wellness activities to prevent illness, as well as identify risk factors that predispose an individual to illness. Risk factors include conditions, situations or age-periods when changes occur in an individual's life[37]. Risk modification strategies can then be used to prevent or minimise the impact of illness. Nurses who understand how clients react to illness 'can minimise the effects of the condition and assist clients and their families in maintaining or returning to optimal health'[38] (p. 2).

In her book on behaviour and illness, Wu[24] describes the social model of illness as the preferred framework for nursing. This model sees illness as the impaired ability to perform social roles and tasks appropriate to that person's status that disrupts the ordinary course of life. Some of the nursing models of health and illness are discussed below. They include clinical; health–illness continuum; health belief; adaptive; health appraisal; and holistic.

CLINICAL MODEL

A clinical model of health views health as a lack of signs and symptoms of pathology. The presence of signs and symptoms supports claims of illness[8]. Indicators of pathology may be solely related to physical symptoms, or may include mental and emotional symptoms[8]. While this model is useful in a scientific sense in studying health and disease, it has been criticised for its limitations in simply viewing health as the absence of signs or symptoms of disease, and not taking into account social and psychological concerns.

While illness is usually seen as something that happens to a person, it is not always a completely static state when one considers how certain factors affect the person's health, such as smoking, lack of exercise, poor diet or stress[27]. These are all modifiable factors that only the individual can change. Therefore, it is important to not simply focus on relieving the signs and symptoms of the illness, particularly if one is interested in preventing further illnesses and promoting health. For instance, a person who smokes, eats fatty foods and does not exercise is likely to have long-term health problems, even though the current signs and symptoms may be absent or have been treated.

HEALTH-ILLNESS CONTINUUM

Thinking about health and illness as relative states rather than as the opposite of each other provides a construct in the form of a health-illness continuum. This model sees health as a dynamic state[39,40] as a person responds to fluctuations in both the internal and external environment to maintain a state of physical, emotional, intellectual, social, developmental, and spiritual well-being[21]. A person's health state moves along the continuum from obvious disease, through the absence of disease, on to a state of optimal functioning in all aspects of life. High-level wellness is at one end of the continuum and severe illness is at the other end. According to Dunn's theory of high-level wellness, it is an integrated method of functioning[21]. In this sense, wellness is a function of personal initiative.

The health-illness continuum model identifies risk factors as being central to the level of health. Risk factors include genetic and physiological variables, such as age, lifestyle and environment. For example, an older person is more likely than a younger person to have heart disease[21]. The model also suggests that attitudes, values, beliefs and perceptions of illness are influences in the experience of illness.

Although this model is useful in comparing a client's current health with previous health, it is difficult to use this model when comparing two clients because of the subjective component to illness. For instance, a person who does not have a physically defined illness may consider themselves unhealthy because they do not feel well, while someone else with a detectable illness may say they are healthy. Another criticism of the model is that it is not actually possible to demonstrate a cut-off point or demarcation between an individual's health state and diseased state.

Wu[24] is critical of placing illness and wellness on one continuum because it tends to focus on the illness aspects of the patient. Wu's approach is to consider illness and wellness as separate entities and behaviours, which enable the nurse to assess and support both the health and disease aspects of the case. An example is the teaching of healthy lifestyles to a client with diabetes[24]. Bartol[41] believes that such teaching could begin with an exploration of what clients find most difficult about living with diabetes and an assessment of their motivation to self-care. This would be followed by teaching and learning about the following six steps:

1. How clients can check their blood glucose levels;
2. The use of glucose monitoring equipment;
3. The significance of exercise, ways of exercising, and how best to include exercise in a daily schedule;
4. Thoughtful planning for eating foods that enhance health; and
5. How diabetes medication can support better body function.

HEALTH BELIEF MODEL

The health belief model[42,43] incorporates the relationship between a person's beliefs and behaviours. It was developed in the 1950s to explain why some people did not utilise preventive health services such as polio vaccinations. According to the model, ways of knowing and behaving are influenced by beliefs and emotions. Factors that influence those beliefs include

- Personal expectations regarding health and illness. The person's perception of susceptibility to an illness is a component of this model. For instance, a person may understand they are at risk of heart disease, given their knowledge that heart disease has a hereditary component, for example, if one of their parents has died of the disease.
- The person's perception of the seriousness of the illness. Earlier experiences with health and illness (e.g., having asthma may increase fear that complications such as pneumonia may develop when a respiratory illness occurs) may be a factor influencing behaviour. This perception is moderated by demographic and sociopsychological variables. The sociocultural context (e.g., personality, peer influence, ethnicity), and age and developmental state (e.g., an older person may be more accepting of an illness than a younger person, realising that they are more susceptible than younger individuals) may be influencing factors.
- The likelihood that the person will take recommended preventive health care measures. Examples of preventive action include lifestyle changes (e.g., improved diet, not smoking, exercise, stress management), increased adherence to medical treatment, or seeking health care advice or treatment.
- Behaviours are also influenced by beliefs related to perceived barriers, such as financial costs, inconvenience or pain, which may interfere with health behaviours. For example, a person may not follow a recommended treatment due to the cost of medication.

This model helps nurses to understand factors influencing client perceptions, beliefs and behaviour in order to plan care that will most effectively assist clients in maintaining or restoring health and preventing illness[44]. Interventions are targeted at changing beliefs or bringing into action those that already exist[45]. However, one of the limitations of this model is that it is value-laden[45]. It is based on Western culture's health belief systems and does not allow for other influences. Furthermore, it proposes that conscious decision-making is based upon attitudes and beliefs[46]. However, it does not account for the fact that individuals sometimes fail to act on their belief systems[45]. It may be that other factors (e.g., physical or emotional) come into play.

ADAPTIVE MODEL

The adaptive model views illness as a failure of adaptation, or maladaptation[7]. According to Dubos[39], adaptive behaviour is that which represents a successful response to stimuli in the environment. Thus, being able to successfully respond to challenging stimuli that may be social, environmental or physical is the adaptive way, or health. In the acute stage of maladaptation, nursing measures are implemented to assist the person's adaptive ability. For example, dressing a wound to minimise infection may allow the person's natural adaptive responses (immunological system) to become effective.

One of the strengths of this model is that it accounts for variables other than the physical that affect health, such as environmental and social factors. One example of adaptive behaviour is to put on warm clothing when the weather is cold[8]. An applied adaptation model developed by Roy[35] proposes that the nurse's role in health promotion is to assist the client to adapt in the areas of physical needs, self-concept, role-mastery and interdependence relations.

HEALTH HAZARD APPRAISAL MODEL

The Health Hazard Appraisal Model[44] lists seven stages of illness:

1. The lowest risk category for severe illness, which tends to coincide with the early years of life;
2. The at-risk stage, with ageing and/or environmental factors placing the person at risk for disease (however, a young person can become severely ill);
3. The stage that occurs due to physical or psychosocial factors placing excessive stress upon the person;
4. The stage that occurs when clinical signs of disease are apparent, although the person is not aware of their existence;
5. The stage that occurs when symptoms are experienced such as pain, blood in urine, lump etc., leading the person to seek health care from a physician;
6. The stage that includes presence of a disability, after the person has sought medical care, and when there is acute pain or disease; and
7. The stage that occurs if the person's condition is not adequately addressed or treated and results in death.

Another way of describing illness in stages is in terms of transition, acceptance and convalescent stages[37]. In the transition phase, the person may have vague, non-specific symptoms. Although the person may not say they are ill, they acknowledge the symptoms of an illness are there. In the acceptance stage, the person takes on a 'sick' role, withdraws from usual responsibilities and roles and takes steps to become well, for example, medications, bed-rest. Medical treatment may be undertaken if the condition worsens. The convalescent stage is the recovery period. If the illness or disease is chronic, recovery is replaced by adaptation.

HOLISTIC MODEL

An holistic approach is one that considers the physical, social, psychological and spiritual aspects and needs of the person. Brallier[46] defines holistic health as

an ongoing sense of finely tuned wellness, which involves not only excellent care of the physical body but also care of ourselves in such a way that we nurture our capacity to be mentally alert and creative as well as emotionally stable and satisfied. It involves the feeling of wholeness we can gain from having defined our philosophy of life and purpose in life (p. 643).

Thus, health is a way of being rather than a state or goal[7]. Western scientific medical models often equate disease with failure, either of medicine or of the person[47]. The holistic view sees the manifestation of disease, and is dependent on how the person integrates the illness into his or her life. Instead of asking 'What's wrong?' the nurse coming from an holistic perspective may ask, 'How are things going for you today?'.

Nurses take an holistic approach to caring for people who are ill and have a commitment to health promotion[47]. Central to the holistic approach is a belief that each person is unique in terms of integration of body, mind and spirit, and the whole combined is more than the sum of its parts[47]. According to the model, 'a change in one aspect of a person's life brings about change in every aspect of his or her being and alters the quality of the whole. Each person has potential for growth in knowledge and skills and in becoming more loving toward himself or herself and others' (p. 17).

The holistic health model of nursing is about promoting optimal health and creating therapeutic environments to achieve this goal[21]. This model requires the nurse to orient care towards the overall well-being of the patient and this includes a will to have close nurse–patient relationships. These relationships lead to an understanding of the patient as a person who can draw on their own knowledge and strength, and that of their family and friends, even when struggling to recover from ill-health[48]. Nurses who provide holistic care respect the patient as the best person to know about their health, given that their subjective experience plays an important role in health and illness. Patients take some of the responsibility for their recovery from illness, particularly in terms of health maintenance[49]. This taking of responsibility can increase perceptions of personal control over one's health[50]. Some holistic nursing interventions include music therapy, relaxation therapy, massage, therapeutic touch, patient advocacy, patient education, counselling, and other health promotion strategies, such as encouraging exercise and appropriate diet. In this context, nurses give quality care when they create comfortable, safe environments that enable their patients to be resilient and confident in their own capacity to get well.

HEALTH PROMOTION

In 1986, the World Health Organization, through the Ottawa Charter, conceptualised health promotion as the means by which people could be enabled to lead productive and satisfying lives, irrespective of their state of health[16]. Health promotion was to include five key activities: building healthy public policy, creating supportive environments, strengthening community action, developing personal skills and reorienting health services[16].

Since the drafting of the Ottawa Charter nurses have concerned themselves with the imperative to incorporate health-promotion activities into their nursing care. A health education and disease prevention focus has been followed by the lifestyle-modification approach[48]. Both approaches reflect a narrow definition of health promotion and do not accommodate some significant concepts such as 'empowerment, equity, collaboration, participation'[48]. Creation of a more appropriate and comprehensive response to the WHO's call for the incorporation of health promotion concepts into the provision of care will be more successful as

- Nurses increase their theoretical understanding of health promotion[51].
- Nurses became more visible in the discourse associated with the development of health promotion. It has been suggested that in its development, nursing theory has incorporated many of the fundamental tenets of health promotion in isolation from the broader public dialogue about health promotion[48].
- Education of nurses provides them with strategies for better incorporating their understanding of the determinants of health into the planning of care.

COPING WITH ILLNESS

The experience of illness is usually a stressful one. Stress refers to a situation where demands require a response or action to be taken[52]. Issues of coping and living with a chronic illness can be complex and overwhelming, and the temporary stress associated with acute illnesses should not be underestimated. Coping behaviours are often influenced by one's family upbringing, attitudes, values and beliefs about health. Factors, such as the use of reason, previous experience with illness, and differential training in respect to symptoms, can explain why some people minimise or deny the experience of symptoms, and avoid seeking medical care; others will react to the slightest symptom by immediately seeking medical treatment[53]. Such differential perceptions, evaluation and actions to symptoms fall under the category of 'illness behaviour' (see Table 1.1).

ILLNESS BEHAVIOUR

When illness does occur, different attitudes about illness cause people to react in different ways. The particular behaviours generally demonstrated by people who are ill are described as illness behaviour. Such behaviours include how people monitor their bodies, define and interpret their symptoms, take remedial actions, and use the health care system[54]. Thus, illness behaviour may include consulting a health professional, taking prescribed medications or changing one's work routine. Illness behaviours can be positive coping mechanisms. Illness behaviour allows for a release from roles and responsibilities, enabling the healing process to occur. However, if the person persists in the 'sick' role after the acute phase, and does not actively facilitate the rehabilitation process, this is seen as abnormal illness behaviour.

TABLE 1.1: EXAMPLES OF COPING BEHAVIOURS DURING ILLNESS	
Coping Behaviour	**Example**
Negative	
Anxiety	Restless behaviour, worrying
Depression	Sad facial expression, no appetite, crying, decreased motivation
Anger	Violent behaviour, impatient, crying
Self-destructive behaviour	Substance abuse (e.g., drugs, smoking, alcohol), poor diet
Denial/Avoidance	Failure to adhere to doctors orders (e.g., failure to take medication)
Helplessness	Dependence on others, decreased motivation
Positive	
Releasing tension	Imagery, rest, massage, talking it out with friends, family or counsellor
Seeking additional information about illness	Asking health professionals for information about illness, reading
Adopting healthy lifestyle	Adhering to healthy diet, exercise within limits of illness, stress management, following doctors orders
Spiritual	Praying, relying on belief in higher power

Variables influencing illness behaviour can be external or internal. External variables include the overt nature of symptoms, social group expectations, ethnicity, accessibility of the health care system, and social support. If the symptoms are visible, the person is more likely to seek health care[21]. Significant other people who make up one's social support, such as family members, friends or work colleagues, can influence a person's likelihood to seek health care assistance for their symptoms. Illness behaviour may be influenced by culture in that one's cultural background teaches the person how to be healthy, how to recognise illness, and how to behave when ill[21]. Financial constraints may prevent an individual following a recommended treatment regime, or even delay seeking health care because of the prohibitive cost of treatment or loss of income.

Internal variables include the perceptions of the symptoms, the nature of the illness and internal perceptions of control. For instance, if the person views the symptoms as serious, they may seek medical assistance. Whether the illness is acute or chronic can influence illness behaviour. An acute illness is more likely to result in the person seeking health care and complying with treatment. A chronic illness may result in less compliance and increased frustration. A person who believes they have control over their illness, is more likely to take an active role in their rehabilitation and cope better with the illness.

IMPACT OF ILLNESS ON THE INDIVIDUAL AND THE FAMILY

Although each person responds uniquely to illness, there are common behavioural and emotional changes experienced by both the individual and family. However, these responses may vary depending on the chronicity and severity of the illness. Although a mild illness may affect the family in minor ways, such as irritability and lack of cohesiveness, a severe life-threatening illness can lead to grief reactions, such as anxiety, shock, denial, anger and withdrawal[21]. Chronic illness may result in families either drawing closer together or drifting apart, the latter occurring as each person is unable to help others within the family.

Illness can also have a negative impact on body image, particularly if changes in physical appearance occur (e.g., burns). The impact on body image may depend upon on the type of physical change (e.g., loss of limb or organ); the person's ability to adapt; the rate of change in physical appearance; and the presence of support services[21].

Some of the possible results of illness are:

- Negative impact on self-concept, or the way one sees oneself in terms of personality strengths and weaknesses. For instance, if the illness results in a person no longer being able to perform certain roles, they may become depressed and have lowered self-esteem.
- Feelings of anxiety, frustration, irritability, bitterness, guilt and depression may occur. This may be particularly the case for chronic illness, where a person may face the prospect of permanent pain, financial insecurity, and/or body disfigurement[29].
- Conflict, because a person may no longer meet family expectations, which can lead to disputes[21].
- Changes in family roles and dynamics. For example, older children may take on adult roles when an adult who is ill is unable to perform their usual roles. If these changes are long term, this can lead to conflict and an adjustment process similar to grieving[21]. As discussed below, the family's coping skills can be enhanced by communication by the nurse in terms of education, support and encouragement of the use of social networks[55].

HOW NURSES HELP PEOPLE COPE WITH ILLNESS AND ACHIEVE HEALTH GOALS

Rather than treating the illness itself, the nurse's role is to help people cope with the response to illness, be it physical, psychological, spiritual, or all three. Nurses seek to help patients utilise their coping abilities (adjusting to or accepting challenges) to an optimal level, and to adapt to conditions that cannot be changed. The patient with a chronic and incurable illness can be helped to minimise its harmful effects, and can be encouraged to continue to set and attain goals in other aspects of their life. Nurses who use a primary health care and social model approach to health promotion will, in collaboration with the patient, create a supportive and enabling environment within which the client can attain personal skills (through education) that assist them achieve optimal health[14]. Successful achievement of the goals of health promotion and disease prevention requires individual patients to accept responsibility for their own health behaviour, if they have the capacity to do so, and requires nurses to advocate and mediate on their behalf[15,37].

Nurses can enhance a person's coping abilities by acting as a resource, and educator, a role model, and a motivator[8]. For instance, they may provide information and educate the patient about their condition. Measures that can help control stress and anxiety are progressive relaxation, prayer, imagery, massage, biofeedback, yoga, meditation and regular exercise. Nurses can promote health by encouraging positive changes to the client's lifestyle, such as diet, exercise, rest, time management and education about health-enhancing behaviours and health risk factors. They can role-model by demonstrating new behaviours, or skills. They can also encourage health promotion by adherence to treatment and undergoing screening tests. In cases where the situation causing stress cannot be changed, such as a chronic illness, the client can be assisted to cope better with the stress by the use of cognitive therapies that involve changing negative, irrational thinking. However, ultimately it is the intrinsic resources of the individual that determines whether the person will be able to cope and reach optimal functioning[37].

THE IMPORTANCE OF FAMILY

Just as the family plays a substantial role in a patient's acquisition of health beliefs and behaviours, it has the potential to contribute to a nurse's health promoting activities[56]. This potential is realised when the family is enabled to contribute to the nurse's understanding of the significance that an illness may have on their family member. Information about the meaning that a patient is likely to place on their illness, and their subsequent response to the illness, can inform the nurse and enable the planning of socially and culturally appropriate care[21]. Families can be a buffer between the patient and the rituals of hospitalisation through their presence in hospital settings. The giving of direct social support is able to diminish the stress that hospitalisation can impose on patients[17,57].

Patients who are chronically ill, but not in hospital, are more likely to experience positive health outcomes if they have sound social relationships with family and friends. 'Positive adjustment to their illness' and compliance with treatment are identified as two important benefits of family support in particular[58].

● Case study

'Diabetes isn't an illness – it's a part of life'[40] (p. 5).

Mr Aboud, 56, works as a psychologist. He appears to be in good health and lives life to the full, but discloses that he has been diagnosed with type 2 diabetes. Mr Aboud reports that his diet is high in carbohydrates and fats and that his professional responsibilities limit his capacity to exercise. Mr Aboud is concerned that the diabetes will cause his apparent good health to deteriorate and he wonders about the need to comply with suggested management strategies.

LEARNING EXERCISES

1. What questions would a nurse need to ask in order to assess the impact that diabetes has had on Mr Aboud?
2. Is it possible for people to normalise diabetes into their lives? How?
3. How could a nurse assist Mr Aboud to see diabetes in a positive light?
4. What positive health outcomes could Mr Aboud experience as a result of the diabetes?
5. What nursing interventions would help Mr Aboud achieve optimal health?

CONCLUSION

By using broader definitions of health and illness, nurses are increasing the scope of nursing practice. The goal of managing a chronic illness is to reduce the occurrence of symptoms or to improve the tolerance of symptoms. A goal of nursing is to foster self-management of illness, encouraging the individual to take charge of his or her own health and to minimise illness through health promotion. However, the goal of incorporating health promotion and disease-prevention strategies, while nursing clients, can be a difficult one to achieve. People who are generally focused on their current condition, may not be in a frame of mind to address risk factors for apparently unrelated, non-existent health problems that may or may not occur in the future. This situation can be addressed by health professionals taking every opportunity to promote healthy behaviours during interactions with clients, rather than the client waiting until an annual health visit. While nurses can enhance a client's coping strategies in dealing with illness, and assist the client reach optimal health, the greatest influence on health outcomes is the inner resources of the individual.

REFLECTIVE QUESTIONS

1. Why is it so difficult to define health and illness?
2. Why is it important for nurses to understand the client's concept of illness?

3. What distinguishes illness from disease?
4. How can illness have a positive impact on people's lives?
5. What limitations does a medical model approach to illness place on the planning of nursing care?
6. Which model of health and illness do you think is best suited to nursing practice? Why?
7. What are some internal and external variables that enable people to stay healthy?
8. What are some internal and external variables related to illness?
9. How does chronic illness affect people's psychosocial well-being?
10. How can nurses enhance the adaptive coping mechanisms of individuals and their families experiencing illness? How does knowledge of health promotion strategies support nurses to plan this aspect of care?

Recommended Readings

Craven, R & Hirnle, C. 2003; 'Health and Wellness' in *Fundamentals of Nursing: Human Health and Function* (4th ed.), Lippincott Williams and Wilkins, Philadelphia, ch. 16.

Freund, PES & McGuire, MB. 1999; *Health, Illness and the Social Body: A Critical Sociology* (2nd ed.), Prentice Hall Inc., New Jersey.

Koch, T, Kralik, D & Taylor, J. 2000; 'Men Living with Diabetes: Minimizing the Intrusiveness of the Disease', *Journal of Clinical Nursing*, 9 (2), 247–254.

Talbot, L. & Verrinder, G. 2005; *Promoting Health: The Primary Health Care Approach* (3rd ed.), Elsevier, Churchill Livingstone, Marrickville, New South Wales.

World Health Organization (WHO). 1986; *The Ottawa Charter for Health Promotion,* World Health Organization, Geneva.

References

1. Andrews, MM & Boyle, JS. 2003; *Transcultural Concepts in Nursing Care* (4th ed.), Lippincott, Philadelphia.
2. Germov, J. 1999; *Second Opinion: An Introduction to Health Sociology,* Oxford University Press, South Melbourne.
3. McLennan, V & Khavarpour, F. 2004; 'Culturally Appropriate Health Promotion: Its Meaning and Application in Aboriginal Communities', *Health Promotion Journal of Australia*, 15 (3), 237–239.
4. National Health and Medical Research Council. 1996; 'Promoting the Health of Indigenous Australians: A Review of Infrastructure Support for Aboriginal and Torres Strait Islander Health Advancement; Final Report and Recommendations', NHMRC, part 2:4.
5. Griffith-Jones, R. 2000; 'Rongoa Maori and Primary Health Care', Masters Thesis, University of Auckland. www.hauora.com/downloads/files/Thesis-Rhys%20Griffit%20Jones-Ronga%20Maori%20and%20Primary%20Health%20Care.pdf. Accessed 16 April 2004.
6. Ministry of Health New Zealand. 2002; 'Maori Health'. www.maorihealth.govt.nz. Accessed 16 April 2004.
7. Freund, PES & McGuire, MB. 1999; *Health, Illness and the Social Body: A Critical Sociology* (2nd ed.), Prentice Hall, New Jersey.
8. Berger, K. 1999; *Fundamentals of Nursing: Collaborating for Optimal Health* (2nd ed.), Appleton & Lange, Connecticut.
9. Macdonald, JJ. 1996; *Primary Health Care: Medicine in Its Place*, Earthscan, London.
10. Baume, F. 1998; *The New Public Health: An Australian Perspective*, Oxford University Press, South Melbourne.
11. Jackson, D & Borbassi, S. 2000; 'The Caring Conundrum: Potential and Perils for Nursing' in J Daly, S Speedy & D Jackson (eds.), *Contexts of Nursing: An Introduction*, McLennan & Petty, Sydney, 65–76.
12. Suchman, E. 1963; *Sociology and the Field of Public Health*, Russell Sage Foundation, New York.
13. Benner, P. 2004; 'Seeing the Person Beyond the Disease', *Journal of Critical Care*, 13 (1), 75.
14. World Health Organization (WHO). 1978; *Declaration of Alma-Ata: International Conference on Primary Health Care*, Alma Ata, USSR, 6–12 September 1978. World Health Organization, Geneva.
15. Wass, A. 2000; *Promoting Health: The Primary Health Care Approach* (2nd ed). W.B. Saunders, Marrickville, New South Wales.

16. World Health Organization (WHO). 1986; *The Ottawa Charter for Health Promotion*, World Health Organization, Geneva.

17. Geary, JA & Hawkins, JW. 1991; 'To Cure, To Care or To Heal', *Nursing Forum*, 26 (3), 5–13.

18. *Macquarie Concise Dictionary.* 2003; Macquarie University, Sydney.

19. *Encyclopedia and Dictionary of Medicine, Nursing, and Allied Health* (2nd ed.), 1978; B Miller & C Keane, W.B. Saunders, Philadelphia.

20. Besson, G. 1967; 'The Health-Illness Spectrum', *American Journal of Public Health*, 57, 1901–1905.

21. Crisp, J & Taylor, C. 2005; *Fundamentals of Nursing* (2nd ed.), Elsevier, Sydney.

22. Jensen, L & Allen, M. 1993; 'Wellness: The Dialectic of Illness, *Image Journal of Nursing Scholarship*, 25 (3), 220.

23. Boorse, C. 1981; 'On the Distinction Between Disease and Illness' in A Caplan, H Englehardt & J McCartney (eds.), *Concepts of Health and Disease: Interdisciplinary Perspectives*, Addison-Wesley Publishing Company, Massachusetts, 546–560.

24. Wu, R. 1973; *Behavior and Illness*, Prentice-Hall, Englewood Cliffs, New Jersey.

25. Weitz, R. 2001; *The Sociology of Health, Illness, and Health Care: A Critical Approach*, Wadsworth, Stamford.

26. Copstead, LC & Banasik, JL. 2000; *Pathophysiology: Biological and Behavioral Perspectives*, W.B. Saunders, Philadelphia.

27. Craven, R & Hirnle, C. 2003: 'Health and Wellness', in *Fundamentals of Nursing: Human Health and Function* (4th ed.), Lippincott Williams and Wilkins, Philadelphia, ch. 16.

28. Simonton, O, Matthews-Simonton, S & Creighton, J. 1978; *Getting Well Again*, Bantam, New York.

29. Phipps, W. 2003; 'Chronic Illness', in W Phipps, *et al.* (eds.), *Medical-Surgical Nursing: Health and Illness Perspectives*, Mosby, St Louis, 71–88.

30. Commission on Chronic Illness. 1956; *Commission on Chronic Illness: Care of the Long-term Patient*, Harvard University Press, Harvard.

31. Kent, T & Hart, M. 1998; *Introduction to Human Disease* (4th ed.), Appleton & Lange, Prentice-Hall, London.

32. Medline Plus. 2003; http://www.nhm.nih.gov/medlineplus/ency/article. Accessed 11 September 2003

33. http://www.ceci.uprm.edu/~ephoebus/id90.htm. Accessed 22 November 2003.

34. Brannon, L & Feist, J. 2004; *Health Psychology: An Introduction to Behaviour and Health* (5th ed.), Wadsworth, Belmont, California.

35. Roy, C. 1980; 'The Roy Adaptation Model' in J Riehl & C Roy, *Conceptual Models for Nursing*

Practice (2nd ed.), Appleton-Century-Crofts, New York.

36. Australian Broadcasting Corporation, 2000; http://www.abc.net.au/science/news/stories/s20342.htm. Retrieved 18 February 2004.

37. De Wit, S. 2001; *Fundamental Concepts and Skills for Nursing*, Saunders, London.

38. Potter, P & Perry, A. 2001; *Fundamentals of Nursing* (5th ed.), Mosby, St Louis.

39. Dubos, R. 1965; *Man Adapting*, Yale University Press, New Haven, Connecticut.

40. Dunn, H. 1973; *High Level Wellness*, Beatty, Arlington, Virginia.

41. Bartol, T. 2002; 'Educating Patients: Diabetes Self-Care', *Nurse Practitioner*, 27, Supplement: *Sourcebook*.

42. Rosenstoch, I. 1974; 'Historical Origin of the Health Belief Model', *Health Education Monograph*, 2, 334.

43. Becker, M & Maiman, L. 1975; 'Sociobehavioral Determinants of Compliance with Health and Medical Care Recommendations', *Medical Care*, 33 (1), 1021.

44. Pelletier, K. 1977; *Mind as Healer, Mind as Slayer*, Delta Publishing Co., Inc., New York.

45. Finfgeld, D, Wongvatunyu, S, Conn, V, Grando, V & Russell, C. 2003; 'Health Belief Model and Reversal Theory: A Comparative Analysis', *Journal of Advanced Nursing*, 43 (3), 288–297.

46. Brallier, L. 1978; 'The Nurse as Holistic Health Practitioner', *Nursing Clinics of North America*, 19, 195–206.

47. Janz, N & Bexler, M. 1984; 'The Health Belief Model: A Decade Later', *Health Education Quarterly*, 11, 1–47.

48. Young, LE & Hayes, V. 2002; *Transforming Health Promotion Practice: Concepts, Issues, and Applications,* F.A. Davis, Philadelphia.

49. Edeman, C & Mandle, C. 1998; *Health Promotion throughout the Life Span* (4th ed.), Mosby, St Louis.

50. Schuster, S. 1997. 'Wholistic Care: Healing a Sick System', *Nursing Management*, 28 (6), 56.

51. Pender, NJ, Murdaugh, CL & Parsons, MA. 2002, *Health Promotion in Nursing Practice* (4th ed.), Prentice Hall, New Jersey.

52. Seyle, H. 1976; *The Stress of Life* (2nd ed.), McGraw-Hill, New York.

53. Mechanic, D. 1981; 'The Concept of Illness Behaviour', in A Caplan, H Engelhardt & J McCartney (eds.), *Concepts of Health and Disease: Interdisciplinary Perspectives*, Addison-Wesley Publishing Company, Massachusetts.

54. Mechanic, D. 1982; 'Sociological Dimensions of Illness Behavior', *Social Science Medicine*, 41 (9), 1207.

55. Engel, J. 1991; 'Disease', in J Cresia & B Parker (eds.), *Conceptual Foundations of Professional Nursing*

Practice, Mosby-Yearbook, Inc., St Louis, 321–329.

56. George, J & Davis, A, 1998; *States of Health: Health and Illness in Australia*, Addison Wesley Longman, Frenchs Forest.

57. Baron, RA & Kalsher, MJ. 2005; *Psychology: From Science to Practice*, Pearson, Boston.

58. Taylor, SE 1999; *Health Psychology* (4th ed.), McGraw-Hill, Los Angeles, 34.

2 | Infectious Disease Health Breakdown

AUTHORS

CECILY HENGSTBERGER-SIMS

JANET FORBER

LEARNING OBJECTIVES

When you have completed this chapter you will be able to
- Define the term 'infection';
- Discuss the process of infection;
- Demonstrate an understanding of the use of infection-control precautions in the health care environment;
- Describe structure, function and broad classification relating to viruses, bacteria, fungi and parasites;
- Discuss pathophysiology and clinical presentation related to a person experiencing health breakdown associated with the infective process; and
- Identify and discuss nursing implications related to prevention, diagnostic testing and therapeutic interventions that affect a person experiencing health breakdown associated with the infective process.

INTRODUCTION

This chapter provides a definition of infection, description of the process of infection and its relationship to the use of fundamental practices for infection control in health care. Together with a general overview of common microorganisms associated with infection, a case study approach is used to demonstrate specific health-breakdown consequences, and to examine nursing implications for specific organisms.

THE CONCEPT OF INFECTION

Human beings, like other animals, play host to a wide variety of microorganisms. These microorganisms are referred to as *commensals* or the 'normal flora' of the body and may be beneficial to the human host[1] (see Table 2.1). Microorganisms assist in metabolising food, production of vitamins (e.g., vitamin K), have a protective function against infection and stimulate the immune response[2]. Microorganisms are found in parts of the body that are exposed to, or communicate with the environment, including, for example, the skin, nose and mouth, intestinal and female genital tracts. These organisms are derived from sources

TABLE 2.1: EXAMPLES OF NORMAL FLORA IN HUMANS	
Area of the Body	**Commensal Organisms**
Mouth and teeth	Bacteria: • Staphylococci • *Streptococcus mutans* Yeasts: • *Candida*
Throat	Bacteria: • *Streptococcus pneumoniae* • *Neisseria* species • *Haemophilus influenzae*
Skin	Bacteria: • Staphylococci • Streptococci • *Corynebacterium*
Bowel	Bacteria: • *Escherichia coli* • Enterobacteriacea • Enterococci • *Clostridium* species
Vagina (adult)	Bacteria: • Lactobaccilli • Streptococci Yeasts: • *Candida*

such as the maternal genital tract at birth, close contacts, the environment and food[3]. The internal organs and tissues of the body, such as the brain, spinal cord and vascular system, are normally sterile, that is, there is an absence of commensal organisms[1].

The term *colonisation* is used to describe the presence of commensal microorganisms where there is no disruption to the normal body function[2]. Colonisation may be transient or permanent. In contrast, microorganisms that are capable of invading the body and causing disease are termed *pathogens*[3]. *Infection* is a disease process caused by a pathogen and occurs when the interaction between the pathogen and the host results in pathological processes and associated tissue damage in the host[3]. The tissue damage associated with infection can result from microbial factors and activities, for example, it can result from a proliferation of the microorganisms and the production of toxins, or from the effects of the host's immune response to the organism.

Some microorganisms are always associated with disease in humans and are termed strict pathogens. Examples include *Salmonella* and *Shigella* (as causes of gastroenteritis) and the rabies virus[2]. However, many infections are caused by opportunistic pathogens, organisms that usually do not cause disease, yet if introduced into sites where they are not typically found, or when host susceptibility is altered, may result in disease[3]. The bacterium, *Escherichia coli* is an example of a microorganism that normally colonises the gastrointestinal tract, but can cause urinary tract infections especially when an indwelling urinary catheter is present. *Pathogenicity* is the organism's ability to cause disease in a susceptible host, while *virulence* refers to the organism's enhanced capacity to cause more severe infection, a quantitative measure of pathogenicity[4].

OBLIGATORY STEPS IN INFECTION

For infectious organisms to perpetuate in nature there needs to be a sequence of interactions between the organism and the potential host. First, the microorganism must gain entry into the body. Humans have many natural barriers such as skin, antibacterial secretions (e.g., lysozyme), and the presence of mucous or ciliated epithelium to prevent organisms accessing the body[5]. However, any breach in these defences, such as a cut to the skin or an invasive device, may allow organisms to enter. Other bodily functions or activities may facilitate access to the body, for example, inhalation or ingestion[6].

Depending on the type of infection, there will be a local effect or a generalised response in the body through the blood or lymphatic system. Once established within the host, the organisms replicate to establish sufficient numbers for continued spread and invasion. Many pathogenic microorganisms have developed strategies that facilitate evasion of immune and other defence mechanisms in the host, so that replication can be completed. Human immunodeficiency virus (HIV) exhibits such an evasion system by killing or interfering with the T-cells of the immune system, which are normally required to eliminate the virus[3,5].

Crucially, in order to perpetuate the infective process, the pathogen must be shed from its current host in a manner – and in sufficient numbers – that enables spread of the pathogen to new hosts. Various mechanisms may assist the pathogen in this process. Viruses that infect the upper respiratory tract, such as the common cold, may induce increased nasal secretions; and they may stimulate coughing and sneezing, with the droplets containing virus particles that can then spread to new potential hosts. For gastrointestinal infections, the combination of diarrhoea and inadequate hygiene practices has been highly successful in spreading diseases such as cholera and typhoid[5].

SIGNS AND SYMPTOMS OF INFECTION

The signs and symptoms associated with infection vary, depending on the causative organism and the site of the infection. One of the most common manifestations of infection is fever and it is believed to be beneficial in combatting the infection process[7]. Pathogens associated with human disease replicate most effectively at temperatures at or below 37°C. The higher temperatures seen in fever may inhibit pathogen replication, and promote phagocytosis, antibody and interferon production, thus aiding the immune response[7].

Many organisms also cause some degree of inflammation with the presence of local heat, swelling, redness and pain at the site of infection. The inflammatory response is a combination of vasodilation, an outpouring of exudate from dilated capillaries, an accumulation of white cells (neutrophils and macrophages) into an area, and the release of immune active chemicals, which regulate the immune response[3].

Rashes are a distinct form of inflammation and their site of origin, form of spread and characteristic type of skin lesion can aid in diagnosing specific infections. Some rashes are evidence of the harmful effects of the interaction between the pathogen and the host's immune system[3].

Other signs and symptoms will be dependent on the infecting organisms and disease caused. Some viruses are cytopathic and cause direct cellular damage, for example, poliovirus, HIV and rhinoviruses (common cold viruses)[5]. *Plasmodium*, the protozoan cause of malaria, causes direct damage to erythrocytes as part of its disease cycle. Toxin-mediated effects are a feature of bacterial infection and are varied and numerous. *Clostridium tetani* releases a neurotoxin causing the spastic paralysis seen in tetanus. *Staphylococcus aureus* may produce a range of toxins, including the toxin responsible for the often-serious toxic shock syndrome. A further example is found in the enterotoxins causing enteritis[2].

THE TRANSMISSION OF INFECTION AND THE PRINCIPLES OF INFECTION CONTROL

The Chain of Infection is represented by a simple model, based on the steps required for the transmission of infection (see Figure 2.1). Each link in the chain must be present and in sequence for an infection to occur. The six components of the Chain of Infection[4] are

1. An infectious agent or pathogen;
2. A reservoir where the infectious agent can survive and/or multiply;
3. A portal of exit – a mechanism or path where the infectious agent can leave the reservoir;
4. A mode of transmission where the infectious agent can transfer from the reservoir to a susceptible host;
5. A portal of entry – a mechanism or path where the infectious agent can gain entry into a susceptible host; and
6. A susceptible host.

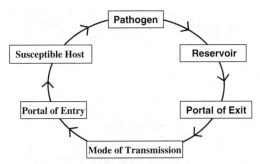

FIGURE 2.1 *Chain of Infection*
Source: Adapted from Lawrence, J & May,
D. 2003; *Infection Control in the Community*,
Churchill Livingstone, Edinburgh, Fig.
2.4, p. 17.

The main groups of pathogens causing infection in humans are viruses, bacteria, fungi, protozoa, helminths (worms) and arthropods[1]. A great diversity for potential reservoirs of these organisms exists, including humans, animals, the environment, and contaminated water and food. For example, the hepatitis A virus may be found in water or food contaminated with sewage (resulting in contaminated shellfish), and *Listeria* can be associated with uncooked meat products, for example, salami and some pâtés (liver spreads). Inanimate sources are environmental, such as dust and contaminated equipment. Humans form a major animate reservoir along with other animals such as cattle, chickens, rodents and some insects[4]. When an organism causing infection arises from these external sources, it is termed *exogenous*. Alternatively, if the organism arises from the patient's own normal microbial flora, it is then considered to be *endogenous* in origin[6].

Portals of exit are the mechanisms by which the microorganisms mobilise from the reservoir at a given time. In considering the human being as a reservoir, potential portals of exit include excretions and secretions, such as faeces, sputum, saliva and the droplets contained within a cough or a sneeze[5].

The potential modes of transmission facilitating the spread of micro-organisms are summarised in Table 2.2. Transmission depends upon several factors including the number of organisms shed and their ability to survive in the environment. There is marked variation in the number of organisms required to infect a new host. Only 10–100 *Shigella dysenteriae* organisms will cause disease in a host. However, 1×10^6 *Salmonella* organisms are necessary to result in *Salmonella* food poisoning[5]. Transmission may be aided by the organism's ability to facilitate spread, such as respiratory illnesses that promotes coughing/sneezing in their host, or those diseases that produce diarrhoea[5].

Portals of entry are the routes that pathogens use to gain entry into the body[6]. Some portals are natural and always present, such as inhalation, ingestion or mucous membranes. Others, especially within health care settings, are temporary portals of entry. Surgical incisions, wound drains, urinary catheters, intravenous lines and endotracheal tubes can significantly increase a person's risk of infection[4].

Many factors influence the susceptibility of a potential host for acquiring infection and this is accentuated within health care settings. These include[4]

- Extremes of age;
- Breaches in the integrity of the skin;
- Underlying disease processes (e.g., diabetes);
- Immunosuppression;
- Aspects of treatment or procedures (e.g., invasive devices, surgery, urinary catheterisation); and
- Antibiotic use.

If all the components of the Chain of Infection are present, then infection can result.

TABLE 2.2: EXAMPLES OF THE MODES OF TRANSMISSION FOR MICROORGANISMS		
Mode of Transmission	**Explanation**	**Examples**
Direct contact	Mostly via human hands, which are easily contaminated by contact with reservoirs of microorganisms, such as other humans, the environment, secretions and excretions.	Bacteria such as methicillin-resistant *Staphylococcus aureus*, vancomycin-resistant enterococci, contagious skin conditions, i.e., scabies, impetigo.
Droplet	Via contact of the mucous membranes of the nose/ mouth or conjunctiva with large particle droplets (>5 nm), which contain the microorganisms created by persons with or carrying the disease.	*Neisseria meningitidis*, whooping cough, rubella.
Airborne	Involves the transmission of small droplets (<5 nm), which contain the microorganism. These droplets can stay suspended in the air for long periods of time.	Tuberculosis, chickenpox.
Ingestion	Ingesting contaminated food, water or ice. Also person-to-person spread by the faecal–oral route.	Cholera, hepatitis A and causes of gastroenteritis, e.g., *Salmonella*.
Parenteral	Injection or inoculation, including needle-stick injury and sharing drug injecting equipment.	Blood-borne viruses, such as hepatitis B, hepatitis C and HIV.
Via vectors	Vectors, including mosquitoes, lice and ticks, transmit a microorganism via biting.	The commonest cause of malaria, the protozoa *Plasmodium falciparum* is transmitted via bites from infected female anopheline mosquitoes.
Vertical	Can be prenatal via the placenta, perinatal via the birth canal, postnatal via breastmilk.	Rubella can cross the placenta, Group B streptococcus birth canal, hepatitis B via breastmilk.

FUNDAMENTAL PRACTICES FOR INFECTION CONTROL

Infection prevention and control centres on practices and procedures aimed at breaking the Chain of Infection. Some of these practices can be pre-emptive, such as the use of vaccination to prevent infectious diseases. Others, such as hand hygiene, can be practised on a regular basis to minimise the spread of infection[4]. Hands can easily become contaminated with microorganisms via contact with people, secretions, excretions, equipment and the environment[8]. Hand hygiene has been repeatedly supported by studies in the literature, and yet there is a continuing lack of compliance among health care workers with this effective infection-control measure[9]. Traditionally, hand hygiene is achieved by hand washing with soap or antiseptic solution and water. However, increasingly in heath care settings, the use of alcohol-based hand rubs/gels are advocated as a means of reducing the number of microorganisms carried on the hands[8].

Other infection-control practices, which break the chain of infection include standard and transmission-based precautions, decontamination of equipment, safe sharps management systems, and the use of environmental and food hygiene practices[4]. The evolution of HIV and AIDS in the 1980s led to the development of *universal precautions* and *body substance isolation*, which are now combined as *Standard Precautions* and form the first tier in many infection control systems[10]. Standard precautions alert health care workers to patient situations that require special barrier techniques and aim to minimise the risk of infection transmission. The barrier techniques utilise personal protective equipment, such as gloves, gowns, nose, mouth and eye protection, when caring for all patients where actual or potential contact with blood or other body fluids may occur. In addition to standard precautions, infection control systems may also use transmission-based precautions when indicated for certain diseases. There are three types of additional precautions for specific infectious diseases spread by the following routes: airborne, droplet, and contact[11,12].

These precautions make use of environmental controls including patient placement in single rooms, and special air handling to minimise transmission from patient to patient and patient to staff. In addition, use of personal protective equipment may be advocated, for example, gloves and aprons are used for patient care and contact with a patient's environment.

Maintenance of clean environments and the decontamination of equipment using cleaning, disinfection and sterilisation are important components of any infection control management plan. In modern health care, there is an increasing role for 'Single Use' disposable items, which negate the need for reprocessing and minimise the risk of transmission. The use of guidelines and practices that promote safe management of indwelling medical devices, including urinary catheters and intravenous equipment, also contributes to the prevention of infection[13,14].

In the following sections, the major groups of microorganisms will be outlined, introducing the key characteristics of viruses, bacteria, fungi and parasites. The range of disease caused by microorganisms is highly diverse and complex. For each group of microorganisms, one disease or condition will be used to illustrate aspects of the infective process associated with that group.

VIRUSES

Viruses infect every form of life from animals and plants to bacteria and other microorganisms. Viruses are small, ranging in size from the poliovirus at 30 nm to large viruses such as vaccinia virus at 400 nm[5]. Structurally, viruses consist of a genome of either DNA or RNA (never both), which is packaged in a protein coat called a *capsid*[2]. The viral protein coat consists of repeating units known as *capsomeres*, and often has distinctive symmetry, such as icosahedral or helical structures[5]. Classification of viruses is based on three determinants: 1) the type of nucleic acid; 2) the structure and symmetry of the capsids of the protein coat; and 3) the presence or absence of an envelope[3]. This outer envelope is derived from the host cell membrane. Enveloped viruses are more susceptible to environmental factors, such as drying and gastric acidity, whereas envelope-free viruses are better able to survive in the environment[5].

Viruses are unable to replicate independently and they rely on the biochemical machinery of their host's cells to replicate – they are termed *obligate intracellular parasites*[2]. The capsid facilitates attachment and entry of the virus to the target host cells. The virus causes the host cells mechanisms to both replicate the viral nucleic acid and to synthesise new proteins for its capsid[5]. Following assembly of these viral components within the host cell, the new virus particle may be released in several ways. Some viruses cause cell lysis, a process where the host cell is destroyed, releasing the new virus[2]. In other infections, such as hepatitis B, the host's cells are not destroyed, but release virus particles at a slow rate over time[5].

The actual name given to viruses may originate from a characteristic of the virus, such as size, or after the locations where they were first isolated. For example, in the picornavirus, 'pico' means small; the poxviruses derive their name from causing conditions referred to as 'poxes' (e.g., smallpox); and the Coxsackie virus was named after Coxsackie, an area of New York[2].

The outcomes of viral infection can vary substantially, ranging from unapparent infection, sub-clinical infection, and disease syndrome leading to death[15].

VIRAL INFECTION: WHAT DOES IT MEAN?

Viruses can cause disease when they enter the body by breaching natural defences via several routes, including direct contact, injection, inhalation, and ingestion. The route of transmission will depend on the source of the virus. For example, the cold virus (rhinovirus) is transmitted via inhaled droplets, and by secretions coming into direct contact with the mucous membranes[2].

The target tissue (tissue tropism) of the virus will determine the disease presentation and associated signs and symptoms. The manifestations of viral infection will vary from host to host and depend on both host and viral factors. Host factors (such as age, prior immunity, effectiveness of the immune response, and any treatment available) will influence the overall outcome. Features of the virus may enhance the virus's ability to invade the host, evade local defences, spread within the host and replicate[2].

● Case Study

Kylie Hancock, 8, lives with her parents. Kylie's mother, Anne, is nine months pregnant with her second child. Kylie has been generally unwell for one day and now has developed a rash, initially appearing on her trunk and spreading to her face, scalp and arms, with no lesions on the feet or hands. The lesions appear as clear vesicles, many of which are oval in shape and with the long axis following creases in the skin. The rash is itchy and Kylie has a temperature of 37.8°C. Kylie has no other symptoms and no medical history of note. The family GP diagnoses Kylie with chickenpox. Anne is unsure if she has previously had chickenpox, so a blood test is arranged for varicella-zoster immunoglobulin (varicella IgG). This is positive, indicating that Anne has previously had chickenpox and is immune. Two weeks later, Anne gives birth to a full-term healthy baby girl, Jessica.

WHAT IS THE PATHOPHYSIOLOGY?

Chickenpox or varicella is a common, highly infectious disease typically of childhood, caused by primary infection with varicella–zoster virus (VZV)[3]. VZV, a member of the herpesvirus family, causes two distinct diseases: varicella (chickenpox), and zoster (shingles). The latter results from reactivation of latent varicella. Varicella is a human disease with worldwide occurrence. Generally, varicella is regarded as a mild self-limiting disease in healthy children. However, complications can occur in children and especially in adults, neonates and immunosuppressed individuals of any age[16].

The herpesviruses are large, double–stranded DNA, enveloped viruses (see Table 2.3)[17–19]. Infections with herpesviruses are common and, while often associated with relatively

TABLE 2.3: FEATURES OF THE HERPESVIRUSES			
Virus	**Abbreviation**	**Diseases**	**Mode of Spread**
Herpes simplex type 1	HSV-1	Generally affects upper part of the body 'Cold-sores'	Virus can be spread in respiratory secretions and saliva. Close contact required (e.g., kissing)
Herpes simplex type 2	HSV-2	Generally affects lower part of the body Genital infections	Requires close contact (sexually transmitted)
Varicella-zoster virus	VZV	Chickenpox Shingles	Airborne spread and close contact
Epstein-Barr virus	EBV	Infectious mononucleosis (glandular fever) Also associated with certain malignancies, e.g., Burkett's lymphoma	Via saliva EBV is one factor, not a direct cause, in development of Burkett's lymphoma
Cytomegalovirus	CMV	Fetal infection in utero can cause morbidity and mortality Often asymptomatic infections in infants and young children May cause infections in transplant recipients	Vertical transmission via the placenta from mother to baby Close contact Transfusions, transplants
Human herpesvirus 6 and 7	HHV-6 HHV-7	Early-childhood roseola	Via oral secretions No diseases associated with HHV-7
Kaposi's sarcoma-related virus	HHV-8	Cofactor in Karposi's sarcoma	Thought to be sexually transmitted via semen, also known to have been transmitted as a result of renal transplantation

mild disease, can cause significant morbidity and mortality, especially in immunosuppressed people. Latency is a feature of herpesviruses, with lifelong carriage of the virus following infection. As noted above, VZV (as a member of the herpesvirus family) establishes a latent infection in the neurons and subsequent reactivation results in a secondary infection, known commonly as shingles[17].

VZV is transmitted from active cases to susceptible host by droplet or airborne spread of secretions from the respiratory tract of varicella cases, and from direct contact with contaminated secretions or the vesicular fluid from skin lesions of varicella or zoster cases. VZV enters via the respiratory tract or conjunctiva[20]. Primary infection with VZV initially begins in the mucosa of the respiratory tract and signs of disease are not present[2,4]. The virus spreads via the blood stream (primary viraemia) and the lymphatic system to the cells of the reticuloendothelial system, where replication of the virus occurs. After 11 to 13 days, a second viraemia spreads the virus primarily to the skin and respiratory tract, but extension to the mouth, conjunctiva and genitourinary tract is also possible[2,4]. VZV is highly infectious and humans are the only reservoir[3].

Following primary infection with VZV and recovery, the virus demonstrates the latency associated with the herpesvirus family and lies dormant in the dorsal root ganglia. Subsequent reactivation of the virus results in the localised cutaneous eruption – herpes zoster or shingles[21]. The rash in herpes zoster is chickenpox. As in nature, it follows a dermatome with small closely placed lesions on an erythematous base[2]. The risk of shingles occurring is associated with changes to specific cell-mediated immune responses, such as may occur with ageing, and in immunosuppression. The rash of shingles is frequently painful in nature and postherpetic neuralgia, (defined as pain, which persists for more than thirty days from onset of rash) is a notable complication, more prevalent with increasing age[21].

WHAT ARE THE CLINICAL MANIFESTATIONS?

The incubation period of VZV ranges from 10 to 21 days, most commonly 14 to 16 days[2,15,20]. There may be a prodromal illness, more frequently seen in adults, with fever, headache, and muscle aches. The rash is characteristic, appearing first on the trunk then the face and scalp. Presence of the rash on the scalp helps distinguish chickenpox from other illnesses[2]. Lesions start as flat macules, which rapidly become raised into small round papules that develop into fluid-filled, blister-like vesicles. Finally, these vesicles become pustular, then break down and crust over[2,15,17].

A feature of the rash is 'cropping' with new lesions appearing in crops over several days, so that lesions of differing stages of development are present at any time. Chickenpox is contagious up to 48 hours before the rash appears and extends until all lesions are crusted and no new lesions occur (usually 5 days)[22]. Generally, chickenpox is a self-limiting illness, but complications can occur. The disease is often more severe in adults and this is believed to be attributable to heightened cell-mediated immune response, which produces greater cell damage[2].

The most common complications are secondary bacterial infection of the vesicles with *Staphylococcus aureus* or *Streptococcus pyogenes*, which may warrant treatment with appropriate antibiotics. Secondary infection increases the risk of scarring from the lesions, as does trauma, such as scratching[2]. Severe disease can be seen in adults, neonates and immunosuppressed individuals, and pulmonary involvement may lead to respiratory failure, requiring mechanical ventilation. In addition, renal impairment, intravascular coagulation and altered liver function can occur and, in such cases, full supportive therapy and intravenous antiviral agents are indicated[3].

Other rare complications include involvement of the neurological system in chickenpox infection (encephalitis), presenting as a cerebellar disturbance with ataxia (affecting coordination and speech) and the visual disturbance, nystagmus. These effects may persist for days or weeks, but are normally self-limiting with a good outcome[3]. A thrombocytopenia with a haemolytic rash and haematuria can occur, and this is usually transient, responding to corticosteroids therapy and platelet transfusion if required[3].

In pregnancy, when the mother is non-immune, chickenpox can lead to severe morbidity in the mother, the fetus and in newborn babies. The complications of varicella pneumonia can occur in 10% of pregnant women with chickenpox, and its severity is greatest in the third trimester[23]. Chickenpox during pregnancy can result in fetal varicella, which occasionally causes 'congenital varicella syndrome'. The effects include skin scarring, congenital malformations and other anomalies[23]. In Australia, the incidence of congenital varicella syndrome is one in 107,000 pregnancies[24]. Chickenpox occurring in pregnancy during the period five days before delivery to two days after delivery may result in severe varicella infection in 17% to 30% of newborns infants[23].

WHAT SHOULD YOU BE LOOKING AT IN THE LABORATORY TESTS?

The diagnosis of chickenpox is usually based upon clinical presentation and laboratory diagnosis is not usually required[20]. If it is necessary to establish a diagnosis, then fluid or scrapings from the lesions can be examined using a fluorescent monoclonal antibody test. This test is sensitive, specific and will confirm the presence of VZV viral particles from the lesions[24].

Laboratory tests are used to establish the presence of immunity to VZV. As the clinical disease is highly distinctive, a reliable history of chickenpox is a good indicator of past exposure and immunity[20]. A range of serological tests is available to detect immunoglobulins (antibodies), both IgG and IgM, to varicella-zoster virus. Recent or current infection is indicated by a positive IgM test. A positive test for varicella antibodies (IgG) indicates past exposure and immunity to VZV[16].

WHAT IS THE TREATMENT?

Uncomplicated varicella infection in an immunocompetent child is a self-limiting disease. The aims of management will be symptomatic relief and prevention of complications. Symptom control may include the use of antipyretics, if pyrexial, and anti-pruritics to soothe itching[25]. Attention should be paid to skin care with bathing and regular changes of clothing and bed linens[26]. Fingernails need to be kept clean and short and itching discouraged to minimise the risk of secondary bacterial infection[26].

While not recommended for routine use in uncomplicated cases of chickenpox, oral or intravenous antiviral therapy may be indicated for immunocompromised patients, and patients with complications including pneumonitis, and adolescents/adults[26]. Viruses, as obligate intracellular parasites, utilise the host cells machinery in order to replicate, complicating antiviral drug designs to limit toxicity to the host cell[2]. Several antiviral drugs, including acyclovir and famciclovir, are active against varicella virus[17,25].

Prevention of varicella infection is possible with use of a live attenuated vaccine, which is approved for use in children over 12 months of age. It is recommended for use in non-immune adolescents and adults, especially those in high-risk occupations, such as health care workers and teachers[20]. The vaccine cannot be given during pregnancy. Vaccines generally contain a component of the microorganism, dead organism or modified live organisms, which stimulate the immune system to produce immunity without resulting in the disease process[6].

In cases of high-risk, non-immune individuals having significant exposure to varicella, including non-immune pregnant women, zoster immunoglobulin (ZIG) may be used to give passive artificial immunity. Passive artificial immunity refers to the administration of antibodies (gamma globulin) derived, in the case of ZIG, from human plasma from blood donors. In contrast, passive natural immunity refers to the transfer of antibodies from mother to baby, across the placenta before birth, which gives protection to the baby for the first few months of life[6]. ZIG must be given to neonates whose mothers develop varicella (chickenpox) from seven days or less before delivery and up to 28 days after delivery, because its use can prevent or lessen the effects of varicella in the newborn period. ZIG must be given as soon as possible, but must be within 72 hours of exposure for optimal effect[23]. Use of ZIG is highly effective but supplies are limited.

NURSING IMPLICATIONS

Chickenpox is highly infectious and transmission-based precautions are required to prevent its spread in hospitals. Patients with chickenpox require a combination of airborne and contact precautions during the period of communicability[11]. When feasible, those with a history of chickenpox, or those who have completed a course of vaccination, should care for patients with chickenpox in preference to staff members who are unsure of their immune status. Nurses should, where possible, establish their immune status. Individuals are considered immune to varicella if they have a history of chickenpox or shingles, or if they have received a full course of vaccination. Those unsure of their immunity can be tested for serological evidence of past infection. If exposed to VZV, susceptible non-immune individuals should be considered potentially infectious 10 to 21 days following exposure[22]. In this circumstance, nurses may need to be reassigned duties that avoid patient contact and patients will need to be nursed in isolation.

When caring for patients with varicella or shingles, it is important to establish if there are high-risk non-immune contacts within family, friends and colleagues because follow-up and possible interventions, including the use of ZIG, may be indicated[16].

LEARNING EXERCISES
1. Outline the main features of viruses.
2. Describe the pathophysiology associated with infection due to varicella-zoster virus.
3. Explain the relationship between chickenpox and shingles.
4. Describe the options available for prevention and treatment of varicella infection.

In this case study, Kylie had a common childhood illness, varicella (chickenpox), which in most cases is self-limiting. Generally there is no specific treatment required, except for symptomatic relief. Chickenpox is highly infectious and can be significant in some people, such as non-immune pregnant women and the immunosuppressed.

When Kylie was found to have chickenpox, a wider assessment of family members and other close contacts was indicated. As Kylie's mother, Anne, was unsure of her own immune status to VZV, serological testing was used to establish her immune status, the positive IgG result indicating immunity to VZV. As Anne was immune, no further action was required for her or her unborn baby. If Anne had been non-immune, zoster immunoglobulin could have been administered to prevent or reduce the severity of the varicella infection, if given within 72 hours of exposure for maximal effect, or up to 96 hours with some benefit[23].

Within health care settings, consideration needs to be given to identifying suspected or known cases of transmissible infections, and to implementing any necessary isolation practices, or contact-tracing activities accordingly. Health care staff should have access within occupationally based screening and vaccination programs, to establish their own immune status and be offered vaccination if indicated[4].

BACTERIA

Bacteria, as a group of microorganisms, are important to nursing because they are one of the most common causes of infectious disease. Bacteria are single cell organisms that are classified as prokaryotic organisms because their DNA is not enclosed in a cellular compartment (i.e., nucleus). Bacteria are classified according to their response to staining, morphology (size and shape), reproduction, respiration, and their genus and species[5,27]. There is a large variance in the shape and size within bacteria. Size varies from 0.5 to 1.0 microns in diameter and length is also variable[27]. Bacteria appear in different shapes, such as: spherical or round (coccus or cocci); rod shape (bacillus or bacilli); and spiral shape (spirellum or spirella)[1].

Bacterial cells have both similar and differentiating structure and inclusions. The cell wall is important because it determines shape, provides support, and depending on its construction and sub-elements, determines whether the bacteria will stain Gram positive or negative. The propensity for how a bacteria stains, depends on the amount of peptidoglycan[1,5,27]. Cells with a thin layer stain Gram negative, while bacteria with a thick cell wall, containing a larger amount of peptidoglycan, stain Gram positive[1,5]. In some bacteria, the presence of a capsule or slime layer, known as glycocalyx, is external to the cell wall. The glycocalyx assists bacteria cells to adhere and attach to a substrate of the host cell[1,3], and to resist phagocytosis, as the engulfing phagocytes are unable to attach to the bacterial cell wall. This promotes the virulence of the bacteria[1].

Bacterial cell walls may also include fine thread or hair-like appendages, attachments such as flagella, pili and fimbriae. Flagella enables motility by a propeller-type motion that pulls the cell along[1]. Pili facilitate the transfer of genetic material between bacterial cells, while the fimbriae assist the bacteria to adhere to other surfaces[1,3]. Within their cell wall, bacteria do not have a defined nucleus, with the DNA and RNA mass lying free in the cytoplasm[1,5]. Also contained within the cytoplasm are the plasmids (small circular inclusions that contain additional genetic material). There are usually a large number of ribosomes scattered throughout the cytoplasm and these are the sites for protein synthesis[1].

Some bacteria are able to form endospores in response to environmental changes or a lack of nutrients. These highly resistant spores allow the bacteria to survive unfavourable conditions. When placed in more favourable conditions, a new bacterial cell can emerge from the spore even after long periods of dormancy[5,27].

Infection relates to an increase in the number of cells, as opposed to the size of the cells. Bacteria normally reproduce via binary fission (cell division and the formation of two identical daughter cells)[1,5]. Bacterial reproduction requires certain environmental or physical factors – temperature, pH, osmotic pressure, and the presence or absence of oxygen. In addition, certain chemical factors, including availability of water, trace elements, nitrogen, carbon, and phosphorus are important. In the right environment, bacteria are able to reproduce by binary fission each half hour. Rapid reproduction means that a single cell can, in a matter of hours, lead to millions of bacteria and serious infection. However, there are differences in growth rates between different types of bacteria[1].

BACTERIAL WOUND INFECTION: WHAT DOES IT MEAN?

The integrity of the skin is an effective barrier against invading microorganisms. Any breach in the skin, including surgical incisions, or skin breakdown leading to changes in skin integrity, may allow microorganisms to gain access to underlying tissues and risk the development of a wound infection[28]. Chronic wounds, including leg ulcers, are open wounds that heal by secondary intention. Colonisation with microorganisms, typically bacteria, is common, and a balance between organism and host factors will influence which wounds remain colonised and heal normally, and which will become infected, delaying healing[29]. Definitions of wound infection vary, although most use four cardinal signs: the presence of swelling, pain, heat and redness in the tissues surrounding the wound[6]. Lipsky[30] defines infection as the presence of purulent secretions (pus), or two or more signs or symptoms of inflammation. Regardless of which definition is applied, the microorganisms contaminating the wound, and the host's resistance to that contamination, will ultimately determine whether a wound becomes infected. Infection in a wound can delay healing, contribute to significant morbidity, and even mortality, for the host person, and result in additional costs to the health care system[29].

● Case study

Harry Davies, 55, has had type 2 diabetes for 12 years. As part of his general diabetes management, Mr Davies regularly attends the foot clinic at his local hospital for inspection and care of his feet. Over the past three weeks, he has developed an area of ulceration on his left heel.

At his latest presentation to the clinic, the ulcer appears enlarged in size and the exudates from the wound are pus-like in nature. There is redness and some swelling around the wound and notable cellulitis to the foot and ankle. The area is warm to the touch yet Mr Davies makes no complaint of pain or discomfort. Swabs are taken for microscopy, culture and sensitivity, and the laboratory identifies a resistant *Staphylococcus aureus*. Mr Davies had previously been found to have methicillin-resistant *Staphylococcus aureus* (MRSA), located from a nasal swab taken as part of a routine screening program within the hospital. Systemically, Mr Davies has a low-grade pyrexia 37.2°C, and his blood glucose levels are less well controlled than normal. He feels tired and more lethargic than usual.

Mr Davies is admitted for antibiotic therapy and surgical debridement of the wound. As he has antibiotic-resistant bacteria, Mr Davies is placed into single-room isolation and staff members are advised to use contact precautions for his care.

WHAT IS THE PATHOPHYSIOLOGY?

There are several general factors that may increase an individual's risk of wound infection[6]:

- Nature of the injury, for example, trauma involving dirt/debris;
- Reduced blood supply that reduces delivery of components of the immune system;
- Presence of devitalised/necrotic (dead) tissue;
- General health – presence of disease that affects immune response, malnourished, immunocompromised;
- Existing skin carriage of a potential pathogen; and
- Drugs that affect immune response (e.g., steroids or antibiotics) may affect bacterial balance.

People with diabetes have a four-fold higher incidence of peripheral vascular disease (PVD) than individuals without diabetes[31]. This contributes to foot ulceration with the subsequent impaired delivery of oxygen, nutrients and antibiotics that affect healing and the ability to combat infection. Poor glucose control predisposes to infection, in particular, with impaired phagocytosis and cell-mediated immunity function[33]. In addition, people with diabetes may have significant peripheral neuropathy, a major contributory factor to ulceration. The combination of repetitive stress, unrelieved pressure on the foot and minor trauma potentiate the development of foot ulcers[31].

Once an area of ulceration has been established, the lack of skin integrity allows for initial colonisation with bacteria and infection may readily ensue. The spread of cellulitis is often indicative of bacterial infection and may be influenced by the nature of the causative organism. *Staphylococcus aureus* has many virulence factors facilitating its ability as a pathogen: one example is that it produces the enzyme hyaluronidase, which hydrolyses hyaluronic acid, enhancing spread through connective tissue[2].

Sources of bacteria causing wound infection can be endogenous or exogenous. As all skin wounds are colonised with microorganisms, it is an area of controversy as to what extent the isolation of bacteria from ulcers is indicative of infection, and so clinical signs and symptoms are important in establishing the presence of infection and its severity[34].

Infection can be associated with health care institutions and the term 'nosocomial' infection is used for infections not incubating or present on admission. Typically for bacterial infections, this means the infection is apparent after 48 hours in hospital[10].

Increasingly, antibiotic resistant bacteria are a feature of infection associated with health care, although resistant bacteria can originate in the community. Methicillin-resistant *Staphylococcus aureus* (MRSA) is one such bacterium prevalent around the world. MRSA is an antibiotic resistant version of *Staphylococcus aureus*, bacteria that can form part of the normal commensal flora of one-third of people[35]. *Staphylococcus aureus* can cause a range of infections from boils and abscesses to wound infection, pneumonia, and septicaemia. MRSA shares the same characteristics as *Staphylococcus* but is resistant to beta-lactam antibiotics, such as methicillin (which is no longer in use,) and flucloxacillin[36]. A range of factors has contributed to the emergence of resistant bacteria. Widespread use of broad-spectrum antibiotics, advances in health care that allow for increasingly complex and high-risk procedures, use of indwelling devices, hospitalisation of immunosuppressed patients, and sub-optimal compliance in infection-control practices are considered to be significant factors in the development of antibiotic resistant strains of bacteria[37]. Colonisation with MRSA can occur in the anterior nares and skin sites, including the groin, axilla and mucous membranes, notably the throat. MRSA can spread endogenously or via cross infection by direct contact[35].

WHAT ARE THE CLINICAL MANIFESTATIONS?

When infection occurs in a wound, such as a diabetic foot ulcer, the underlying pathophysiological processes manifest themselves with a range of signs and symptoms that can be assessed clinically. Tissue injury, including invasion by microorganisms, results in an inflammation response, which has two major components[38]:

1. Vasodilatation and increased capillary permeability; and
2. Infiltration of leucocytes in response to local generation of chemotactic factors.

Several immune mediators contribute to vasodilation and increased vasopermeability, including histamine, leukotrienes and prostaglandins. This increased vasodilation and subsequent fluid infiltration gives rise to the four cardinal signs of inflammation – heat, redness, swelling and pain[39]. Vasodilation of the venuoles with constriction of the arterial bed results in engorging of the vascular network, which gives rise to the redness and localised increase in temperature. Concurrent increased capillary permeability facilitates an influx of cells and fluid, which accumulate as exudates. If these exudates collect in the tissues, they may manifest as oedema. Increasing tissue pressure, as fluid exudates accumulate, can pressurise nerve endings resulting in pain. The direct effects of some inflammatory mediators can also induce pain at the site of injury[40]. The neuropathy typical in diabetes can mask the sensation of pain. The infiltration of the tissues during inflammation includes accumulation of neutrophils at the site of injury. These phagocytose bacteria/other debris and this can result in neutrophil death and release of lysosomal enzymes. This results in tissue damage, liquefaction necrosis and accumulation of tissue debris, dead and dying neutrophils, which collectively are referred to as pus (purulent exudate). The presence of pus as an exudate can be associated with certain strongly chemotactic bacteria, such as *Staphylococcus* species. In addition, the potential of such bacteria to release exotoxins can further contribute to tissue damage, cell death and pus formation[41]. Redness surrounding an ulcer site can also be due to cellulitis. Cellulitis symptoms that include redness or erythema, warmth, pain and swelling is usually secondary to an ulcer formation[42]. In addition to effects on the immune response, normal wound healing processes are impaired in diabetics. Hyperglycaemia is a catabolic state with a resultant negative nitrogen balance, leading to protein breakdown that impairs wound healing[43]. Furthermore, diabetics may have decreased levels of growth factors, such as platelet-derived growth factor (PGDF), which are important in normal wound healing processes.

Mr Davies showed some of the classical signs of infection, with pus coming from the wound, and cellulitis, with redness, swelling and heat around the wound site. However due to the presence of neuropathy, the associated sign of pain or discomfort at the site of infection is masked. While wound infection is localised, systemic signs may also be present, including pyrexia and general feelings of tiredness or lethargy[4].

WHAT SHOULD YOU BE LOOKING AT IN THE LABORATORY TESTS?

A wound swab would be a typical test undertaken in instances of suspected or actual wound infection. The quality of the specimen is vital in achieving useful information and a specimen of pus or tissue (when possible) may yield more accurate findings[28]. With ulcers, specimens that are taken from the base of the ulcer, or contain purulent exudate, will be the most useful in guiding appropriate antibiotic therapy[33]. The standard microbiology request is for *microscopy culture and sensitivity* (MCS). Typical results for this case study are presented in Figure 2.2.

In diabetic foot infection, the most common organisms cultured are aerobic Gram-positive cocci, including *Staphylococcus aureus*, coagulase-negative Staphylococci and Streptococci. In addition, aerobic Gram-negative species including *Eschericia coli* and other enterobacteriaceae species are found. While the results from a wound swab are important in guiding therapeutic options, the clinical presentation must also be taken into consideration because chronic wounds can be colonised with bacteria, but these may not be significant clinically[6].

Alert-based organism surveillance is a minimum standard to observe for antimicrobial-resistant organisms within the laboratory and infection-control services[44]. This system ensures that when resistant organisms are identified from specimens in the laboratory, systems of notification to infection-control teams or ward staff are initiated so that appropriate actions can be taken. In addition, screening programs for MRSA are adopted by many health care organisations. Screening may target inter-hospital transfers, new admissions or specialist high-risk wards and areas, such as intensive care units, transplant units or cardiothoracic units. The specimens taken for screening vary, but suggested sites include the nose, perineum or groin, throat, wounds and manipulated sites (e.g., venous access sites)[44]. Screening for resistant organisms, including MRSA, allows for early detection and the implementation of infection control measures. These measures may include the use of single-room isolation, strict attention to hand hygiene and the use of contact precautions.

Blood tests for white cell count (WCC) and erythrocyte sedimentation rate (ESR) also provide clinical information regarding the patient's infectious status. A differential WCC identifies the numbers of each type of white blood cell. Raised neutrophil and monocyte

	Wound Swab	
Microscopy – uses light microscopy and staining techniques	Gram-positive cocci seen	
Culture – growth of organism on media to determine conditions affecting growth and visualisation of the colonies	100 colonies of *Staphylococcus* species (probably *S. aureus*) isolated	
Antibiotic Sensitivity	*Sensitive to:*	*Resistant to:*
	Fusidic acid Vancomycin Rifampicin	Penicillin Flucloxacillin
Report	Methicillin-resistant *Staphylococcus aureus*	

FIGURE 2.2 *Laboratory findings*

counts are indicative of infection, and lymphocytes can be raised in the convalescent phase of bacterial infection. The ESR is a measure of the time taken for red blood cells to settle within a blood sample. During inflammation and infection, the presence of immune system proteins (acute-phase reactants), increase the time taken for the red blood cells to settle. ESR is presented as a rate of millimetres per hour, and rates of >20 mm/h are indicative of infection[45].

WHAT IS THE TREATMENT?

The over-riding aim in managing an infected wound is to address the 'host-bacterial balance'[46]. This can include debridement of the wound and controlling the bacterial load and inflammation. Surgical debridement may be considered in infected wounds, especially when there are large amounts of devitalised tissue. The principle of debridement is to remove necrotic and infected tissue to leave a clean open wound with a reduced bacterial load, promoting an environment within the wound conducive to healing[33]. The use of topical enzyme treatments, moisture-retentive dressings and vacuum therapy are alternatives to surgical debridement[46].

In some cases, contributory factors predisposing to infection can be eliminated or modified. In this case study, good foot care can prevent the initial development of further ulceration, which may progress and contribute to subsequent infection. Ischaemia may be alleviated by vascular surgery improving blood flow, tissue perfusion, and the delivery of antibiotics and nutrients for wound healing[33].

More novel therapies include the use of hyperbaric oxygen therapy and the use of engineered skin substitutes. Hyperbaric oxygen therapy increases tissue oxygen levels, promoting collagen synthesis, it encourages leucocyte killing of bacteria, and the high levels of oxygen are toxic to anaerobic bacteria[33]. Skin substitutes vary in their composition but are essentially an engineered matrix containing various factors to promote wound healing (e.g., fibroblasts, growth factors). When used in conjunction with more established therapies (debridement, dressing protocols and treatment of infection), skin substitutes are proving to be beneficial in the management of diabetic foot ulcers[33]. Additional therapeutic considerations to facilitate healing include choice of dressing products and dressing technique. Attention to nutritional requirements promoting good nutrition is a further factor significant in wound healing[41].

APPLIED PHARMACOLOGY

Antibiotics first became commonplace within health care in the 1940s. As bacteria have a prokaryotic cell structure, which differs from human cell structure, antibiotics are selective in their toxicity, targeting the bacteria rather than host cells. There are several modes of action for antibiotics and these are broadly grouped as those which: 1) inhibit bacterial cell wall synthesis; 2) inhibit protein synthesis; 3) inhibit nucleic acid; 4) disrupt metabolic pathways; and 5) alter cell membranes[2].

Methicillin-resistant *Staphylococcus aureus* is resistant to many of the common antibiotics used to treat infection with Gram-positive bacteria[44]. This restricts the antibiotics available for use in instances of MRSA infection. Vancomycin, derived from *Streptomyces orientalis*, is the antibiotic of choice for MRSA infection[2]. Vancomycin is a tricyclic glycopeptide antibiotic, which inhibits peptidoglycan formation and therefore disrupts the formation of the cell wall in Gram-positive bacteria[47]. Some species of enterococci bacteria have acquired resistance to vancomycin, which threatens the usefulness of vancomycin in the future[48].

Enterococci have the ability to transfer their resistance to other bacteria, including MRSA. The first incidence of vancomycin-resistant *Staphylococcus aureus* was reported in the USA in 2002[35,49].

NURSING IMPLICATIONS

General considerations when caring for patients with an infection include monitoring vital signs, management of pyrexia as appropriate, ensuring the maintenance of adequate hydration, and maximising patient comfort[50]. Promoting rest reduces metabolic demands and enables body resources and energy to be used for the increased immune response and wound healing. Particular attention to the patient's nutritional requirements, including carbohydrates for energy, proteins and some trace nutrients (vitamin C and zinc), is required for wound healing[50]. Administration of antibiotic therapy must follow required local policies and guidelines.

Although prevalent in bacteria, resistance to pharmacological agents has been observed in all categories of microorganisms[51]. Sometimes referred to as 'superbugs', resistant microorganisms pose a challenge within health care by reducing the therapeutic options available for treatment. In addition, infection caused by resistant organisms generates significant costs to the patient and to the health care system, in terms of increased length of stay, expensive and often toxic drug alternatives, and the associated issues for patients, including loss of earnings.

Various means are used to control the spread of antimicrobial-resistant microorganisms. Screening for resistant organisms may form part of a health care institution's program for infection control. This approach allows for prompt and ongoing identification of patients who are either infected or colonised with MRSA, and care can be aimed at minimising spread of the resistant bacteria within the organisation. Isolation in a single room with additional precautions is an approach that alerts health care staff to take the additional precautions required to minimise spread by direct contact, the mode of transmission for MRSA. When isolation methods are used, the psychosocial well-being of the patient must be considered at all times by maintaining effective staff–patient communication and interaction with the patient[52].

The literature has already noted the next stages in the evolution of MRSA. Heterogenous vancomycin intermediate sensitive *Staphylococcus aureus* (hVISA) is MRSA with reduced susceptibility to vancomycin[48]; and vancomycin-resistant *Staphylococcus aureus* (VRSA)[53] have been reported. These findings limit the treatment choices even further and rely on expensive drugs for which resistance is already documented.

LEARNING EXERCISES

1. Outline the main features of bacteria.
2. Describe factors that may contribute to the development of bacterial infection.
3. Discuss the significance of antimicrobial-resistant microorganisms.
4. Describe some of the nursing considerations in caring for patients with infections.

Infection is a complex interaction between host and microorganism-based factors. Emphasis must always be placed on preventing infection. In this case study, when applied to diabetic foot infection, the identification of, and, where possible, modification of predisposing risk factors (including neuropathy and ischaemia) is also required. The promotion of skin integrity with well-fitting shoes, good foot care and maintenance of a nutritious diet and good glycaemic control are also beneficial.

When infection does occur, there are two facets to management: the treatment of the infection in the individual; and the prevention of potential spread of the infection. Treatment of the individual is aided by accurate diagnosis. As many bacteria are common in the environment, and many are natural commensals for humans, the microbiological reports on specimens must be taken into consideration with the clinical picture, and the signs and symptoms of the patient, bearing in mind that, as in this case study, the neuropathy experienced by many diabetics may mask signs of infection. Preventing the spread of infection requires a range of practices, including hand hygiene, appropriate use of personal protective equipment, such as gloves, and when necessary, patient isolation.

FUNGI (MYCOSES)

Fungi are organisms generally categorised into two major groups – yeasts and moulds. Only about 50 of these cause diseases in humans[1,2]. While fungi vary in morphology or appearance, the cell is surrounded by a cell wall and possesses a nucleus and nuclear membrane. However, they differ from plants in that fungi contain no chlorophyll and, therefore, do not engage in photosynthesis. Fungi are considered more resilient than bacteria[1,2]. Fungal infections are generally opportunistic and seen as an annoyance and not life-threatening, except in individuals with severely compromised immune systems[1].

Yeasts are the more problematic for humans. They are larger than bacteria, unicellular and spherical or ovoid in shape, and contain subcellular organelles. Reproduction is mainly asexual via 'budding'. A small eruption or growth appears on the parent cell that gradually enlarges and then separates, forming a new daughter cell. The daughter cell can separate entirely or help form a chain of yeast cells[1,2]. Pathogenic strains can exhibit 'dimorphism' or the ability to grow in two different forms.

Classification of fungal disease is according to primary sites of infection – superficial mycoses (outer layers of skin and hair); cutaneous mycoses (epidermis and invasive nail and hair diseases); subcutaneous mycoses (dermis, subcutaneous tissue, muscle and fascia); and systemic (often originating in the lung but which spreads to many organ systems)[1,2,27].

Moulds exhibit different structure and some produce chemicals with antibacterial qualities (e.g., penicillin). Moulds are generally not a problem for humans[1].

CANDIDIASIS: WHAT DOES IT MEAN?

Candidiasis or 'thrush' is an infection most commonly caused by the yeast *Candida albicans*[54]. *Candida* is a normal commensal organism of the body, but when the normal body environment is altered, or when the immune system is compromised, it can present as a mild to severe opportunistic infection[2,54–58].

● Case study

Sara Jameson, 19, presents to the Family Planning Clinic for a routine Pap smear. Sara complains that she has been experiencing a thick, white vaginal discharge, extreme irritation (pruritis) in the vulvovaginal region, some burning on micturition, and increasing discomfort during sexual intercourse. She has been taking the oral contraceptive pill for the past six weeks since becoming sexually active with her regular boyfriend. Apart from being 'stressed' about her upcoming university exams, and having had a recent upper respiratory tract infection for which she received the oral antibiotic therapy (amoxycillin), Sara is well and usually leads an active and healthy life.

WHAT IS THE PATHOPHYSIOLOGY?

Candidiasis is typical of opportunistic yeast infections and occurs when the normal body mechanisms keeping these yeasts in control either breakdown or are compromised, allowing the organism to penetrate, colonise and reproduce in the host[2,27]. As part of the normal flora of the body, *Candida* is normally held in check by an intact skin or mucous membrane barrier, the high turnover of skin and mucous membrane cells, competing normal flora, and a competent immune system[1,2,54].

Skin infections are more commonly seen in moist, warm environments, such as skin folds, groin or axillae[1]. Potential vaginal infections are usually controlled by the variety and competition of normal vaginal flora[54]. The most significant factor inhibiting yeast infections in the vaginal region is the lactic acid produced by the lactobacillus that helps maintain the vaginal pH at less than 4.5[54]. This acidic environment discourages the growth of opportunistic microorganisms, such as *Candida albicans*.

Changes to the environment and the subsequent proliferation of yeast (fungal) cells may result from factors including a depressed or immature immune system, pregnancy, use of oral contraceptives, prolonged use of antibiotic therapy or topical or systemic steroids, and the concurrent presence of diabetes mellitus[1,2,27,55,56].

Individuals with severely compromised or immature immune systems become vulnerable for the development of mucocutaneous and systemic infections. Systemic infections (e.g., candidaemia) are often associated with severe pre-existing conditions, such as cancer or leukaemia, or when therapy compromises the immune system, such as in transplant recipients[55]. Invasive procedures that provide an additional portal of entry, for example, intravenous/total parenteral nutrition (IV/TPN) therapy, continuous ambulatory peritoneal dialysis (CAPD), can predispose to systemic infections[1].

Transmission is normally by direct contact with the fungi/spores or via inhalation[1]. Vaginal candidiasis is not classified as a sexually transmitted disease, but can be transmitted sexually by an affected partner to the other partner[54].

WHAT ARE THE CLINICAL MANIFESTATIONS?

Vaginal candidiasis is experienced by nearly 75% of adolescent females and women[54,55,58]. The common symptoms are vulval and vaginal pruritis, accompanied by a thick, white ('cottage cheese-like') vaginal discharge[54,55,57]. There is often associated pain or burning sensation when urinating and there may be discomfort during sexual intercourse, due to the excoriated and inflamed vagina and vulval regions[54,55]. Males who contract the infection may complain of irritation around the glans penis[54].

WHAT SHOULD YOU BE LOOKING AT IN THE LABORATORY TESTS?

The clinical manifestations are usually sufficiently indicative of a candidiasis infection. Diagnostic tests may include vaginal examination where the discharge is usually seen as white plaques covering the vaginal walls and cervix[54]. Vaginal pH using litmus paper testing will typically be less than 4.5 (normal is 3.5–4.5)[41,55,58]. A wet mount slide, using the scrapings from the vaginal wall, may demonstrate the presence of yeast filaments or spores[41,54]. If the wet mount technique is negative, then a culture may be necessary for a definitive diagnosis[41]. Careful collection and processing of specimens is necessary to avoid contamination and falsely attributed cultured growths.

WHAT IS THE TREATMENT?

Antifungal agents are normally prescribed either in oral (e.g., fluconazole) or topical (e.g., nystatin cream or vaginal suppository) preparations. The creams and suppositories are generally available as over-the-counter preparations. These agents interfere with the cellular membranes of the yeasts inhibiting further reproduction[55].

Other treatment is palliative to relieve symptoms and reduce the risk of transference. Attention to general hygiene is important with careful hand washing to prevent transfer of the infection to other areas of the body. The use of warm sodium bicarbonate bathing may alleviate discomfort and also raise the vaginal pH. Avoidance of perfumed soaps and bath products is recommended as these may exacerbate the irritation[54]. Loose clothing and cotton underwear is helpful in minimising further irritation of excoriated and irritated areas in the vulval region[54]. No specific dietary regime but use of acidophilus yoghurt may be helpful[55]. Although not classified as a sexually transmitted disease, the contact between partners during intercourse will provide a vector for re-infection and the partner will also need treatment to reduce the potential for re-infection[1].

NURSING IMPLICATIONS

Among the important issues for nurses is the provision of health care education orientated at prevention and the correct use of treatment regimes. Advice relating to personal hygiene and maintenance of general good health is also important. Sensitivity needs to be applied when providing advice, particularly in relation to personal hygiene, because individuals may easily take offence where personal hygiene is not a contributing factor. The literature varies in its reporting of recurrence (more than four episodes)[54,58] but are universal in recommending that underlying causes, such as immunodeficiency, diabetes and repeated antibiotic use, may be precipitating factors. These should be explored as part of general health assessment in situations of recurrence[55].

In this case study, Sara presents as a fairly typical example of a single-event vaginal yeast infection. Her symptoms are classical and she conforms to the general demographic profile of young adult women who are normally fit and well with no other major illnesses. Compliance with prescribed medication, good general hygiene and the use of palliation to address discomforting symptoms are important health education issues. To prevent potential infection of her partner, or reinfection of herself, the use of condoms and partner treatment compliance during the treatment phase is essential.

PARASITES

Parasites are organisms that derive their source of nutrients from another organism usually referred to as the host[1,27]. They may live on the surface of the host or other organisms (ectoparasites) or within the host (endoparasites)[16,27]. Transmission commonly occurs through two ways: injection; or accidental ingestion[1,5]. Many parasites are capable of forming cysts that form a protective barrier and enable the parasites to survive in adverse environmental conditions and resist destruction[1,5,27]. Parasites often require a mechanical or biological vector for transmission, such as mosquitoes and malaria[1,15,27]. Reproduction is usually asexual (binary fission) although some species are capable of sexual reproduction (e.g., *Cryptosporidium*)[1]. Parasitic infections are a problem worldwide although their severity in Australia is not considered as significant as in developing countries[1]. Populations in Australia most affected by parasites tend to be vulnerable due to their lifestyle and lack of resources (e.g., Aborigines) or immunocompromised (e.g., AIDS patients)[1,27]. There are three major categories of parasites: protozoa; helminths; and arthropods[1,2,27].

Protozoa are mostly free-living unicellular organisms. The main groups and their prominent disease conditions are amoebae (amoebic dysentery), flagellates (giardiasis), ciliates (balantidial dysentery), and sporozoa (malaria and toxoplasmosis)[1,27]. Helminths are commonly referred to as worms. Generally, helminths are larger organisms but may be quite small during developmental stages[1,2,27]. One of the major groups affecting humans is the flatworm, which include tapeworms (Cestoda). Tapeworms can affect humans in their adult form, or in some diseases more severely, when acquired in their larval stage (e.g., hydatid disease). Flukes (Trematoda or Dignea) either penetrate the skin or are ingested. The most significant are the blood flukes or schistosomes, causing schistosomiasis. The other major worm group is the nematodes or roundworms, causing roundworm, hookworm or threadworm infestations[1,5].

Arthropods are insects that form an ectoparasitic relationship with humans and thus a vector for transmission of pathogens, ranging from viruses, bacteria, rickettsias, protozoa and worms. The most common are mosquitoes, ticks, lice, fleas and mites. These insects gain nutrients from human blood and use the same medium to transmit pathogens[1,5].

● Case study

Mrs Gwen Thomas, 80, is a resident in a private nursing home. She has complained of an itchy rash on her hands and forearms for several weeks and was diagnosed with eczema. The skin condition has been unresponsive to traditional eczema treatment. Recently, fellow residents (in the same room) and several of the nursing assistants, who have provided care for Mrs Thomas, are complaining of similar symptoms. Senior nursing staff suspect an outbreak of scabies.

SCABIES: WHAT DOES IT MEAN?

Scabies is a skin infection caused by the mite *Sarcoptes scabiei*[59].

WHAT IS THE PATHOPHYSIOLOGY?

Scabies is a condition caused by the ectoparasite *Sarcoptes scabiei*, also known as the itch mite and related to the mite causing mange in animals. These are very small and not visible to the naked eye, being less than 0.5 mm in length[59,60]. The adult female is larger than the male and following fertilisation, the mites burrow into the upper layers of the epidermis laying thirty to forty eggs that hatch within 3 to 5 days. The larvae excavate and create new burrows and reach maturity in approximately 4 days where the cycle is repeated[60–62]. Scabies is normally transmitted by direct personal contact with the infected person or their clothing or bedding[60–62].

WHAT ARE THE CLINICAL MANIFESTATIONS?

The most significant aspect of presentation is acute pruritis[60–62]. The site of the intense itchiness is dependent on the site of infestation. Commonly, these are the interdigital folds of the skin but may also appear in the groin, elbows, umbilicus, axillae, behind the knee, and under the breasts[60]. Burrows appear as thread-like lines with a vesicle at one end and are often hard to see because of the associated skin disease[60,61]. Excoriation and inflammation around the site of the burrow is a feature and often scabies is misdiagnosed as dermatitis or eczema. The dermatitis reaction (papules, vesicles and nodules,) is usually due to a delayed hypersensitivity reaction[60]. A form of scabies infection with generalised scaling and crusting of the skin is known as Norwegian scabies, and is usually seen in the immunodeficient, such as AIDS patients or the elderly[60,63]. As these patients usually carry a significant mite load, the condition is extremely contagious.

Spread usually occurs due to contact or scratching and this may also predispose to bacterial secondary infections as a breach in the normal skin defence mechanism occurs[60]. The mites are transferred to others by direct contact or through contact with objects or articles including bedding or clothing (i.e., fomites) that may be temporarily housing the mites. The infection may end spontaneously in a few months but chronic cases do exist.

WHAT SHOULD YOU BE LOOKING AT IN THE LABORATORY TESTS?

Definitive diagnosis is by skin scrapings of the infected areas. Although burrows may be seen these are often masked due to the surrounding inflammation. The skin scrapings are microscopically examined and the mites or their eggs are visible if the diagnosis is positive[60,61].

WHAT IS THE TREATMENT?

The application of appropriate topical lotions (permethrin, malathion or maldison, benzyl benzoate, crotamiton, gamma benzene hexachloride and sulphur compounds), and the disinfection of bedding and clothing are the principal treatment agents. The treatment lotion should be applied to all skin surfaces from the top of the head to the soles of the feet and toes for 8 to 12 hours and then washed off. This one dose is usually sufficient, if prepared and administered correctly. The treatment may be repeated in a week if evidence of mites or eggs persists. The pruritic effect of the scabies may persist for several weeks and should be treated palliatively[60–62]. It is important that all those with close personal contact with the patient or their environment are also treated.

APPLIED PHARMACOLOGY

Permethrin cream is considered the most efficient of the scabicides. Aqueous solutions are less irritating to inflamed or excoriated skin than alcohol-based preparations. Gamma benzene hexachloride (Lindane) has been used selectively due to neurotoxic side effects and should not be used in children less than two years of age, or pregnant/lactating women. Crotamiton is suitable for children less than two months, but is less effective than permethrin or Lindane. Sulphur preparations are the least efficacious and have the disadvantage of requiring more than one treatment, an unpleasant smell and may stain clothing or bedding[60,61].

In cases of highly resistant or Norwegian scabies, oral ivermectin 200 µg/kg body weight may be used in one dose or, if persistent, a second dose a week later.

NURSING IMPLICATIONS

The correct application and the prevention of further spread are of critical importance in the treatment of scabies. Prescribed lotions should be checked for currency and appropriately administered to the body with particular attention paid to interdigital and nail-bed areas[61]. Hands that are washed should have the lotion reapplied during the treatment phase. Following application, special care should be taken with children or cognitively impaired to avoid inadvertent ingestion with use of mittens in babies and infants recommended[60,61].

Patients and carers need to be advised that the itchiness will most likely continue after treatment and is not an indication for repeat application. Appropriate staff should assess the need for a repeat application. Symptomatic relief can be assisted by the use of antihistamines, emolient creams or mild topical corticosteroid preparations[60].

All individuals who have had contact with the patient or their direct carers (staff personnel and their families) together with their own bedding or clothing should undergo the treatment to reduce the spread. It is also important that the environment (including patient bedding and clothing) is thoroughly cleaned and disinfected to prevent re-infection and further transmission to others[60,61].

Scabies is one of the re-emergent conditions previously associated with poor personal and environmental conditions. The increase in the number of individuals with immunodeficiency due to physical conditions (e.g., HIV), or as a result of a longer lifespan. The frailties of old age have created a new situation for scabies infestations. In these circumstances, scabies infestations are usually more virulent and the mite load is significantly greater creating a more potent opportunity for transmission and contagion to others who come in contact with the infected individual or their fomites. As scabies is often not suspected, the skin conditions can often be misdiagnosed, as in this case study. Following diagnosis, it would be important for Mrs Thomas to receive the appropriate treatment lotion, disinfection of her fomites, and disinfection of the surrounding area in the nursing home. To prevent recurrence and further spread, all residents, visitors and staff (including their families who complain of skin irritation), and who may have had access to direct contact with Mrs Thomas, or her clothing and bedding, should also receive treatment.

CONCLUSION

During this chapter the concept of infection has been defined and the process of infection described. The importance of infection control and the use of standard and special precautions to prevent infection occurrence or transmission, have been presented as a precursor to subsequent discussion of the major infective agents. For each infective agent, a case history of a typical infection has been used to explore that agent's unique pathophysiology, clinical presentation and related diagnostic testing. Relevant therapeutic interventions have been considered from the nurses' perspective.

Recommended Readings

1. Black, J. 1999; *Microbiology: Principles and Explorations* (4th ed.), Prentice Hall, New Jersey.
2. Horton, R & Parker, L. 2002; *Informed Infection Control Practice*, Churchill-Livingstone, Edinburgh.
3. Lee, G & Bishop, P. 2002; *Microbiology and Infection Control for Health Professionals.* Prentice Hall Health, Frenchs Forest, New South Wales.
4. Mims, C, Playfair, J, Roitt, I, Wakelin, D & Williams, R. 1998; *Medical Microbiology* (2nd ed.), Mosby, London.
5. Murray, PR, Rosenthal, KS, Kobayashi, GS & Pfaller, MA. 2002; *Medical Microbiology* (4th ed.), Mosby, St Louis.

References

1. Lee, G & Bishop, P. 2002; *Microbiology and Infection Control for Health Professionals*, Prentice Hall Health, Frenchs Forest, New South Wales.
2. Murray, PR, Rosenthal, KS, Kobayashi, GS & Pfaller, MA. 2002; *Medical Microbiology* (4th ed.), Mosby, St Louis.

3. Bannister, BA, Begg, NT & Gillespie, SH. 1996; *Infectious Disease*. Blackwell Science, Oxford.

4. Horton, R. & Parker, L. 2002; *Informed Infection Control Practice*, Churchill-Livingstone, Edinburgh.

5. Mims, C, Playfair, J, Roitt, I, Wakelin, D & Williams, R. 1998; *Medical Microbiology* (2nd ed.), Mosby, London.

6. McCulloch, J. 2000; *Infection Control Science: Management and Practice*, Whurr Publishers, London.

7. Rowsey, PJ. 1997; 'Applied Pathophysiology: Pathophysiology of Fever, Part 2: Relooking at Cooling Interventions', *Dimensions of Critical Care Nursing*, 16 (5), 251–256.

8. Centers For Disease Control. 2002; 'Prevention Guideline for Hand Hygiene in Health Care Settings: Recommendations of the Health Care Infection Control Practices Advisory Committee and the HICPAC/SHEA/APIC/ISDA Hand Hygiene Task Force', MMWR 51 (RR 16), CDC, Atlanta.

9. Pittet, D. 2003; 'Hand Hygiene: Improved Standards and Practice for Hospital Care', *Current Opinion in Infectious Disease*, 16, 327–335.

10. Garner, JS. 1996; 'Guidelines for isolation precautions in hospitals', *American Journal of Infection Control*, 24, 24–52.

11. New South Wales Health Department. 2002; *Infection Control Policy*, Circular 2002/45. New South Wales Health Department, Sydney.

12. Queensland Health 2001; *Queensland Health Infection: Control Guidelines*. http://www.health.qld.gov.au/infectioncontrol/documents/pdf/QHICP_WEB.pdf.

13. Pratt, RJ, Pellowe, C, Loveday, HP, Robinson, N, Smith, GW, Barrett, S, Davey, P, Harper, P, Loveday, C & McDougall, C. 2001; 'Guidelines for Preventing Infections Associated with the Insertion and Maintenance of Indwelling Urethral Catheters in Acute Care', *Journal of Hospital Infection*, 47 (Supplement), S39–S46.

14. Pratt, RJ, Pellowe, C, Loveday, HP, Robinson, N, Smith, GW, Barrett, S, Davey, P, Harper, P, Loveday, C & McDougall, C. 2001; 'Guidelines for Preventing Infections Associated with the Insertion and Maintenance of Central Venous Catheters', *Journal of Hospital Infection*, 47 (supplement), S47–S67.

15. Phillips, J & Murray, P. (eds.). 1995; *The Biology of Disease*, Blackwell Scientific Publications, Oxford.

16. The Australian Technical Advisory Group on Immunisation of the Commonwealth Department of Health and Aged Care. 2000; *The Australian Immunisation Handbook* (7th ed.), National Health and Medical Research Council, Canberra.

17. Collier, L & Oxford, J. 2000; *Human Virology: A Text for Students of Medicine, Dentistry and Microbiology* (2nd ed.), Oxford University Press, Oxford.

18. Dukers, N & Rezza, G. 2003; 'Human Herpesvirus 8 Epidemiology: What We Do and Do Not Know', *AIDS*, 17 (12), 1717–1730.

19. Leach, CT. 2000; 'Human herpesvirus–6 and –7 Infections in Children: Agents of Roseola and Other Syndromes', *Current Opinion in Pediatrics*, 12 (3), 269–274.

20. Centers For Disease. 2003; *Epidemiology and Prevention of Vaccine-preventable Diseases* (7th ed.), CDC, Atlanta. http://www.cdc.gov/nip/publications/pink/Full.htm

21. Gnann, JW & Whitley, RJ. 2002; 'Herpes Zoster', *The New England Journal of Medicine*, 347 (5), 340–346.

22. Chin, J. (ed.). 2000; *Control of Communicable Disease Manual* (17th ed.), American Public Health Association, Washington.

23. Heuchan, A & Isaacs, D. 2001; 'The Management of Varicella-Zoster Virus Exposure and Infection in Pregnancy and the Newborn Period', *Medical Journal of Australia*, 174, 288–292.

24. Pagana, KD & Pagana, TJ. 1998; *Mosby's Manual of Diagnostic and Laboratory Tests*, Mosby, St Louis.

25. Mandell, GL, Bennett, JE & Dolin, R. 2000; *Mandell, Douglas and Bennett's Principles and Practice of Infectious Diseases* (5th ed.), vol. 2, Churchill Livingstone, Philadelphia.

26. Hockenberry, MJ, Wilson, D, Winkelstein, ML & Kline, NE. 2003; *Wong's Nursing Care of Infants and Children* (7th ed.), Mosby, St Louis.

27. Black, J. 1999; *Microbiology: Principles and Explorations* (4th ed.), Prentice Hall, New Jersey.

28. Parker, L. 2000; 'Applying the Principles of Infection Control to Wound Care', *British Journal of Nursing*, 9 (7), 397–403.

29. Wysocki, AB. 2002; 'Evaluating and Managing Open Skin Wounds: Colonisation versus Infection', *Advanced Practice In Acute Critical Care*, 13 (3), 382.

30. Lipsky, BA. 2001; 'Infectious Problems of the Foot in Diabetic Patients', in Bowler, JH & Pfeiffer, MA (eds.), *Levin and O'Neal's The Diabetic Foot*, Mosby, St Louis.

31. Wiersema-Bryant, LA & Kraemer, BA. 2000; 'Vascular and Neuropathic Wounds: The Diabetic Wound', in Bryant, RA (ed.), *Acute and Chronic Wounds: Nursing Manual* (2nd ed.), Mosby, St Louis.

32. Reiber, GE, Lisky, BA & Gibbons, GW. 1998; 'The Burden of Diabetic Foot Ulcers', *The American Journal of Surgery*, 176 (supplement 2A), 24 August, 5S–10S.

33. Calhoun, JH, Overgaard, KA, Stevens, CM, Dowling, JPF & Mader, JT. 2002; 'Diabetic Foot Ulcers and Infections: Current Concepts', *Advances in Skin and Wound Care*, 15 (1), 31–42.

34. Boulton, AJM, Connor, H & Cavanagh PR. 2000; *The Foot in Diabetes* (3rd ed.), Wiley & Sons, Chichester.

35. Centres For Disease Control. 2003; *MRSA Fact Sheet*. www.cdc.gov/ncidod/hip/ARESIST/mrsafaq.htm.

36. Rayner, D. 2003; 'MRSA: An Infection Control Overview', *Nursing Standard*, 17, 45–53.

37. Twomey, C. 2000; 'Antibiotic Resistance: An Alarming Health Care Issue', *AORN*, 72 (1), 63–64, 66, 68–80.

38. Stadelmann, WK, Digenis, AG, Tobin, GR. 1998; 'Physiology and Healing Dynamics of Chronic Cutaneous Wounds', *The American Journal of Surgery*, 176 (supplement 2A), 26S–38S.

39. Majno, G & Joris, I. 1996; *Cells, Tissues and Disease*, Blackwell Science, Massachusetts.

40. Woolf, CJ. 2000; 'Pain', *Neurobiology of Disease*, 7 (5) 504–510.

41. Porth, CP & Kunert, MP. 2002; *Pathophysiology: Concepts of Altered Health States*, Lippincott, Williams & Wilkens, Philadelphia.

42. Edmonds, ME & Foster, AVM. 2000; *Managing the Diabetic Foot*, Blackwell Scientific Publications, Oxford.

43. Silhi, N. 1998; 'Diabetes and Wound Healing', *Journal of Wound Care*, 7 (1), 47–51.

44. Report of a Combined Working Party of the British Society for Antimicrobial Chemotherapy, the Hospital Infection Society and the Infection Control Nurses Association. 1998; 'Revised Methicillin Resistant Staphylococcus aureus Infection Control Guidelines for Hospital', *Journal of Hospital Infection*, 39, 253–290.

45. Ignatavicius, DD, Workman, ML & Mishlar, MA. 1999; *Medical–Surgical Nursing: Across the Health Care Continuum* (3rd ed.), vol.1, W.B. Saunders, Philadelphia.

46. Bowler, PG. 2002; 'Wound Pathophysiology, Infection and Therapeutic Options', *Annals of Medicine*, 34 (6), 419–427.

47. Neal, MJ. 2002; *Medical Pharmacology at a Glance* (4th ed.), Blackwell Publishers, Oxford.

48. Chavers, LS, Moser, SA, Benjamin, WH, Banks, SE, Steinhauer, JR, Smith, AM, Johnson, CN, Funkhouser, E, Chavers, LP, Stamm, AM & Waites, KB. 2003; 'Vancomycin-resistant Enterococci: 15 Years and Counting', *Journal of Hospital Infection*, 53, 159–171.

49. Hageman, JC, Pegues, DA & Jepson, C. 2001; 'Vancomycin-intermediate *Staphylococcus aureus* in a Home Health-Care Patient', *Emerging Infectious Diseases*, 7, 1023–1025.

50. Lewis, SM, Heitkempe, MM & Dirksen, SR. 2000; *Medical–Surgical Nursing: Assessment and Management of Clinical Problems* (5th ed.), Mosby, St Louis.

51. Cohen, FL & Tartasky, D. 1997; 'Microbial Resistance to Drug Therapy: A Review', *American Journal of Infection Control*, 25, 51–64.

52. Rees, J, Daies, H, Birchall, C & Price, J. 2000; 'Psychological Effects of Source Isolation Nursing (2): Patient Satisfaction', *Nursing Standard*, 14 (29), 32–36.

53. Centers For Disease Control. 2002; 'Staphylococcus aureus Resistant to Vancomycin: United State', *MMWR* 51, 565–567.

54. Young, F. 2002; 'Vaginal Health', *Nursing Standard*, 16 (23), 47–55.

55. Greenberg, ME, Brook, I, Konop, R, Schleiss, MR, Tolan, RW & Steele, MD. 2002; 'Candidiasis'. http://www.emedicine.com/ped/topic312.htm.

56. Randolph, S. 2002; 'When Candida Turns Deadly', *RN*, 65 (3), 41–45.

57. Becker, KL & Walton-Moss, BJ. 2000; 'Young Woman with Recurrent Yeast Infections', *Lippincott's Primary Care Practice*, 4 (1), 125–131.

58. Bates, S. 2003; 'Vaginal Discharge', *Current Obstetrics and Gynaecology*, 13 (4), 218–223.

59. Greenwood, D, Slack, RCB & Peutherer, JF. 2002; *Medical Microbiology: A Guide to Microbial Infections: Pathogenesis, Immunity, Laboratory Diagnosis and Control* (16th ed.), Churchill-Livingstone, Edinburgh.

60. Markell, EK, John, DT & Krotoski, WA. 1999; *Markell and Voges Medical Parasitology* (8th ed.), W.B. Saunders, Philadelphia.

61. Walker, T. 2001; *Infectious Diseases in Children: A Clinical Guide for Nurses*, Ausmed Publications, Melbourne.

62. Figueroa, J, Hall, S & Ibarra, J. 1998; 'A Guide to Common Parasitic Diseases', *Nursing Standard*, 13 (4), 33–34.

63. Ambrose-Thomas, P. 2000; 'Emerging Parasite Zoonoses: The Role of Host-Parasite Relationship', *International Journal of Parasitology*, 30 (12–13), 1361–1367.

3 | Genetic Health Breakdown

AUTHORS

JANE KOCH

DANIELLA GOLDBERG

LEARNING OBJECTIVES

When you have completed this chapter you will be able to

- Recognise the important structural and functional elements of genetics;
- Understand the pathophysiological processes associated with genetic health breakdown: aetiology, pathogenesis, structure and functional changes leading to the clinical features, course, prognosis and prevention;
- Identify the rationales behind diagnostic, therapeutic and preventive interventions associated with caring for a person with genetic health breakdown, from a pathophysiological perspective; and
- Analyse case studies of clients with Huntington's disease, cystic fibrosis and Duchenne muscular dystrophy, using a pathophysiological approach.

INTRODUCTION

Unless we have an identical twin, we are all genetically different, and the study of human genetics involves looking at these individual differences or variations. Medical genetics applies these principles to the practice of medicine – for example, the fact that children resemble parents, and that certain diseases tend to run in families, has been known for centuries. However, the reasons for these have only become apparent over the past 150 years, and the clinical application of this knowledge is an even more recent development[1].

The many complex events that result in the birth of a new baby usually occur without mishap, and the baby is 'normal' and adjusts successfully to life outside the uterus. Occasionally, a baby is not 'normal', and one of the reasons for this could be a genetic or chromosomal problem (e.g., cystic fibrosis or Down syndrome) and the parents may request advice from a clinical genetics department. However, we are not always 'born with' the problem; genetic health breakdown can be acquired, for example, in the case of some cancers. As a result of the Human Genome Project, many more problems that develop in adult life are known to have a genetic basis, although there is still much basic cell biology to be understood before interventions can be developed that will either prevent or treat these problems[2].

This chapter commences by reviewing the assumed knowledge in the form of a quiz. Unless you understand the implications and applications of Watson and Crick's famous discovery in 1953[3], you will find it difficult to support your client with the many dilemmas that genetic health breakdown can bring. As you will be aware, in this seminal work, James Watson and the late Francis Crick showed that deoxyribonucleic acid (DNA), was the genetic material, and that it was coded for hereditary characteristics.

Some of the basic terminology used in medical genetics will then be introduced, which will be followed by an overview of the various specialties and functions involved in medical genetics. An aspect of this involves genetic counselling, and an important part of the initial consultation involves taking a family history and constructing a pedigree, and so the symbols used in drawing the pedigree will be demonstrated. Some of the common numerical and structural chromosomal disorders will be discussed with explanations as to how they may occur.

The mechanisms that may cause a genetic 'mistake' and the consequences of these will then be described and the common inheritance patterns defined. These inheritance patterns will be demonstrated using case studies, which will also illustrate the many ethical issues involved in chromosome and genetic investigation and testing. The pathophysiology involved in the three case studies will be overviewed to illustrate the nursing implications of genetic health breakdown. The chapter will then be reviewed using questions and a terminology list, followed by a conclusion.

ASSUMED KNOWLEDGE

This section reviews introductory biological science including the structure of nucleic acids and the mechanisms of DNA replication and protein synthesis and how the molecular structure of DNA enables a cell to produce an identical copy of itself (during mitosis), as in skin cells that regrow after an incision, for example. The total DNA in the nucleus of a cell, the genome, comprises many thousands of genes, and one gene contains the code to make one protein. In humans, genes are grouped together to form chromosomes. Also important is an awareness that human reproduction involves the combination of the genetic material from a sperm (spermatozoa) and an egg (oocyte), and an understanding of the sequence of events occurring from fertilisation to birth, including meiosis. Any of these processes may be involved in the specific gene or chromosome problem experienced by a client and thus, it is important to understand the structure and functioning of all of these processes. There are huge volumes of new information involving the area of medical genetics and it is essential that practitioners in the delivery of care in this area have a basic understanding of the research findings.

Complete the following after reviewing the assumed knowledge in appropriate anatomy and physiology texts. See references at the end of the chapter, for example[4,5].

ASSUMED KNOWLEDGE QUESTIONNAIRE

Mark the one answer of the four that you consider the most appropriate.

1. Which statement is most appropriate, regarding nucleic acids.
   a) RNA is a single-stranded molecule made up of the nucleotides G, C, A and T.
   b) DNA is a long, double-stranded molecule made up of the nucleotides G, C, A and T.
   c) There are three forms: DNA, RNA and tDNA.
   d) RNA is transcribed to DNA.
2. The genetic code in DNA is the
   a) Sequence of the nucleotides;
   b) Double helix shape of the molecule;
   c) Hydrogen bonds linking the bases; or
   d) Sequence of sugar and phosphate molecules.
3. The replication of DNA
   a) Is also known as mitosis;
   b) Is also called transcription;
   c) Occurs during interphase of the cell cycle; or
   d) Occurs on the ribosomes.
4. A strand of DNA has the sequence CAGTT. The corresponding messenger RNA sequence would be
   a) CAGTT;
   b) TGCAA;
   c) UGACC; or
   d) GUCAA.
5. The RNA that brings amino acids to the ribosome for protein synthesis is
   a) tRNA;
   b) mRNA;
   c) rRNA;
   d) sRNA; or
   e) nRNA.
6. A gene can best be defined as
   a) The anticodon that specifies the amino acid;
   b) A DNA sequence consisting of introns and exons;
   c) A DNA sequence consisting of exons;

    d) A DNA sequence that carries instructions for a polypeptide or protein; or
    e) Both c and d.
7. The sequence of the phases of mitosis is
    a) Anaphase, prophase, metaphase and telophase;
    b) Prophase, telophase, metaphase and anaphase;
    c) Prophase, metaphase, anaphase and telophase; or
    d) None of the above.
8. The normal phenomenon of 'crossing over' occurs
    a) During meiosis I;
    b) During meiosis II;
    c) In both meiosis and mitosis; or
    d) Both a and b.
9. Gametes are also known as all of the following, except
    a) Germ cells;
    b) Sex cells;
    c) Somatic cells; or
    d) Oocytes and spermatozoa.
10. The process of spermatogenesis forms
    a) Two spermatozoa each with 23 chromosomes;
    b) Four spermatozoa each with 23 chromosomes;
    c) Two spermatozoa each with 46 chromosomes; or
    d) Four spermatozoa each with 46 chromosomes.
11. The sequence of early development of the fetus is
    a) Morula, zygote, blastocyst;
    b) Zygote, blastocyst, morula;
    c) Zygote, morula, blastocyst; or
    d) Morula, blastocyst, zygote.
12. Stem cells
    a) Are the inner cells found in the blastocyst;
    b) Can give rise to every tissue in the body;
    c) Are present in umbilical blood;
    d) Are found in bone marrow; or
    e) May be any of the above.

Circle the correct response, 'T' for true and 'F' for false, in the following:

13. The building blocks of nucleic acids are amino acids.   T F
14. Translation is the process of producing a protein from mRNA.   T F
15. In a DNA molecule, guanine would connect to cytosine.   T F
16. The goal of meiosis is to convert haploid cells to diploid cells.   T F
17. Every cell in the human body, both male and female, contains 46 chromosomes.   T F
18. In the seminiferous tubule, the process of spermatogenesis involves:
    spermatogonium → spermatocytes → spermatids → spermatozoa.   T F
19. The end products of both spermatogenesis and oogenesis are gametes.   T F
20. The fertilised ovum, or zygote, is genetically complete.   T F

(Answers to this assumed knowledge questionnaire are listed at the end of this chapter.)

MEDICAL GENETICS

As with many specialties, the vocabulary of medical genetics becomes increasingly more complex. This section will build on your previous knowledge and help you understand some of the language used by the many professionals involved in medical genetics. Sometimes, you may need to act as an 'interpreter' for your client, although you have probably already realised that access to the Internet has resulted in clients becoming extremely knowledgeable about many aspects of their problem, care and treatment.

WHAT ARE CHROMOSOMES AND GENES?

The human *karyotype*, or set of chromosomes, is made up of 46 chromosomes arranged in recognisable pairs; one member of the pair comes from the mother and the other from the father. Of the 46, 22 pairs are called *autosomes*, which direct many body activities, and the final pair is the *sex chromosomes*. If the sex chromosomes are identical in size (XX), the individual is female; if they are different (XY), the individual is male. All pairs of chromosomes can be identified based on their size, the banding pattern and the position of a constricted portion, called the *centromere* (see Figures 3.1 and 3.2).

The identification and counting ('mapping') of all 46 chromosomes is an important cytogenetic test and is called *karyotyping*. A normal female and male karyotype would be reported as 46, XX or 46, XY respectively[6].

Chromosomes carry our genes and each pair of autosomes is known as a *homologous pair* because they each code for the same features, carrying genes for the same characteristic in the same positions along the chromosome. Some of the larger chromosomes can carry

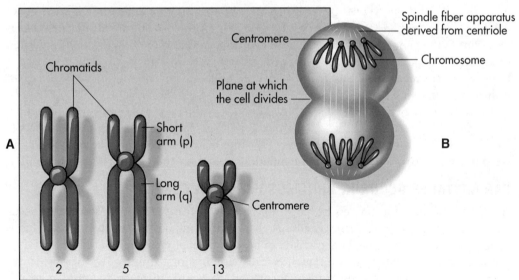

FIGURE 3.1 *Structure of chromosomes A, Human chromosomes 2, 5, and 13. Each is replicated and consists of two chromatids. Chromosome 2 is a metacentric chromosome because the centromere is close to the middle; chromosome 5 is submetacentric because the centromere is set off from the middle; chromosome 13 is acrocentric because the centromere is at or very near the end. B, During mitosis the centromere divides and the chromosomes move to opposite poles of the cell. At the time of centromere division, the chromatids are designated as chromosomes.*

Source: McCance & Huether, Fig. 4.9, p. 124[7].

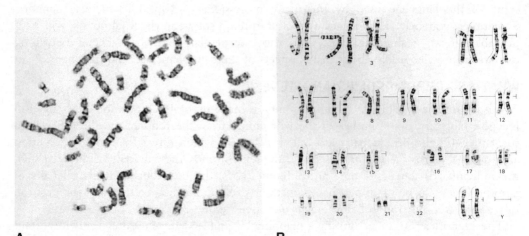

A   **B**

FIGURE 3.2   *A normal female karyotype: A, G-banded metaphase of a normal cell showing the bands of all normal chromosomes. B, G-banded karyotype of a normal female cell showing the banding patterns of the various chromosomes. Identical patterns characterise homologous chromosomes. The chromosomes are arranged from largest to smallest in size.* Source: Damjanov I & Linder J. 1996; *Anderson's Pathology*, (10th ed.), Mosby, St Louis.

more than 4500 genes[4]. These paired genes may be the same or different. Different genes for the same feature are called *alleles* of the gene, for example, tallness and shortness alleles are forms of the gene for height. One allele can be *dominant* to the other, which is referred to as *recessive*. A dominant gene is expressed, whereas recessive genes are only expressed if both copies are recessive alleles. If the alleles are *identical*, they are said to be *homozygous*; if they are different, *heterozygous*.

To summarise then, a gene is a DNA sequence coding for a protein or polypeptide. Our genes characterise us as individuals, one gene from each pair coming from our father and the other from our mother. The *genotype* is the genetic makeup of the individual and the *phenotype* is how a person looks or functions, based on the genotype[4] (see Table 3.1).

CAN MISTAKES OCCUR IN CHROMOSOMES AND GENES?

As you will realise, the process of 'copying' DNA is intricate, and a mistake may occur when the 'copy' is being made, resulting in a permanent change in the DNA. This is commonly called a *mutation*. The mistake can happen during replication of the whole DNA genome prior to producing two daughter cells either prior to mitosis or meiosis. If this happens in germ cells during gamete formation, the 'error' may be transmitted to the offspring and gives rise to an inherited disorder. In somatic cells, (remember these are all body cells, except germs cells), the 'error' will not cause an hereditary disease, but is important in the development of cancer, for example.

Most mutations are either repaired by special 'repair enzymes' or the affected daughter cell will die. If an abnormal protein is produced, 'protein destructor enzymes' or proteases may get rid of it. For some reason, this does not always happen and these mutations can cause problems such as cancer in somatic daughter cells. If the fault occurs in germ cells,

TABLE 3.1: EXAMPLES OF HUMAN PHENOTYPE, DETERMINED BY SIMPLE DOMINANT-RECESSIVE INHERITANCE. (Note: Aa – a capital letter refers to the dominant allele and the small letter to a recessive allele)	
Genotype (Aa or Aa)	**Genotype (aa)**
Free earlobes	Attached earlobes
Far sightedness	Normal vision
Double-jointed thumbs	Normal joint flexibility
Normal skin pigmentation	Albinism

the mutation will be inherited and may lead to an inherited disease. However, there are many mutations that do not cause problems, known as *neutral mutations*.

Most mutations that result in inherited disorders occur in a gene, a *gene mutation*. However, there are mutations that involve the loss or gain of a whole chromosome, for example, Down syndrome (Trisomy 21 or if female, 47, XX, +21) or Turner's syndrome (45, XO). These disorders may occur because of non-disjunction of the chromosomes when dividing to form the egg or sperm and are referred to as *genome mutations*. *Chromosome mutations* occur when genetic material is rearranged leading to visible structural changes.

Simple examples of some of the common gene and chromosome mutations are described in the following sections.

SINGLE GENE MUTATIONS

Examples of single gene mutations include

- Point mutation: A single base is swapped for another. The code is incorrect and therefore a wrong amino acid may be inserted into a protein, which may affect function.
- Frame shift: The codon is read incorrectly. For example, AAC GCA TTA → A ACG CAT TA (a codon is the three-base sequence on DNA, and ultimately mRNA, that provides the 'code' for an amino acid).
- Base sequence repeats: One codon is repeated many times leading to an abnormal form of the normal protein, for example, Huntington's disease (HD).
- Unstable sequence: When there are very many base sequence repeats, for example, in the syndrome of fragile X, which may result in severe learning difficulties.
- Deletion: A large portion of the DNA in a gene is missing, for example, one or more exons are deleted in Duchenne muscular dystrophy (DMD).

VISIBLE CHROMOSOME MUTATIONS

Examples of visible chromosome mutations include

- Translocations: A piece of DNA is switched between two chromosomes. For example, 12:21 means that chromsome 12 and 21 have switched parts of their DNA with each other. This may cause no problems if the switches are complete (a balanced translocation), but there can be serious consequences for the offspring of a person carrying a balanced translocation.
- Deletions: Some DNA is totally lost, that is, many genes and thus vital proteins too.
- Duplication: A sequence of DNA is duplicated and added to the arm of a chromosome.
- Inversion: A DNA sequence is turned upside down.

Single gene disorders commonly follow three patterns of inheritance, autosomal dominant (AD), autosomal recessive (AR) and X-linked. Generally, an AD disorder needs only one parent to have the gene fault; in an AR disorder both parents 'carry' the faulty gene and in an X-linked disorder, males will express the disorder and females will be carrier. These inheritance patterns will be demonstrated in the case studies. For further information, see references[1,7].

WHAT ARE EXAMPLES OF MUTATIONS IN SPECIFIC PROTEINS THAT CAUSE DISEASE?

Genes code for *structural* proteins like collagen, elastin, fibrillin, keratin, dystrophin, actin and myosin, and *functional* proteins, such as enzymes, haemoglobin, albumin, insulin and antibodies (immunoglobulins or Ig).

By understanding the normal roles of these proteins, practitioners are able to predict what could happen when the gene that codes for it is faulty. Elastic fibres are found in tissues requiring elasticity (stretch and recoil) for their normal functioning, such as blood vessels and the uterus. Two proteins present in the fibres, elastin and *fibrillin*, enable this function. A specific defect in the gene coding for fibrillin results in the formation of abnormal elastic fibres and the inherited disorder called *Marfan's syndrome*, where the loss of the elasticity in the aorta, for example, can ultimately lead to the vessel dilating and tearing, sometimes with catastrophic consequences.

Dystrophin is a protein in the cytoplasm of muscle cells that links the inside of the cells with the outside, via proteins in the cell membrane, to provide stability to the cell membrane when the fibre contracts. Dystrophin is absent in *Duchenne muscular dystrophy* (DMD) and as a consequence, the cell membrane tears during contraction. Ultimately, the damage leads to the muscle fibres shrinking and dying, with the tragic consequences in affected boys. *Mutations in enzymes* may result in no enzyme being synthesised, a less active abnormal enzyme or a reduced amount of the normal enzyme. Enzymes are essential for cellular activities and metabolic processes, and a gene fault in an enzyme will affect the particular process catalysed by the enzyme. The consequence could be the build-up of the basic substrate (the initial 'substance' catalysed by the particular metabolic pathway), leading to damage in the tissues, as seen in, for example, *phenylketonuria* (PKU). If the gene fault in the enzyme caused a block in the metabolic process, a decreased amount of end product occurs, for example, in *albinism*, where a reduced amount of melanin is synthesised. *Thalassaemia* and *sickle cell anaemia* result from mutations that affect the synthesis of the polypeptide chains in haemoglobin. One of the case studies will be looking at *cystic fibrosis*, which is a defect in a membrane protein, involved in ion transport into the cell[6].

To recap, there are *genetically inherited disorders* passed on from parent to child, and *genetically acquired disorders* that develop during life. It is also apparent that many disorders involve several genes interacting with the environment to increase the susceptibility to a disease, such as schizophrenia and breast cancer. These are known as *polygenic disorders*. Certain inherited disorders are also more common within specific communities, for example, Tay–Sachs disease in Ashkenazi Jewry, and thalassaemia in the Greek community[6].

CAN GENE PROBLEMS BE CORRECTED?

As more has become known about the basis of gene faults, the obvious question is: Can any of these faults be corrected? From your background knowledge, you will realise the problems implicit in trying to do this; it would involve inserting the correct sequence of DNA into a cell or removing an additional sequence. How could this possibly be accomplished in gametes or somatic cells? There is much research in this area, that is, in gene therapy – the actual transfer of DNA into cells for therapeutic purposes. Advances in molecular technology have led to there being clinical trials in lung diseases (e.g., cystic fibrosis), blood disorders (e.g., haemophilia), neurological and musculoskeletal disorders, as well as cancer[5].

WHAT SERVICES ARE PROVIDED WITHIN MEDICAL GENETICS?

It is apparent that clients with genetic problems need very specific support and information, and this is provided by three main areas or departments involved in medical genetics, each with their own specialist staff. *Clinical genetics* involves counselling, examination, diagnosis and follow-up given by specialist staff, including nurses, doctors and counsellors, to individuals, couples and families concerned about specific genetic disorders. This would include assessment of risks and an explanation of reproductive options to couples at high risk of having a child with a serious genetic disorder. Those who may have chosen not to have children because of a devastating genetic disorder, for example, the female is a carrier for Duchenne muscular dystrophy, now have the possibility of having a healthy child with screening tests, high-resolution ultrasound scanning and prenatal diagnosis (PND), which includes amniocentesis and chorionic villus sampling (CVS). In *molecular genetics*, scientists compare genetic material (DNA), looking for specific mutations in clients undergoing predictive or direct testing. They can also compare genetic material from parents and their fetus to see if the fetus has inherited a serious genetic disorder. If the specific gene fault is not known, they are also able to trace markers through various family members to determine risks to individuals within the family. The scientists in *cytogenetics* look for chromosome abnormalities, and there are now many sophisticated techniques to demonstrate these[1].

Genetic counselling is the communicating of advice about inherited conditions and an important part involves taking a detailed family history and constructing a pedigree. The symbols in Figure 3.3 are used in drawing the pedigree; you will use them when analysing the three case studies.

HUNTINGTON'S DISEASE

WHAT IS HUNTINGTON'S DISEASE?

Huntington's disease (HD) is a rare autosomal dominant (AD) disease that is characterised by progressive movement disorders, very often deterioration in some aspects of mental health, and ultimately dementia. It gradually becomes apparent between the ages of 30 and 55 years, although the age of onset can vary from early childhood until old age. Cognitive impairment may occur before the disease is apparent[8].

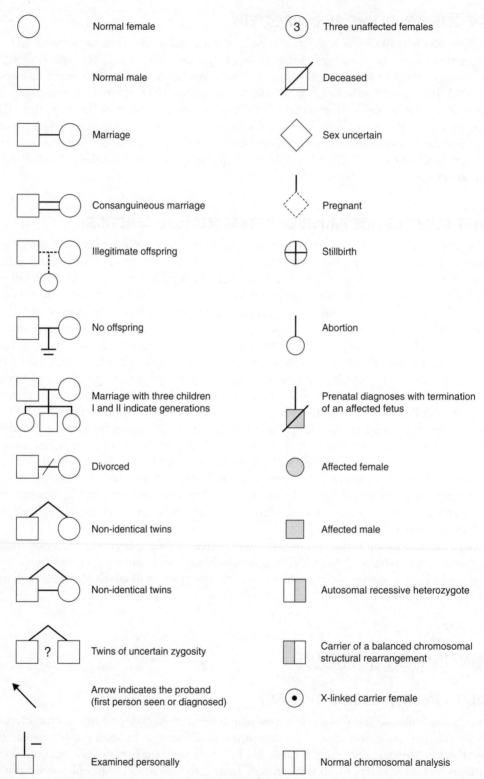

FIGURE 3.3 *Symbols commonly used in pedigree construction*
Source: Adapted from McCance & Huether, 2002; Fig. 4.19, p. 133[7].

● Case study

Jon, 32, has been in hospital for 3 weeks with severe depression. On admission, his wife, Stephanie, indicated that his mood had changed increasingly over the past 2 years and that he has been physically violent towards her over the past few months, which was totally out of character. She put it down to the fact that he was sacked from his job as a watchmaker 6 months ago and was unable to find further employment. He gradually became withdrawn and very 'low' and eventually saw his family doctor, who advised admission to a psychiatric hospital for assessment and treatment. Jon and Stephanie have identical twin boys, 8, a daughter, 3, and Stephanie is now 4 months pregnant.

Jon's father was born in England in 1930 and came to Australia when he was 20. He met and married Jon's mother when he was 25. They had four children, Jon being the eldest, then his sister, Josie, who has a daughter and two sons, an unmarried brother and a younger sister with two daughters. Jon's father died when he was 50 years old. Parkinson's disease (PD) was said to have been the cause of death. He had not kept in contact with his family in England.

During a visit to the hospital, Stephanie becomes very distressed and she discloses the reasons to Jon's registered nurse. Jon's younger sister telephoned her last evening and told Stephanie that she had had a predictive gene test for Huntington's disease (HD) 2 months ago and that it was positive. Last week she had had a termination of pregnancy following prenatal diagnosis (CVS), which confirmed HD. It appears that the family in England had been seen by genetic counsellors following the revelation that a brother and sister of Jon's father had died in their 40s as a consequence of HD. Stephanie had seen a documentary on HD recently and had some understanding of the implications. Apparently, Jon's mother was also aware of the family history in England, but thought that Huntington's disease and Parkinson's disease were the same because they both have 'shaking problems'.

WHAT NEEDS TO BE REVIEWED TO UNDERSTAND HD?

An understanding of HD requires review of the following: AD inheritance; chromosomes; genes and protein synthesis; and structure and function of neurones and the areas of the brain affected – basal ganglia, cerebral cortex; neurotransmitters; normal movement; and stem cells[4,5].

WHAT IS THE CAUSE (AETIOLOGY) OF HD?

The cause of HD is an abnormal gene on the short arm of chromosome 4 (4p16.3), the HD gene, which was discovered in 1993[9]. The normal HD gene codes for a protein called huntingtin. The function of this protein is not known, but it is clearly necessary for normal brain cell function. The normal gene contains 10 to 34 copies of a CAG codon (cytosine-adenine-guanine), which codes for the amino acid glutamine. However, when the disease-causing gene is present, there are many more repeats, the tendency being that the larger the number, the earlier the age of onset of the disease. Most adult-onset clients have repeats ranging from 40 to 50[10]. If the abnormal HD gene is passed from mother to offspring, the number of repeats tends to be the same, but when passed from the father, there is often an increase in the number of repeats, which could lead to an earlier onset of the disease. This phenomenon is known as 'anticipation' and it can be seen when looking at the family tree (pedigree) that the age of onset tends to decrease in successive generations. In the juvenile form of HD, with an age of onset between infancy and 20, the repeats exceed 55[10].

THE CONSEQUENCE OF HAVING THE ABNORMAL HD GENE (THE PATHOGENESIS)

Inheriting the HD gene leads to the abnormal form of the huntingtin protein. Although found in the cytoplasm of all cells of the body, huntingtin selectively kills neurones. There are several theories as to how it does this, but at the simplest level, it may be that the abnormal protein is folded differently and proteases, which would normally remove abnormal proteins, are unable to do so. The abnormal huntingtin then triggers a process leading to protein aggregation and inclusions within the nuclei, which ultimately cause the cells to die. The part of the brain most affected is the basal ganglia, which organises motor movement. The neurones in the caudate nucleus and the putamen, together known as the striatum, are the first to die. Understanding the function of the basal ganglia enables understanding of the effects of HD. The motor cortex is responsible for planning and executing body movement, and there are two pathways between the motor cortex and the basal ganglia. As cells of the striatum die, both pathways are affected. The over-stimulation of one pathway leads to irregular, jerky movements called chorea and under-stimulation of the other leads to slow motor movements. Death of other neurones occurs, especially in the cerebral cortex, affecting the limbic system controlling emotional behaviour, and other areas controlling arousal. As nerve cells die, the neurotransmitters normally secreted by the cells decrease. The neurotransmitter that is depleted most is gamma-amino butyric acid or GABA, which leads to an imbalance of other neurotransmitters[6,11–13].

Thus, the structural change that occurs is the death of neurones and the functional consequences result mainly from a depletion of GABA, which leads to the clinical features.

SUMMARY OF THE CLINICAL FEATURES

Motor symptoms often precede cognitive impairment. However, about 10 years prior to the onset of the motor disorders, mild psychotic and behavioural features may be apparent[14]. The movement disorders include involuntary, jerking movements of limbs, head and trunk (chorea=dance) and slow motor movements (athetosis), and significant problems with speech articulation (dysarthria). There is progressive intellectual decline; memory loss and judgment are impaired. Mental ill health includes depression, neurosis, personality changes, delusions and an increased risk of suicide[15]. Progressive dementia includes loss of inhibition, emotional lability, verbal and emotional outbursts leading, ultimately, to severe dementia.

WHAT IS THE COURSE AND PROGNOSIS OF HD?

Life expectancy is around 10 to 15 years from the age of onset, with intercurrent infection, for example, pneumonia, being the most natural cause of death. At present, the prognosis of HD is poor. However, the discovery of the abnormal gene and therefore the possibility of pre-onset diagnosis and investigation for those carrying the mutation will lead to a deeper understanding of the early, pre-symptomatic changes in the brain. This, together with advances in stem cell research, may lead to a better prognosis in the future.

HOW IS HD DIAGNOSED?

Diagnosis is made by clinical manifestations and family history. The discovery of the HD gene in the short arm of chromosome 4 (4p16.3) led to a definitive genetic test to make or confirm a diagnosis. Using a blood sample, the test analyses the DNA directly for the HD mutation by counting the number of CAG repeats in the huntingtin gene[10]. Individuals who do not have HD usually have 28 or fewer repeats, while individuals with HD usually have 40 or more repeats. Deciding to be tested for HD can be difficult for many reasons. Individuals consider genetic testing to confirm a diagnosis when obvious symptoms are present and there is a confirmed family history of HD. Others, who have a parent with HD, may elect to be tested to resolve uncertainty about their future. A negative test often relieves anxiety and uncertainty. A positive test enables individuals to make decisions about their futures – careers, marriage and families. Some who are at risk choose not to have the test and live with the uncertainty of being at risk. A positive gene test can have significant emotional consequences and also lead to insurance and employment problems. Thus, it is essential that genetic counsellors help individuals make the difficult decisions about testing[16,17].

The structural changes in the brain are seen by magnetic resonance imaging (MRI), which shows significant atrophy ('shrinkage' because of cell death) of the caudate, less atrophy in the putamen, and enlargement of lateral and third ventricles. The frontal and parietal lobes may also be atrophied; occasionally the whole cortex may be decreased in size. A single photon emission tomography scan, or SPECT scan, shows a reduced flow of blood in the affected areas, mainly the caudate, as there would be fewer nerve cells requiring oxygen[7]. The client's clinical features would demonstrate the functional changes; the actual deficits are often localised by neurological examination. The consequences of these changes would be reflected in the nursing assessment, for example, of memory, the ability to perform activities of daily living, the degree of movement problems, mental status, any recent personality change and the ability to attend to a task.

WHAT IS THE TREATMENT OF HD?

At present, there is no cure for HD or any treatment that stops the neurones from dying. Trials are in progress to evaluate the effects of injecting fetal brain cells into the striatum of a person with HD. The rationale is that the fetal cells will divide and replace the damaged tissue, and thus rebuild the damaged neuronal circuits and alleviate symptoms. However, there are ethical issues with this form of treatment, and other sources of stem cells are possible[18,19]. There are other research areas focusing on the abnormal huntingtin protein and aggregates. Scientists also use animal models of HD for various aspects of research, including the testing of potential drugs that could control symptoms or slow the rate of progression of HD, for example[10].

Medical and nursing interventions therefore focus on reducing the clinical features, preventing complications and providing support and assistance to the client and those caring for or close to him.

Thus, the *applied pharmacology* may include

- Antipsychotics drugs (if the client has hallucinations, delusions, violent outbursts), for example, haloperidol, chlorpromazine, olanzapine (contraindicated if the client has dystonia);
- Antidepressant drugs (if the client is depressed, or showing obsessive-compulsive behaviour), for example, fluoxetine, sertraline hydrochloride, nortriptyline
- Tranquilisers (for anxiety and/or chorea), for example, benzodiazepines, paroxetine, venlafaxine, beta-blockers

- Mood-stabilisers (for mania, or bipolar disorder), for example, lithium, valproate, carbamazepine; or
- Botulinum toxin (may be tried if dystonia and/or jaw clenching is severe).

   Because these drugs relate to the effects rather than the cause of HD, the mechanisms of action and possible adverse effects will not be covered here, as most will be elaborated in Chapter 16.

HOW IS HD PREVENTED?

At present, it is highly unlikely that the abnormal gene can be replaced in an affected embryo, and so the only way to prevent HD is to detect the defective HD gene either in the fertilised egg before implantation or in the early stages of pregnancy. Therefore, when one potential parent has been diagnosed with HD, or has been found to carry the gene, the couple may consider either pre-implantation or prenatal testing. This will show whether the potential child will inherit the abnormal HD gene. If pre-implantation testing or genetic diagnosis (PGD) shows that the fertilised egg does not carry the 'faulty' gene, it will be placed into the uterus to implant. However, the success rate of the techniques used (in vitro fertilisation or IVF) is not high. To test the fetus, DNA is extracted from fetal cells via chorionic villus sampling (CVS) or amniocentesis. If the test is positive, the couple can make decisions about whether to terminate the pregnancy[1].

WHAT ARE THE NURSING IMPLICATIONS OF HD?

The general nursing implications of genetic disorders will be discussed at the end of the chapter. However, for HD, this will involve the information and support needed prior to diagnostic, predictive or prenatal genetic testing, and, as has been mentioned earlier, in the later stages of the disease, preventing complications and providing support and assistance to the client and those caring for or close to him.

LEARNING EXERCISES

1. Draw a pedigree of the family history, using the symbols in Figure 3.3.
2. Using your own words, summarise each point in the pathophysiological overview.
3. Write a short paragraph on the impact of HD for Jon and his extended family.

CYSTIC FIBROSIS

 Case study

Barry and Susan Carrington have come to discuss prenatal diagnosis for their pregnancy. They have been to the genetics department on several occasions, initially five years ago to discuss carrier testing when they planned to get married. Barry's older sister died in 1993, aged 17 years, as a consequence of cystic fibrosis (CF). He has a brother aged 33 years with two daughters aged 9 and 7, and a sister aged 26 years, who had a heart and lung transplant three years ago as a result of CF. Barry is the youngest sibling, now aged 25 years.

After their initial consultation five years ago, Barry was shown to have one of the rare CF mutations and, unfortunately, Susan was shown to have the delta F509 mutation. They were initially quite devastated by this. They would not contemplate a termination of pregnancy for religious reasons. Their first child Jake, now aged 3, was shown to have CF after prenatal diagnosis, which they requested so that their child could commence treatment for CF immediately at birth should he be shown to be affected. Also, they wished to be prepared for a diagnosis of CF. Jake is doing well with appropriate interventions and is spending the day with Barry's parents. Susan has an unmarried brother, 21, and a younger sister, Chloe, 17, who wanted to come with them today to discuss carrier testing. Susan's parents insist that the 'genetic problem' is all on David's side of the family and, therefore, have not encouraged their children to investigate their carrier status. Chloe is studying biology at school and has a boyfriend. Susan, 24, is seven weeks pregnant and is very close to her younger sister.

WHAT IS CYSTIC FIBROSIS?

Cystic fibrosis (CF) is an autosomal recessive disorder resulting from defective ion transport in epithelial cells. It is one of the most common genetic diseases in Caucasians, of whom 1 in 25 are carriers of the CF gene[20]. It has widespread effects on multiple organs (exocrine glands and the epithelial lining of the respiratory, gastrointestinal and reproductive tracts) with thick, viscous mucous secretions leading to a range of problems of varying severity. Although the life expectancy of patients with CF has been greatly increased over the past decades with better treatment strategies[21], it can still be fatal in childhood and young adult life.

WHAT DO YOU NEED TO REVIEW TO UNDERSTAND CF?

An understanding of CF requires review of the following: autosomal recessive inheritance; chromosomes; genes and protein synthesis; structure and function of membranes; respiratory, gastrointestinal and reproductive systems; and respiratory tract defence mechanisms.

WHAT IS THE CAUSE (AETIOLOGY) OF CF?

Because this is an autosomal recessive disorder, the cause of CF is an abnormal gene on the long arm of both chromosomes 7, that is, only homozygotes have the disease (for unfamiliar terminology, see earlier section, 'What are chromosomes and genes?'). It is a large and complex gene (over 230,000 bases), and the normal gene codes for a protein called the CF transmembrane conductance regulator (CFTR), which is a membrane protein that transports chloride across the cell membrane. It was located in 1989. The gene is present in every cell in the body but mainly functions in secretory cells, the airways and sinuses, gastrointestinal system (pancreatic, bile duct, small and large bowel epithelium), sweat gland ductal epithelium and the reproductive system (most significantly in the vas deferens). Normally, the CFTR protein regulates the flow of chloride (and sodium) across epithelial surfaces. There are over a thousand different mutations, but the most common mutation, delta F508, accounts for approximately 70% of cases of CF in Australia. There is a spectrum of functioning in the CFTR protein in CF, from no functional protein ('severe' mutation) to some function ('mild' mutation)[22].

THE CONSEQUENCE OF HAVING THE TWO CFTR MUTATIONS (I.E., THE PATHOGENESIS OF CF)

The consequence of the defect in chloride transport differs in various tissues. In the *airway epithelium*, chloride secretion into the lumen is decreased and sodium is actively taken into the cells. This leads to water being absorbed into the cell, which dehydrates the mucous layer and leads to poor movement of cilia. The result is an accumulation of thick, viscous mucus that obstructs the airway and defective mucociliary action, predisposing to infections and inflammation. The airways typically become colonised with bacteria that are difficult to eradicate, particularly *Staphylococcus aureus*, *Pseudomonas aeruginosa* and *Haemophilus influenzae*. This leads to inflammation and bronchitis, damage and dilation of bronchioles and small bronchi (bronchiectasis, often with foul smelling sputum), leading to chronic obstructive pulmonary disease (COPD) with wheezing and air trapping and, ultimately, respiratory failure. The majority of patients die of pulmonary disease. COPD will lead to right-sided heart failure or cor pulmonale. There are several unproven hypotheses that link the CFTR mutation to the initial airway infectious agents, but the result is a protracted inflammatory response to the microorganism antigens, which eventually causes damage[21].

Similarly, in the *pancreatic ducts*, the thick secretions will block the ducts leading to the duodenum. Thus, the pancreatic digestive enzymes do not reach the food in the digestive tract, and maldigestion and malabsorption result in failure to thrive and steatorrhoea. Also, the digestive proenzymes that are retained in the ducts are prematurely activated, leading to inflammation (pancreatitis), tissue damage and fibrosis. The beta cells in the pancreas may be damaged, leading to diabetes mellitus. Viscid mucus in the *biliary tract* will ultimately damage the liver and lead to a poorly functioning gall bladder and gallstones. In the *intestines*, thick mucus in meconium can result in an ileus immediately after birth, and later distal intestinal obstruction and rectal prolapse is possible. Male *reproduction* is affected by absent vas deferens and seminal vesicles. Although spermatogenesis is normal, the sperm cannot be ejaculated, thus leading to infertility (obstructive azospermia). Dehydration of cervical mucus can impair fertility in females. In *sweat gland ducts*, there is decreased reabsorption of sodium chloride from the ducts into the cells leading to an increased concentration of sweat chloride[21]. The gradual salt loss may lead to the consequences of a chronic metabolic alkalosis.

It is probable that there are other genes that modify the severity of CF[23].

SUMMARY OF THE CLINICAL FEATURES

As you have seen, the clinical manifestations are extremely varied and can range from very severe to mild. From the explanation above of how signs and symptoms develop, draw a flow chart to elaborate reasons for the following features found in the major systems affected in severe classic CF, where there is a non-functional CFTR protein[21,23]. Clients are more likely to comply with interventions to reduce their symptoms if they have a good understanding of why they occur.

- Chronic sinusitis; severe chronic productive cough; thick foul-smelling sputum; bronchiectasis; airway obstruction; COPD, a high pCO_2; clubbing of fingers.
- Failure to thrive (protein-calorie malnutrition), oedema with hypoproteinaemia, steatorrhoea; meconium ileus, distal intestinal obstruction, rectal prolapse; malnutrition.
- Pancreatic insufficiency, pancreatitis, diabetes mellitus and related problems.

- Variations in blood pH, both metabolic alkalosis and respiratory acidosis.
- Infertility.

Remember that less severe features, often with a later onset, are seen in patients with non-classic CF, when they have some functional CFTR protein[23].

WHAT IS THE COURSE AND PROGNOSIS OF CF?

In 1938 when CF was first described, 70% of the infants died during their first year of life[23]. Today in developed countries, adults are surviving to well over 30 years of age[23]. This improved mortality is because of improved management in children, particularly airway and nutritional management[23]. Thus, the course and prognosis of CF have changed; the progression of the illness remains as above, and patients still die of pulmonary failure (cor pulmonale), but additionally some now die as a consequence of new treatments, such as lung/heart/liver transplantation or the side effects of drugs used to suppress rejection.

HOW IS CF DIAGNOSED?

Diagnosis is made by clinical manifestations, family history and laboratory tests, such as

- The presence of signs and symptoms;
- A positive family history for CF;
- A positive immunoreactive trypsin test (IRT) in a newborn baby – trypsin will be reduced;
- Laboratory evidence of an abnormality in the CFTR gene;
- A positive sweat test (>60 mmol/L is diagnostic, 40 to 60 is borderline, <40 is negative);
- A raised electrical potential in nasal epithelial cells; or
- DNA identification of the two mutations in the CFTR gene.

It is important that the diagnosis is made as soon as possible because early diagnosis is linked to a better prognosis[21]. Neonatal patients and those in early infancy tend to present with gastrointestinal or nutritional manifestations; lung symptoms tend to develop later. Increasingly, patients with milder forms of CF are presenting in adulthood, maybe as a consequence of seeking advice for infertility.

Nursing implications involve understanding the pathophysiology and genetics in order to support clients and parents through these diagnostic tests.

WHAT IS THE TREATMENT OF CF?

At present, there is no cure for CF or any treatment to correct the defective CFTR channel. Curative treatment would involve restoring the function to the abnormal protein. Thus, this treatment section will summarise treatments aimed to reduce symptoms and potential treatments of the cause[21,23,24].

The *symptomatic supportive therapies* involve the necessity to treat primarily, pancreatic insufficiency, nutrition and liver disease and, secondly, lung disease:

1. Pancreatic insufficiency, nutrition and liver disease
As there is a close relationship between nutrition, lung function and survival, the correction of pancreatic deficiencies to aid adequate nutrition is the rationale behind any interventions. *Oral pancreatic enzymes* are therefore supplemented with food. The nutritional deficiency varies from mildly depleted body fat stores to severe protein malnutrition, and there are specific guidelines implemented in CF centres to ensure adequate nutrition including fat-soluble vitamin and salt supplements as required[23]. Nursing implications

include meticulous observations of the consequences of dietary interventions, encouragement, and explanations of any intervention. Some patients with severe liver problems and less serious lung manifestations may undergo liver transplantation. The interventions for diabetes mellitus are covered in Chapter 4.

2. Lung disease

The pathophysiology of lung disease involves inflammation, infection and thick sputum, and the treatment of these aspects is aimed at slowing down the progression to chronic bronchitis and COPD. These interventions will be included in Chapter 6 while some of the newer therapies in CF will be summarised here[24].

Various *anti-inflammatory therapies* have been shown to reduce inflammation:

- Steroids: Inhaled steroids are used extensively by CF patients, although there is no evidence of benefit and so trials are ongoing[24].
- Non-steroidal anti-inflammatory drugs (NSAID): These inhibit neutrophil migration, adherence and aggregation, although there are concerns about long-term effects and so they are not widely used.
- Macrolide use, such as azithromycin: Macrolides have shown a significant increase in lung function in several trials, although use is not yet widespread[24].

Antimicrobial therapy is needed for infections caused by both *Staphylococcus aureus* and *Pseudomonas aeruginosa*. Prophylactic anti-staphylococcal therapy is controversial although it has been shown to be beneficial in young children less than three years of age, but there are concerns that long-term use of some of the agents may hasten the acquisition of *P. aeruginosa*. Most patients become chronically infected with this organism, which is associated with decline in lung function. Continuous nebulised antimicrobial drugs have been shown to slow this decline in lung function. The treatment for other organisms that emerge in the airway is also necessary[24].

Thick sputum contains mucus, inflammatory cells, dead bacteria and large amounts of DNA from dead neutrophils. An enzyme that breaks down DNA (*DNase*) is used as a *mucolytic* that decreases the viscosity of sputum, making it easier to expectorate. However, in some patients lung function deteriorates, and so most CF centres give trials of the drug before long-term use. *Nebulised hypertonic saline* is also mucolytic and often considered for patients who do not respond to DNase.

Physiotherapy and exercise are also used to aid airway clearance, although research into the appropriate use of both is needed[24].

Lung transplant is the final option for patients with end-stage lung disease, which leads to a significantly improved quality of life. However, most patients die while awaiting transplantation because of lack of donors. This has led to an option of living lobar lung donation, but this has obvious ethical concerns[21].

Several future *curative therapies* are undergoing trials and include

- Gene therapy: This involves the insertion of the DNA gene for the normal CFTR protein into respiratory cells, which will correct the problems caused by the defective protein. There are several vectors being used in an attempt to get the gene into the respiratory tract and one possibility is to insert the gene into a virus (adenovirus) that enters the respiratory epithelium. As Chapter 2 explains, viruses insert their own DNA into the human cell genome and this means that the CFTR gene will be replicated with the viral proteins to produce the normal protein. However, there are many problems associated with this, not least that the respiratory tract's own defence mechanisms will treat the vector as foreign and try to remove it[25].

- Stem cell therapy: It is theoretically possible to insert the normal CFTR gene into a precursor cell.
- CFTR mutations and protein repair: Certain antibiotics affect protein synthesis in various ways and this is being investigated as a method to correct specific CFTR mutations.
- Correction of ion transport: Amiloride is a sodium channel inhibitor that reduces sodium and water absorption into respiratory epithelium. This has led to research into the activation of chloride channels other than CFTR[24].

HOW IS CF PREVENTED?

There are various strategies used to prevent CF. Because approximately 1 in 25 people are carriers of a mutation that will cause CF, that is, they will have one faulty gene or be heterozygous, the likelihood of two carriers having children is 1 in 625 ($1/25 \times 1/25$). Thus, there have been attempts to screen populations for the common mutations, particularly pregnant women. If the woman were shown to be a carrier, then screening would be offered to her partner. As CF is autosomal recessive, there is a one in four chance of the offspring inheriting the gene mutation from both parents. If a couple in this situation chose to have prenatal genetic testing, there are several tests that may be offered. As with the previous case study, the presence of the two genes can be detected either by pre-implantation or prenatal testing. Prenatal diagnosis (PND) is more common where DNA is extracted from fetal cells via chorionic villi sampling (CVS) around 11 weeks gestation or amniocentesis around 14–16 weeks gestation. If the test is positive, the couple can make decisions about whether to terminate the pregnancy. PND is still possible if a couple has a child with CF but the two mutations are not known. Genetic markers near the genes can be used[1].

WHAT ARE THE NURSING IMPLICATIONS OF CF?

The general nursing implications of genetic disorders will be discussed at the end of the chapter. However, for CF, this will involve providing the information and support needed prior to diagnostic, carrier or prenatal genetic testing, and the ongoing, highly specialised interventions and support needed during childhood and, increasingly, the transition to adulthood. Newer treatments have increased life expectancy significantly and it is important that quality of life is also improved. It is therefore acknowledged that far more nursing research is needed to update the clinical, psychosocial, and genetic dimensions of CF[26,27].

LEARNING EXERCISES

1. Summarise each point in the pathophysiological overview, indicating how each relates to Barry and Susan's son, Jake, 3, who is affected with CF.
2. Draw a pedigree of the family history, using the symbols in Figure 3.3.
3. What is the risk of CF in Susan and David's pregnancy?
4. Should they be informed if the CVS indicates a carrier of CF?
5. What is the risk for Chloe of being a carrier of the CF gene?
6. What are the other issues in this pedigree?

DUCHENNE MUSCULAR DYSTROPHY

● Case study

Maria and Paul have been referred by a paediatrician who recently diagnosed their first son, Peter, 4, with Duchenne muscular dystrophy (DMD). Maria, 26, is seven weeks pregnant with her second child and has come to discuss the option of prenatal genetic diagnosis. Both Maria and Paul have been very distressed since Peter was diagnosed, and have gained much support from the local Duchenne muscular dystrophy group. They are aware that DMD is usually passed on from the maternal side, but did not realise that it could occur because of a new (de novo) mutation occurring during the formation of the egg, sperm or the early zygote.

Maria's mother Abbie, 65, is still alive but her father died five years ago after a 'heart attack' at age 63. She has an older half-sister, Anne, 35, who has one child, Tony, 3, and Anne is planning to have more children very soon. Maria also has a younger unmarried sister, Bronwyn, 26, and brother, John, 24. While the family history is being discussed, she reveals that she had a half-brother Bob who was in a wheelchair and died at age 18. Maria was only four years old when he died and she did not remember much about him. Her mother said that Bob had died of pneumonia, but would not talk about any aspect of his illness. Abbie also has two sisters but they are not close.

It is explained to Maria that her half-brother may have had DMD and that, if this were true, both her mother and she would be obligate carriers of the DMD mutation. Maria and Paul are informed that their son could have a blood test to obtain DNA to identify the DMD mutation responsible for his disease. Maria is made aware of the implications of the family history and the genetic test result for other family members.

On their second consultation a week later, the couple decides to allow their son to have the genetic test so that the DMD mutation can be identified. Prenatal genetic testing can then be used to see if the current pregnancy is male and, if so, whether he has the mutation and would, therefore, be affected with DMD. The first step is to identify the specific DMD mutation in Peter using a genetic screening process.

On the next consultation, Maria and Paul are told that their son's mutation could not be identified, as it is not one of the common forms of the mutation. It is explained that there is another way to identify the chromosome that has the mutation, called DNA linkage analysis, which involves both the mother and son having genetic tests.

By their fourth consultation, the molecular genetics laboratory has successfully identified the X chromosome that carries the mutation in Maria's family. As Maria is now 12 weeks pregnant, the couple decides to have prenatal tests to determine the sex of the fetus. There would be no further tests needed for a girl, but further genetic tests would be needed for a boy to confirm if the fetus has inherited the mutation. An appointment is made with Maria's obstetrician for a CVS in two day's time, as the molecular genetics laboratory has sufficient information to screen the sample. They are aware of the risks of CVS, particularly that of a miscarriage. They are also aware that, although they feel at present that they would terminate the pregnancy should the fetus be an affected male, they will have a further consultation to be given the results before the termination would be performed. Thus, they will be have an opportunity for further discussion regarding the pregnancy and should be given the appropriate support whatever their ultimate decision.

It is also suggested that Maria contact her sister and half-sister as they too are at risk of carrying the DMD mutation and passing it on to future offspring and therefore, they may appreciate a genetic consultation.

WHAT IS DUCHENNE MUSCULAR DYSTROPHY?

Duchenne muscular dystrophy (DMD) is a genetic disease that affects only males, with rare exceptions. It follows the mendelian pattern of X-linked inheritance, that is, the genetic mutation is passed on from mother to son. In Australia, DMD affects about 1 in 3000 births. The disease is characterised by progressive muscle weakness that affects walking at an early age (2–4 years) and normally confines the boy to a wheelchair by the age of 12. As the boy reaches his teens, he often suffers progressive damage to the respiratory and heart muscles, which often becomes life threatening. Most do not live past their early 20s.

WHAT DO YOU NEED TO REVIEW TO UNDERSTAND DMD?

X-linked inheritance; chromosomes, genes and protein synthesis, structure and function of muscle, muscle fibres (muscle fibre membrane – the sarcolemma), myofibrils, actin, myosin and muscle contraction; respiratory muscles and the mechanics of respiration; the heart[4,5].

WHAT IS THE CAUSE (AETIOLOGY) OF DMD?

The cause of DMD is an inherited abnormality in the dystrophin gene, a large gene (2.5 kb) on the short arm of the X chromosome (Xp21.2). The size of the genetic mutation ranges from a single point mutation to a deletion of a large portion of DNA. Two-thirds of mutations encompass one or many exons. There is some correlation between the extent of the deletion and the severity of the disorder, but knowledge is limited[28]. Mutations in the dystrophin gene are also responsible for the much milder form of DMD called Becker's muscular dystrophy[29].

In the majority of affected boys, DMD is inherited. However, in about one-third of cases, the genetic fault occurs in a family for the first time and this is called a de novo or new mutation.

THE CONSEQUENCE OF HAVING THE ABNORMAL DYSTROPHIN GENE (PATHOGENESIS)?

The normal dystrophin gene codes for the dystrophin protein that is essential for the muscle fibre (myocyte) stability and integrity. Dystrophin is a protein that is found in the cytoplasm near the muscle fibre membrane that acts as an anchor between the internal cytoskeleton and the external matrix, linked by proteins in the membrane. It helps to hold the myocytes together, protecting against mechanical injury during muscle contraction. Males with DMD have little of no dystrophin and, thus, the stress of muscle contraction ultimately damages the membranes, which results in the muscle fibres breaking down[7].

In muscular dystrophy, the muscle looks 'dystrophic'[6]. This means that there is degeneration and regeneration of muscle fibres occurring in the muscle, and the fibres are of varying sizes and some of them have been replaced by connective or 'scar' tissue. The structural changes in the dystrophic muscle are clearly different from normal muscle, where there are bundles of fibres that are uniform in size, and tightly packed[6]. The muscles become enlarged but weak and feel hard and rubbery, known as 'pseudohypertrophy'.

The functional consequence is a typical pattern of progressive weakness in the muscles – legs, pelvis, pectorals and shoulders – that leads to the clinical features and ultimately death because of the consequences of respiratory or heart muscle involvement.

SUMMARY OF THE CLINICAL FEATURES

The most distinctive, early features of DMD are a progressive proximal muscle weakness, clumsiness, falling, a typical style of walking described as a waddling gait and enlargement of the calf muscles in toddlers. Later, between ages 6–12 years, walking becomes increasingly difficult, with a tendency to stand and walk on the ball of the foot with the heels off the ground. This is because the Achilles tendons have tightened because the calf muscles are weak. The boys also have lordosis (or swayback), an exaggerated forward curve of the lower part of the back, which develops because of weakening pelvic and shoulder muscles and the boy trying to keep balance by sticking out his abdomen and throwing back his shoulders when walking. They also get up from the floor in an unusual manner (Gower's manoeuvre)[30]. Gradually, progressive weakness makes lifting and walking impossible, usually between 8–14 years, with additional spine deformity (scoliosis). Additional problems include impaired intellectual development, retinal impairment and, less common, gastrointestinal and urinary tract problems[30]. By their teen years, boys with DMD often begin to develop serious complications, in particular, the damage done by DMD to the heart and the muscles involved in respiration can become life threatening.

WHAT IS THE COURSE AND PROGNOSIS OF DMD?

The onset of Duchenne muscular dystrophy usually occurs before age 3, and the person is confined to a wheelchair by age 12 and usually does not survive past their early 20s.

HOW IS DMD DIAGNOSED?

Generally, the diagnosis of DMD is confirmed by a combination of clinical manifestations, family history and laboratory tests including gene testing. DMD is usually diagnosed after age 3 when a doctor is consulted because of abnormal posture, gait and enlarged calf muscles.

Any suspicion of muscular dystrophy is investigated by a combination of diagnostic tests, including serum creatine phosphokinase (CPK, CK or SCK), electromyography and muscle biopsy[30]. If a boy presents with the typical clinical features of DMD, a blood test (CK) is carried out first to support or exclude the suspicion. CK, present inside muscle fibres, is highly elevated because it leaks out of the damaged muscle fibres and is therefore found in increased amounts in the blood. If there is an elevated CK, further testing is done to confirm the diagnosis[30].

Muscle biopsy is usually the confirmatory test for a diagnosis. It reveals the structural changes associated with the disease and shows muscle fibre degeneration with fibrosis and fatty infiltration[6], which explains the pseudohypertrophy. Chemical analysis, using techniques including immuno-histochemistry and Western blot, shows the lack of dystrophin protein in muscle[28]. The biopsy requires general anaesthetic and surgical incision. Electromyography will display the functional muscle changes resulting from DMD and exclude any other causes of weakness, for example, nerve disorders[28]. Electromyography involves observing the electrical activity generated in muscle when it contracts, through a needle inserted in the muscle. If a boy is known to be at risk of DMD because of a family history, the disease can be diagnosed before the age of 3, by genetic testing and/or CK measurements.

Since the identification of the abnormal dystrophin gene in 1987, DNA testing for dystrophin gene abnormalities is routinely carried out in molecular genetics laboratories to confirm clinically suspected cases of DMD. In about 60% of DMD cases, the inherited DNA deletion is identified, confirming the diagnosis. When *direct* gene testing cannot reveal a new genetic mutation, an *indirect* genetic test approach, DNA polymorphism or DNA linkage analysis, can be used[1]. If no deletion is detected using either form of genetic testing, a muscle biopsy is taken to see if there is an abnormally low amount of dystrophin in the muscle fibres.

In addition, genetic testing is a useful diagnostic tool to differentiate DMD from other myopathies that may have similar clinical manifestations, but are caused by a mutation in other genes (e.g., autosomal recessive limb girdle muscular dystrophy)[28].

A diagnosis of DMD has genetic implication for other family members. It is important that all females of reproductive age are offered genetic counselling and testing if they wish to determine their carrier status. If they are gene carriers (heterozygotes), they will be made aware that the prenatal diagnosis is possible.

WHAT IS THE TREATMENT FOR DMD?

There is presently no cure for DMD. However, scientists are pursuing potential therapies that may halt or reverse the muscle destruction. Researchers are working on a gene therapy approach that involves creating a dystrophin gene without the DMD mutation and transferring it into weak DMD muscle cells to restore the strength in the muscles. Gene therapy studies in mice models are promising but human clinical trials are still a long way off[32]. Stem cells (from muscle and bone marrow) are also being investigated as a potential source for regenerating muscle cells, again only in animal models to date[32]. Myoblast transfer is another approach whereby early muscle cells from a close relative are grown in culture and then injected in a boy with DMD; however, research is still in an early phase[33]. Many other therapeutic approaches are being investigated, including the use of utrophin and myostatin blockade[34,35].

For now, proper multidisciplinary team management, ideally at special clinics for muscle diseases, is essential and includes comprehensive professional input directed at maximising independence, physical capabilities, general health and quality of life of affected people and their families.

Glucocorticoids, e.g., *prednisone* or *prednisolone*, have been shown to slow the loss of muscle and increase strength, although studies to provide evidence-based guidelines for use are still in progress. The adverse effects of long-term use are significant, for example, osteoporosis, so research to develop similar new drugs with less severe side effects is ongoing[36].

Treatment for DMD focuses mostly on reducing the clinical features and preventing complications as well as providing support. Complications include:

- Joint contracture: Physiotherapy is essential to slow down the development of contractures, which restrict the range of movements, although with the progression of muscle weakness, lower limb contractures are inevitable. Physiotherapy is continued and surgery may be used to release the Achilles tendon, although extensive surgery is not routinely performed[31].
- Scoliosis: Curvature of the spine is a serious complication that can be treated surgically by inserting metal rods into the vertebral column. There are obviously potential complications with this treatment.
- Cardiomyopathy: Heart muscle weakness is evaluated by a cardiologist and often angiotensin converting enzymes (ACE) inhibitors are used, combined with diuretics and digoxin if cardiac failure develops.
- Weakened respiratory system: Respiratory muscles are weakened reducing lung function. Difficulty in coughing can become life threatening and thus, the respiratory system must be closely monitored so that a minor chest infection, for example, does not develop into pneumonia. Mechanical assistance may also be used, for example, nocturnal nasal intermittent positive-pressure ventilation[31].

CAN DMD BE PREVENTED?

Pre-implantation genetic diagnosis (PGD) can detect the abnormal gene in the fertilised egg before implantation, although this requires the use of in vitro fertilisation (IVF) techniques. More commonly, prenatal diagnosis (PND) in the early stages of pregnancy is performed. PND involves extracting the DNA from fetal cells obtained by chorionic villus sampling (CVS) or amniocentesis.

In both PGD and PND, a couple choose to have a genetic test to determine if the fetus carries the gene for DMD. If it is a male with the faulty gene, he will have the disease, but in females, there is a 50% chance she will be a carrier of the disease. Prenatal genetic testing allows couples to make the choice whether to terminate the pregnancy, if a fetus has the gene for the disease.

WHAT ARE THE NURSING IMPLICATIONS OF DMD?

The general nursing implications of genetic disorders will be discussed at the end of the chapter. However, for DMD, this will involve the information and support needed prior to diagnostic, carrier or prenatal genetic testing, and the ongoing, highly specialised interventions and support needed to support the child and family, including psychological, social and often financial. Both parents should participate in all care decisions. Modification in housing, transport, schooling and lifestyle for the family is needed to help all involved adapt to this protracted, fatal disease[31]. Some of the boys may even live long enough to benefit from the potential new treatments.

LEARNING EXERCISES
1. Draw a pedigree of the family history, using the symbols in Figure 3.3.
2. What other information is necessary from Maria's mother?
3. What are the implications of the genetic test results for Anne and her family?
4. Do Maria and Anne have the same gene mutation even though they are half-sisters? Explain.
5. Maria and Paul wish to know the carrier status of their girl fetus. Should they be given this information?
6. Summarise each point in the pathophysiological overview.

SUMMARY OF KEY CONCEPTS

Following is a summary of the pathophysiology relevant to these case studies:

- The disorder was *defined*;
- The *aetiology* (cause) was discussed;
- The events that lead to the *structural*, and therefore *functional*, changes were discussed (this is often referred to as the *pathogenesis*);
- The *consequences* for the client were outlined; that is, the *clinical features, course, and prognosis* of the disorder; and
- The *diagnosis, treatment* (therapeutic interventions − *medical and nursing*) and *prevention* were summarised.

This chapter has emphasised the reasons for the genetic problem, the consequences for the client, and some applied pharmacology. However, there are many links between the above components and genetic nursing practice. A *definition* provides a concise, succinct overview necessary for client explanations, whether child or adult. It also provides a cue for you to reflect on any background knowledge you may need to review, for example, normal structure and function. *Aetiology* is pertinent to prevention, for example, we may not be able to prevent germ cell mutations, but it is apparent that lifestyle changes may indeed prevent the genetic change that leads to cancer. Knowledge that there is a cause often helps parents 'come to terms' with a diagnosis, and a possible future therapy offers them hope. Clients often ask why they or their children have problems associated with the particular disorder, and for you to be able to explain this simply, it is necessary to have some knowledge of the *pathogenesis*. Interventions will increasingly be targeted at this process, stem cell therapy and other current research focuses. It is essential to try to understand the *structural changes* that occur, not only to be able to predict the functional changes but also to explain to the client the importance and consequences of diagnostic procedures, for example, how a gene fault is detected for diagnosis. A clear understanding of the normal physiology (*functional changes*) is essential to explain the clinical features or problems experienced by the client, and functional diagnostic tests and interventions to the client and family. Parents often blame themselves or each other when there is a genetic disease. This often compromises family dynamics, and to understand, simply, about the mechanism of the specific gene fault may help them lose the sense of guilt they feel. Understanding of the problems experienced by the client is essential, too, in order to assess, plan, implement and evaluate care in all of the case studies used in this chapter. Clients need to know the normal *course of their disease*; this is also necessary for you when planning care and educating the client and family. The outcome of the disorder, the *prognosis*, is necessary again when planning and educating. In all three case studies, the impact of the prognosis is very apparent. Your empathy and awareness of the psychological, social, economic, cultural and lifestyle implications of the disorder for the client and family are fundamental to a good therapeutic relationship. *Diagnosis* involves the methods used to confirm the effects of the structural and functional consequences and the nurse's role in these, for example, genetic tests, blood tests and radiology. *Treatment* includes the rationales behind therapeutic and nursing interventions. There is no curative treatment for genetic diseases at present, and most applied pharmacology will have been covered in other chapters. Highly empathetic skills are involved in the area of genetics as well as the nurse's role in any procedures (prenatal diagnosis), medications (the mechanisms of action, observations for intended and adverse effects) and an awareness of other therapies (physiotherapy, occupational and alternative). Your role in the *prevention* is possible if lifestyle changes may affect the cause, that is, the genetic change. Prevention also includes the anguish of prenatal diagnosis for couples and the possible termination of an affected fetus. It is so important that couples have enough information to make their own decision, as some feel that a child with a severe genetic disease has enriched their life, although the child's life may have been short, and others seek a prenatal diagnosis to be prepared for a child with a genetic disorder.

CHAPTER SUMMARY QUESTIONNAIRE

Complete the following review questions by marking the one answer you consider to be correct.

1. Characteristics determined on inspection of an individual are known as the
   a) Phenotype;
   b) Genotype;
   c) Polygene; or
   d) Polysperm.
2. Recessive genes are usually expressed in humans only
   a) When coding for skin colour;
   b) When coding for genetic diseases;
   c) In an embryo; or
   d) When both alleles are the same, or homozygous.
3. If an individual has only an X chromosome ('XO'), then that person is genetically
   a) Male;
   b) Female;
   c) Neither male nor female; or
   d) The condition of 'XO' can never occur.
4. A group of symptoms called Down syndrome results from
   a) Trisomy 15;
   b) Trisomy 19;
   c) Trisomy 21; or
   d) Trisomy 23.
5. If a boy inherits a disease that is autosomal recessive, he inherited it from his
   a) Father;
   b) Mother;
   c) Father and mother; or
   d) Paternal grandmother.
6. Gene mutations in the sex chromosomes of a human would tend to become visibly expressed
   a) More frequently in males;
   b) More frequently in females;
   c) Equally frequently in both sexes; or
   d) None of the above is correct.
7. A chromosomal abnormality in which part of a chromosome is lost is known as
   a) Inversion;
   b) Deletion;
   c) Translocation; or
   d) Crossing over

8. Huntington disease is an example of a(n) _____ gene.
   a) Incomplete dominant;
   b) Recessive;
   c) X-linked; or
   d) Dominant.
9. Which of the following statements is INCORRECT regarding a de novo mutation that has occurred in a boy with Duchenne muscular dystrophy (DMD)?
   a) His mother is a carrier of the mutation.
   b) The mutation occurred during spermatogenesis (sperm production).
   c) The mutation occurred during oogenesis (egg production).
   d) The mutation occurred in the zygote.
10. The most clinically useful technique for prenatal diagnosis of chromosomal or genetic abnormalities at 11 weeks gestation is:
   a) Blood chemistry;
   b) Amniocentesis;
   c) A DNA probe; or
   d) Chorion villus sampling (CVS).

Circle the correct response, 'T' for true and 'F' for false, in the following:

11. Cystic fibrosis is an autosomal dominant disease.	T	F
12. An error in which homologous chromosomes fail to separate during meiosis is termed translocation.	T	F
13. A genetically normal male is always homozygous for genes on the X chromosome.	T	F
14. Environmental factors can influence the expression of a trait.	T	F
15. The manner in which the genotype is expressed is called the phenotype.	T	F
16. All congenital disorders are inherited disorders.	T	F
17. DMD is an X-linked condition caused by a recessive gene.	T	F
18. An allele that completely masks the expression of the other alleles is called recessive.	T	F
19. The daughters of a mother who carries the gene mutation for DMD will always be carriers.	T	F
20. Cystic fibrosis is commonly caused by inheriting one delta F508 faulty gene.	T	F

(Answers are this chapter summary questionnaire are listed at the end of this chapter.)

TERMINOLOGY

Following is an extended list of terms found in this chapter:

Nucleic acid; DNA replication; genome; gene; extrons; transcription; translation; structural protein; functional protein; chromosomes; mitosis; meiosis; 'crossing over'; gametes; oogenesis; spermatogenesis; zygote; stem cells; fertilisation; implantation; embryo; fetus; karyotype; autosomes; centromere; homologous pair; allele; genotype; phenotype; mutation; point mutation; base sequence repeat mutation; dystrophin; phenylketonuria (PKU); cytogenetics; pedigree; autosomal dominant (AD) disease; glutamine; huntingtin; caudate nucleus; chorea; GABA; SPECT scan; PND; gene carrier; CFTR; deltaF508; Pseudomonas aeruginosa; COPD; obstructive azospermia; steatorrhoea; meconium ileus; sweat test; NSAID; antimicrobial therapy; DNase; mucolytic; gene therapy; stem cell therapy; paediatrician; de novo mutation; obligate carrier; X-linked inheritance; Xp21.2; deletion; lordosis; creatine kinase; electromyography; hypertrophy; heterozygotes; predictive genetic testing; prednisolone; contracture, Achilles tendon; cardiomyopathy; ACE inhibitor; intermittent positive pressure ventilation; chorionic villus sample; structure; function; aetiology; pathogenesis; clinical features; prognosis.

CONCLUSION

This chapter has looked at genetic health breakdown from a pathological orientation, that is, why 'faults' in genes and chromosomes result in illness or disorder. In many genetic disorders, the reason for the problem is known, but much research is ongoing to understand the consequences of the problem and also how to rectify them. However, because of the complexities involved, 'cures' remain elusive and may never be possible; pharmacological and other therapeutic approaches can only, at present, be directed towards the consequences of the health breakdown.

The case studies have overviewed a pathophysiological process to help you 'organise' three genetic disorders and, hopefully, to apply to others. The pathophysiology has emphasised the functional consequences of the disorder important to a nurse because these changes will lead to the problems a client experiences[7]. However, it is impossible to understand how function is affected without knowing the structure upon which function occurs. Also 'being healthy' involves far more than the structure and functioning of the body and includes, for example, interpersonal relationships and social and cultural networks[37]. Genetic ill health can often lead to a breakdown in these networks for clients and carers and, thus, a breakdown in other aspects of their health, and one aspect of genetic nursing practice aims to prevent this occurring. Other links have been made between the components of the pathophysiological process and genetic nursing practice.

The authors have deliberately viewed genetic health breakdown from a pathological orientation, that is, the disorder produced, but there is now evidence that some genetic problems are preventable, for example, some cancers, and emphasis therefore should be placed on education to help clients develop a lifestyle and support networks to enable them to remain well[38].

'Evidence based practice' and the extending roles of nurses have necessitated a greater understanding of biological sciences involved in pathophysiology. Nurses need to feel comfortable using the medical terminology involved in the 'illness' and 'disease' caused by genetic problems, to allow communication with both clinicians and clients. There have been huge advances in genetics as well as biochemistry, molecular biology, pharmacology and imaging techniques, and professional nurses need to be able to understand the significance of these scientific developments. Recent developments mean that this previously specialised area is now essential knowledge for all nurses[39]. It also means that nurses must be aware of the significant implications of genetic testing, both in children and in adults, with potential effects on their future insurance and employment possibilities[40,41].

ANSWERS TO ASSUMED KNOWLEDGE QUESTIONNAIRE

1b; 2a; 3c; 4d; 5a; 6e; 7d; 8a; 9c; 10b; 11c; 12e, 13F; 14T; 15T; 16F; 17F; 18T; 19T; 20T.

ANSWERS TO CHAPTER SUMMARY QUESTIONNAIRE

1a; 2d; 3b; 4c, 5c; 6a; 7b; 8d; 9a; 10d; 11F; 12F; 13F; 14T; 15T; 16F; 17T; 18F; 19F; 20F.

Recommended Readings

Connor, IM & Ferguson-Smith, MA. 1997; *Essential Medical Genetics* (5th ed.), Blackwell Scientific Publications, London.

Cotran, RS, Kumar, V & Collins, T. 1999; *Robbins Pathologic Basis of Disease* (6th ed.), ch. 6, W.B. Saunders, Philadelphia.

Jorde, LB. 2002; 'Genes and Gene-Environment Interactions', in KL McCance & SE Huether (eds.), *Pathophysiology: The Biologic Basis for Disease in Adults and Children* (4th ed.), Mosby, St Louis, ch. 4, 104–117, ch. 33, ch.34.

Thibodeau, GA & Patton, KT. 2003; *Anatomy and Physiology* (5th ed.), Mosby, St Louis.

Marieb, EN. 2004; *Human Anatomy and Physiology* (6th ed.), Pearson Benjamin/Cummings, San Francisco, ch. 3, 95–113, ch. 28, ch. 29.

References

1. Connor, IM & Ferguson-Smith, MA. 1997; *Essential Medical Genetics*, (5th ed.), Blackwell Scientific Publications, London.

2. Austin, CP. 2003; 'The Completed Human Genome: Implications for Chemical Biology', *Current Opinion in Chemical Biology*, 7, 511–515.

3. Watson, JD & Crick, FHC. 1953; A Structure for Deoxyribose Nucleic Acid', *Nature*, 171, 737–738.

4. Marieb, EN. 2003; *Human Anatomy and Physiology*, (6th ed.), Pearson Benjamin/Cummings, San Francisco.

5. Thibodeau, GA & Patton, KT. 2003; *Anatomy and Physiology* (5th ed.), Mosby, St Louis.

6. Cotran, RS, Kumar, V & Collins, T. 1999; *Robbins Pathologic Basis of Disease*, (6th ed.), W. B. Saunders, Philadelphia.

7. McCance, KL & Huether, SE. 2002; *Pathophysiology: The Biologic Basis for Disease in Adults and Children* (4th ed.), Mosby, St Louis.

8. Squitieri, F, Cannella, M, Giallonardo, P, Maglione, V, Mariotti, C & Hayden, MR. 2001; 'Onset and Pre-Onset Studies to define the Huntington's Disease Natural History', *Brain Research Bulletin*, 56 (3–4), 233–238.

9. The Huntington's Disease Collaborative Group. 1993; 'A Novel Gene Containing a Trinucleotide Repeat That Is Expanded and Unstable on Huntington's Disease Chromosomes', *Cell*, (72), 1–20.

10. Rubinsztein, DC. 2002; 'Lessons from Animal Models of Huntington's Disease', *Trends in Genetics*, 18 (4), 202–209.

11. Harper, PS. 1996; *Huntington's Disease*, W.B. Saunders, London.

12. Ross, CA & Margolis, RL. 2001; 'Huntington's Disease', *Clinical Neuroscience Research*, 1 (1–2), 142–152.

13. Petersen, A, Mani, K & Brundin, P. 1999; 'Recent Advances on the Pathogenesis of Huntington's Disease', *Experimental Neurology*, 157 (1), 1–18.

14. Berrios, GE, Wagle, AC, Markova, IS, Wagle, SA, Ho, LW, Rubinsztein, *et al.* 2001; 'Psychiatric Symptoms and CAG Repeats in Neurologically Asymptomatic Huntington's Disease Gene Carriers', *Psychiatry Research*, 102 (3), 217–225.

15. Naarding, P, Kremer, HPH & Zitman, FG. 2001; 'Huntington's Disease: A Review of the Literature on Prevalence and Treatment of Neuropsychiatric Phenomena', *European Psychiatry*, 16 (8), 439–445.

16. Taylor, SD. 2004; 'Predictive Genetic Test Decisions for Huntington's Disease: Context, Appraisal and New Moral Imperatives', *Social Science & Medicine*, 58 (1), (January), 137–149.

17. Chapman, E. 2002; 'Ethical Dilemmas in Testing for Late Onset Conditions: Reactions to Testing and Perceived Impact on Other Family Members', *Journal of Genetic Counseling*, 11 (5), 351–367.

18. Shannon, KM & Kordower, JH. 1996; 'Neural Transplantation for Huntington's Disease', *Cell Transplantation*, 5 (2), 339–352.

19. Tabar, V & Studer, L. 2002; 'Novel Sources of Stem Cells for Bain Rair', *Clinical Neuroscience Research*, 2, 2–11.

20. Sheppard, MN & Nicholson, AG. 2002; 'The Pathology of Cystic Fibrosis', *Current Diagnostic Pathology*, 8 (1), 50–59.

21. Ratjen, F & Doring, G. 2003; 'Cystic Fibrosis', *The Lancet*, 361 (9358), 681–689.

22. Hull, J. 2003; 'Basic Science of Cystic Fibrosis', *Current Paediatrics*, 13 (4), 253–258.

23. Jackson, R & Pencharz, PB. 2003; 'Cystic Fibrosis', *Clinical Gastroenterology*, 17 (2), 213–235.

24. Spencer, H & Jaffe, A. 2003; 'Newer Therapies in Cystic Fibrosis', *Current Paediatrics*, 13 (4), 259–263.

25. Davies, JC, Geddes, DM & Alton, EW. 2001; Prospects for Gene Therapy in Lung Disease', *Current Opinion in Pharmacology*, 1 (3), 272–278.

26. Sigmon, HD & Grady, PA. 2002; 'Increasing Nursing Research in Cystic Fibrosis', *Heart & Lung: The Journal of Acute and Critical Care*, 31 (2), 81–84.

27. Pfeffer, PE, Pfeffer, JM & Hodson, ME. 2003; 'Psychosocial and Psychiatric Side of Cystic Fibrosis in Adolescents and Adults', *Journal of Cystic Fibrosis*, 2, 61–68.

28. Emery, AEH. 2002; 'The Muscular Dystrophies', *The Lancet* 359, 687–695.

29. Dalkilic, I & Kunkel, LM. 2003; 'Muscular Dystrophies: Genes to Pathogenesis', *Current Opinion in Genetics & Development*, 13 (3), 231–238.

30. Metules, T. 2002; 'Duchenne Muscular Dystrophy', *RN*, 65 (10), 39–48.

31. Manzur, AY & Muntoni, F. 2002; 'The Management of Duchenne Muscular Dystrophy', *Current Paediatrics*, 12 (4), 261–268.

32. Kapsa, R, Kornberg, AJ & Byrne, E. 2003; 'Novel Therapies for Duchenne Muscular Dystrophy', *The Lancet Neurology*, 2, 299–310.

33. Smythe, GM, Hodgetts, SI & Grounds, MD. 2000; 'Immunotherapy and the Future of Myoblast Transfer Therapy', *Molecular Therapy*, 1 (4), 304.

34. Perkins, KJ & Davies, KE. 2002; 'The Role of Utrophin in the Potential Therapy of Duchenne Muscular Dystrophy', *Neuromuscular Disorders*, 12 (1), 78–89.

35. Bogdanovich, S, Krag, TOB, Barton, ER, Morris, LD, Whittemore, L, Ahima, RS & Khurana, TS. 2002; 'Functional Improvement of Dystrophic Muscle by Myostatin Blockade', *Nature*, 420, 418–421.

36. Muntoni, F, Fisher, I, Morgan, JE & Abraham, D. 2002; 'Steroids in Duchenne Muscular Dystrophy: From Clinical Trials to Genomic Research', *Neuromuscular Disorders*, 12 (1), 162–165.

37. Wass, A. 2000. *Promoting Health: The Primary Care Approach* (2nd ed.), Harcourt Brace, Sydney.

38. Antonovsky, A. 1987; *Unravelling the Mystery of Health*, Jossey-Bass, San Francisco.

39. Skirton, H & Patch, C. 2000; 'The "New Genetics" and Nursing: What Does It Have to Do with Me?' *Nursing Standard*, 14 (19), 42–46.

40. Jacobs, L. 1999; 'The Individual, the Family, and Genetic Testing', *Journal of Professional Nursing*, 15 (5), 313–324.

41. Twomey, JG. 2002; 'Genetic Testing of Children: Confluence or Collision between Parents and Professionals?' *AACN Clinical Issues*, 13 (4), 557–566.

4 | Disorders of the Endocrine System

AUTHORS

KATHLEEN DIXON

YENNA SALAMONSON

LEARNING OBJECTIVES

When you have completed this chapter you will be able to
- Describe the function of the endocrine system and identify the endocrine glands;
- Describe the role of hormones in the body;
- Discuss the pathophysiology of specific thyroid, pancreatic and adrenal disorders – diabetes insipidus, diabetes mellitus, hypothyroidism, hyperthyroidism, adrenal insufficiency and Cushing's syndrome;
- Describe and discuss the treatment options with particular emphasis on pharmacological management of these disorders; and
- Discuss the specific nursing implications of caring for people with diabetes, or with disorders of the thyroid and adrenal glands.

INTRODUCTION

This chapter explores some of the more commonly experienced endocrine disorders. Common endocrine disorders, such as those of the pancreatic islet cells, thyroid and adrenal glands, are discussed in relation to nursing practice. Case studies are used to explore the pathophysiology, treatment options, pharmacological management, and related nursing care for these endocrine disorders.

THE ENDOCRINE SYSTEM

The endocrine system is made up of endocrine glands (and some endocrine tissue), which are widely dispersed throughout the body[1]. The major endocrine glands are the hypothalamus, the pituitary gland, the pineal gland, the thyroid gland, the parathyroid glands, the thymus gland, the pancreatic islets, the adrenal glands, and the ovaries and testes[1,2]. Unlike the exocrine glands that transport their non–hormonal chemical secretions within ducts and ultimately to the exterior of the body, the endocrine glands are ductless glands that secrete hormones directly into tissue fluid. Some hormones are secreted into the bloodstream and transported to distant sites where they exert their action[1]. Other hormones not secreted into the bloodstream act locally. Each hormone binds to specific hormone receptors located on target cells throughout the body. Hormones may have paracrine or autocrine action; in paracrine signalling, the hormone acts on nearby target cells and in autocrine signalling, the hormone acts on the same cells that produce it[3].

Hormones are either amino acid–based or steroid-based[1]. Most hormones are of the amino acid type[1]; they are water soluble with relatively short half-lives[4] and are carried to the target cell dissolved in plasma. Steroid hormones are derived from cholesterol[1], they are insoluble in plasma and are transported to their target cell bound to a carrier protein, resulting in a longer half-life[3,4].

Hormones exert their effect by binding to receptor sites, which are located on the inside or outside of the target cells[3]. Steroid hormones bind to specific receptors inside target cells. This interaction can stimulate or inhibit genetic transcription, which modifies protein production in the target cell[4,5]. Water-soluble hormones bind to protein receptors located on the outside of the target cell membrane, activating distinctive types of cellular molecules called second messengers. Second messengers trigger a series of molecular reactions, which alter the physiological state of the cell[5]. By either method of binding, hormones act as chemical messengers to influence the metabolic activity of the target cell[3,4].

Hormone production by each endocrine gland is finely balanced. Endocrine disorders are usually manifested by an overproduction or an underproduction of a specific hormone, which alters the function of various body systems. Hormones have multiple and wide ranging influences on body processes including reproduction, growth and development, stress responses, maintenance of fluid and electrolyte balance and nutrients in the blood, and regulation of metabolism[1]. Some common endocrine disorders are discussed below.

DIABETES

The most obvious sign of diabetes is excessive urination or polyuria. Diabetes was given its name by the Greeks after their word for siphon or 'to flow through'. There are two distinct types of diabetes: diabetes insipidus and diabetes mellitus. The word *insipidus* is derived from the Latin word meaning 'having no flavour' whereas *mellitus* means 'sweetened or honey-like' to indicate the urine was sweet. Although these two types of diabetes are distinctly different, they have a number of similarities. Hormonal deficiencies or hormonal resistance causes both types of diabetes and common symptoms include excessive thirst and frequent urination[6]. Diabetes mellitus is a relatively common condition, whereas diabetes insipidus is relatively rare[7].

DIABETES INSIPIDUS

There are two main types of diabetes insipidus (DI): central (neurogenic) and nephrogenic. In central DI, there is a deficiency of antidiuretic hormone (ADH), also called vasopressin[8]. The deficiency of ADH production by the ADH secretory neurones in the hypothalamus may be a primary disorder (e.g., congenital), or a secondary disorder (e.g., head trauma, tumours, inflammation or haemorrhage)[9]. In nephrogenic diabetes insipidus there is normal production of ADH. However, the kidney's ability to respond to ADH is impaired. This may also be a primary disorder (e.g., genetic disorder), or secondary to renal disease, hypokalaemia, hypercalcaemia or to drugs that inhibit the peripheral action of ADH, such as lithium[9].

● Case study

Stefan Smolcic, 70 years of age, who has a history of bipolar disorder, presented to the emergency department of the hospital with polyuria and polydipsia. His routine medication included lithium prescribed for his psychiatric condition. Mr Smolcic complained that he was always thirsty, he drank at least twenty glasses of fluid a day and passed large amounts of urine, 'all the time, day and night'. He was especially bothered about having to get up frequently throughout the night to urinate.

Laboratory results on admission were serum sodium 150 mmol/L (normal range 137 to 146 mmol/L). His serum osmolality was 305 mOsmol/kg (normal range 280 to 295 mOsmol/kg), and his urine osmolality was 125 mOsmol/kg (normal range 500 to 800 mOsm/kg). He passed 10 litres of very dilute urine in the first 24 hours of hospital admission. The urine specific gravity was low, less than 1.005 (normal range 1.006 and 1.030).

Mr Smolcic has nephrogenic DI related to lithium. Lithium is frequently prescribed for the treatment of psychiatric conditions, and may result in lithium-induced DI, which is the most common cause of DI. In view of the hypernatraemia (high serum sodium), Mr Smolcic was commenced on a dietary restriction of sodium. He was given 4 mcg of desmopressin acetate intravenously, which was associated with a modest decrease in serum sodium and in urine output. For long-term management, Mr Smolcic was prescribed a daily dose of amiloride HCl 5 mg, a daily dose of hydrochlorothiazide 50 mg, and indomethacin 25 mg three times daily[9].

PATHOPHYSIOLOGY

Diabetes insipidus is caused by ineffective or deficient secretion of ADH[10]. Normally ADH increases solute-free water reabsorption through the tubular cells of the kidneys. The water is returned to the circulation, leading to a decrease in plasma osmolality, an increase in urine osmolality and low urine volumes. Individuals who are deficient in ADH (central DI) and those whose renal tubules are insensitive or resistant to the effects of ADH (nephrogenic DI) are compromised in their ability to conserve solute-free water[8-10].

CLINICAL MANIFESTATIONS

The clinical manifestations of DI include an excessive and dilute urine output, which may range from 3 to 18 litres per day[7-9]. Other clinical features include polydipsia (excessive thirst), which is an attempt to compensate for the excessive water loss. Nocturia is a common symptom, which can lead to sleep deprivation and fatigue[7-9]. If the patient does not have an adequate fluid intake, dehydration and hypernatraemia may ensue.

DIAGNOSTIC TESTS

DI may be diagnosed by a urine specific gravity of less than 1.005 and a urine osmolality of less than 200 mOsm/kg[7]. Serum osmolality may be within the normal range (280 to 295 mOsm/kg). There will, however, be a noticeable rise in serum osmolality if water is not readily available or if the patient's thirst mechanisms are inadequate. A water deprivation test may be used in the diagnosis of DI, and may also be used to differentiate between central and nephrogenic forms of DI[9,11]. Careful monitoring is necessary during this diagnostic procedure due to the risk of severe dehydration. The test involves withholding fluid intake and testing urine and plasma osmolality[10]. This is followed by the administration of desmopressin and further testing of urine and plasma osmolality. In the patient with central DI, urine osmolality is lower than plasma osmolality. However after the administration of desmopressin, urine osmolality increases dramatically[10]. In nephrogenic DI, urine osmolality is also less than plasma osmolality, with only a slight increase in urine osmolality after the administration of desmopressin[12].

TREATMENT AND APPLIED PHARMACOLOGY

The treatment of the patient with DI requires fluid replacement as well as correction of hypernatraemia and other electrolyte abnormalities. For patients with central DI, the treatment of choice is desmopressin, a synthetic analogue of ADH[13]. In nephrogenic DI, the effectiveness of desmopressin is usually limited[14], as the underlying problem is not ADH deficiency but an impaired renal response to ADH. Both central and nephrogenic DI will partially respond to the use of thiazide diuretics, such as hydrochlorothiazide or amiloride. These drugs act by depleting total body sodium and thus increasing the isotonic absorption of water in the proximal tubule of nephrons[7]. In addition to the promotion of sodium loss by the use of thiazide diuretics, dietary sodium restriction is also recommended for the correction of hypernatraemia. Non-steroidal anti-inflammatory drugs (NSAIDs) such as indomethacin are sometimes used in the treatment of nephrogenic DI during the acute phase[15]; these act through inhibiting prostaglandin synthesis, which regulates glomerular blood flow and reduces urine output[12].

NURSING IMPLICATIONS

The implications of caring for a patient with DI involve

- Monitoring fluid intake and output;
- Monitoring urine and serum osmolality, and serum electrolytes;
- Observing for signs and symptoms of dehydration;
- Administering medications used in the treatment of DI, understanding dosage, actions and side effects; and
- Educating the patient about the signs and symptoms of their disease, and the actions of medications.

DIABETES MELLITUS

Diabetes mellitus (DM) is broadly described as a chronic, metabolic disorder characterised by abnormalities in carbohydrate, protein and fat metabolism resulting from defects in insulin secretion, insulin action, or both[16]. The three most common forms of DM are type 1, type 2 and gestational diabetes. The classification of type 1 DM as juvenile onset and type 2 DM as mature onset is not an accurate reflection of the epidemiology of this group of disorders. Hence, the use of these terms or 'insulin-dependent diabetes mellitus' and 'non-insulin-dependent diabetes mellitus' and their acronyms 'IDDM' and 'NIDDM' is obsolete as these terms can be inaccurate and misleading[16,17].

Diabetes mellitus is a serious and growing global public health issue contributing to significant premature mortality, morbidity, disability and loss of potential years of life[18]. More than 7% of the Australian adult population have DM. However, the prevalence increases to 23% in those aged 75 years or older and is estimated to be 10 to 30% among the indigenous communities and people from the Pacific Islands and some Asian countries[19]. In New Zealand, the rate of DM among adults of European descent is 3.1% but more than 8% among those of Māori and Pacific Island descent[20]. Australia experiences very high rates of type 1 DM compared with most countries of the world, and it is ranked as one of the most common serious childhood diseases[21]. Type 2 DM is the major form of diabetes in Australia and is a common disorder among people over the age of 40 years[19]. With the increase in paediatric obesity, Type 2 DM is also emerging to be a health issue among children and adolescents.

Type 1 DM is primarily caused by immune-mediated destruction of beta cells of the pancreas, resulting in minimal or no insulin production[22]. Hence the person with type 1 DM requires life-long treatment with insulin. Type 2 DM results from a combination of insulin resistance and a defect in insulin secretion; the person with type 2 DM may not require insulin administration. There is a strong association between type 2 DM and excess body fat, with an estimated 80–90% of people with type 2 DM being overweight or obese[23]. It has been suggested that the problems of obesity and type 2 DM, share some of the same causative factors, for example, excessive energy intake and low physical activity[24]. There is evidence that type 2 DM can be prevented in high-risk individuals by lifestyle interventions, such as weight loss through diet and exercise[25,26].

Gestational diabetes mellitus (GDM) is defined as any degree of glucose intolerance during pregnancy[16]. Gestational diabetes is similar to type 2 DM in that it also occurs at higher rates in some populations, including the indigenous populations of Australasia, America, Asia and the Pacific Islands. Although glucose tolerance usually returns to normal shortly after delivery, up to 50% of those who develop gestational diabetes will develop type 2 DM within ten years[27].

● Case study – type 1 diabetes mellitus

Penny Parker, 18, presented to the emergency department with a four-day history of feeling unwell. She had been experiencing polyuria, abdominal pain, nausea and vomiting. Her medical history was unremarkable. Vital signs taken on admission were recorded as BP 102/72 mmHg, heart rate 100 beats per minute, temperature 37.8°C, respiratory rate 24 breaths per minute and pulse oximetry 100% on room air. Penny weighed approximately 55 kilograms and responded to questions monosyllabically. Her mucous membranes were very dry and lungs were clear. Laboratory results on admission were

- Serum potassium 5.2 mmol/L (normal range 3.5 to 5.0 mmol/L); all the other serum electrolytes were within the normal range;
- Serum glucose 50.5 mmol/L (normal range 3 to 8 mmol/L);
- Arterial blood gas (ABGs) results were as follows, pH 7.34 (normal range 7.35 to 7.45), PaO_2 93 mmHg (normal range 75 to 100 mmHg), $PaCO_2$ 37 mmHg (normal range 35 to 45 mmHg), base excess −3 (normal range −2 to +2), bicarbonate 20 mmol/L (normal range 21 to 28 mmol/L);
- Full blood count results showed the white cell count (WCC) was 11.7×10^9/L (normal range 4 to 11×10^9/L), haemoglobin 153 g/L (normal range 115 to 165 g/L) and haematocrit of 48.1% (normal range 36% to 48%);
- Urinalysis showed large glucose and small ketones (normal: no detectable glucose or ketones); and
- Blood was taken for anti-GAD antibodies (see Diagnostic Tests below) and blood and urine cultures were sent to the laboratory.

Penny has type 1 DM and is experiencing an acute complication known as diabetic ketoacidosis (DKA). She was commenced on an intravenous infusion of normal saline, followed by an insulin infusion. Regular monitoring of serum glucose, urea, creatinine, electrolytes and ABGs was undertaken. Once stabilised, Penny was transferred to the high dependency unit for further management. Both DKA and hyperosmolar hyperglycaemic state (HHS) are hyperglycaemic emergencies that are acute complications of diabetes mellitus[28]. The magnitude of metabolic acidosis is usually more pronounced in DKA whereas the magnitude of dehydration is usually more severe in HHS. DKA is most often seen with type 1 DM, whereas HHS is more likely to occur with type 2 DM. The most common precipitating factor in both DKA and HHS is infection[29]. Other precipitating factors include pancreatitis, cardiovascular events, trauma and drugs. DKA has a mortality rate of 5% compared to HHS, which has a mortality rate of 15%[29].

PATHOPHYSIOLOGY OF DKA AND HHS

The pathophysiological basis of DKA and HHS is shown in Figure 4.1. The underlying pathophysiological mechanism in both DKA and HHS is a deficiency in insulin resulting in an increase in the release of counter-regulatory hormones (glucagon, catecholamines, cortisol and growth hormone)[28,30]. Insulin deficiency and increased counter-regulatory hormones cause hyperglycaemia by accelerating gluconeogenesis (production of glucose), glycogenolysis (breakdown of glycogen) and through decreased peripheral glucose use. As blood glucose levels increase there is a corresponding rise in serum osmolality, which creates an osmotic gradient, causing fluid to shift from the intracellular fluid compartment to the intravascular fluid compartment resulting in intracellular dehydration[28,30].

In DKA, the counter-regulatory hormones activate lipolysis (fat breakdown). Hormone-sensitive lipase causes the breakdown of triglycerides releasing free fatty acids. The liver takes up the free fatty acids and converts them to ketone bodies, a process predominantly stimulated by glucagon[28]. Ketone bodies are buffered by bicarbonate. However, the production of ketone bodies is in excess to bicarbonate levels resulting in ketosis, which is a state of metabolic acidosis[28].

Ketosis is not a hallmark of HHS. The reason for the absence of ketosis remains unclear, although factors including lower levels of free fatty acids and higher levels of endogenous insulin reserve are two proposed explanations[28].

CLINICAL MANIFESTATIONS

The clinical manifestations of both DKA and HHS include glycosuria, polyuria and altered mental status[29]. As blood glucose increases, the amount being filtered by the glomeruli in

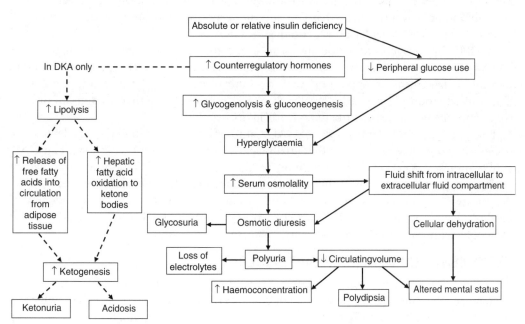

FIGURE 4.1 *Pathophysiology of hyperglycaemic crises in diabetes mellitus.*

the kidneys exceeds the capacity of the renal tubule to reabsorb glucose. The consequence is urinary glucose loss, known as glycosuria. The high glucose content also exerts an abnormally high osmotic pressure within the renal filtrate, causing an osmotic diuresis, which induces excessive water and electrolyte loss. Dehydration, both intracellular and intravascular, occurs as a result of fluid shifts from the intracellular compartment, and hyperglycaemia-induced osmotic diuresis. Dehydration results in an increase in thirst leading to polydipsia (excessive water intake). However, this may be absent in elderly patients with HHS. Other presenting features of severe dehydration include dry mucous membranes, sunken eyeballs and poor skin turgor. Dehydration also increases haemoconcentration, which may lead to embolic complications such as deep vein thrombosis (DVT) and pulmonary embolism[31]. Neurological manifestations of dehydration include lethargy, stupor, confusion, aggression and coma. An altered mental status is more likely to occur in HHS because of the magnitude of hyperglycaemia-induced osmotic fluid loss.

In DKA only, the presence of ketone bodies results in the excretion of ketoacids in the urine (ketonuria). The presence of metabolic acidosis in DKA induces hyperventilation through the stimulation of central as well as peripheral chemoreceptors, which decreases the partial pressure of carbon dioxide in plasma. This type of laboured respiration is known as Kussmaul respiration. Abdominal pain and vomiting are frequently reported in patients with DKA but these are not typical manifestations of HHS[29].

The clinical manifestations which result from the long-term complications of type 1 DM are the same as those which occur in type 2 DM. Refer to the section on clinical manifestations in type 2 DM for a description of long-term complications.

DIAGNOSTIC TESTS

Both clinical manifestations and laboratory tests are necessary to confirm the diagnosis of DKA and HHS. In DKA, plasma glucose levels are usually 14 mmol/L or greater[30]. The arterial blood pH is usually less than 7.3 and the serum bicarbonate is usually 15 mmol/L or less[30]. There is also evidence of ketonuria in DKA.

In HHS, hyperglycaemia is usually more severe than in DKA, with a plasma glucose level of 34 mmol/L or greater[28]. The profound hyperglycaemia that is experienced in HHS induces an hyperosmolar syndrome, with a serum osmolality of at least 320 mmol/kg[29]. The arterial blood pH is usually greater than 7.3 and there are either no ketones or only trace amounts in the urine of patients with HHS[28].

The glutamic acid decarboxylase (GAD) antibodies test and the C-peptide test are sometimes used to assist in the differential diagnosis of type 1 and type 2 DM. The GAD antibodies test detects antibodies to insulin-producing beta cells[16]. These autoantibodies are elevated in people with type 1 DM, and are evidence of an autoimmune disorder. The C-peptide test is a blood test for a hormone produced in conjunction with endogenous insulin[32]. People with type 1 DM have low to unmeasurable levels of C-peptide, whereas in people with type 2 DM the levels are normal[33].

TREATMENT AND APPLIED PHARMACOLOGY

The treatment of acute hyperglycaemic crisis aims to restore perfusion and improve circulatory volume, decrease serum glucose, correct acidosis, reverse lipolysis and proteolysis, correct electrolyte deficits, and avoid treatment complications including hypoglycaemia, cerebral oedema and hypokalaemia[28–30]. As a result of osmotic diuresis, patients with DKA and HHS usually present to hospital in a dehydrated state. Intravenous fluid therapy is necessary to restore both intravascular and intracellular volume. The initial fluid therapy is usually an infusion of normal saline. Subsequent fluid replacement depends on the state of hydration, serum electrolyte and glucose levels, and urinary output. In addition to correcting dehydration, fluid therapy will also improve hyperglycaemia, hyperosmolality and acidosis[28–30].

The administration of insulin therapy is usually by means of continuous intravenous infusion via an automated infusion pump. Insulin therapy facilitates intracellular transport of glucose and the movement of water and electrolytes, such as potassium, magnesium and phosphate into the cell. It is important to aim for a gradual and steady fall in plasma glucose levels, as this decreases the risk of hypoglycaemia, hypokalaemia and cerebral oedema. In DKA, hyperglycaemia is usually corrected before ketoacidosis, therefore it is important to continue with insulin therapy to reverse and inhibit ketogenesis. A glucose infusion is commonly administered in conjunction with insulin therapy to avoid the complication of hypoglycaemia[30].

During therapy for DKA or HHS, capillary blood glucose levels are measured every one to two hours at the bedside. Blood is also sampled regularly for laboratory measurements of serum electrolytes, glucose, urea and creatinine[29,30]. Regular monitoring of blood pH and serum bicarbonate is also recommended for patients with DKA[29,30].

NURSING IMPLICATIONS

The implications of caring for a patient with acute hyperglycaemic crisis involve monitoring

- Vital signs including temperature, heart rate, respiration rate and blood pressure;
- Fluid intake and output to evaluate adequacy of fluid replacement;
- Blood glucose levels to ensure steady and progressive normalisation of blood glucose;
- Serum electrolytes, glucose, urea and creatinine to check the adequacy of fluid and electrolyte replacement;
- Serum bicarbonate and arterial or venous pH in DKA patients to ensure steady and progressive normalisation of blood acid-base balance; and
- Other signs and symptoms of improvement or deterioration in the patient's condition (e.g., improvement or alteration in mental status).

LEARNING EXERCISES

1. Name the two different disorders in which the term diabetes is used.
2. Describe the hormone deficiencies that occur in both disorders.
3. Explain why polyuria is a symptom that occurs in both disorders.
4. Why are people with type 1 DM treated with exogenous insulin?
5. Explain the differences in the pathophysiology of diabetic ketoacidosis and hyperglycaemic hyperosmolar syndrome.

● Case study – type 2 diabetes mellitus

Asok Dass, 60, from Fiji, presented to the local hospital four days ago and was diagnosed and treated for an acute myocardial infarction (MI). He was previously diagnosed with type 2 DM, but had no previous history of coronary artery disease. He has been taking glibenclamide 5 mg daily for the past two years. He does not smoke or drink alcohol and has no other medical problems. He works as an accountant and leads a sedentary lifestyle. In addition to the routine laboratory tests performed for a patient with acute MI, further laboratory tests included the following fasting serum levels:

- Glycosylated haemoglobin (HbA_{1c}) 11.5% (normal range 4% to 6%);
- Blood glucose level 13 mmol/L (normal range 3.0 to 5.5 mmol/L);
- Total cholesterol 6.5 mmol/L (normal range <5.5 mmol/L); and
- Triglyceride 2.40 mmol/L (normal range 0.10 to 2.10 mmol/L).

During hospitalisation, Mr Dass was prescribed routine medications for management of his MI (see Chapter 5). He was also commenced on subcutaneous insulin injections.

The MI experienced by Mr Dass is one of the major complications of type 2 DM. The most common cause of death in people with DM is from macrovascular disease, with coronary artery disease (CAD) the most prevalent[34]. The cardiovascular risk factors that are more common among people with type 2 DM include dyslipidaemia and hypertension[34].

PATHOPHYSIOLOGY OF CHRONIC COMPLICATIONS OF DM

Diabetes mellitus is characterised by a number of chronic complications associated with metabolic dysfunction[35]. These complications can be broadly classified as *macrovascular* and *microvascular* complications. Macrovascular complications develop as a consequence of atherosclerotic disease of the large vessels, including cardiac, cerebral and peripheral vascular disease[36]. Microvascular complications usually only become evident in people with overt diabetes mellitus[35]. Examples of microvascular complications include diabetic retinopathy, nephropathy and neuropathy.

Macrovascular disease is usually evident during the pre-diabetic stage, as insulin resistance develops – a disorder associated with excess weight, ageing, infection and pregnancy[37,38]. Insulin resistance is the pre-diabetic stage of impaired glucose tolerance[39] where there is decreased sensitivity of insulin receptors in the liver, adipose tissue and skeletal muscles. Patients with insulin resistance become hyperinsulinaemic to overcome the underlying defect of insulin resistance[34]. The association between insulin resistance, hyperinsulinaemia, hypertension, obesity, dyslipidaemia, the procoagulant state and cardiovascular disease is now well recognised[34].

There is no single pathophysiological mechanism in the development of the chronic complications of DM. The postulated pathophysiological processes can be categorised as vascular abnormalities (e.g., endothelial dysfunctions, glucose-induced abnormalities, excessive glycation of circulating and membrane-bound proteins), and other mechanisms (e.g., abnormalities in growth factors and platelet dysfunction)[34,36,40].

There is good evidence that the pathogenesis of the atherogenic lesion in macrovascular disease is endothelial cell dysfunction[41]. The causes of endothelial abnormalities include insulin resistance and hyperglycaemia[41]. High blood glucose levels inhibit the production of vasodilatory nitric oxide, which contributes to the procoagulant state in the blood[34,41]. A deficiency in nitric oxide promotes platelet aggregation, proliferation of smooth muscle and an increase in monocyte adhesiveness[34,41]. These alterations accelerate the formation of atherosclerosis and alter the structure and function of blood vessels.

Microvascular disease involves structural changes in the capillaries and small vessels and most commonly affects the retina causing diabetic retinopathy, the kidneys causing diabetic nephropathy, and the peripheral nerves causing diabetic neuropathy[36]. Risk factors for microvascular complications include poor glycaemic control, duration of diabetes, hypertension and microalbuminuria[41]. The pathogenesis of microvascular complications is multifactorial with metabolic and vascular involvement. There is evidence that glycation of body proteins results in the release of cytokines and other inflammatory mediators[41]. In neuropathy, the diminished blood supply to nerves results in axonal and myelin sheath damage. Oxidative stress, as a result of an increase in substances such as reactive oxygen species (ROS), is another pathogenic mechanism of diabetic complications[42]. ROS oxidise and damage deoxyribose nucleic acid (DNA), proteins and lipids resulting in tissue damage[42].

CLINICAL MANIFESTATIONS

Symptoms of polyuria, polydipsia and unexplained weight loss, in type 1 DM only, are strongly suggestive of DM. The clinical manifestations of the chronic complications of DM result from impairment of macrovascular and microvascular circulation.

Macrovascular disease results in cardiac, cerebral and peripheral vascular disease. Clinical manifestations of cardiac complications include chest discomfort or pain and shortness of breath associated with nausea or diaphoresis (see Chapter 5 for further discussion). Some people with DM may not experience chest pain despite having severe coronary artery disease[34]. Manifestations of cerebral complications may include blindness in one eye, weakness on one side of the body, tingling sensations, speech difficulties, confusion, or double vision[41]. Consciousness is usually normal. Signs and symptoms of peripheral vessel disease include leg cramping after walking, a condition known as intermittent claudication and loss of sensation with no detectable pulse on the affected limb[43].

As noted earlier, manifestations of microvascular disease include diabetic retinopathy, nephropathy, and peripheral neuropathy. Diabetic retinopathy manifests as blurred vision and is caused by altered permeability of the blood vessels in the retina resulting in oedema. Patients may also complain of seeing spots or floaters, caused by blood leaking into the retina and vitreous humour. The late phase of the disease may cause a sudden loss of vision from serious problems such as glaucoma and retinal detachment[44].

Diabetic nephropathy affects glomerular filtration rate (GFR), which is followed by a progressive increase in urinary albumin excretion. However, diabetic nephropathy may be functionally silent for many years as signs and symptoms will not arise until a significant percentage of renal tissue has been destroyed. The clinical manifestations of severe renal damage include peripheral oedema, nausea and vomiting, fatigue, itching and unintended weight gain due to fluid accumulation[36,44].

Diabetic neuropathy may manifest soon after the diagnosis of DM. Autonomic neuropathy is a serious form of diabetic neuropathy that may result in impotence, gastrointestinal disturbances, bladder dysfunction and orthostatic hypotension. Pain is another serious problem associated with autonomic neuropathy. Pain may be intermittent or continuous and is usually worse at night[44].

DIAGNOSTIC TESTS

A fasting plasma glucose level of 7 mmol/L or higher on at least two occasions confirms a diagnosis of diabetes mellitus[17,45]. Other tests may include a random plasma glucose level of 11.1 mmol/L or higher, or an oral glucose tolerance test with a plasma glucose of level 11.1 mmol/L or higher, on at least two occasions[17,45].

Glycosylated haemoglobin (HbA$_{1c}$ or A1C) is now widely used as a measurement of glycaemic control. This test measures the amount of glucose that is bound to haemoglobin and is directly related to the concentration of glucose in the blood over the preceding 1 to 3 months[35]. Good glycaemic control reflects an HbA1c of less than 7% and is associated with a significant reduction in diabetic complications[17,45]. The incidence of CAD in people with DM increases with increasing HbA$_{1c}$ levels[35].

TREATMENT

A number of studies have demonstrated that intensive management delays the onset and progression of diabetic complications[46–50]. The emphasis is on strict blood glucose control through a combination of lifestyle interventions and pharmacological therapies. Lifestyle interventions focus on dietary changes and an exercise regimen, as weight loss is pivotal in controlling blood glucose levels in people with type 2 DM.

Pharmacological therapy centres on the use of antihyperglycaemic medications including sulfonylureas, biguanides, thiazolidinediones, alpha–glucosidase inhibitors and insulin[35]. In type 2 DM, these agents can be used as monotherapy or combination therapy[34]. In type 1 DM, insulin is the only effective drug treatment[30].

SULFONYLUREAS

There are several different types of sulfonylureas available. They are the most commonly used class of antihyperglycaemic agents[35,37]. These drugs work mainly by stimulating the pancreas to release more insulin. Some of the most common adverse effects are hypoglycaemia and weight gain[35].

BIGUANIDES

The only antihyperglycaemic agent in this class is metformin. It lowers blood glucose by lowering hepatic glucose production and improving glucose uptake in peripheral tissues[35,51]. Although metformin is not usually associated with hypoglycaemia or weight gain, this drug can cause gastrointestinal disturbances such as nausea, flatulence and diarrhoea. In rare cases, metformin is associated with lactic acidosis[51], although the causative link between metformin and lactic acidosis has now been challenged[52]. This drug should not be administered to patients with renal problems as metformin is excreted by the kidney and the risk of metformin accumulation and lactic acidosis increases in renal impairment[51].

THIAZOLIDINEDIONES

Two antihyperglycaemics, rosiglitazone and pioglitazone, belong to this class of agents. They reduce insulin resistance by increasing the insulin-responsive genes responsible for glucose uptake[35,53]. Like metformin, thiazolidinediones are not associated with hypoglycaemia. However, they can cause weight gain by increasing peripheral subcutaneous fat content[54], and cause fluid retention and oedema, although the aetiology is unclear[51,53,54].

ALPHA-GLUCOSIDASE INHIBITORS

This group of agents acts by inhibiting the ability of enzymes to break down oligosaccharides and disaccharides into monosaccharides, thus delaying carbohydrate absorption in the small intestine[35]. Alpha-glucosidase inhibitors reduce postprandial hyperglycaemia. An example of this group of drugs is acarbose. This drug is poorly absorbed and is rarely associated with systemic adverse effects, although flatulence is an adverse effect that may result in poor patient compliance[51,53].

INSULIN

The replacement of insulin is necessary where there is an absolute deficiency of endogenous insulin as in type 1 DM. Although not all people with type 2 DM require insulin therapy, it can be used in the management of both type 1 and type 2 DM. Excellent glycaemic control can be achieved with insulin therapy. However it requires specialised patient education and training in insulin use and dose adjustment[53]. Common adverse effects of insulin therapy include hypoglycaemia and weight gain[53].

NURSING IMPLICATIONS

The nursing implications of caring for a patient with chronic complications of DM involve

- Regularly monitoring blood glucose levels;
- Monitoring HbA$_{1c}$ to determine glycaemic control over the past three months;
- Observing for signs and symptoms of macrovascular and microvascular complications; and
- Providing information and education for patients about their disorder to enable effective self-care.

LEARNING EXERCISES

1. Explain why some people with type 2 DM can control their disorder with lifestyle modification.
2. Describe the mode of action of antihyperglycaemic drugs.
3. Identify the long-term complications of DM.
4. Describe insulin resistance.
5. Explain the tests used to diagnose DM.

DISORDERS OF THE THYROID GLAND

Thyroid hormones are responsible for regulating oxygen use, the basal metabolic rate, cellular metabolism and growth and development[4]. Disorders result from underactivity, overactivity, or abnormal anatomy of the thyroid gland. Women are affected by thyroid disorders more commonly than men[55] and there is a tendency for familial clustering[4] (occurring in families). The thyroid gland secretes thyroid hormone in the form of thyroxine (T_4) and triiodothyronine (T_3). The hypothalamic–pituitary axis controls the production of thyroid hormone. The hypothalamus secretes thyroid-releasing hormone (TRH) that stimulates the thyrotroph cells in the anterior pituitary to secrete thyroid-stimulating hormone (also known as thyrotrophin or TSH) which in turn, increases the production and secretion of thyroid hormone by the thyroid gland[56]. TSH synthesis and secretion is controlled by T_3 concentrations within the thyrotroph cells. Negative feedback occurs when high levels of T_3 shutdown TSH secretion by decreasing the responsiveness of TSH to TRH[4].

HYPOTHYROIDISM

Hypofunction or underactivity of the thyroid gland is known as *hypothyroidism* (decreased production of thyroid hormone) or as mild thyroid failure[57]. Severe hypothyroidism in adults is known as myxoedema, which can progress to myxoedematous coma[55]. In children the manifestations of untreated congenital hypothyroidism are known as cretinism[57]. The most common cause of hypothyroidism is an autoimmune disorder known as Hashimoto's thyroiditis[58,59]. The other causes of hypothyroidism include thyroidectomy (surgical removal of the thyroid gland), iodine deficiency, defective hormone synthesis, antithyroid drugs or large amounts of iodine that block thyroid hormone production[57]. Hypothyroidism is the second most common endocrine disease in older people[60].

● Case study

Janice Cohen, 54, is the mother of four children. She confides in a friend who is a nurse that she is concerned about her lack of energy and weight gain of more than 12 kilograms (despite a reduction in appetite), which has occurred over the past couple of months. She says she is always constipated and complains of feeling 'sluggish'. On closer questioning, the nurse discovers that Janice feels the cold and that she thinks she is mildly depressed. The nurse also notes the presence of a goitre (enlarged thyroid gland).

When she presents for a medical check-up on the nurse's advice, Janice is diagnosed as having Hashimoto's thyroiditis, a condition that manifests as hypothyroidism and goitre. If severe, myxoedema (commonly presenting as nonpitting oedema or thickened skin) is present. It is the most common form of hypothyroidism[3] and predominantly occurs in middle-aged and older women[3]. Diagnosis is confirmed by thyroid function tests and an antithyroid antibody test. Janice is commenced on oral thyroid hormone replacement therapy.

PATHOPHYSIOLOGY

Hashimoto's thyroiditis (also known as primary hypothyroidism) is an autoimmune disorder that destroys the thyroid gland[3]. Autoimmunity results from the production of immune cells that are directed against host tissues or antigens[3]. In Hashimoto's thyroiditis, it is thought that T cells destroy the thyroid epithelial cells[61]. The subsequent underactivity of the thyroid gland causes a decreased production of thyroid hormones T_3 and T_4 and results in failure of the normal negative feedback control of TSH leading to elevated levels of TSH[60].

CLINICAL MANIFESTATIONS

The clinical manifestations of hypothyroidism include goitre, hypometabolism and myxoedema. Goitre is an increase in thyroid gland size[58], resulting from excess levels of TSH (secreted in order to enhance the uptake and concentration of iodine by the thyroid gland)[56,57]. Hypometabolism results from thyroid hormone deficiency and is characterised by a slow onset of weight gain, lack of appetite, weakness, fatigue, cold intolerance, dry skin and coarse, brittle hair. There is a reduction in gastrointestinal motility leading to constipation and flatulence and an increase in the amount of circulating lipids leading to atherosclerosis. Lethargy, depression and slowed mental processes including impaired memory result from nervous system involvement. Myxoedema is the result of fluid accumulation and is characterised by a puffy face and eyes, and a swollen tongue[3,58]. Fluid can collect in any organ and may lead to pleural or pericardial effusion, an enlarged heart, bradycardia and decreased cardiac output[3].

Myxoedematous coma is a severe form of life-threatening hypothyroidism, which most often occurs in older women with chronic hypothyroidism[3]. It is precipitated by cold weather and is characterised by coma and an extreme manifestation of the signs and symptoms of hypothyroidism[3].

DIAGNOSTIC TESTS

Hypothyroidism can be diagnosed using thyroid function tests, blood tests for levels of serum TSH, T_4, FT_4 (free thyroxine, the metabolically active form of T_4)[5] and T_3. In primary hypothyroidism, TSH is increased and T_4 and T_3 levels are low, as is FT_4[58]. An increased level of serum TSH is the most significant diagnostic feature of primary hypothyroidism[56]. To confirm Hashimoto's thyroiditis, thyroid peroxidase antibody levels should be measured[59].

TREATMENT

The treatment of hypothyroidism requires life-long replacement therapy with oral thyroid hormone[57]. Therapy is with levo-thyroxine (L-thyroxine)[60], a synthetic preparation of T_4 identical to the naturally occurring hormone[57]. The goal is to eliminate symptoms and restore a euthyroid state (restore thyroid hormone levels to normal and decrease levels of TSH)[57]. Plasma concentrations of TSH are measured at 2, 4 and 10 months after the commencement of therapy, if TSH levels fall within the reference interval of 0.4–5.0 mIU/L, they can be measured annually thereafter[62].

NURSING IMPLICATIONS

The implications of caring for a patient with hypothyroidism involve

- Providing education to the patient about the signs and symptoms of hypothyroidism;
- Monitoring the patient's fluid intake and encouraging the patient to keep hydrated to prevent constipation;
- Providing a warm environment;
- Monitoring thyroid hormone levels and understanding the implications for medication administration;
- Being aware of possible drug toxicities associated with the patient's slowed metabolism;
- Monitoring the hospitalised patient for signs and symptoms of myxoedematous coma;
- Encouraging the patient to have a well-balanced, low-calorie, high-fibre diet and to monitor their weight. It may be helpful to refer the patient to a dietitian;
- Encouraging the patient to undertake physical activity to prevent constipation and to reduce weight gain once appetite has improved;
- Ensuring the patient has a good understanding about the importance of taking their medications and the rationale for medication use; and
- Encouraging the patient to see their doctor if they become unwell.

HYPERTHYROIDISM

Hyperfunction or overactivity of the thyroid gland is known as *hyperthyroidism* (excessive secretion of thyroid hormone) or thyrotoxicosis[59]. The main form of hyperthyroidism is Grave's disease[55,56,63]. Other causes include toxic nodular goitre, cancer of the thyroid and rarely, excessive ingestion of thyroid hormone[3]. A severe exacerbation of this condition is known as thyrotoxic crisis or thyroid storm, which results from extremely high levels of thyroid hormone[3].

● Case study

Jeannie Tsardos, 38, has been admitted to hospital with partial thickness burn injuries to both hands. She presented to the emergency department during the morning having sustained chemical burns to both hands from oven cleaner. She told the nursing staff that she had been cleaning her oven without gloves. Her burns were washed and treated with silver sulfadiazine cream and encased in plastic bags. Both hands were elevated and she was given IV tramadol hydrochloride for pain prior to being transferred to a ward.

On admission to the ward, Jeannie is quite agitated and restless. She talks rapidly and non-stop, so the nurse has difficulty getting a history from her. Her observations are: pulse 110 beats per minute, temperature 37.7°C, respirations 24 breaths per minute, blood pressure 150/100 mmHg. While taking Jeannie's observations the nurse notes that she is mildly diaphoretic and is complaining of feeling hot. She asks for the window to be opened to let in fresh air. Jeannie is quite thin and the nurse suspects she is underweight. The nurse also notes the presence of a goitre, that Jeannie has bulging eyes, and that her hair is thin and patchy. Jeannie says that she lives on her own, having recently separated from her husband and that she lost a lot of weight around the time of her marriage breakup. The nurse is concerned about Jeannie's vital signs and her level of agitation and requests an urgent review by the medical officer.

After careful examination, the medical officer makes a provisional diagnosis of Grave's disease. Urgent thyroid function tests, including thyroid antibody tests, are ordered, the results of which confirm the diagnosis. Jeannie is commenced on propranolol 40 mg tds and carbimazole 10 mg tds.

Grave's disease is a condition that manifests as hyperthyroidism, goitre and exophthalmos (protrusion of the eyes). It is the most common cause of hyperthyroidism and predominantly occurs in women[55,60], frequently between 20 to 40 years of age[3,56,63].

PATHOPHYSIOLOGY

Grave's disease is an autoimmune disorder[55]. The thyroid gland is abnormally stimulated by thyroid-stimulating immunoglobulins (TSIs)[56]. TSIs are antibodies which are directed against the TSH receptor site in the thyroid follicles. They stimulate the receptors for thyroid stimulating hormone (TSH)[3,59] on the thyroid gland and cause overactivity of the thyroid gland resulting in overproduction of thyroxine. In effect, TSIs mimic the effect of TSH on the thyroid gland. The normal negative feedback regulatory controls on TSH do not work on TSIs and so the thyroid gland becomes overactive, leading to excess thyroid hormone production.

CLINICAL MANIFESTATIONS

The clinical manifestations of hyperthyroidism can be mild or severe[55]. The excess production of thyroid hormone results in increased metabolism leading to increased heat production, increased appetite, weight loss (which occurs if caloric intake does not match metabolic rate), diarrhoea, sweating, heat intolerance and shortness of breath. Increased sympathetic nervous system activity that causes excessive stimulation of the beta-adrenergic receptors in the cardiovascular system, leads to tachycardia, palpitations, increased cardiac output and increased peripheral blood flow[55,57].

Increased central nervous system stimulation results in tremor, restlessness, nervousness, insomnia and mental health problems ranging from depression to delirium. Exophthalmos results from excess tissue growth behind the eyeball[3]. Goitre results from continuous stimulation of the thyroid gland by TSIs[56].

Thyroid storm is an extreme and life-threatening form of hyperthyroidism[3]. It is precipitated by physiological stressors, such as infection, myocardial infarction, and surgery[55] and is characterised by an extreme manifestation of the signs and symptoms of hyperthyroidism.

DIAGNOSTIC TESTS

Hyperthyroidism can be diagnosed by measuring serum levels of free thyroxine, TSH levels and also by measuring an increased uptake of radioactive iodine by the thyroid gland[4]. The blood results expected in primary hyperthyroidism include reduced serum levels of TSH, increased levels of T_4 (thyroxine), FT_4 (free thyroxine, the metabolically active form of T_4)

and T$_3$ (triiodothyronine)[58,60,63]. Thyroid antibody testing involves testing for cytoplasmic antibodies, such as antithyroglobulin and antimicrosomal antibodies (which will be positive in both Grave's disease and Hashimoto's thyroiditis)[63]. Tests to detect the presence of TSIs[64] can also be undertaken.

TREATMENT

The treatment of Grave's disease is aimed at decreasing the level of thyroid hormone production and blocking the effects of excess thyroid hormone[60]. This can be achieved by eradication of the thyroid gland with radioactive iodine (RAI), with surgical removal of the thyroid gland[63], or drugs to either decrease thyroid function or to block the effects of thyroid hormone[4,60].

Radioactive iodine (^{131}I) is a radioactive isotope of stable iodine. It is chemically identical to iodine but has radioactive properties[4,60]. Administered orally it is taken up and concentrated in the thyroid gland, where emission of radioactive beta particles destroys thyroid tissue. There is minimal damage to other tissues, as the beta particles do not travel outside the thyroid gland[57]. Hypothyroidism will result if too much of the thyroid tissue is destroyed[60]. RAI is principally used for people who are debilitated or elderly[60].

Surgery may involve partial removal of the thyroid gland (subtotal thyroidectomy)[63]. High doses of non-radioactive iodine solution containing a mixture of 5% elemental iodine and 10% potassium iodide in water, is used pre-operatively to reduce the function and vascularity of the thyroid gland[60,63]. Although small amounts of iodine are necessary for normal thyroid gland function, paradoxically large amounts of iodine such as those found in iodine solution, depress TRH and TSH release. Iodine solution suppresses the thyroid gland by decreasing iodine uptake and inhibiting thyroid hormone synthesis and the release of thyroid hormone[57,60]. The effect of iodine solution weakens over time and so it cannot be used for sustained suppression of thyroid function[60].

Drugs to decrease thyroid function are the thioureas, which include carbimazole and propylthiouracil[56,60,63]. These drugs concentrate in the thyroid gland and inhibit the synthesis of thyroid hormone. Drugs to block the effects of thyroid hormone are beta-blockers. Overproduction of thyroid hormone, causes an up regulation (increase in the number) of beta-adrenergic receptors, which makes target tissues more sensitive to stimulation by the sympathetic nervous system. Propranolol is a beta-adrenergic blocking agent, which blocks the effects of increased sympathetic nervous system activity on the beta-adrenergic receptors[3,56,63].

NURSING IMPLICATIONS

The implications of caring for a patient with Grave's disease involve

- Providing education to the patient about the signs and symptoms of Grave's disease;
- Monitoring the patient's fluid intake and encouraging the patient to keep hydrated;
- Encouraging the patient to get plenty of rest in a cool environment and to wear lightweight clothing;
- Monitoring the hospitalised patient for signs and symptoms of thyroid storm;
- Ensuring the patient has a good understanding about the importance of taking their medications and the rationale for medication use;

- Encouraging the patient to have a well-balanced high-calorie diet and to monitor their weight. It may be helpful to refer the patient to a dietitian[55]; and
- For the patient with exophthalmos, encouraging the use of artificial tears to protect the cornea[55].

LEARNING EXERCISES

1. Discuss the differences in the clinical manifestations of hypothyroidism and hyperthyroidism.
2. What are the reasons for the presence of goitre in both hypothyroidism and hyperthyroidism?
3. Discuss the reasons for the development of heart disease in Grave's disease.
4. Explain why TSH is elevated in primary hypothyroidism and decreased in primary hyperthyroidism.
5. Discuss the pharmacological management of Grave's disease.

DISORDERS OF THE ADRENAL GLANDS

Adrenal disorders result from either underactivity or overactivity of the adrenal gland. The adrenal cortex secretes three types of steroid hormones; glucocorticoids, mineralocorticoids, and androgens[4]. Cortisol is the principal glucocorticoid hormone. Secretion of the glucocorticoids and androgens is controlled by adrenocorticotrophic hormone (ACTH), secreted by the anterior pituitary gland[3]. The blood levels of glucocorticoids are controlled by negative feedback mechanisms. Corticotrophin-releasing hormone (CRH), secreted by the hypothalamus, stimulates the secretion of ACTH, which increases the level of cortisol secretion by the adrenal cortex. Negative feedback occurs when high levels of cortisol inhibit CRH secretion from the hypothalamus and ACTH secretion from the anterior pituitary gland[4].

ADRENAL INSUFFICIENCY

Hypofunction or underactivity of the adrenal gland is known as *adrenal insufficiency* (decreased production and secretion of glucocorticoids and mineralocorticoids)[55]. Primary adrenal insufficiency is termed Addison's disease. Secondary adrenal insufficiency results from lack of adrenocorticotrophic hormone (ACTH) from the anterior pituitary gland[55], commonly caused by the rapid withdrawal of therapeutically administered steroids.

 Case study

Jonathon Tan, 61, presented to the emergency department in a markedly unwell state. He complained of progressive development of symptoms that included feeling generally unwell, with marked weakness and fatigue. He felt dizzy most of the time, which became worse when standing. He also commented on unintentional weight loss, increased frequency of urination and the progressive development of darkening of his skin much 'like a suntan'. On taking his observations, the nurse noted that he was tachycardic with a pulse of 110 beats per minute and that he had orthostatic hypotension. His blood pressure when lying down was 95/55 mmHg, and when standing was 80/40 mmHg. Blood tests revealed that he had hyponatraemia, hyperkalaemia, mildly raised urea and creatinine levels and hypoglycaemia.

On the basis of Mr Tan's history and clinical manifestations, he was diagnosed with primary adrenal insufficiency or Addison's disease. The diagnosis was confirmed with an ACTH stimulation test[4]. Treatment was commenced with glucocorticoid replacement therapy consisting of cortisone acetate 25 mg at 7am and 12.5 mg at 5pm.

Addison's disease is a condition in which the manifestations result from mineralocorticoid and glucocorticoid deficiency and ACTH excess. It is a rare disorder that can progress to acute adrenal crisis[3]. The disorder occurs in people of either sex and affects all age groups[55]. The most common cause is autoimmune destruction of the adrenal gland[55].

PATHOPHYSIOLOGY

Addison's disease is an autoimmune disorder[65] in which all the layers of the adrenal cortex are destroyed by inflammation[3]. Other causes include tuberculosis (which can result in spread of the tubercle bacillus from the lungs via blood or lymph), breast, lung or gastrointestinal cancer (which results in metastatic spread) and heparin administration causing bilateral adrenal haemorrhage[3,66].

CLINICAL MANIFESTATIONS

The clinical manifestations of Addison's disease develop slowly and progressively[55]. More than 90% of the gland is destroyed before manifestations occur[55]. Mineralocorticoid (aldosterone) deficiency results in an inability to retain salt and water leading to hyponatraemia (low serum sodium), orthostatic hypotension (a drop in blood pressure when standing up) and decreased cardiac output[3,66]. There is reduced excretion of potassium by the kidneys leading to hyperkalaemia and cardiac arrythmias[4,67]. Glucocorticoid (cortisol) deficiency results in an inability to maintain blood glucose levels causing hypoglycaemia[3]. Symptoms resulting from these deficits include weakness, fatigue, dehydration, weight loss, anorexia, nausea and vomiting. Excess levels of ACTH stimulate the production of melanin leading to hyperpigmentation of the skin in general, with a particular bronze discolouration of skin folds, pressure points, fingers and toes[3].

Acute adrenal crisis is a life-threatening consequence of adrenal insufficiency. Where a person has pre-existing Addison's disease, any situation of stress, such as trauma or illness, can precipitate a sudden or progressive increase in the symptoms leading to confusion, decreased level of consciousness and shock[65].

DIAGNOSTIC TESTS

Primary adrenal insufficiency can be diagnosed by measuring serum levels of cortisol and ACTH[64]. The blood results expected include decreased levels of cortisol and elevated levels of ACTH. If the person has secondary adrenal insufficiency from hypopituitarism, then decreased levels of ACTH would be expected. In addition, the ACTH stimulation test is performed to test the ability of the adrenal glands to respond to ACTH administration by injection[65]. An increase in plasma cortisol levels after ACTH administration indicates the adrenal glands are able to function when stimulated, thus the problem of adrenal insufficiency is of pituitary origin. Failure of cortisol levels to rise after ACTH administration indicates failure of the adrenal glands[64].

TREATMENT

Addison's disease is a chronic endocrine disorder, which requires life-long replacement therapy with an oral glucocorticoid and a mineralocorticoid[57]. The usual glucocorticoid is hydrocortisone, a synthetic steroid identical to cortisol (the naturally occurring hormone)[57]. Hydrocortisone has some mineralocorticoid activity. However, if this is insufficient to alleviate symptoms, a mineralocorticoid such as fludrocortisone is also taken[60]. The adequacy of replacement therapy is evaluated by improvement of the patient's clinical symptoms.

NURSING IMPLICATIONS

The implications of caring for a patient with Addison's disease involve

- Providing education to the patient about the signs and symptoms of Addison's disease, in particular the need to see a doctor if they experience increased levels of stress or become unwell;
- Maintaining a record of fluid balance;
- Monitoring potassium levels for hyperkalaemia;
- Monitoring the hospitalised patient for signs and symptoms of acute adrenal crisis, including blood glucose levels for hypoglycaemia, and serum sodium and urea levels for dehydration;
- Ensuring the patient has a good understanding about the importance of taking their medications and the rationale for medication use. Glucocorticoids are given at times that mimic normal diurnal variation of cortisol secretion. The larger dose is given in the morning and the second, smaller dose is given in the late afternoon rather than in the evening to prevent insomnia[57];
- Ensuring the patient understands the need to increase their hydrocortisone dose during times of stress and to carry an emergency supply of injectable hydrocortisone[57]; and
- Encouraging the patient to monitor their weight.

CUSHING'S SYNDROME

Hyperfunction or overactivity of the adrenal gland is known as *Cushing's syndrome* or Cushing's disease[55]. Overproduction or excessive amounts of the glucocorticoid hormone cortisol either produced by the adrenal gland or administered therapeutically is known as Cushing's syndrome[55,66]. Excess production of cortisol that is caused by the pituitary gland, is called Cushing's disease.

● Case study

Maudie Fitzsimmons, 28, has been admitted to hospital for investigation of gastrointestinal bleeding. Maudie was diagnosed with ulcerative colitis when she was 18 years old. She has been hospitalised on numerous occasions for exacerbations of the disease. Her current treatment regimen involves 20 mg of prednisone daily; she has been taking this dose since her last hospitalisation 4 months ago. On admission to the ward, the nurse notes that Maudie has a typical cushingoid appearance, she is hypertensive with a blood pressure of 145/100 mmHg and her random blood glucose level is 10 mmol/L.

On the basis of her history and clinical presentation, Maudie is diagnosed with iatrogenic Cushing's syndrome. Her treatment will involve a gradual reduction in dose of prednisone and surgical resection of the rectum and colon.

Cushing's syndrome is a condition in which the manifestations result from the exaggerated effects of the action of cortisol[3]. The disorder most frequently occurs in adults between the ages of 20 to 50 years[55], although iatrogencic Cushing's syndrome resulting from long-term therapy with high–dose glucocorticoids can occur in any age group.

PATHOPHYSIOLOGY

There are four main causes of Cushing's syndrome. The first cause is iatrogenic and is due to the therapeutic administration of large doses of exogenous glucocorticoids, most commonly used for the treatment of inflammatory diseases such as asthma or rheumatoid arthritis[57]. The remaining causes are non–iatrogenic, but all result in the excess production of endogenous glucocorticoids. The second cause is from adrenal tumors, which are either benign or malignant, leading to excessive cortisol secretion. The third is ectopic, and is caused by non-endocrine ACTH secreting tumors, such as small-cell carcinoma of the lung which secretes ACTH. The fourth, known as Cushing's disease, is caused by a pituitary tumor leading to excessive production of ACTH by the pituitary gland[3,66].

CLINICAL MANIFESTATIONS

The clinical manifestations of Cushing's syndrome are wide ranging and can include a cushingoid appearance[55] which presents as central obesity or a protruding abdomen, buffalo hump and moon face, all of which result from excess lipolysis (fat breakdown) and redistribution of adipose tissue[3]. The subsequent excess in circulating lipids causes atherosclerosis[3]. Limbs are thin, there is muscle wasting and weakness, and thin weakened skin resulting from protein catabolism (breakdown)[3]. Osteoporosis and fractures tend to occur from bone demineralisation[55]. Renal calculi also result from excessive mobilisation of calcium from bone. Demineralisation occurs because excess cortisol decreases calcium absorption from the gastrointestinal tract leading to a fall in blood levels of calcium. The resultant hypocalcaemia stimulates the parathyroid hormones to increase serum calcium levels through reabsorption from bone[3]. Purple or red striae (stretch marks) may appear over breasts, abdomen and thighs from loss of elastic and subcutaneous tissue. Salt and water retention occur because cortisol has some mineralocorticoid effect[57]. Hypertension results from a combination of the mineralocorticoid effect and from vasoconstriction (which occurs because cortisol increases vascular sensitivity to catecholamines). Hyperglycaemia results from the conversion of fatty acids and amino acids into glucose, or the release of glucose from glycogen storage[55]. Excess cortisol depresses immune function leading to increased susceptibility to infection and also increases gastric acid secretion causing gastric ulcers. Excess androgen levels are significant in females and may accompany increased levels of cortisol resulting in hirsutism, acne and irregular menstruation[3]. Androgen over-production in males does not result in clinical manifestations because testosterone produced by the testes has the major androgenic effect in men. Alterations in mental status are due to the effects of excess levels of glucocorticoids and may vary from mild fluctuations in mood to psychosis[3].

DIAGNOSTIC TESTS

Cushing's syndrome can be confirmed by measuring excess levels of cortisol, either by 24-hour urinary cortisol or plasma cortisol levels[4,64]. A dexamethasone suppression test may also be used, where dexamethasone (a synthetic steroid) is administered to suppress ACTH secretion. Under normal conditions ACTH suppression will suppress the secretion of cortisol[4,64].

TREATMENT

The treatment of Cushing's syndrome depends on the cause and may involve surgery, pharmacological or radiation therapy[57]. The treatment of choice for iatrogenic Cushing's syndrome is slow withdrawal of glucocorticoids[66], because high doses of exogenous glucocorticoids suppress the production of cortisol by the adrenal cortex and sudden withdrawal of glucocorticoids can lead to adrenal insufficiency and adrenal crisis. For adrenal tumors, an adrenalectomy may be performed and for ectopic ACTH and pituitary tumors, removal of the tumor, irradiation or chemotherapy may be used. Adrenal steroid synthesis inhibitors, such as aminoglutethimide and metyrapone may be given[64].

NURSING IMPLICATIONS

The implications of caring for a patient with Cushing's syndrome involve

- Providing education to the patient about the signs and symptoms of Cushing's syndrome, in particular the need to protect themselves from injury or infection;
- Assessing vital observations regularly, particularly monitoring for hypertension;
- Checking blood glucose levels for hyperglycaemia;
- Assisting with 24-hour urine collection for urinary cortisol levels[55];
- Maintaining a record of fluid balance.
- Monitoring serum potassium levels for hypokalaemia and serum sodium levels for hypernatraemia;
- Involving a dietitian in planning meals with the patient;
- Reassuring the patient about mood lability[55]; and
- Ensuring the patient with iatrogenic Cushing's syndrome understands the need to slowly withdraw from their medication to prevent the onset of an adrenal crisis.

LEARNING EXERCISES

1. Explain why a patient with primary adrenal insufficiency would show decreased levels of cortisol and increased levels of ACTH.
2. Describe the clinical manifestations of mineralocorticoid deficiency in a patient with primary adrenal insufficiency.
3. Describe the pathophysiology of iatrogenic Cushing's syndrome.
4. Explain why a patient with Cushing's syndrome would have elevated blood glucose levels.
5. Explain why a patient with iatrogenic Cushing's syndrome cannot abruptly cease taking their medication.

Recommended Readings

Bryant, B, Knights, K & Salerno, E. 2003; *Pharmacology for Health Professionals*, Elsevier, Sydney.

Dunstan, DW, Zimmet, PZ, Welborn, TA, De Courten, MP, Cameron, AJ, Sicree, RA, *et al*, 2002; 'The Rising Prevalence of Diabetes and Impaired Glucose Tolerance: The Australian Diabetes, Obesity and Lifestyle Study', *Diabetes Care*, 25 (5), 829–834.

Kettyle, WM & Arky, RA. 1998; *Lippincott's Pathophysiology Series: Endocrine Pathophysiology*, Lippincott-Raven, Philadelphia.

Pagana, KD & Pagana, TJ. 2002; *Mosby's Manual of Diagnostic and Laboratory Tests* (2nd ed.), Mosby, St Louis.

Porth, CM. 2002; *Pathophysiology Concepts of Altered Health States* (6th ed.), Lippincott Williams & Wilkins, Philadelphia.

References

1. Marieb, EN. 2001; *Human Anatomy and Physiology* (5th ed.), Benjamin Cummings, San Francisco.
2. Mulvihill, ML, Zelman, M, Holdaway, P, Tompary, E & Turchany, J. 2001; *Human Diseases: A Systemic Approach* (5th ed.), Prentice Hall, New Jersey.
3. Porth, CM. 2005; *Pathophysiology Concepts of Altered Health States* (6th ed.), Lippincott Williams & Wilkins, Philadelphia.
4. Kettyle, WM & Arky, RA. 1998; *Lippincott's Pathophysiology Series: Endocrine Pathophysiology*, Lippincott-Raven, Philadelphia.
5. Goldberg, S. 2001; *Clinical Physiology Made Ridiculously Simple*, McGraw-Hill, Singapore.
6. Birnbaumer, M. 2002; 'V2R Structure and Diabetes Insipidus', *Receptors & Channels*, 8 (1), 51–56.
7. Adam, P. 1997; 'Evaluation and Management of Diabetes Insipidus', *American Family Physician*, 55 (6), 2146–2153.

8. Bell, TN. 1994; 'Diabetes Insipidus', *Critical Care Nursing Clinics of North America*, 6 (4), 675–685.
9. Nickolaus, MJ. 1999; 'Diabetes Insipidus: A Current Perspective', *Critical Care Nurse*, 19 (6), 18–30.
10. Holcomb, SS. 2002; 'Diabetes Insipidus', *DCCN – Dimensions of Critical Care Nursing*, 21 (3), 94–97.
11. Blevins, LS. Jr & Wand, GS. 1992; 'Diabetes Insipidus', *Critical Care Medicine*, 20 (1), 69–79.
12. MacGregor, DA. 1995; 'Hyperosmolar Coma Due to Lithium-induced Diabetes Insipidus', *Lancet*, 346 (8972), 413–417.
13. *MIMS Online version 1.1.* (1 May 2003–31 July 2003 ed.); MIMS, Australia.
14. Singer, I, Oster, JR & Fishman, LM. 1997; 'The Management of Diabetes Insipidus in Adults', *Archives of Internal Medicine*, 157 (12), 1293–1301.
15. Stone, KA. 1999; 'Lithium-induced Nephrogenic Diabetes Insipidus', *Journal of the American Board of Family Practice*, 12 (1), 43–47.
16. Report of a WHO Consultation. 1999; 'Definition, Diagnosis and Classification of Diabetes Mellitus and Its Complications', Department of Noncommunicable Disease Surveillance, World Health Organization, Geneva.
17 Meltzer, S, Leiter, L, Daneman, D, Gerstein, HC, Lau, D, Ludwig, S, *et al* 1998; '1998 Clinical Practice Guidelines for the Management of Diabetes in Canada', *Canadian Medical Association Journal*, 159 (supplement 8), S1–29.
18. Harris, MI, Flegal, KM, Cowie, CC, Eberhardt, MS, Goldstein, DE, Little, RR, *et al.* 1998; 'Prevalence of Diabetes, Impaired Fasting Glucose, and Impaired Glucose Tolerance in US Adults: The Third National Health and Nutrition Examination Survey, 1988–1994', *Diabetes Care*, 21 (4), 518–524.
19. Dunstan, DW, Zimmet, PZ, Welborn, TA, De Courten, MP, Cameron, AJ, Sicree, RA, *et al.* 2002; 'The Rising Prevalence of Diabetes and Impaired Glucose Tolerance: The Australian Diabetes,

Obesity and Lifestyle Study', *Diabetes Care*, 25 (5), 829–834.

20. Moore, MP & Lunt, H. 2000; 'Diabetes in New Zealand', *Diabetes Research & Clinical Practice*, 50 (2), S65–71.

21. Colagiuri, S, Colagiuri, R & Ward, J. 1998; *National Diabetes Strategy and Implementation Plan*, Diabetes Australia, Canberra.

22. Bednar-Auldridge, HL & Calhoun, BC. 2001; 'Pancreas Transplantation for Type 1 Diabetes Treatment', *Physician Assistant*, 25 (5), 32–34.

23. Campbell, L & Rossner, S. 2001; 'Management of Obesity in Patients with Type 2 Diabetes', *Diabetic Medicine*, 18 (5), 345–354.

24. Astrup, A & Finer, N. 2000; 'Redefining Type 2 Diabetes: "Diabesity" or "Obesity Dependent Diabetes Mellitus"?' *Obesity Reviews*, 1 (2), 57–59.

25. Tuomilehto, J, Lindstrom, J, Eriksson, JG, Valle, TT, Hamalainen, H, Ilanne-Parikka, P, *et al.* 2001; 'Prevention of Type 2 Diabetes Mellitus by Changes in Lifestyle Among Subjects with Impaired Glucose Tolerance', [see comment], *New England Journal of Medicine*, 344 (18), 1343–1350.

26. Hu, FB, Manson, JE, Stampfer, MJ, Colditz, G, Liu, S, Solomon, CG, *et al.* 2001; 'Diet, Lifestyle, and the Risk of Type 2 Diabetes Mellitus in Women', *New England Journal of Medicine*, 345 (11), 790–797.

27. Dornhorst, A & Frost, G. 2002; 'The Principles of Dietary Management of Gestational Diabetes: Reflection on Current Evidence', *Journal of Human Nutrition & Dietetics*, 15 (2), 145–156.

28. Umpierrez, GE, Khajavi, M & Kitabchi, AE. 1996; 'Diabetic Ketoacidosis and Hyperglycemic Hyperosmolar Nonketotic Syndrome', *American Journal of the Medical Sciences*, 311 (5), 225–233.

29. Kitabchi, AE, Umpierrez, GE, Murphy, MB, Barrett, EJ, Kreisberg, RA, Malone, JI, *et al.* 2003; 'Hyperglycemic Crises in Patients with Diabetes Mellitus', *Diabetes Care*, 26 (1), S109–117.

30. Chiasson, JL, Aris-Jilwan, N, Belanger, R, Bertrand, S, Beauregard, H, Ekoe, JM, *et al.* 2003; 'Diagnosis and Treatment of Diabetic Ketoacidosis and the Hyperglycemic Hyperosmolar State', *Canadian Medical Association Journal*, 168 (7), 859–866.

31. Lavis, VR, D'Souza, D & Brown, SD. 1994; 'Decompensated Diabetes: New Features of an Old Problem', *Circulation*, 90 (6), 3108–3112.

32. Berger, B, Stenstrom, G & Sundkvist, G. 2000; 'Random C-Peptide in the Classification of Diabetes', *Scandinavian Journal of Clinical & Laboratory Investigation*, 60 (8), 687–693.

33. Wright-Pascoe, R, Mills, J, Choo-Kang, E & Morrison, EY. 2000; 'The Role of C-Peptide in the Classification of Diabetes Mellitus', *West Indian Medical Journal*, 49 (2), 138–142.

34. Ghosh, J, Weiss, M, Kay, R & Frishman, W. 2003; 'Diabetes Mellitus and Coronary Artery Disease: Therapeutic Considerations', *Heart Disease*, 5 (2), 119–128.

35. Gerich, JE. 2001; 'Matching Treatment to Pathophysiology in Type 2 Diabetes', *Clinical Therapeutics*, 23 (5), 646–659.

36. Bell, DS. 2002; 'Chronic Complications of Diabetes', *Southern Medical Journal*, 95 (1), 30–34.

37. Goldstein, BJ. 2002; 'Insulin Resistance as the Core Defect in Type 2 Diabetes Mellitus', *American Journal of Cardiology*, 90 (5A), 3G–10G.

38. Sivan, E & Boden, G. 2003; 'Free Fatty Acids, Insulin Resistance, and Pregnancy', *Current Diabetes Reports*, 3 (4), 319–322.

39. Sherwin, RS, Anderson, RM, Buse, JB, Chin, MH, Eddy, D, Fradkin, J, *et al.* 2003; 'The Prevention or Delay of Type 2 Diabetes', *Diabetes Care*, 26 (1), S62–S69.

40. Quinn, L. 2002; 'Mechanisms in the Development of Type 2 Diabetes Mellitus', *Journal of Cardiovascular Nursing*, 16 (2), 1–16.

41. Vinik, A & Flemmer, M. 2002; 'Diabetes and Macrovascular Disease', *Journal of Diabetes & Its Complications*, 16 (3), 235–245.

42. Bonnefont-Rousselot, D. 2002; 'Glucose and Reactive Oxygen Species', *Current Opinion in Clinical Nutrition & Metabolic Care*, 5 (5), 561–568.

43. Bailes, BK. 2002; 'Diabetes Mellitus and its Chronic Complications', *AORN Journal*, 76 (2), 266–276, 278–282.

44. Nathan, DM. 1993; 'Long-term Complications of Diabetes Mellitus', *New England Journal of Medicine*, 328 (23), 1676–1685.

45. Barr, RG, Nathan, DM, Meigs, JB & Singer, DE. 2002; 'Tests of Glycemia for the Diagnosis of Type 2 Diabetes Mellitus', *Annals of Internal Medicine*, 137 (4), 263–272.

46. Lonneville, YH, Ozdek, SC, Onol, M, Yetkin, I, Gurelik, G & Hasanreisoglu, B. 2003; 'The Effect of Blood Glucose Regulation on Retinal Nerve Fiber Layer Thickness in Diabetic Patients', *Ophthalmologica*, 217 (5), 347–350.

47. Mehler, PS, Coll, JR, Estacio, R, Esler, A, Schrier, RW & Hiatt, WR. 2003; 'Intensive Blood Pressure Control Reduces the Risk of Cardiovascular Events in Patients with Peripheral Arterial Disease and Type 2 Diabetes', *Circulation*, 107 (5), 753–756.

48. Manley, S. 2003; 'Haemoglobin A1c – a Marker for Complications of Type 2 Diabetes: The Experience from the UK Prospective Diabetes Study (UKPDS)', *Clinical Chemistry & Laboratory Medicine*, 41 (9), 1182–1190.

49. Viberti, G. 2003; 'The Need for Tighter Control of Cardiovascular Risk Factors in Diabetic Patients', *Journal of Hypertension Supplement*, 21 (1), S3–6.

50. American Association of Diabetes, E. 2002; 'Intensive Diabetes Management: Implications of the DCCT and UKPDS', *Diabetes Educator*, 28 (5), 735–740.

51. Luna, B & Feinglos, MN. 2001; 'Oral Agents in the Management of Type 2 Diabetes Mellitus', *American Family Physician*, 63 (9), 1747–1756.

52. Lalau, JD & Race, JM. 2001; 'Lactic Acidosis in Metformin Therapy: Searching for a Link with Metformin in Reports of "Metformin-associated Lactic Acidosis"', *Diabetes, Obesity and Metabolism*, 3 (3), 195–201.

53. DeFronzo, RA. 1999; 'Pharmacologic Therapy for Type 2 Diabetes Mellitus', *Annals of Internal Medicine*, 131 (4), 281–303.

54. Zangeneh, F, Kudva, YC & Basu, A. 2003; 'Insulin Sensitizers', *Mayo Clinic Proceedings*, 78 (4), 471–479.

55. Gutierrez, KJ & Peterson, PG. 2002; *Pathophysiology*, W. B. Saunders, Philadelphia.

56. Holcomb, SS. 2002; 'Thyroid Disease: A Primer for the Critical Care Nurse', *DCCN – Dimensions of Critical Care Nursing*, 21 (4), 127–133.

57. Lehne, RA. 2001; *Pharmacology for Nursing Care*, (4th ed.), W. B. Saunders, Philadelphia.

58. Higgins, C. 2000; *Understanding Laboratory Investigations: A Text for Nurses and Healthcare Professionals*, Blackwell Science, Oxford.

59. Topliss, DJ & Eastman, CJ. 2004; 'Diagnosis and Management of Hyperthyroidism and Hypothyroidism', *Medical Journal of Australia*, 180 (4), 186–193.

60. Bryant, B, Knights, K & Salerno, E. 2003; *Pharmacology for Health Professionals*, Elsevier Science, Harcourt Australia, Marrickville, New South Wales.

61. Farley, A & Hendry, C. 2002; 'Autoimmune Disorders', *Nursing Standard*, 16 (41), 38–40.

62. Royal College of Pathologists of Australia, RCPA Manual. 2004; 'Thyroid Stimulating Hormone (TSH)-Serum', Retrieved from http://www.rcpamanual.edu.au/

63. Boyages, SC. 2000; 'Thyrotoxicosis'. Retrieved from E-MIMS, May 2002, MIMS Australia, St Leonards, New South Wales.

64. Pagana, KD & Pagana, TJ. 2002; *Mosby's Manual of Diagnostic and Laboratory Tests* (2nd ed.), Mosby, St Louis.

65. Sabol, VK. 2001; 'Addisonian Crisis: This Life-threatening Condition May Be Triggered by a Variety of Stressors', *American Journal of Nursing*, 101 (7), 24–28.

66. Stiel, JN. 2002; 'Adrenal Disorders'. Retrieved from E-MIMS, May 2002, MIMS Australia, St Leonards, New South Wales.

67. Nayback, AM 2000; 'Hyponataemia as a Consequence of Acute Adrenal Insufficiency and Hypothyroidism', *Journal of Emergency Nursing*, 26 (2), 130–133.

5 | Cardiac Health Breakdown

AUTHORS

PATRICIA DAVIDSON

DOMINIC LEUNG

JOHN DALY

LEARNING OBJECTIVES

When you have completed this chapter you will be able to
- Describe the anatomical and physiological features of the heart and cardiovascular system;
- Appreciate the pathophysiological changes associated with cardiovascular dysfunction;
- Appreciate the importance of accurate patient history and symptom assessment in patients with cardiac dysfunction;
- Identify key cardiac diagnostic and therapeutic techniques;
- Describe key pharmacological agents used in cardiology practice and considerations for nursing management; and
- Evaluate the appropriateness of nursing interventions for people with heart disease.

INTRODUCTION

Cardiovascular disease (CVD) is a leading cause of disability in Australia, New Zealand and other developed countries. CVD and its manifestation in conditions, such as acute myocardial infarction, stroke and heart failure, are responsible for significant disease burden globally[1-3]. This chapter focuses on cardiac health breakdown, but it is important to consider the impact of other systems on the aetiology, presentation and progression of heart disease. In particular, you should consider the potential for respiratory dysfunction (Chapter 6), renal dysfunction (Chapter 7), and haematological disturbances (Chapter 12). Although cardiovascular dysfunction can manifest in numerous conditions, this chapter will focus on the discussion of the diagnosis and management of the commonly encountered clinical problems of acute coronary syndromes, heart failure and atrial fibrillation. As you work through this chapter, it is important to remember that cardiac health breakdown often occurs in the elderly and is often only one of their co-morbid chronic diseases. This increases the complexity of management, and, particularly, the potential for drug interactions. For example, a patient may be prescribed a non-steroidal anti-inflammatory medication for osteoarthritis, but this may have a deleterious effect on the renal function of a patient with chronic heart failure.

CVD, manifested as acute coronary syndrome (ACS) – unstable angina pectoris, or acute myocardial infarction – and heart failure (HF) is a major cause of morbidity and mortality in industrialised societies. Australians aged over 60 years account for 70% of acute myocardial infarctions (AMIs), 61% of percutaneous coronary interventions (PCI) and 73% of coronary artery bypass graft surgery (CABG)[4]. By 2020 it is estimated that in developed countries, up to 80% of disease burden with be a result of chronic diseases such as cardiovascular disease[3]. Therefore, when assessing and managing a patient, it is important not to only consider other actual or potential co-morbid conditions and the potential for drug interactions, but also the importance of promotion of self-management in the treatment plan.

Although conditions manifesting as cardiac health breakdown are chronic in nature, initial manifestations often present as acute deteriorations such as acute myocardial infarction or acute pulmonary oedema. It is disastrous that the initial presentation for many individuals may be a sudden cardiac death or a catastrophic stroke. Unfortunately, many people ignore the signs of a potential heart attack[5,6]. This delay in seeking treatment and the concept that cardiac health breakdown is largely preventable are the motivation behind widespread public health campaigns to urge individuals to look at modifiable risk factors such as high blood pressure, obesity and physical inactivity[7-10].

Due to the high prevalence of heart disease, cardiology is the focus of substantive research and is a dynamic and evolving science. Consequently, clinical practice changes rapidly and it is important for the clinician to keep abreast of changes and recent developments in detection, management and prevention. A good way to do this is to access the web sites of key professional bodies that are responsible for the development of best practice guidelines. These include the Heart Foundation of Australia; National Heart Foundation of New Zealand, Cardiac Society of Australia and New Zealand; Australian College of Critical Care Nurses, American Heart Association; American College of Cardiology; Heart Failure Society of America and European College of Cardiology. A list of these web sites is given at the end of this chapter.

ANATOMY AND PHYSIOLOGY OF THE HEART

A detailed understanding of normal and abnormal cardiac anatomy and physiology, and how these relate more broadly to the cardiovascular system, is fundamental to understanding diagnostic and management strategies for patients with heart disease. A comprehensive description of this information is beyond the scope of this chapter. It is important to review cardiac anatomy and physiology in depth before reading this chapter. Following is a summary of the key anatomical features of the heart.

The heart is a four-chambered muscular organ responsible for circulating blood around the body. These chambers are known as the *right atrium*; the *right ventricle*; the *left atrium* and the *left ventricle*. Blood enters the heart via the atria. There are two large veins, which enter the heart on the right hand side and bring deoxygenated blood into the right atrium. The *superior vena cava* brings in deoxygenated blood from the upper extremities of the body and the head while the *inferior vena cava* brings in blood from the body and the lower extremities. This deoxygenated blood is fed into the right ventricle and taken to the lungs where gas exchange occurs (see Chapter 6), before returning to the left atrium through the right and left pulmonary veins. The oxygen-rich blood enters the left side of the heart and is pumped out into the systemic circulation by the larger left ventricle. Blood leaves the heart via the *aorta*, the largest artery in the body, into the upper body via the arteries branching off the aortic arch and into the thorax, trunk and lower body via the descending aorta. These anatomical features are shown in Figure 5.1.

VALVES

Valves separate the chambers of the heart and are designed to prevent backflow of blood. As the heart contracts, the valves open and blood is pumped from one chamber to the adjoining chamber. The right atrium and right ventricle are separated by the tricuspid valve, named because it consists of three leaflets. The mitral valve functions similarly on the left side of the heart, and has two leaflets. The pulmonary valve and aortic valve are located at the outlets of the right and left ventricles respectively. If the valves do not close properly backflow occurs (e.g., mitral valve regurgitation). In some cases the valves don't open properly (e.g., aortic valve stenosis).

CORONARY ARTERIES

The right and left coronary arteries branch off the aorta (see Figure 5.1). If the coronary arteries become narrowed by deposits of cholesterol in the lining of the arteries (atherosclerosis) then the flow of blood to the myocardium (heart muscle) may be restricted. This is a common cause of ischaemia and subsequent myocardial infarction.

CARDIAC OUTPUT

The term cardiac output (CO) is defined as the amount of blood, in litres, that is ejected by the heart each minute. The calculation of CO is based on the product of heart rate and stroke volume. Stroke volume is defined as the amount of blood ejected from the heart with each heartbeat. It is determined by factors including preload, afterload and contractility. Preload is the amount of volume or pressure in the ventricle at end-diastole while afterload is the resistance the heart has to overcome in order to eject the blood. Simplistically, contractility is the ability of the heart to stretch and contract[11].

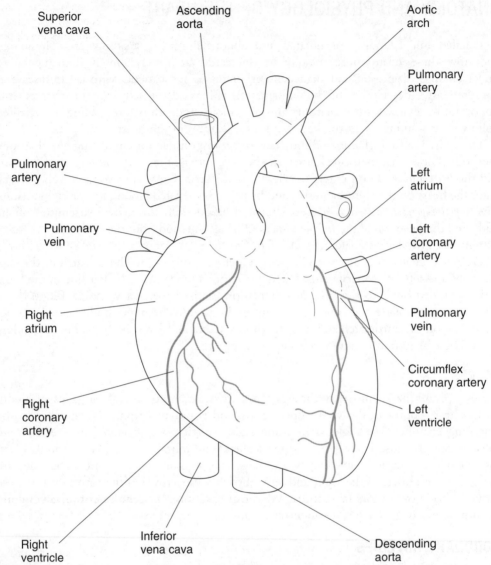

FIGURE 5.1 *External features of the heart, major vessels and coronary arteries*

PREVENTION, DIAGNOSIS AND MANAGEMENT OF CARDIAC HEALTH BREAKDOWN

Regardless of the causes and nature of cardiac health breakdown, the following principles should guide prevention, diagnosis and management:

• Wherever possible, preventive measures should be implemented. This ranges from primary prevention strategies, such as smoking cessation and physical activity programs, to secondary prevention strategies, such as beta blocker therapy in acute coronary syndromes, to strategies to minimise preventable admissions to hospital for patients with heart failure.

- High-risk groups (such as diabetic and indigenous populations) warrant closer vigilance and higher levels of intervention, including health promotion and secondary prevention strategies.
- Interventions and treatments are based on the best available evidence and guidelines developed by key professional groups such as the National Heart Foundation of Australia and the Cardiac Society of Australia and New Zealand.
- Care should be patient-centred, tailored to the needs, capacity and preferences of individual patients. Service delivery systems and models of care should be designed to optimise continuity of care and should be guided by systematic review of patient outcomes and reflective practice. These models of care should consider management aspects from primary prevention strategies through to palliative care.
- Self-management strategies and non-pharmacological strategies, such as an optimal diet, exercise and stress-management techniques, should be incorporated in all treatment plans.
- The risks and complications of all diagnostic and management strategies (including costs) should be carefully weighted against the potential benefits to the individual.
- Models of nursing care should be based upon: the best available evidence; assessment of patient and health provider needs; measurement of health-related and intervention outcomes; a multidisciplinary approach where applicable; optimal and equitable utilisation of health care resource; and include interventions that are culturally sensitive and appropriate.

SELF-CARE AND SELF-MANAGEMENT IN CARDIAC HEALTH BREAKDOWN

Adjustment to a diagnosis of cardiac health breakdown has implications for self-care[12]. In order to promote self-care in patients, information, systems, processes and support are required to maximise risk-factor modification and adherence to lifestyle modifications[13]. Self-care strategies need to be customised to the individual and optimally incorporates family members and significant others in care planning. The growing burden of chronic disease accentuates the importance of self-management principles in chronic-disease management. Given the cultural diversity of contemporary society, it is important that treatment plans are appropriate to culturally and linguistically diverse groups[14,15].

KEY ELEMENTS OF DIAGNOSIS OF CARDIAC HEALTH BREAKDOWN

Key elements of a complete cardiac diagnosis include consideration of anatomic and physiological disturbances, functional status and disease aetiology[16]. Key aspects in taking a focused history include[17]

- Previous health history, including immunisations, prior intravenous drug use, history of rheumatic heart disease, medical and surgical procedures, pregnancies, menopause;
- Family history of heart disease, stroke, diabetes and sudden death in family members. Many forms of heart disease are genetically acquired, for example hypertrophic cardiomyopathy and coronary atherosclerosis. Therefore, taking a family history is an important strategy in assessing risk and prognosis;
- Risk factor profile, including hypertension, family history, obesity, diabetes, physical inactivity and depression;
- Medication history, including prescribed, over-the-counter and illegal (in particular amphetamine and cocaine)[18] drug use;
- Onset and nature of symptoms assessing the individual's activity pattern, and symptoms associated with exertion is important. Standardised measures of functional status are used to communicate functional status and monitor therapeutic management and disease progression;
- Health-seeking beliefs and disease attributions[14,19]; and
- Presence of depression, social isolation and lack of social support.

In 2003, the National Heart Foundation of Australia (NHF) released a position statement, informed by a systematic review, that clearly identified these issues as significant risk factors for coronary heart disease (CHD)[20]. This review concluded that there is evidence of an independent causal association between depression, social isolation and lack of quality social support and the aetiology and outcome of CHD.

DETERMINING A DIAGNOSIS OF CARDIAC HEALTH BREAKDOWN

Determining a cardiac diagnosis is dependent on a comprehensive history and physical examination of the patient. Despite the myriad technological investigations available to the health professionals (see Table 5.1), clinical assessment remains the basis for the diagnosis of many conditions and the development of a plan for diagnostic testing and cardiovascular therapeutics. Clinical examination and history are facilitated by diagnostic tests including: 1) the electrocardiogram; 2) chest X-ray; 3) echocardiogram; 4) radionuclide and imaging techniques; 5) coronary angiography; and 6) laboratory tests. The chest X-ray can help differentiate patients with a normal-sized heart from patients with an enlarged cardiac silhouette, suggesting acute exacerbation of some underlying form of chronic heart failure, or identify pulmonary oedema (suggesting heart failure secondary to acute myocardial infarction, or valvular insufficiency, or pulmonary congestion)[16]. Pathophysiological presentations of cardiac health breakdown are numerous and diverse and texts discussing these can be found in the list of recommended readings.

GUIDING PRINCIPLES IN THE MANAGEMENT PLAN OF CARDIAC HEALTH BREAKDOWN

Once a diagnosis of heart disease is made, the therapeutic regimen is developed. Key factors to consider in the development of the treatment plan are the use of evidence-based strategies with consideration of the following factors:

TABLE 5.1: COMMON DIAGNOSTIC TESTS IN SUSPECTED CARDIAC HEALTH BREAKDOWN	
Diagnostic Test	**Description**
Echocardiography Transoesophageal echocardiography Intravascular ultrasound Stress echocardiography	Using ultrasound technology these tests show the structure and function of the heart, in particular, the heart valves and muscle function
Electrocardiography Holter monitoring Electrophysiological studies Holter monitoring	These tests monitor the electrical function of the heart and diagnose cardiac arrhythmias
Coronary angiography Magnetic resonance imaging (MRI) Gated heart pool scans Positron emission tomography (PET) Scan	These diagnostic tests assess circulation in the coronary system and the pumping function of the heart

- Lifestyle and behavioural risk factor management (e.g., dietary modification);
- Biomedical risk factors and medical management (e.g., revascularisation in acute myscardial in farction);
- Pharmacological intervention (e.g., warfarin therapy to prevent embolic events in atrial fibrillation);
- Non–pharmacological intervention (e.g., exercise in heart failure); and
- Psychological and social issues management (e.g., management of depression and cardiac rehabilitation).

COMMON SCENARIOS FOR CARDIAC HEALTH BREAKDOWN

Acute coronary syndromes (ACS), heart failure (HF) and atrial fibrillation (AF) are common presentations of cardiac health breakdown. It is important not to consider these as 'discrete' entities. It is possible for a patient to present with an ACS with AF and in HF. The ageing of our society has increased the complexity of cardiology management with co–morbidities common in clinical presentations.

MYOCARDIAL ISCHAEMIA

Myocardial ischaemia can occur as a result of:

- Obstruction to blood flow or inadequate myocardial perfusion; or
- Cardiac rhythm or rate alterations disturbing cardiac output;

Symptoms of myocardial ischaemia are often described as angina and manifest frequently as chest discomfort. In addition, reduction of cardiac output can lead to symptoms such as weakness and fatigue. Chest discomfort, however, may result from a variety of causes other than myocardial ischemia. Conversely, many individuals with myocardial ischaemia may not experience any chest pain or discomfort[21,22].

ACUTE CORONARY SYNDROMES

Coronary heart disease is the most common form of heart disease in adults and may manifest as angina, heart failure, arrhythmias, acute myocardial infarction (AMI) and sudden cardiac death[21,23]. Coronary heart disease continues to be the leading cause of death among adults in the Australia and New Zealand, and remains so despite improvements in prevention and treatment of disease[24,25]. The treatment of AMI has evolved dramatically over the past 20 years from bed rest, and management of associated complications, to aggressive reperfusion strategies (primary angioplasty and thrombolytic therapy) and other measures to minimise myocardial damage[26]. *Acute coronary syndrome* (ACS) refers to a set of clinical symptoms that result from rupture of vulnerable plaques in the coronary arteries[21]. Conceptually, ACS is viewed as a continuum representing the relationship between the vulnerable plaque and coronary artery[22]. The vulnerability of plaque and subsequent clot formation and impairment of coronary artery blood flow, represented schematically in Figure 5.2, dictates the therapeutic management strategies of ACS.

Occasionally, concomitant conditions, such as atrial fibrillation (see Figure 5.3), complicate clinical management. From clinical, diagnostic and therapeutic perspectives, this continuum ranges from *unstable angina pectoris (UAP)*, where ischaemic symptoms can occur at rest and be protracted, *non-ST-segment elevation MI (NSTEMI)*, where symptoms are associated with electrocardiographic changes and elevation of cardiac markers, through to *ST-segment elevation MI (STEMI)*, as illustrated in Figure 5.4, and *sudden cardiac death*. The result of ruptured atherosclerotic plaque and decrease of coronary blood flow may lead to development of heart failure or sudden cardiac death. Unfortunately, sudden cardiac death can be the initial, disastrous manifestation of ACS[21]. A key diagnostic tool in ACS is the electrocardiogram (ECG). An ECG measures and records the electrical activity (depolarisation and repolarisation) of the heart muscle. The configuration of the ECG reflects the patterns of contraction and relaxation throughout the heart. Abnormalities of the ST segment are reflecting changes in the repolarisation pattern of the ventricles. This can be due to myocardial ischaemia or infarction, pericarditis or ventricular hypertrophy. When ST segments are elevated this is highly suggestive of an acute myocardial infarction and is usually termed a ST-segment elevation myocardial infarction (STEMI). ST segment elevation in association with symptoms of ischaemia, such as chest pain and shortness of breath, requires urgent treatment to unblock affected arteries. A depressed or horizontal ST wave suggests impaired blood flow to the myocardium. If this finding occurs within the context of ischaemic symptoms and elevated cardiac markers this may be termed *non-ST-segment elevation MI* (NSTEMI).

The precipitator of an ACS event is thought to be rupture or erosion of an atherosclerotic plaque in a coronary artery due to inflammation followed by thrombosis. Several factors

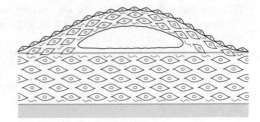

Stable plaque

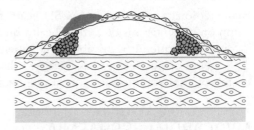

Unstable plaque: Thrombus formation

FIGURE 5.2 *Atherosclerotic plaque*

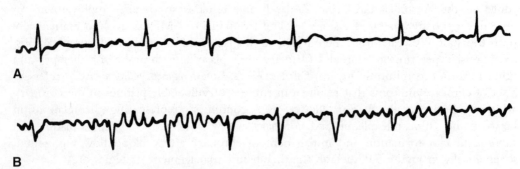

A

B

FIGURE 5.3 *Rhythm strip identifying atrial fibrillation*
Source: Hampton, J. 2002; *The ECG Made Easy* (5th ed.), Churchill Livingstone, Edinburgh, 79.

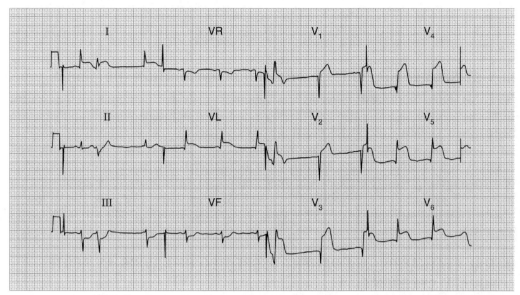

FIGURE 5.4 *ECG demonstrating ST segment changes of acute anterolateral myocardial infarction. This ECG was recorded from a 60-year-old woman who had had severe chest tightness for 1 hour*
Source: Hampton, J. 2003; *150 ECG Problems* (2nd ed.), Churchill Livingstone, New York, 195.

may precipitate the rupture of vulnerable plaque. This rupture leads to the activation, adhesion, and aggregation of platelets and the activation of the clotting cascade, resulting in the formation of an occlusive thrombus. Local thrombosis, occurring after plaque disruption, results from complex interactions between clotting factors, the lipid core of the plaque, exposed smooth-muscle cells, macrophages, and collagen. In response to the disruption of the endothelial wall, platelets aggregate and release their granular contents, which further propagate platelet aggregation and promote vasoconstriction and thrombus formation. If this process leads to complete occlusion of the artery, then acute myocardial infarction with ST-segment elevation occurs. Alternatively, if the process leads to severe stenosis but the artery nonetheless remains patent, then unstable angina occurs. Coronary vasospasm may also contribute to vascular instability by altering pre-existing coronary plaques, which causes intimal disruption and penetration of macrophages or aggregation of platelets. Rapid proliferation and migration of smooth-muscle cells in response to endothelial injury may lead to narrowing of the coronary arteries and ischaemic symptoms[22].

UNSTABLE ANGINA PECTORIS

The diagnosis of UAP may be based on any of the following clinical presentations:

- *Angina (symptoms of myocardial ischaemia)* occurs without any exertion and generally lasts for 20 minutes or longer.

• *Increasing angina* occurs in a patient with a prior diagnosis of angina pectoris. This is when episodes increase in frequency, are longer in duration, are precipitated by less than usual exertion, or occur at rest.

NON-ST-SEGMENT ELEVATION MYOCARDIAL INFARCTION (NSTEMI)

NSTEMI differs from UAP in terms of diagnosis, therapy and prognosis on the basis of ECG changes. These two differential diagnoses are often indistinguishable at presentation based upon clinical history. NSTEMI involves ischaemia severe enough to result in myocardial damage, although cardiac markers (cardiac markers such as troponins and enzymes, e.g., creatinine kinase MB) may not be elevated until several hours after onset of ischaemic symptoms. Therapeutically, interventions are aimed at arresting the progression of the ACS presentation from NSTEMI to STEMI where there is greater risk of loss of myocardium and subsequent complications. The complications of STEMI are listed in Table 5.2.

INITIAL EVALUATION IN A PATIENT SUSPECTED OF HAVING AN ACUTE CORONARY SYNDROME

When evaluating a patient with suspected myocardial ischaemia the following factors should be considered:

• Clinical presentation;
• Previous clinical history, particularly previous ACS presentations;
• Comprehensive risk factor profile including family history. Important risk factors that can be modified by nursing intervention are listed in Table 5.3;
• Current medications;
• Co-morbid conditions;
• Patient's age;
• Patient's gender; and
• Patient's appreciation of risk and benefits of therapeutic options.

TABLE 5.2: COMPLICATIONS OF STEMI[16,80–82]
Recurrent ischaemia
Pericarditis
Reinfarction
Acute heart failure
Chronic heart failure
Thromboembolism
Ventricular septal rupture
Reinfarction
Infarct extension
Left ventricular aneurysm
Arrhythmias
Mitral valve dysfunction

TABLE 5.3: PREVENTABLE RISK FACTORS FOR CARDIAC HEALTH BREAKDOWN
Tobacco smoking
High blood pressure
High blood cholesterol
Obesity
Insufficient physical activity
High alcohol intake
Type 2 diabetes
Stress and other psychosocial factors

This information will assist the clinician in developing a diagnostic and therapeutic plan. For example, it is futile to perform a coronary angiogram with the associated risks on a patient who has previously declined coronary artery bypass surgery unless they are prepared to follow through with invasive therapeutic options. Similarly it is important that patients appreciate the risks and benefits associated with thrombolytic therapy and primary angioplasty. The factors above also help the clinician to assess prognosis and risk. This will guide diagnostic, therapeutic and management decisions. For example, it will dictate whether the patient should undergo an immediate percutaneous coronary intervention (PCI) and where the patient is best managed. That is, whether the patient is best managed in a coronary care unit (CCU) or a step-down or sub acute unit. As the risk of complications increases with treatment delays, clinicians must make certain clinical decisions, concerning the appropriate level of care, immediately after obtaining the ECG[27,28].

MAKING A DIAGNOSIS OF ACS AND DEVELOPING A MANAGEMENT PLAN

The presentation of a patient with ACS can be varied, ranging from people with diabetes who do not experience typical 'chest pain' associated with heart attack (because of impaired autonomic function), through to the crushing central chest pain we view as 'typical chest pain'. All patients who present with chest tightness, pressure or pain (which may radiate to the jaw, the neck, or either or both arms) must be assumed to have possible ACS. In addition, people who have symptoms of 'indigestion', shortness of breath, extreme fatigue, or dizziness should also be systematically assessed for the presence of heart disease. Dyspnoea, diaphoresis, nausea, and/or vomiting should also increase the index of suspicion of ACS. Older patients may present with syncope, or dyspnoea without experiencing chest pain. Women are more likely than men to present with symptoms considered to be 'atypical'[29]. This makes the diagnosis of ACS complex, particularly in busy emergency departments. In the USA, failure to diagnose ACS is the most common cause of litigation for emergency physicians. However, following the steps listed below decreases the likelihood of 'missing' a diagnosis of ACS in the clinical setting.

The important inverse relationship between delay from onset of ischaemic symptoms to reperfusion strategies and prognosis underscores the importance of early presentation and the important role of effective triage[30]. The ECG remains an accessible and effective screening tool in conjunction with an astute physical assessment. Localised pain in the absence of other symptoms; a low-risk profile and a normal ECG may assist in ruling out ACS. Many diagnostic algorithms exist to assist clinicians in making these decisions based on clinical symptoms.

Key elements of making a diagnosis of ACS are the

- 12-lead electrocardiogram (ECG);
- clinical history, including onset and nature of symptoms and risk factors, such as family history, illegal drug use, smoking, diabetes, hypertension, psychological factors, hyperlipidemia; and
- biochemical cardiac markers.

ELECTROCARDIOGRAM

For all patients *with* suspected ACS, an electrocardiogram (ECG) should be performed within 5 to 10 minutes of presentation to hospital. Many aspects of the clinical history can be undertaken concurrently with the ECG. Importantly, the ECG should be interpreted by a senior clinician and compared with prior recordings, if any are available. Serial ECGs should be taken as necessary, for example if there is any recurrence of chest pain and if continuous ST segment monitoring is available, it should be used. Electrocardiograms with ST segment changes strongly suggest acute ischaemia. Clinicians should be aware that a 'normal' ECG does not rule out ACS, but alters the probability to make it less likely. Patients with T-wave inversion, new bundle branch block, or left ventricular hypertrophy on their ECG are at an increased risk of ACS and associated complications.

CLINICAL HISTORY AND PHYSICAL EXAMINATION

A systematic approach to the clinical examination is important in making a clinical diagnosis. Vital signs should be documented, including blood pressure in each arm, heart rate, temperature and pulse oximetry. The heart and lungs should be auscultated in particular for the presence of abnormalities, such as an S3 gallop in heart sounds, a cardiac murmur or the presence of rales in the chest. Acute dyspnoea, pleuritic chest pain, and differential breath sounds may indicate pneumothorax or pulmonary embolus. A complete cardiovascular assessment should be performed to detect bruits or pulse deficits. For example, identification of aortic regurgitation on auscultation and unequal pulses may indicate aortic dissection.

CARDIAC MARKERS AND ENZYMES

Cardiac enzymes or markers are protein molecules released into the blood stream from heart muscle damaged by a blocked artery. The most common enzymes or markers monitored in clinical practice are *troponin I, troponin T* and *creatine kinase MB (CKMB)*.

The troponin complex regulates the contraction of striated muscle and consists of three types:

1. Troponin C, which binds to calcium ions;
2. Troponin I, which binds to actin and inhibits actin-myosin interactions;
3. Troponin T, which binds to tropomyosin, thereby attaching the troponin complex to the thin filament[31,32].

Under usual conditions, cardiac troponin T and cardiac troponin I are not detectable in the blood of healthy persons. Release of these substances occurs when myocytes are damaged by conditions such as trauma, inflammation, and impairment of blood flow due to ACS. Following necrosis of myocardial tissue creatinine kinase (CK) is released. Skeletal muscle contains less than 3% CKMB, whereas the muscle of the heart contains up to 20% of CKMB, therefore CKMB has increased specificity for myocardial damage. Troponin I and T are commonly used as they show earlier elevated levels in the presence of myocardial injury (median 3.8 hours for troponin T versus 4.8 hours for CKMB[31,33]).

RISK ASSESSMENT DETERMINES TREATMENT IN CARDIAC HEALTH BREAKDOWN

In ACS, the level of risk determines the management strategy and level of intervention. Following are listed the characteristics of high, intermediate and low-risk factors[34]:

HIGH-RISK FEATURES
1. Prolonged (>10 min) ongoing chest pain/discomfort;
2. ST elevation or depression (>0.5 mm) or deep T wave inversion in three or more; leads;
3. Elevated serum markers of myocardial injury (especially cardiac troponin I or T);
4. Syncope;
5. Heart failure, mitral regurgitation or gallop rhythm; and
6. Haemodynamic instability.

INTERMEDIATE-RISK FEATURES
1. Prolonged but resolved chest pain/discomfort;
2. Nocturnal ischaemic symptoms;
3. New onset grade III or IV chest pain in the previous two weeks;
4. Age over 65 years;
5. History of myocardial infarction or revascularisation;
6. Electrocardiography (ECG) normal or pathologic Q waves; and
7. Non-significant (<0.5 mm) ST deviation, or minor T wave inversion in less than three leads.

LOW-RISK FEATURES
1. Increased frequency or severity of angina;
2. Angina provoked at a lower threshold;
3. New onset angina more than two weeks before presentation; and
4. Normal ECG and negative serum troponin.

It is a chilling fact that more than 50% of all heart attack deaths occur before the patient reaches hospital[6]. This underscores the importance of early symptom recognition and public access to automated defibrillators[5,35–37]. The great majority of AMI patients currently do not receive the benefit of thrombolytic and other treatments within the first hour of symptom onset[6,30]. Both acute mortality and subsequent prognosis are related to the extent to which the myocardium is damaged by the infarction. Strategies focusing on early reperfusion can prevent myocardial necrosis, and clinical trials with thrombolytic agents demonstrating a significant reduction in AMI mortality have dramatically improved outcomes for AMI patients. The case study below gives a scenario of a usual or common presentation and management of a patient with a diagnosis of ACS.

● Case study

Maggie Jordan, 67, has been experiencing increasing shortness of breath and generalised chest discomfort over the past six months. She has attributed her increased shortness of breath to getting older and recent weight gain. She has been taking an antacid for her chest discomfort, which wakes her up in the early hours of the morning with what she described as indigestion.

One morning, Maggie wakes at 3 am gasping for air. In addition to her shortness of breath, she feels nauseous and light-headed. This is the worst episode Maggie has had to date and she feels frightened. She calls her general practitioner's after-hours service, which orders an ambulance to go to her house immediately. The paramedics apply an ECG monitor, which demonstrates widespread ST segment changes, tachycardia (heart rate 120 beats per minute) and hypotension (systolic blood pressure 85 mmHg). On the basis of their clinical knowledge and protocols, they treat Maggie as a suspected case of ACS. They administer oxygen via mask, aspirin (orally), glyceryl trinitrate (sublingually) and morphine sulphate (intravenously). As they continue their assessment, they strongly suspect acute myocardial infarction. They know that if this is the case, Maggie will require urgent treatment so they alert the local emergency department and send her ECG via facsimile.

When Maggie reaches the emergency department, she is assessed by the emergency staff specialist and clinical nurse specialist, who confirm the suspicions of the paramedics. They alert the cardiology team who prepare to take her to the cardiac catheter laboratory for urgent revascularisation. Maggie subsequently has an angioplasty performed on the left anterior descending coronary artery. At angiogram, it is also noted that she has some impairment of ventricular function and blockages in other coronary arteries. Key management strategies are administration of anti-platelet agents (aspirin and clopidogrel) and anti-thrombin agents (heparin) to arrest thrombin formation. Other therapies include strategies to modulate the renin angiotensin system (ACE inhibitors), sympathetic nervous system (beta blockers) and lipid metabolism (statin therapy). While reading the discussion of ACS management that follows, keep Maggie's clinical scenario in mind to help place these key management strategies in a clinical context.

Initial actions for management of an ACS event[22] are as follows:

1. **Antiplatelet therapy:** Administration of aspirin for platelet aggregation inhibition should be given to all patients with no history of aspirin sensitivity. Those who cannot take aspirin may be given clopidogrel.
2. **Oxygen therapy:** Oxygen therapy should only be given to patients with documented hypoxaemia or respiratory dysfunction as there is no evidence of physiological benefit.
3. **Glyceryl trinitrate (GTN):** Through its peripheral and coronary artery dilating effects, GTN reduces preload and myocardial oxygen consumption. This potential benefit may, however, be offset in part by reflex heart rate increases unless a β-blocker is also prescribed. This medication can cause hypotension because of its vasoldilatory properties.

4. **Morphine:** This is recommended only for patients who fail to respond to oral/sublingual nitroglycerin. The anxiolytic and analgesic effects of morphine are useful, however clinicians need to be aware of the potential adverse effects of hypotension and/or respiratory depression.
5. **Intravenous access:** All patients with suspected ACS should have an intravenous (IV) cannula inserted as soon as practical.
6. **Anticoagulation therapy:** Antiplatelet therapy should be followed by anticoagulation therapy with *unfractionated IV heparin* or subcutaneous *low-molecular weight heparin*. *Platelet GP IIb/IIIa inhibitors* are then administered to patients with high-risk features or continuing ischaemia, and to patients awaiting invasive treatment such as angioplasty.
7. **Beta (β) blocker therapy:** β-blockers reduce myocardial oxygen consumption through their action on the sympathetic nervous system and negative chronotropic and negative inotropic effects. β-blocker therapy may reduce progression from ACS to MI by approximately 13%[7,13]. Angiotensin receptor blockers should also be prescribed to counteract the effects of the renin–angiotensin system on ventricular remodelling.

ONGOING MANAGEMENT OF ACS

Following risk stratification, patients with UAP/NSTEMI are generally managed according to one of two different strategies:

1. **Early conservative strategy:** Treatment with low-molecular weight heparin and GP IIb/IIIa inhibitors can help prevent adverse outcomes, and is preferred in low-risk patients. Only patients with recurrent ischaemia or a strongly positive stress test should undergo coronary angiography, as this invasive procedure is costly and confers potential risks such as bleeding and stroke.
2. **Early invasive strategy:** For patients without obvious clinical contraindications to coronary revascularisation, early angiography provides an invasive means of risk stratification. Ventricular function as assessed by echocardiography, co-morbidities, prior history and patient preferences are all considered in the decision to perform percutaneous coronary interventions (PCI). Coronary revascularisation can improve prognosis, relieve symptoms, prevent ischaemic complications, and improve function. The outcomes of PCI have been enhanced by stenting and adjunctive treatment with GP IIb/IIIa inhibitors[38]. Coronary artery bypass grafting (CABG) may be appropriate for high-risk patients with left ventricular systolic dysfunction, diabetes, or certain forms of two- or three-vessel disease[39].

LONG-TERM MANAGEMENT STRATEGIES

Management strategies for the long term include:

1. **Statin therapy:** This should be considered in all patients following unstable angina or non-ST elevation myocardial infarction. Aspirin and beta-blockers should be recommended for all patients with coronary artery disease unless contraindicated.
2. **Angiotensin converting enzyme (ACE) inhibitors:** These should be prescribed in the absence of significant contraindication such as renal failure.
3. **Prevention:** All patients with a diagnosis of unstable angina or myocardial infarction should be referred to, and encouraged to participate in secondary prevention programs, such as cardiac rehabilitation[40,41].

HEART FAILURE

Heart failure (HF), both acute and chronic, represents a complex constellation of pathophysiological processes resulting in a syndrome precipitated by inadequate cardiac output and abnormal neurohormonal activation[42]. The primary cause of HF is cardiac muscle dysfunction due to a range of aetiologies, the most common being ischaemic heart disease (manifested as ACS) and hypertension. Co-morbidities, both organic (e.g., renal dysfunction and sleep apnoea) and psychological (e.g., depression and cognitive dysfunction), often accompany HF, increasing the complexity of assessment and management. Clinical criteria for diagnosis of HF are given in Table 5.4[43] and the New York Heart Association Classification[44] commonly used to categorise severity and function limitation is shown in Table 5.5. Heart failure has significant physical and psychosocial impact upon the individual and their carers and is responsible for a significant burden to health care systems internationally. In Australia and New Zealand, along with other developed countries, heart failure is responsible for significant disease burden[15,45–47].

ACUTE HEART FAILURE

Acute heart failure is may be associated with cardiogenic shock resulting from acute myocardial infarction (AMI), myocarditis, acute valvular dysfunction or de-compensated

TABLE 5.4: FRAMINGHAM CRITERIA FOR THE DIAGNOSIS OF HEART FAILURE[43]
Diagnosis is made in the presence of *two major* or *one major and two minor* criteria (provided symptoms are not attributable to any other condition)

Major Criteria	Minor Criteria
Paroxysmal nocturnal dyspnoea	Ankle oedema
Neck vein distension	Night cough
Rales	Hepatomegaly
Cardiomegaly	Pleural effusion
Acute pulmonary oedema	Vital capacity ≤ one third of maximum
S3-gallop	Tachycardia ≥120 beats per minute
Increased venous pressure (>16 cm H_2O)	Major or minor
Circulation time ≥25 s	Weight loss >4.5 kg over 5 days of treatment
Hepatojugular reflex	

TABLE 5.5: NEW YORK HEART ASSOCIATION CLASSIFICATION OF HEART FAILURE[44]	
Class I	No limitation: ordinary physical exercise does not cause undue fatigue, dyspnoea or palpitations
Class II	Slight impairment of physical activity: comfortable at rest but ordinary activity results in fatigue, palpitations
Class III	Marked limitation of physical activity: comfortable at rest but less than ordinary activity results in symptoms.
Class IV	Unable to carry out any physical activity without discomfort: symptoms of CHF are present even at rest with increased discomfort with any physical activity.

chronic heart failure. Acute heart failure requires immediate treatment based upon relieving pulmonary congestion, reducing myocardial oxygen demand and augmenting blood flow. The goals of treatment of cardiogenic shock are to enhance cardiac output and reverse the shock syndrome. In many patients, the use of diuretics and vasodilators is insufficient to relieve symptoms and achieve a stable haemodynamic status. Inotropic support, mechanical ventilation and intra-aortic balloon pump strategies may be required[48]. Specific goals of treatment include maintaining oxygen saturation above 90%, mean arterial pressure above 60 mmHg, cardiac index greater than 2.2 L/min/m^2, urine output greater than 30 mL/h, and normal acid-base balance and body temperature[11].

CHRONIC HEART FAILURE

In countries such as Australia, New Zealand, the USA and the United Kingdom, the incidence and prevalence of chronic HF is increasing faster than any other cardiovascular disorder[49]. This is despite the decline in age-adjusted mortality from coronary disease in these countries. Chronic HF is estimated to affect 1% of the general population. This means that 3–5% of people over the age of 65 years, and 10% of those older than 75 years will have HF[50].

Chronic HF is caused by dysfunction of the ventricles of the heart. Impairment of function can be caused by conditions that

- Directly impair cardiac muscle function (e.g., myocardial infarction, or cardiomyopathies);
- Cause pressure overload (e.g., aortic stenosis, chronic hypertension, acute elevation of blood pressure); and
- Cause volume overload (e.g., mitral incompetence, or fluid overload), uncontrolled arrhythmias, either chronic or acute, and diseases involving the pericardium.

The National Heart Foundation of Australia and the Cardiac Society of Australia and New Zealand guidelines discriminate between HF of systolic and diastolic aetiologies. Systolic HF is the inability of the heart to pump properly, and is the most common form of HF. Ischaemic heart disease and hypertension are the most significant contributors to the development of *systolic heart failure*[34].

The term *diastolic heart failure* refers to the inability of heart to fill at normal filling pressures, despite normal ventricular contraction. Leading causes of impaired diastolic function are hypertension, coronary artery disease, diabetes, obesity, and aortic stenosis. Diastolic HF is more common in the elderly, where combined ischaemia, hypertrophy and age-related fibrosis may produce increased myocardial stiffness or delayed relaxation[51-53]. As discussed previously, the New York Heart Association Class is the most commonly used system for classifying the severity of HF and is detailed in Table 5.5.

The European Study Group of the European Society of Cardiology[54] proposes criteria for establishing the diagnosis of diastolic HF. Primarily, a diagnosis of diastolic heart failure is made upon the evidence of clinical HF with normal or near normal left ventricular systolic function.

Patients with advanced HF have a 12-month survival rate of 25–50%, and a 2-year survival rate of <10%[47]. Although the condition of some of these patients may respond to intervention, such as pharmacotherapy and revascularisation, many still have a poor long-term prognosis[50]. This underscores the importance of incorporation of a palliative approach to care.

The following factors have been attributed to the high hospitalisation rates for HF:

• Non-adherence with treatment regimens;
• Inadequate discharge planning and follow-up;
• Poor social support;
• Depression;
• Failure of patients and/or their carers to seek prompt attention when exacerbations of symptoms occur;
• Biochemical markers such as raised creatinine, anaemia, and low serum sodium and albumin;
• Presence of co-morbidities such as diabetes, dementia and sleep apnoea syndrome;
• Advanced age;
• Prolonged admission to hospital; and
• Physical inactivity and functional decline[46,55-59].

DIAGNOSTIC INVESTIGATIONS

The diagnosis of HF and the assessment of severity are based on

• Clinical signs, such as raised jugular venous pressure and peripheral oedema;
• Symptoms derived from the clinical history, in particular exercise tolerance or capacity to carry out activities of daily living[15];
• Specific diagnostic investigations, in particular echocardiography[60]. Types of echocardiographic investigations are listed in Table 5.6; and
• Response to specific treatment, such as diuretics[61].

TABLE 5.6: ECHOCARDIOGRAPHIC INVESTIGATIONS
Transthoracic two-dimensional/Doppler echocardiography
Transoesophageal echocardiography
Intra-operative echocardiography
Stress echocardiography
Contrast echocardiography
Intracardiac and intravascular ultrasound

Source: ACC/AHA Echocardiography Guidelines Accessed at http: www.aha.org

The purposes of diagnostic investigations are to confirm the clinical diagnosis, identify a cause or causes, precipitating factor(s), exacerbating factor(s), assess severity, guide therapy, and determine prognosis. Initial investigations include

- Electrocardiogram;
- Chest X-ray;
- Haematology – full blood count;
- Biochemistry – electrolytes and liver function tests; and
- Echocardiography.

The following investigations are often performed, based on the index of suspicion of aetiology and precipitation, after considering the risks and benefits for the individual:

- Serum B-type natriuretic peptide assays;
- Thyroid function tests and iron studies;
- Genetic testing and profiling in suspected inherited conditions;
- Viral studies in patients with suspected cardiomyopathy;
- Coronary angiography in suspected ischaemic syndromes;
- Haemodynamic measurements;
- Endomyocardial biopsy, to determine a cause for cardiomyopathy; and
- Gated radionuclide scans.

PHARMACOLOGICAL MANAGEMENT OF HEART FAILURE

Advances in pharmacological therapy have remarkably improved the management of HF. Key pharmacological strategies are outlined in the following sections.

ANGIOTENSION CONVERTING ENZYME (ACE) INHIBITORS

ACE inhibitors or angiotensin converting enzyme inhibitors reduce peripheral vascular resistance via inhibition of the angiotensin-converting enzyme. This action reduces the myocardial oxygen consumption, thereby improving cardiac output and subsequently minimising left ventricular and vascular hypertrophy. In large-scale clinical trials, ACE inhibitors have consistently shown beneficial effects on mortality, morbidity, and quality of life for people with systolic heart failure[62,63]. However, the beneficial effects of ACE inhibitors for diastolic heart failure have not yet been proven, and clinical trials are currently in progress.

ANGIOTENSIN II RECEPTOR ANTAGONISTS

These agents block the actions of angiotensin II at its type I receptor. Angiotensin II receptor antagonists, as their name suggests, block the binding of angiotensin II to the AT1 receptor. The CHARM trial evaluating candesartan, demonstrated a reduction in cardiovascular deaths and hospital admissions for heart failure regardless of ejection fraction[64]. There is no good evidence that hypotension and renal dysfunction are a less frequent problem with angiotensin II receptor antagonists than with ACE inhibitors[65-67].

LOOP AND THIAZIDE DIURETICS

Diuretics increase fluid loss through the kidneys by decreasing water reabsorption[68]. Despite the widespread use of loop and thiazide diuretics, there are no randomised controlled trials demonstrating their impact on improved survival of patients with HF. Clinical experience and small trials reveal that loop and thiazide diuretics improve the symptoms of heart failure (e.g., dyspnoea and oedema)[68]. This relief of congestive symptoms can improve exercise capacity. However, diuretics should never be prescribed as monotherapy in patients with chronic HF[58].

BETA-BLOCKERS

Left ventricular systolic dysfunction is associated with activation of a host of interconnected neurohormonal 'adaptive' mechanisms, most notably the sympathetic and renin-angiotensin-aldosterone systems. Chronic activation of these mechanisms exerts deleterious haemodynamic and direct cardiotoxic effects and contributes to the progressive deterioration of ventricular function. Attenuation of these mechanisms is associated with improvement in survival. Numerous randomised clinical trials have shown that when appropriately prescribed and initiated, long-term treatment with beta-blockers can lessen the symptoms of chronic HF, improve the clinical status of patients, enhance their sense of well-being, reduce admissions, and reduce mortality[58]. Beta-blockers are also known to have an additive effect with ACE inhibitors and are recommended best practice[57,61,69].

SPIRONOLACTONE

Spironolactone acts as an aldosterone inhibitor (prevents salt retention), and is used to treat advanced heart failure when symptoms persist after other drug therapies are maximised. In the RALES trial, the addition of low doses of spironolactone (an aldosterone antagonist) to an ACE inhibitor reduced the risk of death and hospitalisation in patients with NYHA class III or IV HF[70]. In the EPHESUS trial, a selective aldosterone blocker was found to be advantageous in patients with left ventricular dysfunction after myocardial infarction[71,72].

DIGITALIS

Digoxin is one of the cardiac (or digitalis) glycosides, a closely related group of drugs having in common specific effects on the myocardium. Clinical trial findings demonstrate that digoxin reduces the symptoms and signs of heart failure and improves exercise capacity when used alone or in combination with diuretics, but does not have any net effect on mortality. It appears that patients with more severe HF benefit most from digoxin added to other pharmacotherapy[69].

HYDRALAZINE AND ISOSORBIDE DINITRATE (H-ISDN)

These agents cause release of nitric oxide (NO). In the body NO signals smooth muscle to relax by activating guanylate cyclase, increasing cGMP, and decreasing calcium ion levels in the cell causing vasodilation. H-ISDN has been reported to increase exercise capacity and reduce mortality when added to diuretic and digoxin therapy However, trial evidence suggests that enalapril (an ACE inhibitor) is more effective than H-ISDN as adjunctive treatment to diuretics and digoxin, and is better tolerated[73,74].

NON-PHARMACOLOGICAL MANAGEMENT OF HEART FAILURE

Non-pharmacological management strategies include technological devices and behavioural strategies. Devices such as biventricular pacing and implantable defibrillators have improved outcomes for patients with HF[75–77]. However, these strategies are only available to the minority of patients with HF because of access and cost.

Behavioural strategies aimed at optimal physical functioning and self-management of risk factors include activity and exercise, dietary salt intake, weight management and smoking cessation[78]. Controlled trials have demonstrated that HF patients who increase their exercise tolerance have a better prognosis, in addition to having positive effects on physiological well being, severity of dyspnoea, peak capacity and quality of life[79–81]. Exercise also has positive effects on peripheral vasodilator responses[79]. Best practice guidelines recommend restricting dietary salt intake to limit dietary sodium to <2 g/day in order to minimise fluid retention[61]. The reduction in body weight and levels of obesity has been shown to lower blood pressure, reduce cardiac effort and improve patients' lipid profile. New evidence also suggests that obesity is an independent risk factor for heart failure[82]. Smoking cessation programs should be tailored to the individual and utilise nicotine replacement therapy where it is not contra-indicated in order to prevent vasoconstriction and maximise pulmonary function[83]. Research has demonstrated that immunisation against influenza may reduce admissions to hospital for chronic HF[84]. It is recommended best practice.

As discussed above self-monitoring and management is important in chronic disease and in particular HF. Thus interventions that increase patients' and/or their carers' confidence in their ability to manage their own disease and make appropriate decisions have been more successful at improving patient outcomes and reducing the use of health services than interventions that merely provide patients with information but do not alter patients' perceptions of their capacity to manage their disease[85–87]. People who develop chronic conditions such as HF often take some time to come to terms with their disease and adapt their behaviour and lifestyle to accommodate it[88,89]. There remains a need for greater integration of educational techniques from social and behavioural sciences[90], and for multi-disciplinary team efforts that recognise and accommodate differences in patients' cultural, environmental and social characteristics[15,91].

● Case study

Doris Williams, 87, lived alone in a first floor unit. She complained of being isolated with no nearby relatives and few friends. Following an admission with heart failure, a nurse coordinated heart failure outreach program and followed up on Doris' treatment. The history of deterioration in Doris' clinical condition was quickly addressed and a referral was made to a cardiologist who optimised her pharmacological therapy to include an ACE inhibitor, and beta-blocker in addition to her usual diuretic and digoxin regime. In collaboration with the cardiologist, a flexible diuretic regimen was implemented with the heart failure nurse specialist successfully titrating Doris's diuretic dose, according to her symptoms and body weight. Key strategies in the nursing care plan were: 1) the instigation of self-care principles that would help maintain her mobility and independence; and 2) implementation of a daily weight chart to monitor her volume status. As Doris was frail and at risk of falling, this task was shared by the general practitioner, heart failure nurse and family members on a common chart.

ATRIAL FIBRILLATION

Atrial fibrillation is the most common sustained cardiac rhythm disturbance. The prevalence of AF in the adult population is 0.5%, rising to 10% among people aged over 75 years and is associated with a five times increase in the incidence of stroke[92,93]. The cumulative incidence of stroke among patients 60 years or younger with lone AF is not significantly different from that in a control population matched for age and sex – a rate of 0.5% per year. In the elderly, however, risk is much higher, often exceeding 10% per year. Non-valvular atrial fibrillation (NVAF) is a significant predictor for both a higher incidence of stroke and increased mortality[94]. In patients who also have rheumatic mitral stenosis, the risk of stroke is 17 times higher[94,95].

On ECG, AF is characterised by the presence of rapid, irregular, fibrillatory waves that vary in size, shape, and timing. This set of findings is usually associated with an irregular ventricular response as illustrated in Figure 5.4. Key management strategies relate to chemical and/or electrical cardioversion to achieve rhythm and rate control. Common pharmacological agents for the management of atrial fibrillation are described in Table 5.7.

Transoesophageal echocardiography (TOE) is a useful strategy in stratifying the risk of embolic complications in atrial fibrillation. TOE is the most sensitive clinical tool available for detecting left atrial thrombus and spontaneous echo contrast. These factors occur as a consequence of reduced atrial flow velocities and left atrial contraction dysfunction caused by atrial fibrillation. Spontaneous echo contrast (SEC), is characterised by a swirling mass of fine echoes, also described as echo 'smoke' and indicates blood stasis and the thrombus and is a predictor for increased risk of thrombo-embolism[96]. This is illustrated in Figure 5.5. Spontaneous echo contrast is not easily imaged by transthoracic echocardiography because the surface echocardiogram has a limited view of the left atrial appendage where most atrial thrombi form in patients with atrial fibrillation. However, an absence of left atrial thrombus or spontaneous echo contrast does not necessarily infer a lower risk in patients with atrial fibrillation[96].

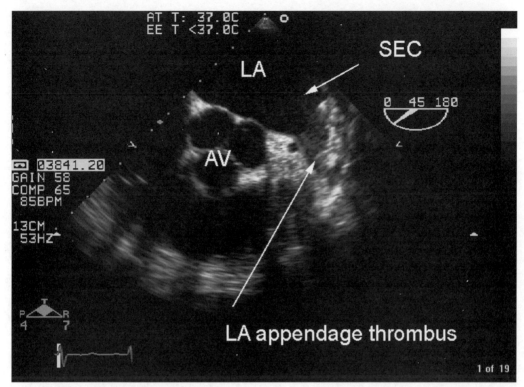

FIGURE 5.5 *Spontaneous echo contrast*
LA (left atrium); SEC (spontaneous echo contrast); and AV (atrioventricular)

TABLE 5.7: COMMON PHARMACOLOGICAL AGENTS FOR THE MANAGEMENT OF ATRIAL FIBRILLATION

Medication Vaughn Williams Classification	Action	Nursing Considerations
Type IA Procainamide Quinidine	1. Lengthens depolarisation 2. Decreases automaticity	• Monitor for atrioventricular block • Monitor electrolytes, particularly magnesium and potassium
Type IC Flecainide Propafenone	1. Slows conduction 2. Inhibits sodium channels	• May be proarryhthmic, particularly in patients with left ventricular dysfunction • Monitor renal function closely with flecanide
Type III Sotalol Dofetilide Ibultide Amiodarone	1. Increase action potential duration and refractory period 2. Sotalol and amiodarone have some beta blocking properties	• Care with sotalol in patients with reactive airways disease and left ventricular dysfunction; sotalol is more useful for rate control than cardioversion • Consider potential for torsade de pointe with ibultide • *Amiodarone*: monitor for hepatic, pulmonary and thyroid toxicity; inform patient regarding potential for photosensitivity

Source: Davidson PM, Rees DM, Brighton TA, Enis J, Cockburn J, McCrohon J, Elliott D, Paull G, Daly J. 2004; 'Non-Valvular Atrial Fibrillation and Stroke: Implications for Nursing Practice and Therapeutics', *Australian Critical Care*, 17 (2),65–73.

● **Case study**

Arthur Collins, 56, presents to his general practitioner (GP) complaining of palpitations in his chest. His GP notes that Arthur's pulse is irregular and he is hypertensive (190/90 mmHg). The GP performs an ECG that documents atrial fibrillation and refers Arthur to a cardiologist for further investigation and management, which may involve elective cardioversion. Atrial fibrillation occurs when the atria do not contract in a coordinated systematic way and is thought to occur because of increased atrial stretch and multiple re-entrant circuits in the atrial myocardium precipitating an irregular, variable pattern[72]. The GP explains to Arthur that he has a number of modifiable risk factors: obesity (body mass index 38), hypertension, smoking, and physical inactivity. Arthur is commenced on an ACE inhibitor for his hypertension and commenced on warfarin for thrombo-prophylaxis. Arthur and his GP negotiate a plan to address risk-factor management in order to prevent subsequent cardiovascular events.

LEARNING EXERCISES
1. List the factors that contribute to the development of atrial fibrillation. Explain the role of anti-thrombotic agents in the management of atrial fibrillation.
2. Review risk factors contributing to cardiac health breakdown.
3. Describe the role of electrical cardioversion in the management of atrial fibrillation.

LONG-TERM MANAGEMENT OF PATIENTS WITH CARDIAC BREAKDOWN

Promotion of self-management and risk-reduction strategies is important in the management of cardiac dysfunction. To address these issues, cardiac rehabilitation is often recommended. Different models of cardiac rehabilitation exist, from home-based to group classes. Evidence indicates that cardiac rehabilitation programs are effective in reducing cardiac risk and are safe for patients. The benefits of exercise include positive effects on haemodynamics, functional capacity, psychological and social well-being. Table 5.8 describes a summary of the Secondary Prevention Guidelines of the Heart Foundation of Australia and the Cardiac Society of Australia and New Zealand[40].

Education and information programs help patients and their families

- Recover and adjust from an acute event;
- Make lifestyle adjustments and promotion of treatment adherence;
- Alleviate anxiety and distress associated with their diagnosis; and
- Make informed decisions and increase their sense of control.

Psychological and social problems can have a significant adverse effect on recovery and adjustment for individuals and their families. In particular, social isolation and depression

TABLE 5.8: SUMMARY OF KEY RECOMMENDATIONS FROM THE REDUCING RISK IN HEART DISEASE GUIDELINES FOR THE PREVENTION OF CARDIOVASCULAR EVENTS IN THOSE WITH CORONARY HEART DISEASE (NHFA/CSANZ 2005)

LIFESTYLE / BEHAVIOURAL RISK FACTORS AND MANAGEMENT	
Smoking	*Goal:* Complete cessation and avoidance of passive smoking. • Refer to Quitline 131 848. • Consider pharmacotherapy for patients smoking > 10 cigarettes per day.
Nutrition	*Goal:* Establishment/maintenance of healthy eating patterns, with saturated & trans fatty acid intake ≤ 8% of total energy intake. • Refer to Heart Foundation 'Enjoy Healthy Eating' messages, Heartline 1300 36 27 87 or www.heartfoundation.com.au.
Alcohol	*Goal:* Low risk alcohol consumption in those who drink. • Advise those with hypertension to limit alcohol intake to no more than 2 standard drinks per day (men), 1 standard drink per day (women).
Physical activity	*Goal:* At least 30 minutes of moderate intensity physical activity on five or more days per week (150 mins per week minimum). • Begin at low intensity and gradually increase over several weeks, particularly in the post-acute event period.
Weight management	*Goal:* Waist measurement ≤ 94 cm (males) or ≤ 80 cm (females); BMI < 25 kg/m^{2*}. • Set intermediate achievable goals.
BIOMEDICAL RISK FACTORS AND MEDICAL MANAGEMENT	
Lipids	*Goal:* TC < 4.0 mmol/l; LDL-C < 2.5 mmol/L; HDL-C > 1.0 mmol/L; Triglycerides < 2.0 mmol/L. • All patients should receive healthy eating advice. • Statin therapy is recommended for patients with coronary heart disease unless contraindicated, and in hospitalised patients, should be initiated during that admission.

Blood pressure (BP)	*Goal:* Dependent on age and presence of diabetes; proteinuria; renal insufficiency:
	  Adults ≥ 65 (unless there is diabetes and/or renal insufficiency and/or proteinuria ≥ 0.25 g/day), BP < 140/90 mm Hg;
	  Adults < 65; and all adults with diabetes and/or renal insufficiency and or proteinuria 0.25–1 g/day, BP < 130/85 mm Hg; and
	  Adults with proteinuria > 1 g/day (with or without diabetes), BP < 125/75 mm Hg.
	• Generally ACEI are recommended as first line antihypertensives in patients with CVD.

TABLE 5.8 (cont'd)	
Diabetes	*Goal:* Identify undiagnosed type 2 diabetes; maintain optimal blood glucose levels in those with diabetes (HbA1c ≤ 7%). • Screen all patients with CHD for diabetes. • Manage hyperglycaemia with lifestyle interventions and pharmacotherapy if indicated.
PHARMACOLOGICAL MANAGEMENT	
Antiplatelet agents	• Use aspirin 70–150 mg/day for all unless contraindicated. • Additional role for clopidogrel in patients with recurrent cardiac ischaemic events; stent implantation.
ACE inhibitors (ACEI)	• Consider in all patients, especially those at high risk, unless contraindicated. Start early post-myocardial infarction. • Use angiotension II receptor antagonists for patients who develop unacceptable side effects on ACEIs.
Beta-blockers	• For most patients post acute coronary syndrome, unless contraindicated, and continue indefinitely especially in high-risk patients.
Statins	• For all patients with CHD unless contraindicated. • In hospitalised patients, therapy should be initiated during that admission.
Anticoagulants	• Use warfarin in patients at high risk of thromboembolism post-myocardial infarction. • Warfarin may sometimes by combined with aspirin – monitor closely for signs of bleeding.
NON-PHARMACOLOGICAL MANAGEMENT	
Secondary prevention/cardiac rehabilitation programs	• All patients to have access to and be actively referred to a comprehensive secondary prevention/cardiac rehabilitation service.
Chest pain action plan	• All patients to have written action plan to follow in event of chest pain, including advice on use of antianginal medication and emergency action (dial 000 for ambulance) if chest pain/discomfort is not completely relieved in 10–15 minutes.
PSYCHOLOGICAL FACTORS AND ASSESSMENT	
Psychological management	• Assess all patients for co-morbid depression and, if present, initiate appropriate psychological and medical management. • SSRIs are safe and efficacious for management of depression in patients with CHD (note potential interaction with warfarin). • Avoid use of tricyclic antidepressants in patients with CHD due to class III antiarrhythmic effect. • Cognitive-behavioural therapy (alone or in combination with medication) is also efficacious in depression management.

TABLE 5.8 (cont'd)	
Social management	• Assess all patients for level of social support and provide follow-up for those considered at risk through referral to cardiac rehabilitation services and/or to social worker or psychologist. Consider role of patient support groups.

Key points:

- The guidelines were developed using a consensus approach which involved an independent assessment of key Australian and international evidence-based clinical guidelines, scientific articles and trial data[1], which are incomplete in some areas.

- Recommendations are not necessarily congruent with current PBS criteria for eligibility for subsidy in all areas.

- The guidelines provide a general framework for appropriate practice, to be followed subject to the practitioner's judgement in each individual case. All treatments should be individualised according to the patient's comorbidities, drug tolerance, lifestyle/living circumstances and wishes.

- For all medications observe usual contraindications, be mindful of the potential for significant and possibly adverse drug interactions and allergies, and carefully monitor and review patients regularly.

- Where drug therapy is recommended for indefinite use, these recommendations have been based on the extrapolated findings of clinical trials which are by their nature of limited duration.

- Patients are often discharged from hospital after an acute coronary event on low doses of medications such as beta-blockers, ACE inhibitors and statins. In the majority of cases, it is recommended that the dose of each individual medication be increased to the recommended maximum target dose as required and tolerated.

- Any improvement in risk factors and movement towards the ideal risk factor 'goals' and 'targets' will be beneficial. Risk-factor modification should be considered as a total package so that, for example, attention is not diverted from addressing smoking cessation while treating dyslipidaemia, hypertension and diabetes.

- Diabetes, renal impairment, and non-coronary heart disease manifestations of atherosclerosis such as cerebrovascular disease or peripheral vascular disease indicate higher risk for coronary events. Patients with coronary heart disease should be screened for these conditions and managed appropriately.

- It is important to monitor and support patients' adherence to lifestyle advice and medications on an ongoing basis – where appropriate consider using ancillary measures (e.g. special clinics, telephone support, 'coaching').

Note: This guide can also be used for those with other manifestations of atherosclerosis (e.g., aortic, carotid and peripheral vascular disease).
* Weight management goals based on studies of European populations. These may not be appropriate for all ages and ethnic groups.
Source: National Heart Foundation of Australia.

can have a negative impact upon recovery of functional capacity and adherence to medications, lifestyle changes and exercise regimens. Patients with anxiety and/or depression can benefit from professional counselling and/or group therapy.

PALLIATIVE CARE

The chronic nature of cardiac disease means that patients die as part of their disease trajectory, and, therefore, palliative care principles should be incorporated in care plans where the prognosis is poor (e.g., end-stage HF). Effective communication with the patient and the patient's family and carers about the expected course of the illness and final treatment options is strongly emphasised. Discussions regarding treatment preferences should cover responses to a potentially reversible exacerbation of CHF, a cardiac arrest, a sudden catastrophic event, such as a severe cerebrovascular accident, and worsening of major non-cardiac co-morbidities. It is important to have these discussions with patients during periods of stability and not leaving these to episodes of crisis[97–100].

CONCLUSION

This chapter has provided an overview of some common presentations of cardiac health breakdown. Nurses play an important role in the care of patients with actual and potential cardiac breakdown. These roles range from the primary prevention setting to tertiary care in clinical, policy and research settings. Nurses have traditionally been at the forefront of holistic cardiovascular health care and have pioneered many cardiac rehabilitation and other secondary prevention programs[59, 101–103]. There is now increasing evidence to support the importance of non-pharmacological strategies and nursing models of care in preventing and treating cardiac health breakdown. These strategies underscore the important role of nurses in both the independent and dependent spheres of practice.

USEFUL WEB SITES

The web sites listed below are those of prominent professional bodies that collectively, through their members, develop guidelines and recommendations in response to changes in treatment, procedures and pharmacological agents. As medical and nursing knowledge is a dynamic and evolving process, readers of this article are strongly encouraged to access these frequently for the most up-to-date knowledge:

- Heart Foundation of Australia: http://www.heartfoundation.com.au
- National Heart Foundation of New Zealand: http://www.nhf.org.nz/
- Cardiac Society of Australia and New Zealand: http://www.csanz.edu.au
- American College of Cardiology: http://www.acc.org
- American Heart Association: http://www.aha.org
- Heart Failure Society of America: http://www.hfsa.org
- European Society of Cardiology: http://www.escardio.org
- Australian College of Critical Care Nurses: http://www.acccn.com.au
- American Association of Critical Care Nurses: http://www.aacn.org

Recommended Readings

Bunker, SJ, *et al.* 2003; 'Stress and Coronary Heart Disease: Psychosocial Risk Factors', *Medical Journal of Australia*, 178 (6), 272–276.

Thompson, PL. 1997; *Coronary Care Manual*, Churchill Livingstone, New York.

Goldston, K & Davidson, PM. 2003; 'Clinical Update – Guidelines for Reducing Risk in Heart Disease: Implications for Nursing Practice and Research', *Australian Nursing Journal*, 11.

Davidson, P, Macdonald, P, Paull, G, Rees, D, Howes, L, Cockburn, J & Brown, M. 2003; 'Diuretic Therapy in Chronic Heart Failure: Implications for Heart Failure Nurse Specialists', *Australian Critical Care*, 16, 59–69.

Grady, KL, Dracup, K, Kennedy, G, Moser, DK, Piano, M, Stevenson, LW & Young, JB. 2000; AHA scientific statement. 'Team Management of Patients with Heart Failure: A Statement for Healthcare Professionals from the Cardiovascular Nursing Council of the American Heart Association', *Circulation*, 102, 2443–56.

References

1. National Heart Foundation of New Zealand. 2004; 'Mortality Facts'. http://www.nhf.org.nz. Accessed 16 August 2004.

2. Yusuf, S, Reddy, S, Ounpuu, S & Anand, S. 2001; 'Global Burden of Cardiovascular Diseases, Part II: Variations in Cardiovascular Disease by Specific Ethnic Groups and Geographic Regions and Prevention Strategies', *Circulation*, December 4, 104 (23), 2855–2864.

3. Kelly, D. 1997; 'Our Future Society: A Global Challenge', *Circulation*, 95.

4. Australian Institute of Health and Welfare (AIHW). 2004; 'Heart Stroke and Vascular Diseases: Australian Facts', AIHW, Canberra.

5. Dracup, K, McKinley, S & Moser, D. 1997; 'Australian Patients Delay in Response to Heart Attack Symptoms', *Medical Journal of Australia*, 166, 237–247.

6. Dracup, K, Moser, DK, McKinley, S, Ball, C, Yamasaki, K, Kim, C, *et al.* 2003; 'Clinical Scholarship: An International Perspective on the Time to Treatment for Acute Myocardial Infarction', *Journal of Nursing Scholarship*, 35, 317–323.

7. Bett, N, Aroney, G & Thompson, P. 1993; 'Delays Preceding Admission to Hospital and Treatment with Thrombolytic Agents of Patients with Possible Heart Attack', *Australian & New Zealand Journal of Medicine*, 23 (3), 312–313.

8. Veitch, J, Salmon, J, Clavisi, O & Owen, N. 1999; 'Physical Inactivity and Other Health Risks Among Australian Males in Less-skilled Occupations', *Journal of Occupational & Environmental Medicine*, 41 (9), 794–798.

9. Hoy, WE, Wang, Z, Baker, PR & Kelly, AM. 2003; 'Secondary Prevention of Renal and Cardiovascular Disease: Results of a Renal and Cardiovascular Treatment Program in an Australian Aboriginal Community', *Journal of the American Society of Nephrology*, 14 (7, supplement 2) S178–S185.

10. Dalton, M, Cameron, AJ, Zimmet, PZ, Shaw, JE, Jolley, D, Dunstan, DW, Welborn TA & AusDiab Steering Committee. 2003; 'Waist Circumference, Waist-Hip Ratio and Body Mass Index and Their Correlation with Cardiovascular Disease Risk Factors in Australian Adults', *Journal of Internal Medicine*, 254 (6), 555–563.

11. Holcomb, SS. 2002; 'Cardiogenic Shock: A Success Story', *DCCN – Dimensions of Critical Care Nursing*, 21, 232–235.

12. Jaarsma, T, Halfens, R, Huijer Abu-Saad, H, Dracup, K, Gorgels, T, van Ree, J, *et al.* 1999; 'Effects of Education and Support on Self-Care and Resource Utilization in Patients with Heart Failure', *European Heart Journal*, 20, 673–682.

13. Rockwell, J & Riegel, B. 2001; 'Predictors of Self-Care in Persons with Heart Failure', *Heart & Lung: Journal of Acute & Critical Care*, 30, 18–25.

14. Daly, J, Davidson, P, Chang, E, Hancock, K, Rees, D & Thompson, DR. 2002; 'Cultural Aspects of Adjustment to Coronary Heart Disease in Chinese-Australians: A Review of the Literature', *Journal of Advanced Nursing*, 39, 391–399.

15. Davidson, P, Stewart, S, Elliott, D, Daly, J, Sindone, A & Cockburn, J. 2001; 'Addressing the Burden of Heart Failure in Australia: The Scope for Home-based Interventions', *Journal of Cardiovascular Nursing*, 16, 56–68.

16. Braunwald, E, Fauci, A, Isselbacher, K, Kasper, D, Hauser, S, Longo, D & Jameson, L. 2003; 'Disorders of the Cardiovascular System (Part 8)', Harrisons Online. Accessed 20 January 2004.

17. Thompson, P. 1997; 'Patient History', *Coronary Care Manual* (P. Thompson, ed.). Churchill Livingstone, New York, 97–103.

18. Zickler, P. 2003; 'Cocaine's Effect on Blood Components May Be Linked to Heart Attack and Stroke', *NIDA Notes*, 17, 5.

19. Davidson, PM, Daly, J, Hancock, K, Moser, D, Chang, E & Cockburn, J. 2003; 'Perceptions and Experiences of Heart Disease: A Literature Review and Identification of a Research Agenda in Older Women', *European Journal of Cardiovascular Nursing*, 2, 255–264.

20. Bunker, S, *et al.* 2003; 'Stress and Coronary Heart Disease: Psychosocial Risk Factors', *Medical Journal of Australia*, 178, 272–276.

21. Braunwald, E, Antman, E, Beasley, J, *et al.* 2000; 'ACC/AHA Guidelines for the Management of Patients with Unstable Angina and Non-ST-Segment Elevation Myocardial Infarction: A Report of the American College of Cardiology/American Heart Association Task Force on Practice Guidelines (Committee on the Management of Patients With Unstable Angina)', *Journal of American College of Cardiology*, 36, 970–1062.

22. Braunwald, E, Antman, E, Beasley, J, *et al.* 2002; 'ACC/AHA 2002 Guideline Update for the Management of Patients with Unstable Angina and Non-ST-Segment Elevation Myocardial Infarction: A Report of the American College of Cardiology/American Heart Association Task Force on Practice Guidelines'.

23. Braunwald, E. 2003; 'Application of Current Guidelines to the Management of Unstable Angina and Non-ST-Elevation Myocardial Infarction', *Circulation*, 108 (supplement III), 28–37.

24. Williams, M. 2003; 'Risk Assessment and Management of Cardiovascular Disease in New Zealand', *New Zealand Medical Journal*, 116 (1185), U661.

25. Milne, R, Gamble, G, Whitlock, G & Jackson, R. 2003; 'Framingham Heart Study Risk Equation Predicts First Cardiovascular Event Rates in New Zealanders at the Population', *New Zealand Medical Journal*, 116 (1185), U662.

26. Sharpe, N & Doughty, R. 1998; 'Epidemiology of Heart Failure and Ventricular Dysfunction', *Lancet*, 352 (supplement 1), SI3–S17.

27. Gibler, WB, Armstrong, PW, Ohman, EM, Weaver, WD, Stebbins, AL, Gore, JM, *et al.* 2002; 'Persistence of Delays in Presentation and Treatment for Patients with Acute Myocardial Infarction: The GUSTO-I and GUSTO-III Experience', *Annals of Emergency Medicine*, 39, 123–130.

28. Yeghiazarians, Y, Braunstein, JB, Askari, A & Stone, PH. 2000; 'Medical Progress: Unstable Angina Pectoris', *New England Journal of Medicine*, 342, 101–114.

29. Davidson, PM, Daly, J, Hancock, K & Jackson, D. 2003; 'Australian Women and Heart Disease: Trends, Epidemiological Perspectives and the Need for a Culturally Competent Research Agenda', *Contemporary Nurse*, 16, 62–73.

30. Dracup, K, Alonzo, AA, Atkins, JM, Bennett, NM, Braslow, A, Clark, LT, *et al.* 1997; 'The Physician's Role in Minimizing Prehospital Delay in Patients at High-risk for Acute Myocardial Infarction: Recommendations from the National Heart Attack Alert Program', *Annals of Internal Medicine*,

126, 645–51.31; and Antman, EM. 2002; 'Decision Making with Cardiac Troponin Tests', *New England Journal of Medicine*, 346, 2079–2082.

31. Casey, PE. 2004; 'Markers of Myocardial Injury and Dysfunction', *AACN Clinical Issues*, 15 (4), 547–557.

32. Thompson, P. 1997; 'Biochemical Markers of Myocardial Necrosis', in *Coronary Care Manual* (P. Thompson, ed.), Churchill Livingstone, New York, 129–136.

33. Aviles, RJ, Askari, AT, Lindahl, B, Wallentin, L, Jia, G, Ohman, EM, *et al.* 2002; 'Troponin T Levels in Patients with Acute Coronary Syndromes, with or without Renal Dysfunction', *New England Journal of Medicine*, 346, 2047–2052.

34. National Heart Foundation of Australia (NHF) and Cardiac Society of Australia and New Zealand (CSANZ). 2002; *Heart Failure Guidelines*.

35. Groeneveld, PW, Kwong, JL, Liu, Y, Rodriguez, AJ, Jones, MP, Sanders, GD & Garber, AM. 2001; 'Cost-Effectiveness of Automated External Defibrillators on Airlines', *Journal of the American Medical Association*, 286, 1482–1489.

36. Balady, GJ, Chaitman, B, Foster, C, Froelicher, E, Gordon, N, Van Camp, S, American Heart Association & American College of Sports Medicine. 2002; 'Automated External Defibrillators in Health/Fitness Facilities: Supplement to the AHA/ACSM Recommendations for Cardiovascular Screening, Staffing, and Emergency Policies at Health/Fitness Facilities', *Circulation*, (5 March), 105 (9), 1147–1150.

37. Takata, TS, Page, RL & Joglar, JA. 2001; 'Automated External Defibrillators: Technical Considerations and Clinical Promise', *Annals of Internal Medicine*, 135 (11), 990–998.

38. Topol, EJ. 2003; 'A Guide to Therapeutic Decision-making in Patients with Non-ST-Segment Elevation Acute Coronary Syndromes', *Journal of the American College of Cardiology*, 41 (supplement S), 123S–129S.

39. Topol, EJ. 2003; 'Current Status and Future Prospects for Acute Myocardial Infarction Therapy', *Circulation*, 108 (supplement III) 6–13.

40. National Heart Foundation of Australia & Cardiac Society of Australia and New Zealand. 2005; *Reducing Risk in Heart Disease 2004. Guidelines for Preventing Cardiovascular Events in People with Coronary Heart Disease*. National Heart Foundation of Australia.

41. Parks, D, Allison, M, Doughty, R, Cunningham, L & Ellis, CJ. 2000; 'An Audit of Phase II Cardiac Rehabilitation at Auckland Hospital', *New Zealand Medical Journal*, 113 (1109), 158–161.

42. Macdonald, P. 1997; Pathophysiology of Cardiac Failure', in *Coronary Care Manual* (P. Thompson,

ed.), Churchill Livingstone, New York, 87–93.

43. McKee, P, Castelli, W, PMM & Kannel, W. 1971; 'The Natural History of Congestive Heart Failure: The Framingham Study', *New England Journal of Medicine*, 285, 1441–1446.

44. Kossman, C. 1964; *Diseases of the Heart and Blood Vessels: Nomenclature and Criteria for Diagnosis* (6th ed.), Little Brown, Boston.

45. Doughty, R, Yee, T, Sharpe, N & MacMahon, S. 1995; 'Hospital Admissions and Deaths Due to Congestive Heart Failure in New Zealand, 1988–91', *New Zealand Medical Journal*, 108 (1012), 473–475.

46. Doughty, R, Andersen, V & Sharpe, N. 1997; 'Optimal Treatment of Heart Failure in the Elderly', *Drugs & Aging*, 10 (6), 435–443.

47. Stewart, S, MacIntyre, K, Hole, D, Capewell, S & McMurray, J. 2001; 'More "Malignant" than Cancer? Five-Year Survival Following a First Admission for Heart Failure', *European Journal of Heart Failure*, 3, 315–322.

48. Frazier, OH & Delgado, RM. 2003; 'Mechanical Circulatory Support for Advanced Heart Failure: Where Does It Stand in 2003?' *Circulation*, 108 (25), 3064–3068.

49. McMurray, J & Stewart, S. 2000; 'Epidemiology, Aetiology, and Prognosis of Heart Failure', *Heart*, 83, 596–602.

50. Zannad, F, Briancon, S, Juilliere, Y, Mertes, PM, Villemot, JP, Alla, F & Virion, JM. 1999; 'Incidence, Clinical and Etiologic Features, and Outcomes of Advanced Chronic Heart Failure: The EPICAL Study – Epidemiologie de l'Insuffisance Cardiaque Avancee en Lorraine', *Journal of the American College of Cardiology*, (March), 33 (3), 734–742.

51. Andrew, P. 2003; 'Diastolic Heart Failure Demystified', *Chest*, 124, 744–753.

52. Bollinger, K & Sadar, AM. 2003; 'Care and Management of the Patient with Right Heart Failure Secondary to Diastolic Dysfunction: An Advanced Practice Perspective and Case Review', *Critical Care Nursing Quarterly*, 26, 22–27.

53. Paul, S. 2003; 'Diastolic Dysfunction', *Critical Care Nursing Clinics of North America*, 15, 495–500.

54. European Study Group on Diastolic Heart Failure. 1998; 'How to Diagnose Diastolic Heart Failure', *European Journal of Heart Failure*, 1 (19), 990–1003.

55. Wolk, R, Kara, T & Somers, VK. 2003; 'Sleep-Disordered Breathing and Cardiovascular Disease', *Circulation*, 108, 9–12.

56. Welsh, JD, Heiser, RM, Schooler, MP, Brockopp, DY, Parshall, MB, Cassidy, KB & Saleh, U. 2002; 'Characteristics and Treatment of Patients with Heart Failure in the Emergency Department', *Journal of Emergency Nursing*, 28, 126–131.

57. Packer, M, Coats, AJS, Fowler, MB, Katus, HA, Krum, H, Mohacsi, P, et al. 2001; 'Effect of Carvedilol on Survival in Severe Chronic Heart Failure', *New England Journal of Medicine*, 344, 1651–1658.

58. Gibbs, CR, Davies, MK & Lip, GYH. 2000; 'ABC of Heart Failure: Management: Digoxin and other Inotropes, Beta Blockers, and Antiarrhythmic and Antithrombotic Treatment', *British Medical Journal*, 320, 495–498.

59. Stewart, S, Marley, J & Horowitz, J. 1999; 'Effects of a Multidisciplinary, Home-based Intervention on Unplanned Readmissions and Survival Among Patients with Chronic Congestive Heart Failure: A Randomised Controlled Study', *Lancet*, 354.

60. Vitarelli, A, Tiukinhoy, S, Di Luzio, S, Zampino, M & Gheorghiade, M. 2003; 'The Role of Echocardiography in the Diagnosis and Management of Heart Failure', *Heart Failure Reviews*, 8, 181–189.

61. Krum, H, et al, Cardiac Society of Australia & New Zealand Chronic Heart Failure Clinical Practice Guidelines Writing Panel 2001; 'Guidelines for Management of Patients with Chronic Heart Failure in Australia', *Medical Journal of Australia*, 174, 459–466.

62. Latini, R, Maggioni, AP, Flather, M, Sleight, P & Tognoni, G. 1995; 'ACE Inhibitor Use in Patients with Myocardial Infarction: Summary of Evidence from Clinical Trials', *Circulation*, 92 (10), 3132–3137.

63. Yusuf, S. 1999; 'Randomised Controlled Trials in Cardiovascular Medicine: Past Achievements, Future Challenges', *British Medical Journal*, 319 (7209), 564–568.

64. Mielniczuk, L & Stevenson, LW. 2005; 'Angiotensin-converting Enzyme Inhibitors and Angiotensin II Type I Receptor Blockers in the Management of Congestive Heart Failure Patients: What We Have Learned from Recent Clinical Trials?' *Current Opinion in Cardiology*, 20 (4), 250–255.

65. Borghi, C & Ambrosioni, E. 1998; 'Evidence-based Medicine and ACE Inhibition', *Journal of Cardiovascular Pharmacology*, 32 (supplement 2), S24–S35.

66. Baruch, L, Anand, I, Cohen, IS, Ziesche, S, Judd, D & Cohn, JN. 1999; 'Augmented Short- and Long-Term Hemodynamic and Hormonal Effects of an Angiotensin Receptor Blocker Added to Angiotensin Converting Enzyme Inhibitor Therapy in Patients with Heart Failure: Vasodilator Heart Failure Trial (V-HeFT) Study Group', *Circulation*, 25, 99 (20), 2658–2664.

67. Moser, DK & Biddle, MJ. 2003; 'Angiotensin-Converting Enzyme Inhibitors and Angiotensin II Receptor Blockers: What We Know and Current Controversies', *Critical Care Nursing Clinics of North America*, 15, 423–437.

68. Davidson, P, Macdonald, P, Paull, G, Rees, D, Howes, L, Cockburn, J & Brown, M. 2003; 'Diuretic Therapy in Chronic Heart Failure: Implications for Heart Failure Nurse Specialists', *Australian Critical Care*, 16, 59–69.

69. Krum, H & Liew, D. 2003; 'Clinical Practice: Therapeutic Review: Recent Advances in the Management of Chronic Heart Failure', *Australian Family Physician*, 32, 39–43.70.

70. Pitt, B, Zannad, F, Remme, W, *et al.* 1999; 'The Effect of Spironolactone on Morbidity and Mortality in Patients with Severe Heart Failure', *New England Journal of Medicine*, 34, 709–717.

71. Pitt, B, Remme, W, Zannad, F, *et al.* 2003; 'Eplernone, a Selective Aldosterone Blocker in Patients with Left Ventricular Dysfunction after Myocardial Infarction', *New England Journal of Medicine*, 348, 1309–1321.

72. Coats, AJ. 2001; 'Exciting New Drugs on the Horizon: Eplerenone, a Selective Aldosterone Receptor Antagonist (SARA)', *International Journal of Cardiology*, (August), 80 (1), 1–4.

73. McKelvie, RS, Benedict, CR & Yusuf, S. 1999; 'Evidence based Cardiology: Prevention of Congestive Heart Failure and Management of Asymptomatic Left Ventricular Dysfunction', *British Medical Journal*, 318 (7195), 1400–1402.

74. Carson, P, Johnson, G, Fletcher, R & Cohn, J. 1996; 'Mild Systolic Dysfunction in Heart Failure (Left Ventricular Ejection Fraction >35%): Baseline Characteristics, Prognosis and Response to Therapy in the Vasodilator in Heart Failure Trials (V-HeFT)', *Journal of the American College of Cardiology*, 27 (3), 642–649.

75. Abraham, WT & Hayes, DL. 2003; 'Cardiac Resynchronization Therapy for Heart Failure', *Circulation*, 108 (21), 2596–2603.

76. Kerwin, WF & Paz, O. 2003; 'Cardiac Resynchronization Therapy: Overcoming Ventricular Dyssynchrony in Dilated Heart Failure', *Cardiology in Review*, 211 (4), 221–239.

77. Wilkoff, BL, Cook, JR, Epstein, AE, Greene, HL, Hallstrom, AP, Hsia, H, *et al.* 2002; 'Dual-Chamber Pacing or Ventricular Backup Pacing in Patients with an Implantable Defibrillator: The Dual Chamber and VVI Implantable Defibrillator (DAVID) Trial', *Journal of the American Medical Association*, 288 (24), 3115–3123.

78. Grady, KL, Dracup, K, Kennedy, G, Moser, DK, Piano, M, Stevenson, LW & Young, JB. 2000; 'AHA Scientific Statement – Team Management of Patients with Heart Failure: A Statement for Healthcare Professionals from the Cardiovascular Nursing Council of the American Heart Association', *Circulation*, 102, 2443–2456.

79. Brubaker, P. 1997; Exercise Intolerance in Congestive Heart Failure: A Lesson in Exercise Physiology', *Journal of Cardiopulmonary Rehabilitation*, 17, 217–221.

80. Brubaker, PH, Marburger, CT, Morgan, TM, Fray, B & Kitzman, DW. 2003; 'Exercise Responses of Elderly Patients with Diastolic versus Systolic Heart Failure', *Medicine & Science in Sports & Exercise*, (September), 35 (9), 1477–1485.

81. Sindone, A, Sammel, NL, Keech, A & Macdonald, P. 1998; 'Exercise Training Improves Symptoms, Exercise Capacity and Neurohumoral Abnormalities in Moderate to Severe Heart Failure', (Abstract), *Journal of American College of Cardiology*, 32, 509.

82. Kenchaiah, S, Evans, JC, Levy, D, Wilson, PWF, Benjamin, EJ, Larson, MG, *et al.* 2002; 'Obesity and the Risk of Heart Failure', *New England Journal of Medicine*, 347, 305–313.

83. Jay, SJ, Critchley, J & Capewell, S. 2003; 'Passive Smoke Exposure and Risk of Death from Coronary Heart Disease; and Mortality Risk Reduction Associated with Smoking Cessation in Patients with Coronary Heart Disease: A Systematic Review.' *Journal of the American Medical Association*, 290, 86–97; 290, 1708–1709.

84. Ayanian, J, Weissman, J, Chasan-Taber, S & Epstein, A. 1999; 'Quality of Care by Race and Gender for Congestive Heart Failure and Pneumonia', *Medical Care*, 37, 1260–1269.

85. Carlson, B, Riegel, B & Moser, DK. 2001; 'Self-Care Abilities of Patients with Heart Failure', *Heart & Lung: Journal of Acute & Critical Care*, 30, 351–359.

86. Lorig, K. 2002; 'Partnerships Between Expert Patients and Physicians', *Lancet (North American Edition)*, 359, 814–815.87; Lorig, K, Holman, H, Sobel, D, Laurent, D, Gonzalez, V & Minor, M. 2000; *Living a Healthy Life with Chronic Conditions: Self-Management of Heart Disease, Arthritis, Diabetes, Asthma, Bronchitis, Emphysema & Others*, Bull Publishing Company, Boulder, Co., 2.

87. Hamner, JB. 2005; 'State of the Science: Posthospitalization Nursing Interventions in Congestive Heart Failure', *Advances in Nursing Science*, 28 (2), 175–190.

88. Stull, DE, Starling, R, Haas, G & Young, JB. 1999; 'Becoming a Patient with Heart Failure', *Heart & Lung: Journal of Acute & Critical Care*, 28, 284–292.

89. Stull, DE, Clough, LA & Van Dussen, D. 2001; 'Self-Report Quality of Life as a Predictor of

Hospitalization for Patients with LV Dysfunction: A Life Course Approach', *Research in Nursing & Health*, 24, 460–469.

90. Moser, DK. 2002; 'Psychosocial Factors and their Association with Clinical Outcomes in Patients with Heart Failure: Why Clinicians Do Not Seem to Care', *European Journal of Cardiovascular Nursing*, 1, 183–188.

91. Moser, DK. 2001; 'Heart Failure Management: Optimal Health Care Delivery Programs', *Annual Review of Nursing Research*, 126.

92. Hankey, G. 2001; 'Non-Valvular Atrial Fibrillation and Stroke Prevention', *Medical Journal of Australia*, 174, 234–238.

93. Kannel, W, Abbott, R, Savage, D, *et al.* 1983; Coronary Heart Disease and Atrial Fibrillation: The Framingham Study', *American Heart Journal*, 106, 389–396.94

94. Fuster, V, Reiden, L, Asinger, R, *et al.* 2001; 'ACC/AHA/ESC Guidelines for the Management of Patients with Atrial Fibrillation', *Journal of American College of Cardiology*, 38, 1266ii–1266lx.

95. Davidson, P, Rees, D, Brighton, T, Enis, J, Cockburn, J, McCrohon, J, *et al.* 2004; 'Non-Valvular Atrial Fibrillation and Stroke: Implications for Nursing Practice and Therapeutics', *Australian Critical Care*, 17 (2), 65–73.

96. Leung, DY, Davidson, PM, Cranney, GB & Walsh, WF. 1997; 'Thromboembolic Risks of Left Atrial Thrombus Detected by Transesophageal Echocardiogram', *American Journal of Cardiology*, 79, 626–629.

97. Davidson, PM, Introna, K, Cockburn, J, Daly, J, Dunford, M, Paull, G & Dracup, K. 2002; 'Synergising Acute Care and Palliative Care to Optimise Nursing Care in End-Stage Cardiorespiratory Disease', *Australian Critical Care*, 15, 64–69.

98. Lynn, J & Goldstein, NE. 2003; 'Advance Care Planning For Fatal Chronic Illness: Avoiding Commonplace Errors And Unwarranted Suffering', *Annals of Internal Medicine*, 20, 138(10), 812–818.99; Lynn, J, Nolan, K, Kabcenell, A, Weissman, D, Milne, C, Berwick, DM, *et al.* 2002; 'Reforming Care for Persons Near the End of Life: The Promise of Quality Improvement', *Annals of Internal Medicine*, 137 (2), 117–122.

99. Goodlin, SJ, Hauptman, PJ, Arnold, R, *et al.* 2004; 'Consensus Statement: Palliative and Supportive Care in Advanced Heart Failure', *Journal of Cardiac Failure*, 10 (3), 200–209.

100. Teno, JM, Stevens, M, Spernak, S & Lynn, J. 1998; 'Role of Written Advance Directives in Decision Making: Insights from Qualitative and Quantitative Data', *Journal of General Internal Medicine*, 13 (7), 439–446.

101. Stewart, S & Horowitz, JD. 2002; 'Home-Based Intervention in Congestive Heart Failure: Long-Term Implications on Readmission And Survival', *Circulation*, 105 (24), 2861–2866.

102. Harris, DE & Record, NB. 2003; 'Cardiac Rehabilitation in Community Settings', *Journal of Cardiopulmonary Rehabilitation*, 23, 250–259.

103. Ahmed, A. 2002; 'Quality And Outcomes of Heart Failure Care in Older Adults: Role of Multidisciplinary Disease-Management Programs', *Journal of the American Geriatrics Society*, 50, 1590–1593.

6 | Respiratory Health Breakdown

AUTHORS

FIONA COYER

JOANNE RAMSBOTHAM

LEARNING OBJECTIVES

When you have completed this chapter you will be able to
- Recognise the important anatomical and physiological features of the respiratory system;
- Describe the pathophysiological changes associated with respiratory health breakdown;
- Understand the nursing application of diagnostic and therapeutic techniques associated with caring for a person with a respiratory health breakdown;
- Identify the common pharmacological agents utilised in managing respiratory health breakdown; and
- Consider nursing interventions required for people with respiratory health breakdown.

INTRODUCTION

This chapter reviews the key aspects of respiratory system anatomy and physiology. Using a case study approach, the chapter examines respiratory health breakdown from three clinical categories: infective, traumatic and chronic problems. Important nursing considerations are discussed in relation to the case studies. Early recognition and intervention in the sequelae of respiratory problems are essential to improve patient outcomes and reduce morbidity and mortality. Table 6.1 highlights the breakdown of patient problems into clinical categories and common respiratory conditions. Continued deterioration in any of these conditions can lead to respiratory failure, which may develop rapidly even in the patient with little or no pre-existing lung pathology.

Lung cancer is also a common disease of the respiratory system – it is the leading cause of male deaths and the second leading cause of female deaths from malignant disease in the world. Cigarette smoking is the predominant cause of lung cancer (80–90%), and is dose-response related. The common lung cancers include squamous cell; adenocarcinoma; small cell (oat cell) carcinoma; mesothelioma; and Kaposi's sarcoma. Further discussion about cancers is provided in Chapter 14.

WHAT MAKES UP THE RESPIRATORY SYSTEM?

The primary function of the respiratory system is to provide oxygen (O_2) for all metabolic processes to the body's cells and tissues (oxygenation), and to remove carbon dioxide (CO_2) from the gaseous waste products of metabolism (ventilation)[1].

TABLE 6.1: RESPIRATORY HEALTH BREAKDOWN	
Clinical Category	**Common Conditions**
Traumatic	• Pneumothorax • Haemothorax • Tension pneumothorax • Pulmonary contusion • Rib fractures
Infective	Upper respiratory tract problems: • Common cold • Rhinitis • Sinusitis • Pharyngitis • Laryngitis Lower respiratory tract problems: • Bronchiolitis • Bronchitis • Pneumonia (viral, bacterial or fungal) • Severe acute respiratory syndrome (SARS) • Tuberculosis
Chronic	• Asthma • Emphysema • Bronchitis

Anatomically, the respiratory system is divided into the upper and lower respiratory tracts. The key structures in the upper respiratory tract include the nasal cavities, the pharynx and the larynx, within the head and neck. The main function of the upper respiratory tract is to warm, filter and humidify inspired air. The nasal cavities are comprised of highly vascularised tissue consisting of pseudo-stratified, ciliated columnar epithelium. These structures provide a large surface area for heat and water exchange[2]. The pharynx is a funnel-shaped passageway and is shared by the respiratory and digestive systems. The larynx (voice box) connects the pharynx with the trachea, and contains cartilages with the epiglottic cartilage at the top. The epiglottis serves to create the cough reflex and protect the lower respiratory tract from aspiration of anything other than air. The largest cartilage is the thyroid cartilage (sometimes called the Adam's apple). Three pairs of cartilage comprise the vocal cords. The last cartilage is the cricoid cartilage, which connects the thyroid cartilage and the trachea.

The lower respiratory tract includes the trachea and lungs (which include the bronchi, bronchioles and alveoli). A large portion of the lower respiratory tract is encased in and protected by the thoracic cage, and the muscles of ventilation, namely the diaphragm and the intercostal muscles (see Figure 6.1).

The adult trachea averages 2.0–2.5 cm in diameter and ranges from 10–12 cm in length. It is made of 16–20 C-shaped pieces of cartilaginous rings known as hyaline cartilage. This C shape provides support to the airway, but allows changes in airway diameter to accommodate the oesophagus posteriorly. The trachea divides into the right and left main bronchi at the anatomical point called the carina. The main bronchi continue to divide and segment into smaller and smaller airways. This is representative of the branches of a tree fanning out into every portion of the lung. The alveoli are cup-like structures found in a cluster at the terminal bronchioles. Adult lungs have approximately 300 million alveoli. This provides a vast surface area for gas exchange averaging $70\,m^2$.

The thorax or chest cavity contains the lungs, pleura and muscles of respiration. The lungs are cone-shaped organs, located on either side of the heart within the chest cavity. They contain part of the trachea, the main bronchi and bronchioles and alveoli. There are three distinct lobes of the right lung, and two lobes in the left lung. The pleura are serous membranes that cover the lungs and line the thoracic cavity. The function of the pleura is to act as a lubricating surface to enable the lungs to expand easily with respiration. The primary muscles of respiration are the diaphragm and the external intercostal muscles. The diaphragm is supplied by the phrenic nerve, which originates from the spinal cord at the level of the third cervical vertebrae. The diaphragm accounts for 75% of the change in thoracic volume during inspiration[1]. The external intercostal muscles are located between the ribs. Contract of these muscles during inspiration elevates the ribs, increasing thoracic volume.

PULMONARY BLOOD SUPPLY

The lungs have two different types of blood supply: pulmonary and bronchial. In pulmonary blood supply the lungs receive the body's entire circulation volume each minute. The blood supply to the lungs begins at the pulmonary trunk, which stems from and receives deoxygenated venous blood from the right side of the heart. The pulmonary artery divides into the right and left main pulmonary arteries to supply the right and left lungs. These arteries continue to divide and subdivide until they form a pulmonary capillary network around each alveolus. It is here that diffusion of gases occurs. Following

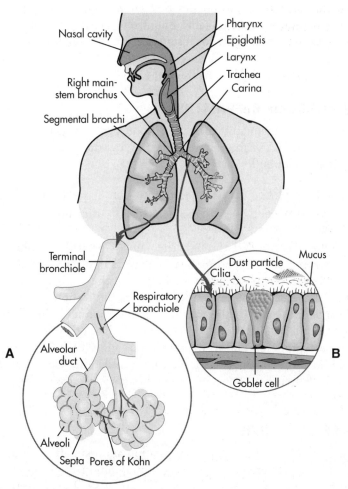

FIGURE 6.1   *Structures of the respiratory tract*
Source: Redrawn from Price, SA & Wilson, LM. 2003; *Pathophysiology: Clinical, Concepts of Disease Processes* (6th ed.), Mosby, St Louis, Fig. 35.1, p. 542.

gas exchange, oxygenated blood is returned to the left side of the heart through the pulmonary veins[2]. Bronchial blood supply to the lungs commences with the bronchial arteries, which arise from the thoracic aorta. The bronchial arteries supply oxygenated blood to the bronchi and lung parenchyma. The majority of bronchial venous return is via the azygos vein to the left atrium.

NERVOUS CONTROL OF RESPIRATION

Respiration is an automatic function needing no conscious awareness. The respiratory centres in the medulla oblongata and upper pons in the brain stem control the stimulus to determine the rhythm of breathing. Neurones in the medulla oblongata control the cyclical pattern of inspiration and expiration. Excitatory impulses are transmitted to the diaphragm and external intercostal muscles to contract and commence inspiration. Two other areas in the respiratory centre of the brain stem assist in modifying the rhythm of breathing – the apneustic centre extends inspiration and the pneumotaxic centre limits or controls the time for inspiration. These centres work together to control the depth of respiration in response to the body's needs[3].

CHEMICAL CONTROL OF RESPIRATION

The respiratory system maintains normal amounts of oxygen, hydrogen ions and carbon dioxide within a dynamic state reflected by the following equation of the bicarbonate–carbonic acid buffer system[2]:

$$CO_2 \quad + \quad H_2O \quad \leftrightarrow \quad H_2CO_3 \quad \leftrightarrow \quad HCO_3^- \quad + \quad H^+$$

Carbon dioxide Water Carbonic acid Bicarbonate Hydrogen ion

This equilibrium is controlled through the rate of breathing. Abnormal states such as hypoxia, acidaemia and hypercapnoea act to stimulate central and peripheral chemoreceptors. Central chemoreceptors are located in the respiratory centre in the brain stem and peripheral chemoreceptors are located in the bifurcation of the common carotid arteries and the arch of the aorta[3]. The primary chemical stimuli in breathing are hydrogen ions and CO_2. Central chemoreceptors respond to hydrogen ion concentration and peripheral chemoreceptors respond to hydrogen ions and CO_2. Chemoreceptors transmit impulses to the medulla oblongata to increase ventilation. Consequently, ventilation increases when hydrogen ion concentration rises and decreases when hydrogen ion concentration falls[4].

MECHANICS OF BREATHING

Air moves in and out of the lungs during inspiration and expiration because of a pressure difference between the pressure inside the lungs (intrapulmonary pressure) and the pressure outside (atmospheric pressure)[1]. Atmospheric pressure at sea level is 760 mmHg standard temperature and pressure, dry (STPD). For inspiration to commence, the respiratory centre sends an excitatory stimulus to the diaphragm and the external intercostal muscles to contract. Contraction of the diaphragm lengthens the thoracic cavity. Contraction of the external intercostal muscles widens the thorax. This creates a pressure difference, as the thorax is now larger and intrapulmonary pressure has decreased to 758 mmHg. Air moves into the lungs from the higher external area of pressure to a lower area of internal pressure. At the end of inspiration, the muscles relax and the thorax becomes smaller. This increases the intrapulmonary pressure to 762 mmHg, which exceeds atmospheric pressure and air moves out of the lungs from a higher area of internal pressure to a lower area of external pressure.

GAS EXCHANGE AND TRANSPORT

The function of respiration is twofold: to achieve oxygen (O_2) delivery to the tissues and to remove carbon dioxide (CO_2) from the tissues into the atmosphere. This is achieved by two processes: gas exchange (at the lungs and cellular level) and gas transport.

Oxygen and carbon dioxide are exchanged at the alveolar capillary membrane by the process of diffusion. Oxygen moves from an area of high concentration (alveolar gas or atmospheric air) to an area of lower concentration (pulmonary capillary). Carbon dioxide moves from an area of high concentration (pulmonary capillary) to an area of lower concentration (alveoli). At cellular level O_2 moves from the capillary to the tissues (cells) down a diffusion gradient. The pressure of O_2 within the capillary is approximately 40 mmHg and within the cells is approximately 5 mmHg. The CO_2 diffusion gradient is opposite to that of O_2. At cellular level, CO_2 moves from the tissues (cells) to the capillary. The pressure of CO_2 within the cells is approximately 60 mmHg and within the capillary is approximately 1 mmHg.

Oxygen is transported in two ways: 97–99% is bound to haemoglobin (Hb), which is measured clinically by oxygen saturation (SaO_2); 1–3% is dissolved in plasma[5], which is measured clinically by arterial blood gas analysis (ABG) specifically the partial pressure of oxygen dissolved in arterial blood (PaO_2). The oxygen-haemoglobin dissociation curve reflects the affinity of oxygen to the haemoglobin molecules. The curve demonstrates that there is not a linear relationship between PaO_2 and haemoglobin-oxygen saturation (SaO_2). This is particularly important at the critical level where PaO_2 drops dramatically when compared to the SaO_2 – while a 95% SaO_2 equates to a PaO_2 level of 80 mmHg, an SaO_2 of 90% reflects a clinically significant drop in PaO_2 to 60 mmHg (a state of hypoxaemia)[2]. The nursing considerations related to this issue are discussed later in the chapter. The PaO_2 level is important for optimal oxygenation as it exerts a pressure to enable O_2 to diffuse across capillary membranes to the cell[6].

SUMMARY OF ANATOMY AND PHYSIOLOGY

Following are the key concepts:

- The lungs are the organs responsible for maintaining ventilation and oxygenation.
- Respiration is an automatic function needing no conscious awareness. The respiratory centre in the medulla oblongata and upper pons in the brain stem control the stimulus to determine the rhythm of breathing.
- The respiratory system maintains normal amounts of oxygen, hydrogen ions and carbon dioxide through chemical stimulus.
- Air moves in and out of the lungs during inspiration and expiration because of a pressure gradient difference.
- O_2 and CO_2 move across the alveolar capillary membrane and into the cells by the process of diffusion. O_2 is transported around the body to the cells by being dissolved in plasma and bound to haemoglobin.

ACUTE RESPIRATORY FAILURE

Urden, Stacy and Lough define acute respiratory failure (ARF) as

a clinical condition in which the pulmonary system fails to maintain adequate gas exchange[4] (p. 551).

WHAT DOES ACUTE RESPIRATORY FAILURE MEAN?

The degree of failure is most commonly measured by continuous SaO_2 bedside monitoring or through ABG analysis. If acceptable values of pH, $PaCO_2$ and PaO_2 are not maintained, the respiratory system is said to be in failure. Unlike other body system failures, it can be clinically difficult to offer definitive laboratory values on when respiratory failure does and does not commence – any deterioration is along a continuum, and the patient's clinical presentation and underlying or pre-existing condition will be the best guides. All data, including subjective clinical history, clinical assessment and objective laboratory values, must be taken into account. As a guide for the clinician, the following values for respiratory failure are suggested:

- PaO_2 is less than or equal to 60 mmHg; or
- $PaCO_2$ is equal to or greater than 45 mmHg[4].

Other laboratory criteria that may be helpful in determining acute respiratory failure are pH levels indicating acidaemia and an SaO_2 of less than 90%[7,8].

CAUSES OF ACUTE RESPIRATORY FAILURE

Failure of the respiratory system may be attributed to a variety of causes, some common, others uncommon. In order to breathe effectively and oxygenate tissues, a number of key systems need to be working effectively. To recall all the varied causes of respiratory failure, it is helpful to relate the causes to the anatomical reference points involved in respiration. Table 6.2 summarises some of the common causes of acute respiratory failure by linking clinical conditions to a location of the injury or malfunction.

TYPES OF ACUTE RESPIRATORY FAILURE

Failure of the respiratory system may occur with or without impairment of carbon dioxide elimination. Consequently, respiratory failure has been divided into two main types, hypoxaemic failure and hypercapnoeic hypoxaemic failure:

1. **Type 1 Hypoxaemic respiratory failure:** This failure has been described as abnormal oxygenation of the blood. As the name implies, in this type of failure, the patient's PaO_2 may be low (60 mmHg or less), the SaO_2 will be low (less than 90%), yet the $PaCO_2$ may be normal to low. Thus, the primary mechanism of this type of failure is that of inadequate oxygenation or hypoxaemia[3].

TABLE 6.2: CAUSES OF ACUTE RESPIRATORY FAILURE	
Location of Injury/ Malfunction	**Clinical Condition**
Respiratory centre in the brain stem	Direct trauma, infection, vascular lesions, brainstem lesions, drug overdose, central sleep apnoea
Spinal cord	Cervical lesion or trauma
Motor nerves	Guillain-Barré syndrome
Neuromuscular junction	Myasthenia gravis, botulism
Chest wall	Kyphoscoliosis, ankylosing spondylitis
Pleura	Pneumothorax, haemothorax, tension pneumothorax, pleural effusion, rib fractures, flail segment
Lung parenchyma (bronchioles, alveoli)	Pulmonary infection [viral, bacterial, fungal], aspiration, inhalation of toxins [smoke, chemicals], pulmonary oedema, cancer, acute respiratory distress syndrome (ARDS)
Pulmonary circulation	Pulmonary embolism, primary pulmonary hypertension

Source: Adapted from Wilkins, Stoller & Scanlan[3]; Urden, Stacy & Lough[4].

2. **Type 2 Hypercapnoeic hypoxaemic respiratory failure:** This failure suggests abnormal oxygenation of the blood, as well as an inability of the respiratory system to eliminate carbon dioxide. In this type, the patient's PaO_2 may be low (60 mmHg or less), and the patient's $PaCO_2$ may be elevated (greater than 45 mmHg). Type 2 failure is, therefore, a combination of CO_2 retention (hypercapnoea) and inadequate oxygenation (hypoxaemia)[3].

WHAT IS THE PATHOPHYSIOLOGY OF ACUTE RESPIRATORY FAILURE?

There are four essential mechanisms identified in the pathophysiological sequelae of acute respiratory failure: alveolar hypoventilation; ventilation/perfusion (V/Q) mismatch; physiological shunt; and diffusion impairment[9]:

1. **Alveolar hypoventilation:** The average person at rest breathes about 12 to 20 breaths per minute. Each breath exchanges approximately 500 mL of air. This is called the tidal volume (V_T). The total volume of gas exchanged each minute is represented as follows:

$$V_E \text{ (minute ventilation)} = f \text{ (frequency or breaths per minute)} \times V_T \text{ (tidal volume)}.$$

Not all gas inspired with each breath reaches the alveoli to participate in gas exchange. A portion is contained in the larger airways and upper respiratory tract and does not participate in gas exchange – this is called anatomical dead space. Anatomical dead space is estimated at 150 mL per 500 mL inspired breath. This dead space needs to be taken into account when estimating alveolar ventilation, or the amount of gas participating in gas exchange[10]. Alveolar minute ventilation can be represented as follows:

$$V_A \text{ (alveolar minute ventilation)} = f \times (V_T - V_D)$$
(where V_D is anatomical dead space volume)

Alveolar hypoventilation occurs when either the respiratory rate (f) or the V_T is reduced resulting in insufficient gas exchange to meet the metabolic demands of the body. This is usually associated with hypercapnoea. An elevation in $PaCO_2$ indicates inadequate alveolar ventilation. This is usually seen in patients whose respiratory drive is suppressed (e.g., over-medication with narcotics or head trauma), or in patients who underventilate due to pain with breathing (e.g., any thoracic trauma or postoperatively following thoracic and upper abdominal surgery).

2. **Ventilation/perfusion (V/Q) mismatch:** The lung is said to be functioning optimally when ventilation (V = alveolar ventilation) is proportional to perfusion (Q = pulmonary circulation). Alveolar ventilation is approximately 4 L/min. As the cardiac output can be estimated at 5 L/min, pulmonary blood flow should also be 5 L/min, all things being equal. Thus, the average ratio of alveolar ventilation to pulmonary perfusion is said to be 4 L to 5 L or 4:5 or about 0.8[3].

However, the relationship of alveolar ventilation to pulmonary perfusion varies considerably throughout the lung and is dependent upon a number of factors, such as pressure gradients affecting both ventilation and perfusion, and patient position (erect, supine or prone). In the upright adult person, the apices of the lung receive moderate ventilation but little perfusion (the V/Q here is > 0.8). Conversely, the bases of the lung in this scenario receive more perfusion and less ventilation (therefore, the V/Q is < 0.8). This is more balanced in the mid portion of the lung where, due to pressure equalising, ventilation and perfusion are evenly distributed[2,10].

The pathophysiology of a mismatch in ventilation and perfusion results in systemic hypoxaemia. The types of V/Q imbalances that may occur include: 1) low-ventilation/ perfusion ratio – where perfusion exceeds ventilation, a physiological shunt is said to be present (see next section for further discussion); and 2) high ventilation/perfusion ratio – when ventilation exceeds perfusion, dead space develops since there is an overabundance of gas that is not able to participate in gas exchange – this can be caused by pulmonary embolism.

3. **Physiological shunt:** When pulmonary perfusion exceeds alveolar ventilation, a physiological shunt is said to be present. A physiological shunt occurs when deoxygenated blood returns to the left side of the heart, and to the systemic circulation, after passing through non-ventilated alveoli. Consequently, deoxygenated blood is shunted from the right side of the heart to the left side of the heart. This causes an admixture of deoxygenated and oxygenated blood returning to the left side of the heart to be pumped out to the tissues and organs. The pathophysiological result is systemic hypoxaemia from this venous admixture. The severity of the shunt is calculated by the difference between the tension of O_2 in the alveoli (PAO_2) and the systemic arterial circulation (PaO_2); this is called the alveolar-arterial (A-a) gradient[11].

   Theoretically, the tension of oxygen leaving the pulmonary capillary (PaO_2) would be equal to the tension of oxygen in the alveoli (PAO_2). However, physiologically the PAO_2 (alveolar oxygen tension) is approximately 110 mmHg and the PaO_2 (arterial oxygen tension) is 100 mmHg. This normal physiological difference of 10 mmHg is attributed to an anatomical shunt due to: 1) exiting of blood from lung regions with low ventilation in proportion to perfusion; 2) drainage of venous blood from the bronchial circulation into the pulmonary veins; and 3) drainage of some coronary venous blood directly into the left atrium by the thebesian veins[4].

   Clinically, a normal A-a gradient is less than 15 mmHg. If the A-a gradient is greater than 15 mmHg, this indicates underlying respiratory pathology, such as: 1) intracardiac shunts (atrial septal defects and ventricular septal defects); 2) pulmonary arteriovenous (AV) malformations; and 3) pulmonary disease when the alveoli are filled with fluid or exudate (pulmonary oedema, pneumonia, aspiration)[11].

4. **Diffusion impairment:** The main principle governing gas exchange in the alveoli and between the blood and body cells is that of diffusion. Diffusion can be defined as the movement of molecules from an area of high concentration to an area of low concentration until concentration is equal throughout. The principle of diffusion also relates to Dalton's gas law of partial pressure, where gas molecules that are dissolved exert a partial pressure (PaO_2 = partial pressure of oxygen in the artery) in the liquid (plasma) to enable diffusion to take place. This partial pressure is also essential for O_2 molecules to bind or saturate to haemoglobin[11].

   The alveolar diffusion membrane is comprised of four layers: alveolar epithelial wall; basement membrane of alveolus; capillary basement membrane; and endothelial cells of capillary.

   For diffusion to take place rapidly and effectively the diffusion membrane must have certain characteristics: 1) be very thin to facilitate rapid diffusion of molecules – all four layers of the alveolar capillary membrane are only 0.2–0.6 mcm thick[2]; 2) cover sufficient area to allow for enough exchange of gases – each lung contains 350 million alveoli, providing a surface area of $70 m^2$ for gas exchange; and 3) present a minimal diffusion pathway – the integrity of the diffusion membrane[9] requires it to be free from accumulation of fluid or other substances that may impair gas exchange. The alveoli contain alveolar macrophages, which are phagocytic cells inside the alveoli that clear bacteria and other material invading the alveoli. Some causes of diffusion impairment are fluid accumulation from pulmonary oedema, and mucous and inflammation from pneumonia[9].

WHAT DIAGNOSTIC INVESTIGATIONS ARE APPROPRIATE?

A thorough health history and physical assessment of the respiratory system often uncovers problems worthy of further investigation or confirmation[8]. The recommended reading by Finesilver (2001) offers a thorough overview of respiratory health history and physical assessment. Adjunctive assessment tools, such as pulmonary function tests, pulse oximetry, arterial blood gas results and chest X-rays, can often provide valuable quantitative information regarding the respiratory system.

PULMONARY FUNCTION TESTS

Pulmonary function tests are designed to quantify respiratory function according to gender, age and body size, and form an essential part of respiratory assessment. Pulmonary function tests serve many purposes, such as preoperative evaluation, evaluating lung mechanics, diagnosing and monitoring pulmonary diseases, and monitoring response to therapy[12]. There are four areas to a complete set of pulmonary function tests: lung volumes (this covers spirometry and vital capacity); mechanics of breathing (measures flow of gas and lung compliance and resistance); diffusion of gases (refers to ventilation/perfusion scanning); and arterial blood gases. Commonly, bedside spirometry includes assessment of forced expiratory volume in 1 second (FEV_1) and forced vital capacity (FVC), to evaluate respiratory status or in response to treatment. Other lung mechanics are usually measured in specific pulmonary function laboratories.

ARTERIAL BLOOD GASES

The goal of interpreting arterial blood gas (ABS) analysis is to assess how effectively the body is maintaining homeostasis, keeping the pH of the body within normal limits. Table 6.3 reviews the normal values for each of the ABG components.

Changes differing from these normal values will reflect changes in the acid–base balance[6]. For example, a pH less than 7.4 indicates acidosis; whereas a pH greater than 7.4 indicates alkalosis. The $PaCO_2$ represents the partial pressure of carbon dioxide dissolved in arterial blood. Arterial carbon dioxide levels are indicative of ventilation. Thus $PaCO_2$ levels are used to measure respiratory acid–base balance. Bicarbonate (HCO_3^-) is the main chemical buffer in plasma. Bicarbonate levels are used to measure metabolic acid–base balance. Base excess refers to the quantity of strong acid or base required to restore the pH to 7.4. A positive value of BE (e.g., >+2) indicates an excess of base (or deficit of acid), while a negative value (e.g., <−2) indicates a deficit of base (or excess of acid).

The steps in interpretation of ABGs are[13]:

1. Evaluate pH level: acidaemia (pH < 7.35) or alkalaemia (pH > 7.45). The pH level reflects primary disorder if there is more than one imbalance;
2. Evaluate ventilation (PCO_2): ventilatory failure (PCO_2 > 45 mm Hg) or alveolar hyperventilation (PCO_2 < 35 mm Hg);
3. Evaluate metabolic processes (HCO_3^-): metabolic acidosis (<22 mmol/L) or metabolic alkalosis (>26 mmol/L). Abnormal bicarbonate levels reflect a primary metabolic disorder (non-respiratory causes), or metabolic compensation to a respiratory disorder;
4. Determine primary compensatory disorder(s): relate the abnormal levels of the PCO_2 or HCO_3^- to the direction of the pH abnormality;

TABLE 6.3: ABG ACID-BASE VALUES				
	Normal Values	**Median**	**Acidosis**	**Alkalosis**
pH	7.35–7.45	7.4	⇓	⇑
$PaCO_2$	35–45 mmHg	40 mmHg	⇑	⇓
HCO_3^-	22–26 mmol/L	24 mmol/L	⇓	⇑
base excess (BE)	−2 to +2	0	⇓	⇑

5. Evaluate oxygenation: mild hypoxaemia (60–80 mm Hg), moderate hypoxaemia (40–60 mm Hg), severe hypoxaemia (<40 mm Hg); and
6. Interpret: include the primary disorder, compensation and oxygenation status, for example, partially compensated respiratory acidosis with moderate hypoxaemia.

OXYGEN SATURATION (SAO₂)

The use of pulse oximetry has become a standard tool in most clinical settings[14]. A pulse oximeter measures the percentage of haemoglobin molecules saturated with oxygen (SaO_2). The normal value for SaO_2 is 95–99% on room air[15]. As noted earlier, a limitation of pulse oximetry is that the SaO_2 does not always accurately reflect oxygenation (PaO_2), particularly when SaO_2 falls below 90%. A number of clinical and technical factors also affects the accuracy of pulse oximetry: 1) poor peripheral pulsatile states (mean BP ≤ 50 mmHg, narrow pulse pressure, vasoconstriction); 2) other physiological states (e.g., anaemia, carboxyhaemoglobin); and 3) technical factors (e.g., motion artifact, external light interference, intravenous dyes)[15].

CHEST RADIOGRAPHY

Chest radiography (X-ray) is an important and very common diagnostic tool for any patient presenting with respiratory or thoracic problems. Radiographic examination of the chest is indicated in any patients having breathing difficulties, or those patients who may develop breathing difficulties later[16]. Radiological findings can be diagnostic and also may suggest a differential diagnosis[17].

Chest X-ray interpretation utilises the following sequential steps[18]:

1. Check the patient's name and the date of the X-ray.
2. Check the technical quality of the film:
   a) *Projection.* This is determined by the direction of the X-ray beam in relation to the patient. Check to see if the film is anterior-posterior (AP), where the film is behind the patient's back and the X-ray taken from the front, or if the film is posterior-anterior (PA), where the film is in front of the patient and the X-ray taken from the patient's back. Check if the patient was erect or supine;
   b) *Orientation.* Generally check the anatomical right-to-left markers, ensuring the apex of the heart is on the left. Check the film is marked right and left;
   c) *Rotation.* Check the positioning or rotation of the patient on the film. The patient's chest should be in the middle of the film. This is verified by determining that the medial ends of the clavicles are equidistant from the vertebrae;
   d) *Penetration.* The vertebral bodies should be just visible through the cardiac shadow. If they are too visible, the film is over-penetrated. If they are not visible the film is under-penetrated; and
   e) *Degree of inspiration.* Poor inspiration will make the heart appear larger on the X-ray. The degree of inspiration is judged by counting the number of ribs above the diaphragm. The sixth anterior rib should be visible above the diaphragm; and
3. Use a logical approach to assess the X-ray. The follow steps commence at the trachea and move systematically downwards through the film and then outward through the chest wall and lung fields:
   a) *Trachea.* The trachea should be central and should appear as narrow translucent midline bands;
   b) *Mediastinum.* The maximum transverse diameter of the heart is less than 15.5 cm in males and less than 14.5 cm in females. The largest projection of the heart is seen with the one third of the shadow to the right of midline of the thorax;

c) *Diaphragm.* The diaphragm should appear as two convex domes. The right diaphragm is approximately 1–3 cm higher;

d) *Chest wall.* Check the bone shadows of the ribs and clavicle. Breast tissue may appear as diminished translucency over the lower half of the lung fields;

e) *Lung fields.* The hemi-thorax should be of equal size. The lungs should be equidistant from the vertebral processes. There should be similar and equal distribution of vasculature, which is more pronounced in the lower fields. The bronchi are not usually visible, but may be seen as small opacities near blood vessels;

f) *Pleura.* The costo-phrenic angle (located in the corner between the pleura and the diaphragm) should be well defined and acute. The clarity of pleural markings should be noted.

TRAUMATIC RESPIRATORY HEALTH BREAKDOWN

Chest injuries contribute to morbidity and mortality in more than 60% of patients with multiple injuries[19]. The mechanism of chest trauma is by shearing, compression, torsion and acceleration/deceleration forces[20].

● Case study

Paul Tomasavic, 19, presented to the emergency department after a sudden onset of left-sided chest pain and difficulty in breathing. Paul is 190 cm tall and weighs approximately 85 kg. Paul had been playing basketball when the pain started. On presentation, Paul's vital signs were: blood pressure 125/85 mmHg; heart rate 105 beats/minute (sinus tachycardia); and respiratory rate 32 breaths per minute. Paul described himself as 'fit and healthy' and was on no medications.

Paul was examined by medical staff. Percussion of the chest demonstrated hyperresonant sounds on the left side, while auscultation showed decreased breath sounds also on the left side on the chest. Paul was commenced on oxygen via simple face mask at 4 L/min and an intravenous line was inserted with 0.9% saline running at 30 mL/h to keep the vein open. A 12-lead electrocardiograph and chest X-ray were ordered. A left-sided pneumothorax was suspected.

PNEUMOTHORAX

A pneumothorax is the accumulation of air in the intrapleural space[21]. This may occur spontaneously or traumatically. Typically, it occurs in patients with underlying respiratory problems, such as asthma, chronic obstructive lung disease or malignancies. A pneumothorax may occur as a result of direct chest trauma by blunt (e.g., motor vehicle accident, fall or assault with blunt object) or penetrating forces (e.g., knife, gunshot or other missiles). However, it can also occur spontaneously in otherwise healthy people, particularly thin, young males[20]. Table 6.4 highlights the types of pneumothorax and the associated causes.

TABLE 6.4: TYPES, DESCRIPTION AND CAUSES OF PNEUMOTHORAX		
Type	**Description**	**Cause**
Spontaneous	Disruption of the pleura allowing air from lung to enter pleural space	May occur with or without underlying lung disease. Predisposing lung diseases are asthma, chronic airflow limitation (CAL), pneumonia, tuberculosis, cystic fibrosis and connective tissues disorders such as Marfan's syndrome
Traumatic		
Open	Laceration of the pleura allowing atmospheric air to enter pleural space	Occurs as a result of penetrating chest trauma
Closed	Laceration of the pleura that allows air from the lung to enter the pleural space	May occur as a result of blunt chest trauma
Iatrogenic	Laceration of the pleura that allows air from the lung to enter the pleural space	May occur as a result of therapeutic or diagnostic procedures, such as central line insertion, needle biopsy and aspirations, and mechanical ventilation
Tension	Laceration of the pleura that allows air into the pleural space but does not allow it to exit. Pressure/tension increases in the intrapleural space causing the affected lung to collapse and the mediastinal contents to be squeezed and shifted to the unaffected side	May be the result of a spontaneous or traumatic pneumothorax

Source: Adapted from Wilkins, Stoller & Scanlan[3]; Urden, Stacy & Lough[4].

WHAT IS THE PATHOPHYSIOLOGY?

The pathophysiological mechanisms of pneumothorax are subtle[22]. When air is present in the intrapleural space, the dynamics of lung pressures change. Air in the intrapleural space causes terminal airway closure. This is compounded by the patient's experience of pain on inspiration that causes them to hypoventilate[23]. This causes regional differences in pulmonary ventilation and represents a V/Q inequality. At the effected site ventilation is less than normal, indicating a low V/Q. In areas with a low V/Q, the PAO_2 is lower and the PCO_2 is higher than normal. Venous blood entering these regional areas of low V/Q cannot pick up O_2 and offload CO_2, so no gas exchange occurs. As this deoxygenated blood returns to the left side of the heart it mixes with other oxygenated blood. This has the effect of diluting the oxygen content of arterial blood in the left heart and is called a right to left shunt. Consequently the patient will become hypoxic. Thus, for a patient with a large untreated pneumothorax, the pathophysiological mechanisms of hypoventilation,

ventilation/perfusion mismatch and shunt create the overall effect of hypercapnoeic hypoxaemic respiratory failure.

WHAT ARE THE CLINICAL MANIFESTATIONS?

The clinical manifestations are dependent on the size of the pneumothorax[24]. With a small pneumothorax, the patient may be asymptomatic. With a larger pneumothorax, the patient may present with sudden onset of dyspnoea and description of a sharp pleuritic chest pain that is usually worse on inspiration. There will be hyperresonance on percussion on the affected side. Auscultation of the patient's chest may evidence diminished or absent breath sounds. The patient may have a history of trauma, heavy exertion or a previous occurrence of a pneumothorax[22].

WHAT DIAGNOSTIC INVESTIGATIONS ARE APPROPRIATE?

A thorough history and examination is essential for diagnosing pneumothorax. As patients classically present with a history of chest pain and shortness of breath, it is essential to rule out any cardiac problems first. A 12-lead electrocardiograph may be taken, but this will be normal in a patient with a pneumothorax.

ABGs may be taken. These may show an initial respiratory alkalosis caused by a decrease in $PaCO_2$ as a result of tachypnoea. Later ABGs will show hypoxaemia with decreased to low PaO_2 levels, and acidaemia with elevated $PaCO_2$ levels. SaO_2 may decrease at first, but will usually be greater than 90%[19]. Pulmonary function tests would show a decrease in vital capacity.

A chest X-ray is essential to determine the presence, size and extent of the pneumothorax. Vascular shadows and lung tissue markings in a normal lung field will disappear if there is air in the intrapleural space[18]. Sequential chest X-rays will confirm whether treatment has been effective[21].

WHAT IS THE TREATMENT?

The management of a pneumothorax is dependent upon the size as diagnosed on chest X-ray. A pneumothorax of 15% or less is managed conservatively with supplemental oxygen, which rapidly accelerates reabsorption of trapped air by the pleura[24]. Symptoms often resolve within 24 hours[21].

A pneumothorax of greater than 15% requires the insertion of a chest tube. An intercostal chest tube is inserted in the intrapleural space to remove fluid or air and consequently, re-instate the intrapleural pressure and reexpand the collapsed lung. Once inserted in the intrapleural space, the chest tube is connected to an underwater seal drainage (UWSD) system. The water seal chamber (see Figure 6.2 and 6.3) acts as a one-way valve, allowing air to escape from the pleural space but not to reenter[4]. The patient is monitored by chest auscultation and chest X-ray for re-expansion of the lung.

Surgical intervention for spontaneous pneumothorax is rarely required and is only considered when the air leak persists for greater than 4 days. The clinical decision to use sclerosing agents such as talc, to prevent recurrent episodes, is variable[24]. Talc pleurodesis prevents the accumulation of fluid in the pleural space by causing fusion of the pleura and obliterating the pleural space[25]. However, it is noted that primary spontaneous pneumothorax has a recurrence rate of 30%[3].

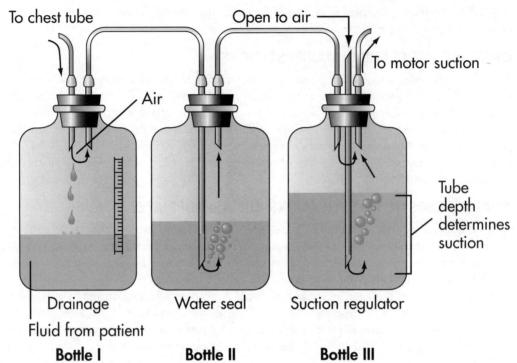

To chest tube   Open to air

To motor suction

Air

Tube
depth
determines
suction

Drainage   Water seal   Suction regulator

Fluid from patient

Bottle I   **Bottle II**   **Bottle III**

FIGURE 6.2 *Under water seal chest drainage. Three-bottle water seal suction*
Source: Lewis, SM, *et al.* 2004; *Medical-Surgical Nursing* (6th ed.), Mosby, St Louis, Fig.
27.9, p. 623.

LEARNING EXERCISES

1. Describe the different types of pneumothorax.
2. Outline the pathophysiology associated with a spontaneous pneumothorax.
3. Outline the clinical manifestations of a patient with a pneumothorax.
4. Explain the nursing management of a patient with a spontaneous pneumothorax.

In this case study, Paul's history and examination suggest he has had a spontaneous
pneumothorax. He classically fits the category of spontaneous pneumothorax in young,
thin males. In many patients with spontaneous pneumothorax, the signs, symptoms and
chest X-ray findings are subtle and may be overlooked. It is important to note that
all chest pain should be treated as cardiac in origin until it is definitively proved
otherwise.

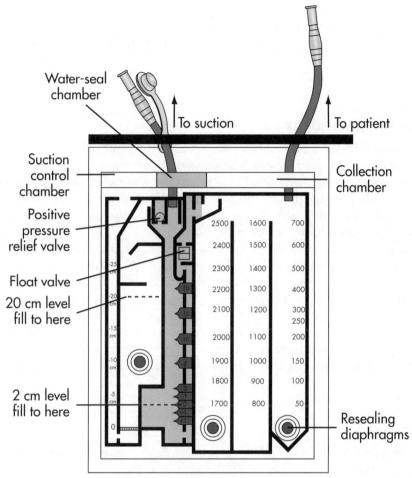

FIGURE 6.3 *Pleur-evac disposable chest drainage system*
Source: Courtesy Deknatel, Inc., Fall River, MA.

Paul is displaying some evidence of hypoventilation. His pathophysiological mechanisms are V/Q mismatch and, consequently, shunt. He would progress to type 1 hypoxaemic acute respiratory failure, and if untreated, he would fatigue and then progress to type 2 hypercapnoeic hypoxaemic acute respiratory failure.

Paul's chest X-ray revealed a 50% pneumothorax on the left side. The mediastinal structures were in their normal position and no tracheal deviation was evident. As this was a moderate pneumothorax, Paul needed a chest tube to re-expand his lung. Paul was given 5 mg of midazolam intravenously and a 28-gauge chest tube was inserted in the fifth intercostal space midaxillary line and placed apically in the thorax. The chest tube was connected to a UWSD system. Paul's vital signs improved and remained stable. He was transferred to a medical ward. No air leak was noted and the chest tube was removed 24 hours later. Chest X-ray following removal was normal. Paul's nursing care focussed on assessment of his respiratory status, management of the chest tube and underwater seal drainage and education about recurrent spontaneous pneumothorax. Paul was discharged home after 48 hours.

TENSION PNEUMOTHORAX

A tension pneumothorax occurs when a laceration of the pleura allows air into the pleural space but does not allow air to exit. The pressure or tension increases and builds in the intrapleural space causing the affected lung to collapse and the mediastinal contents to be squeezed and shift to the unaffected side[20]. This dramatically increasing pressure and mediastinal shift causes the heart and great vessels to be compressed until there is no space for blood to be pumped into or out of the heart.

Tension pneumothorax is a life-threatening problem. Clinical manifestations are severe dyspnoea, tachypnoea, decreased or absent breath sounds on the affected side, tracheal deviation to the unaffected side. Clinical deterioration can progress to absent palpable blood pressure and pulse and profound hypoxia. Emergency treatment by rapid needle decompression of the tension pneumothorax[26] is required, using a large-bore needle (greater than 16 gauge) inserted in the second intercostal space, mid-clavicular line on the affected side. Decompression is immediate, with rapid return of heartbeat and blood pressure. Later a chest tube is inserted and attached to a UWSD system as discussed earlier.

HAEMOTHORAX

A haemothorax is a collection of blood in the intrapleural space. Blunt or penetrating injury to the chest wall may cause local vessels, such as the internal mammary arteries or intercostal arteries, to rupture. A large haemothorax is defined as a collection of greater than 1.5 L of blood in the pleural space[26]. Clinical manifestations will be as for pneumothorax, but in addition percussion of the chest elicits a dull sound. A haemothorax may also include symptoms of shock from blood loss, such as decreased blood pressure, tachycardia, pale, cool or clammy skin, poor capillary refill and flat neck veins. Diagnosis is made through clinical presentation, history and chest radiograph. Treatment is the insertion of a chest drain into the 5–6th intercostal space, midaxillary line on the affected side for drainage of the blood and then fluid resuscitation is given for any signs of shock[19].

PULMONARY CONTUSION

A pulmonary contusion is a bruising of lung tissue and often results from blunt trauma such as a rapid compression/decompression injury[19]. The haemorrhagic and resulting oedematous effects of the bruising may be mild or severe. Clinical manifestations include haemoptysis, tachycardia, tachypnoea and dull chest pain, localised over the site of the contusion. If the contusion is severe, the patient may progress to type 2 hypercapnoeic hypoxic respiratory failure. Treatment is aimed at supporting oxygenation and ventilation with supplemental oxygen, analgesia and non-invasive ventilation (NIV) strategies, such as continuous positive airways pressure (CPAP) or biphasic positive airway pressure (BiPAP). Severe pulmonary contusion may require supportive invasive mechanical ventilation[4,27].

RIB FRACTURES

Fractures of the ribs are most commonly caused by blunt trauma[20]. Ribs 5–10 are most commonly fractured. Rib fractures may potentially rupture the intercostal arteries, which lie in the groove of the inferior margin of each rib. Although the blood loss from intercostal artery rupture does not compromise the young and fit, it can be a potential problem for the older adult and patients with pre-existing clinical compromise. Clinical manifestations of rib fractures include chest wall pain that worsens with deep breathing or coughing, localised tenderness, shallow, rapid respirations, tachycardia and possible raised blood pressure. Diagnosis is confirmed by chest X-ray. Simple rib fractures may be treated with intercostal nerve block, oral analgesia and incentive spirometry. Extensive rib fractures (e.g., flail segment) may require invasive supportive therapy, such as mechanical ventilation and sedation[26,27].

INFECTIVE RESPIRATORY HEALTH BREAKDOWN

As a person breathes and the respiratory system filters air, there is exposure to many airborne irritating particles and infective agents. This section discusses upper and lower respiratory tract infections. Infections of the upper airways are predominately minor in nature and are managed in a primary care setting. Lower respiratory tract infections can be more complex, and may alter the function of other body systems and the health of the whole individual.

UPPER RESPIRATORY TRACT INFECTIONS
VIRAL RHINITIS
Upper respiratory tract infections are among the most common diseases of humans, with viral rhinitis (common cold) being the most prevalent[28]. It is spread by airborne droplet, and symptoms include sneezing, local itching and copious nasal secretions leading to obstruction, all due to local inflammation. Systemic symptoms of the immune system response, such as elevated temperature and malaise, may also be present. Treatment focuses on symptom relief while the virus is self-limiting.

ALLERGIC RHINITIS
Similar local symptoms to viral rhinitis occur in allergic rhinitis; however, the local reaction is due to an allergen rather than a virus (e.g., pollens, dust, pet hair, moulds). Treatment of symptoms involves application of anti-inflammatory agents by nasal spray, or use of antihistamines and decongestants, as well as identification and elimination of triggers[3].

SINUSITIS

Sinusitis occurs when the exit from the sinuses becomes narrowed or blocked due to inflammation or hypertrophy, and secretions accumulate behind the ostia providing a medium for bacterial growth. The resulting collection and inflammation cause local pain, headache and systemic symptoms of infection. Sinusitis can be of an acute or chronic nature, and is a common complication of both allergic and viral rhinitis. Treatment may include antibiotics and symptom management with analgesics, decongestants and nasal sprays to reduce local oedema and loosen purulent secretions[3].

PHARYNGITIS AND TONSILLITIS

Pharyngitis is an acute inflammation of the pharyngeal walls and may include the tonsils, palate and uvula. A viral agent is frequently the cause of acute episodes[28]. Tonsillitis is an acute inflammation and infection of the palatine tonsils and is commonly bacterial in nature. *Group A beta-hemolytic streptococcus* is a common causative organism in both pharyngitis and tonsillitis (commonly called strep throat)[28]. Local infection and inflammation cause lymph node enlargement, swelling, erythema and pain. Systemic symptoms include fever and arthralgia. Treatment with antibiotics is warranted if the source is thought to be bacterial. Dysphagia due to local pain may be treated with analgesics to facilitate hydration and nutrition[3].

LARYNGITIS

Laryngitis is acute inflammation of the larynx and is often associated with either upper or lower respiratory infections, or local irritation due to pollutants, or excessive use of the voice. A change in the voice pitch and tone is due to the localised inflammation and swelling altering the airflow through the larynx[3].

LOWER RESPIRATORY TRACT PROBLEMS
BRONCHIOLITIS

Bronchiolitis is an acute lower respiratory viral infection of the bronchioles that is commonly caused by the respiratory syncytial virus (RSV)[29]. It frequently occurs in children, particularly infants under 2 years of age. It is the most common pathogen linked to respiratory illness and hospitalisation of infants and young children. In adults, RSV presents as a minor upper respiratory tract infection. In children with RSV, the bronchiole mucosa swells in response to infection and inflammation, the small airways fill with mucous and exudate, and acute respiratory distress rapidly follows. Treatment for infants is supportive and primarily focuses on supplemental oxygen, humidification to loosen secretions, rest and nasogastric feeds if distress is severe[29].

ACUTE BRONCHITIS

Acute bronchitis is an inflammation of the bronchi in the lower respiratory tract. It can be caused by bacteria, viruses or exposure to inhaled irritants[30]. It is often associated with smoking or an existing upper respiratory tract infection. Acute bronchitis is usually self limiting and of a short nature. It should be differentiated from chronic bronchitis, which is usually associated with chronic obstructive pulmonary disease (refer to section later in this chapter).

Clinical manifestations of acute bronchitis consist of productive cough, fever, headache and dyspnoea. Management is usually based on symptomatic treatment for clinical manifestations and includes antibiotics, adequate fluid intake, rest and supplemental oxygen if required.

PNEUMONIA

Pneumonia is defined as acute inflammation of the lung parenchyma (bronchioles and alveoli). It can be infective in nature due to bacterial, viral or fungal agents. Before the discovery of penicillin and sulpha-based drugs, bacterial pneumonia was a leading cause of death among children and adults[31].

In a healthy person, the airway below the trachea is sterile due to many protective mechanisms (e.g., the cough reflex, the epiglottis, ciliary action and microscopic action of the immune system)[2]. A person with pneumonia acquires organisms below the trachea by three main mechanisms: 1) aspiration of organisms from the nasopharynx or oropharynx; 2) inhalation of organisms that are airborne; and 3) haematogenous spread from a primary source of infection elsewhere in the body. Once the infectious agent reaches the lung tissue, multiplication takes place in the warm, moist environment and the infection spreads to other local lung tissue. The inflammatory response is initiated and mediators are released which cause dilation of capillaries, resulting in diffusion impairment and accumulation of various blood cells, exudate and serous fluid. The infected lung parenchyma functions poorly and acute respiratory failure may follow.

Clinical manifestations include localised symptoms of inflammation such as coughing, and increased mucous production. On auscultation, breath sounds may be diminished or even absent over the affected areas, and crackles (rales) may also be heard. Systemic symptoms include dyspnoea, tachypnoea, orthopnoea, tachycardia and elevated temperature. Pain on inspiration may also be present due to inflammation, and the patient may be fatigued due to an increased work of breathing.

Treatment involves supportive therapies, such as supplemental oxygen and physiotherapy, to manage symptoms. Antibiotic therapy is specific to the infective agent and is determined by microscopic culture and sensitivity of sputum[3,32].

SEVERE ACUTE RESPIRATORY SYNDROME

Severe acute respiratory syndrome (SARS) is a viral respiratory illness caused by a coronavirus, called SARS-associated Coronavirus (SARS CoV)[33]. The first cases of SARS emerged in November, 2002 from Guangdong Province, China. Following the global outbreak (February–June 2003), data from the World Health Organization Ad Hoc Working Group on the Epidemiology of SARS[34] noted a cumulative total of 8422 probable cases, with 916 patient deaths reported from 29 countries, and 63% of cases from mainland China.

It would appear that SARS is transmitted through exposure to infected respiratory droplets during close person-to-person contact. The pathophysiology of SARS is not fully understood. It is postulated that destruction of lung tissue is as a result of an exacerbated immune response rather than from the direct effects of viral replication[35]. The exacerbated immune response is initiated and the pathophysiological sequela follows that of pneumonia. The infected lung parenchyma functions poorly, and severe acute respiratory failure may follow.

SARS presents as an atypical pneumonia. Clinical manifestations of SARS include initial presentation of fever (>38.0°C), headache and overall malaise. Some patients also present with mild respiratory symptoms such as dyspnoea. Within 2–7 days, patients develop a dry cough. Between 10–20% of patients also complain of diarrhoea. The majority of patients with SARS have a clear history of either exposure to a case of SARS or to a setting where SARS transmission was occurring[34]. Patients with SARS appear to be most infectious at days 7–9 of illness. At this point some patients recover, whereas others appear to rapidly deteriorate to severe respiratory failure[35].

There is no specific treatment for SARS itself. Treatment focuses on symptom management of acute respiratory failure. Patients with severe respiratory failure may require mechanical ventilation support[34,35].

TUBERCULOSIS

Tuberculosis is an infectious disease caused by *Mycobacterium tuberculi*, which usually infects the lungs. Tuberculosis is an opportunistic, infective agent and people at risk include those in poor health (e.g., immunosuppression), those who are homeless, or those who reside in close proximity to others (e.g., refugee camp residents)[3]. The World Health Organization estimates that worldwide over 8 million new cases of tuberculosis are diagnosed each year and approximately 3 million people die from the disease annually[36].

The bacilli are inhaled during close contact with an infected individual and multiply with little initial resistance from the host[9]. Most patients with tuberculosis are asymptomatic when diagnosed. Specific manifestations may include fatigue, weight loss, low-grade pyrexia, and night sweats. Pulmonary tuberculosis manifests in a moist and productive cough which is sometimes accompanied by generalised dull chest pain[36]. A combination pharmacological therapy (e.g., isoniazid, rifampicin, pyrazinamide, streptomycin, ethambutol) is the mainstay of management of tuberculosis[37].

CHRONIC RESPIRATORY HEALTH BREAKDOWN

Chronic respiratory problems are those that persist for a long time, often the person's remaining life span, for which there is no curative option. A common term currently utilised is chronic airflow limitation (CAL). CAL encompasses both the obstructive and restrictive components that exist in chronic respiratory disease. Asthma and chronic obstructive pulmonary disease (COPD), the two key health breakdown areas to be addressed in this section, are both characterised by airflow obstruction. These problems can be minor in nature or quite debilitating. Treatment aims to eliminate exacerbations, minimise the impact on lifestyle by symptoms experienced, and slow or stop the progression of the disease[38,39].

ASTHMA

The prevalence of asthma is rising worldwide[40]. Asthma is a chronic, inflammatory disorder of the tracheobronchial tree, in which the patient experiences recurrent episodes of wheezing, breathlessness, coughing and feelings of chest tightness. Asthma is the most common chronic disease of childhood, and a significant proportion of children will continue to experience it into adulthood[29]. Status asthmaticus is a severe, life threatening asthma attack that is resistant to usual treatment[7].

Case study

Jason Nguyen, 23, presents to the emergency department complaining of shortness of breath and appears quite pale and anxious. The history he gives to the nurse includes working casually in the building trade as a labourer. He says he gets hay fever sometimes but is otherwise healthy, and has no known food or drug allergies. He reports one hospitalisation as a 4-year-old for asthma, but thought he had grown out of it and has not taken any drugs for asthma for years. On examination of his chest, he has extensive accessory muscle use on inspiration and bilateral expiratory wheezing. Vital signs are respiratory rate 32 breaths/min, blood pressure 147/86 mmHg, pulse 108 beats/minute, temperature 37.0°C and oxygen saturation of 86% on room air. An arterial blood gas sample reveals pH – 7.33 (7.35–7.45), PaO_2 – 70 mmHg (80–100 mmHg), $PaCO_2$ – 52 mmHg (35–45 mmHg), and HCO_3 – 24 mmol/L (22–26 mmol/L). Jason is initially given 6 L/min of supplemental oxygen via a facemask and sat upright in a chair. The doctor prescribes 2 puffs of salbutamol inhaler via a spacer, to be repeated three times over the next 15 minutes.

WHAT IS THE PATHOPHYSIOLOGY OF ASTHMA?

Asthma is triggered by exposure to triggers that activate a complex interaction of inflammatory cells, including mast cells, eosinophils, lymphocytes, epithelial cells, neutrophils and platelets. Known extrinsic triggers include dust mites, environmental tobacco smoke, pet hair or intrinsic triggers such as a respiratory infection or exercise[3,41]. Air flow during an episode is limited by the inflammatory process stimulating the parasympathetic nerves in the lung tissues, causing constriction of the smooth muscle in the bronchioles, narrowing the airway lumens and increasing airway resistance. The intensity of this bronchoconstriction is directly related to the severity of the inflammatory process[41]. The inflammatory response also results in histamine release and vasodilation, causing swelling of the airways and increased mucous production that further obstructs the airways. These factors result in hyperinflation of the lungs, ventilation-perfusion abnormalities, and changes in arterial blood oxygen and carbon dioxide levels.

WHAT ARE THE CLINICAL MANIFESTATIONS OF ASTHMA?

The patient may experience recurrent episodes of asthma with an onset either abrupt onset (within minutes) or gradual onset (over a period of hours or days). Table 6.5 summarises the clinical manifestations and associated arterial blood gas changes.

WHAT DIAGNOSTIC INVESTIGATIONS ARE APPROPRIATE?

The diagnosis of asthma requires a thorough patient history and physical assessment and the use of adjunctive diagnostic investigations[3]. The characteristic symptoms suggestive of asthma are: wheeze, chest tightness, shortness of breath and cough. These symptoms may be recurrent, worse at night or in the early morning, or triggered by exercise, irritants, allergens or viral infections. However, the symptoms of asthma vary widely from person

TABLE 6.5: CLINICAL MANIFESTATIONS AND ASSOCIATED ARTERIAL BLOOD GAS CHANGES

Time Frame	pH	PaCO₂	PaO₂	Clinical Manifestations
Early in episode	⇧ or normal	⇩ or normal	⇩	Dyspnoea, coughing, feelings of chest tightness, wheezing, prolonged expiration, accessory muscle use, tachycardia
Progressing episode				Fatigue, worsening dyspnoea leads to speaking in broken sentences or single words, harsh breath sounds from oedematous airways
Prolonged attack or status asthmaticus	⇩	⇧	⇩	Exhaustion, diminished breath sounds due to severe obstruction, change in level of consciousness due to hypercapnoea

to person and it is important to note that absence of typical symptoms does not exclude the diagnosis of asthma.

The primary diagnostic investigation of pulmonary function for asthma is spirometry. Spirometry measures the maximal volume of air forcibly and quickly exhaled by the patient following a maximal inhalation (forced vital capacity, FVC) and the maximum volume of air the patient can exhale during the first second of the FVC (forced expiratory volume in 1 second, FEV_1) [1]. The aim of spirometry is to assess the degree of the patient's airflow obstruction (manifested by decreased FEV_1 and FEV_1 to FVC ratio), and to measure the extent of airflow obstruction compared to predicted normal values (where a 12% and 200 mL improvement in FEV_1 is expected after the administration of bronchodilator therapy, e.g., reversible airflow obstruction)[42].

Spirometry is generally recommended over measurements by a peak flow meter[40,43]. The peak flow meter is a home-use device. It is used to detect and measure a patient's variation from their predetermined best peak flow and so indicate the presence and degree of airflow obstruction as an aid to self-management.

A diagnosis of asthma can be made when a patient has the following criteria:

- Variable symptoms (especially cough, chest tightness, wheeze and shortness of breath);
- Forced expiratory volume (FEV_1) increases by 15% or more in adults and children after bronchodilator medication (provided that in adults the baseline FEV_1 is more than 1.3 L);
- Peak expiratory flow (PEF) increases by 20% after bronchodilator medication, provided the adult baseline peak flow is more than 300 L per min; and
- PEF in adults varies by 20% within a day on more than one occasion[42].

Additional diagnostic investigations are not routine for the diagnosis of asthma. However, other investigations may be considered as no single investigation is appropriate for every patient. The following investigations may be useful when considering alternative diagnoses, identifying precipitating factors for asthma, assessing asthma severity, and investigating potential complications: chest X-ray, bronchial challenge tests (e.g., histamine, methacholine, hypertonic saline) and allergy testing utilising skin prick tests or a radioallergoabsorbent test (RAST)[42].

APPLIED PHARMACOLOGY

The two main goals of medication use in asthma are to prevent and control symptoms while reducing the frequency and severity of episodes. The first goal is to prophylactically reduce the sensitivity of airways to allergens by reducing the inflammatory reactivity with long-term use of corticosteroid-based inhalations, such as beclomethasone and budesonide. As a group, these pharmacological agents are commonly called preventers. If the episode is severe, systemic corticosteroids (e.g., prednisolone) may also be used to combat the inflammatory aspect of the acute episode. The second goal of treatment is the use of inhaled beta$_2$ adrenoreceptor agonists to relieve the bronchoconstriction and open the airways, commonly called relievers. Short-acting beta$_2$ adrenoreceptor agonists, such as salbutamol or terbutaline, act in approximately five minutes and their effect lasts three to four hours[37]. Three sequential treatments in one hour are often used in the acute phase to relieve symptoms[41]. These drugs are delivered directly to the lung tissue via inhaler devices. Knowledge of how to operate the inhaler devices is important to ensure a high percentage of the drug actually reaches the target tissue. Anticholinergic agents (e.g., ipratropium) also produce bronchial dilation; however, their effect and action makes them more suitable for maintenance treatment or combination therapy rather than acute symptom relief[32,37]. While these pharmacological agents take effect, the maintenance of oxygenation through use of supplemental oxygen and prevention of fatigue or exertion is a priority in an acute episode.

NURSING IMPLICATIONS
ACUTE EPISODE OF ASTHMA

Health treatment for a patient with an acute episode of asthma health treatment aims to reduce the airway inflammation, hyper-reactivity and hyper-responsiveness of the lower respiratory system, while maintaining adequate systemic oxygenation. The nurse's role is twofold in: (1) administering oxygen therapy and medications, and (2) monitoring the effectiveness of treatments and severity of the exacerbation. Repeated doses of inhaled B$_2$ adrenergic agonists such as Ventolin are used and corticosteroids may also be prescribed[42]. The choice of drug therapy often depends on the severity of asthma symptoms. The monitoring role consists of frequent nursing assessment of respiratory and cardiovascular systems including peak expiratory flow rate, lung sounds, respiratory rate and the work of breathing, e.g., accessory muscle use, heart rate and blood pressure. The degree of wheezing a patient has during an acute episode of asthma does not correlate to the severity of an asthma attack. Many patients with severe obstruction are not able to expel enough air to generate a loud wheeze. Oximetry is part of monitoring and is also used to titrate oxygen therapy. If the attack is severe ABGs may also be used in monitoring.

HEALTH TEACHING

Skilled home self-management by the individual, in conjunction with regular and ongoing health professional review, provides the best outcome for patients who have asthma. The use of a written asthma management plan, developed in conjunction with the patient and family, can resolve confusion when multiple medications and monitoring regimes are needed[42]. Patients should be taught to recognise individual asthma triggers and avoid them.

Correct use of inhalation devices, such as spacers and metered dose inhalers, understanding of the use and action of medications and daily peak expiratory flow monitoring are key areas of patient teaching[42]. This is achieved through patient education within a partnership approach where the nurse facilitates the patient's knowledge development and collaborates with the patient in monitoring and establishing asthma preventative management behaviours, for example using a B_2 adrenergic agonist 20 minutes before exercise. These strategies reduce the frequency of asthma symptoms, exacerbations and the impact of asthma on lifestyle, for example sick leave from work.

LEARNING EXERCISES

1. Describe the risk factors for the development of asthma.
2. Outline the pathophysiology of the signs and symptoms associated with asthma.
3. Outline the clinical manifestations of a patient with asthma.
4. Explain the nursing management of a patient with poor oxygenation related to asthma.
5. Explain the goals of patient education related to the prevention of exacerbation of asthma signs and symptoms.

In this case study, Jason's history of childhood asthma and hay fever indicate airway reactivity to allergens. Observed clinical data on the respiratory system includes wheezing, accessory muscle use and respiratory rate of 28 breaths/min – this clearly indicates that Jason is using physiological compensatory mechanisms to combat the effects of poor air flow from bronchoconstriction due to asthma. The low oxygen saturation of 86% indicates hypoxia, and the observed tachycardia, pallor and anxiety also support this. The ABGs indicate Jason may then be classified as having type 1 hypoxaemic respiratory failure. However, if his condition worsens or he becomes fatigued, he may also progress to type 2 hypercapnoeic respiratory failure. The mechanism of respiratory failure in asthma is primarily *alveolar hypoventilation* as the bronchospasm limits expiratory airflow. As the episode progresses or if it becomes severe, there may also be diffusion limitation due to oedema and obstruction of the small airways with mucus. His blood pressure and pulse are both high and are being influenced by the *stress response* of the sympathetic nervous system, as well as his anxiety. The ABGs indicate respiratory acidosis, hypoxia, and carbon dioxide is beginning to be retained as Jason's level is at the higher end of the normal range. These changes are a result of poor ventilation. Treatment with supplemental oxygen will support Jason's oxygenation and combat the symptoms of acute respiratory failure; positioning will support ventilation while the salbutamol takes effect to relieve the bronchoconstriction. After these initial treatment measures, Jason's response will be evaluated and further clinical data collected to guide additional interventions.

CHRONIC OBSTRUCTIVE PULMONARY DISEASE

Chronic obstructive pulmonary disease (COPD) is characterised by airflow obstruction that is caused by either emphysema or chronic bronchitis, or a combination of both disease processes[39,41]. COPD is a largely preventable disease that is a leading cause of mortality and morbidity worldwide, for which the rates of both are rising. It characteristically affects middle-aged and elderly people, and its aetiology is strongly associated with cigarette smoking, and it is progressive in those who continue to smoke[44]. The mechanisms by which smoking tobacco causes COPD are complex, as each cigarette contains thousands of individual chemicals that stimulate inflammation and tissue breakdown. Tobacco products overwhelm normal respiratory system defences, stimulating inflammation and increased numbers of neutrophils and macrophages, which release enzymes that destroy alveolar tissue and contribute to the breakdown of connective tissue[28]. Smoking also decreases ciliary activity and causes hyperplasia of the goblet cells, resulting in excessive mucous production and narrowed airways.

PATHOPHYSIOLOGY OF EMPHYSEMA

Emphysema is characterised by breakdown of elastin and collagen, resulting in hyperinflation of the alveoli, destruction of the alveoli walls, and formation of large air spaces (lobules), which have less surface area than normal alveoli[11]. These spaces have reduced pulmonary circulation through destruction of the alveoli capillary walls, resulting in less alveolar-capillary diffusion and therefore decreased gas exchange. To compensate for this, the person with emphysema subconsciously increases their respiratory rate to increase alveolar ventilation. Emphysema can be centrilobular, where the primary area of involvement is the central portion of the bronchioles (often associated with chronic bronchitis), or panlobular, where the destruction and distension is distal to the bronchioles[2]. The clinical manifestations of emphysema and chronic bronchitis are summarised in Table 6.6.

PATHOPHYSIOLOGY OF CHRONIC BRONCHITIS

Chronic bronchitis is characterised by over-production of mucus in the bronchi accompanied by a recurrent cough. The over-supply of mucus is related to hyperplasia of the mucous-secreting glands in the trachea and bronchi, and an increase in the number of goblet cells in the lower respiratory tract[10]. Normal defence mechanisms function poorly as cilia are eroded, alveolar macrophages function inadequately and inflammatory changes narrow the small airways. Consequently, alveolar diffusion is impaired, and there may also be a physiological shunt due to mucus preventing gas exchange. Lower respiratory tract infections are common, as the over-production of mucus and lowered defences provide an ideal environment for microorganisms to flourish[44].

WHAT DIAGNOSTIC INVESTIGATIONS ARE APPROPRIATE?

The diagnosis of COPD also requires a thorough patient history, physical assessment and use of further diagnostic investigations[3]. The characteristic symptoms suggestive of COPD are: shortness of breath (typically on exertion), cough and sputum production. Other common symptoms may include: chest tightness and wheezing (although this is often absent in severe, stable COPD).

The primary diagnostic investigation of pulmonary function for COPD is spirometry. COPD diagnosis is determined by the presence of irreversible airflow obstruction. Unlike asthma, the obstructive element of COPD is not able to be reversed by medications or other treatments. Airflow obstruction is non-reversible when, after the administration of

TABLE 6.6: CLINICAL MANIFESTATIONS OF CHRONIC OBSTRUCTIVE PULMONARY DISEASE

Feature	Emphysema	Chronic Bronchitis
Health history	Generally healthy, but a smoker	Recurrent chest infections, exacerbation of symptoms by irritants and cold air, smoker
Cough/sputum	Minor/negligible	Significant/copious purulent
Physical examination and general appearance	Cachectic, history of weight loss and protein-calorie malnutrition	Tendency towards obesity, cyanotic, polycythaemia, oedematous, distended neck veins, and other symptoms of right heart failure
Dyspnoea	Slowly progressive	Variable, often late in illness
Breath sounds	Quiet or diminished	Scattered wheezing, gurgles (rhonchi), crackles (rales)
Chest appearance	Increase in anteroposterior diameter, barrel chest, prominent accessory muscles of respiration, limited diaphragmatic excursion	Slight to marked increase in anteroposterior diameter, pulmonary hypertension
ABGs	Near normal, $\downarrow PaO_2$, normal or $\downarrow PaCO_2$, hypercapnia in late disease	$\downarrow PaO_2$, $\uparrow PaCO_2$
Chest X-ray	Hyperinflation, flat diaphragm, widened intercostal margins	Congested lung fields, cardiac enlargement

Many people with COPD may have one dominant disease process. However, some may also have elements of both emphysema and chronic bronchitis.

bronchodilator therapy, the ratio of FEV_1 to FVC is less than 70% and the FEV_1 is less than 80% of the predicted "normal" value. The ratio of FEV_1 to vital capacity (VC) is a sensitive indicator for mild COPD[45].

The following additional investigations may be useful when considering the diagnosis of COPD, alternative diagnoses, assessing COPD severity, and investigating potential complications:

• Chest X-ray (although not sensitive in the diagnosis of COPD, it is useful to exclude other conditions such as lung cancer);
• High resolution computed tomography (HRCT) scanning (gives precise images of the lung tissue and mediastinal structures so the presence of emphysema and the size and number of bullae can be determined);
• ABG measurement (should be considered in all patients with severe respiratory disease and those patients whose dyspnoea is disproportional to their clinical status);
• Sputum examination (this is recommended for patients with an acute exacerbation of COPD);
• Complex lung function tests (to measure of airways resistance, static lung volumes and compliance);
• Exercise testing (to identify other causes of exercise limitation such as hyperventilation and musculoskeletal disorders); and
• Sleep studies (where overnight pulse oximetry may be indicated for COPD patients receiving long-term domiciliary oxygen therapy to assess its efficacy)[45].

APPLIED PHARMACOLOGY

Medications useful in preventing exacerbations and managing chronic symptoms of COPD include agents that dissolve mucus (mucolytics), and a combination regimen of inhaled short-acting (salbutamol) and long-acting (salmeterol) beta$_2$ agonists and anticholinergics, such as ipratropium[44,46] which reduce the inflammation and reactivity of the airways. Acute exacerbation of COPD symptoms are commonly caused by viral or bacterial (70%) infection[44]. Antibiotic agents and short-term use of corticosteroids are also effective in reducing infection, inflammation and airway reactivity, reducing the patient's symptoms and promoting recovery[46].

NURSING IMPLICATIONS

Acute exacerbation of COPD leading to acute respiratory failure is a common complication of this disease. Due to the chronic nature of COPD, patients may delay seeking treatment for exacerbation from the health team, allowing symptoms and physiological compromise to worsen. Symptoms of exacerbation of the chronic state of COPD include systemic symptoms of fever and increasing fatigue as well as respiratory symptoms such as increasing dyspnoea, worsening cough, wheezing indicating bronchospasm and an increase in sputum production or purulence[46]. In 70% of patients with acute exacerbations of COPD a bacterial infection is the primary cause. Exacerbations are also commonly caused by viral infections and airborne irritants such as pollution[44]. Health treatment of acute exacerbation focuses on minimisation of symptoms with medications, lifestyle adaptations that limit exertion and supplemental oxygen to support oxygenation.

In the past, there has been concern over administering high-flow oxygen to patients with COPD. Normally CO_2 accumulation is the stimulant that drives the respiratory centre however, some patients with COPD retain CO_2 due to their disease and develop a tolerance for high levels of CO_2; consequently loosing their sensitivity to CO_2. These patients theoretically rely on hypoxaemia as their respiratory centre stimulus and when supplemental oxygen is administered, this stimulus may be removed and the respiratory drive suppressed. In practice, if oxygen is titrated to the lowest effective dose using ABG data and the patient closely monitored, respiratory centre suppression with an over supply of oxygen is not a serious threat. It is important to note supplying adequate oxygen to support all aspects of body tissue function takes priority over potential CO_2 retention.

HEALTH TEACHING

Health teaching is an important dimension of the nurse's role in providing nursing care for patient's with COPD. Teaching centres on increasing patient knowledge of medications and treatment devices to promote self-care management and preserve functional capacity. Assisting the patient to learn new adaptive behaviours that improve their day-to-day functioning and decrease the individual impact of their disease symptoms is also a priority, for example using home oxygen while undertaking energy consuming activities like hygiene. It is useful to consider referral to a structured respiratory rehabilitation program that addresses strategies to enhance cardiovascular fitness, exercise endurance and psychosocial coping. These programs may decrease individual disability and have a positive effect on quality of life[47].

CONCLUSION

The respiratory system is comprised of the upper and lower respiratory tracts. The primary function of the respiratory system is to provide oxygen for all metabolic processes in cells and tissues and to remove carbon dioxide, the gaseous waste products of metabolism. Knowledge of respiratory anatomy and physiology is the foundation from which the nurse develops an understanding of the impact of respiratory disease and makes clinical decisions regarding nursing strategies to enhance the person's oxygenation and ventilation.

Respiratory health breakdown can be categorised as traumatic, infective and chronic. Nursing practice interventions to address traumatic and infective respiratory health breakdown include: symptomatic support with patient positioning and administration of supplemental oxygen, management of pain, management of chest drains, administering bactericidal agents, and education regarding self-management of therapies and lifestyle modifications.

Nursing patients with chronic respiratory dysfunction can be complex. The effect of respiratory disease on an individual's physical functioning and lifestyle is often limiting, and can become debilitating as the condition progresses. The primary nursing activities in caring for a person with chronic respiratory dysfunction in the acute setting, initially focus on minimising and controlling acute exacerbations. This is achieved using systemic and inhaled medications and various oxygen-delivery devices, limiting physical activity, and supporting the psychological status of the patient and their significant others. Ongoing practice focuses on patient education and support concerning self-care, monitoring and medication management.

Recommended Readings

Chen, E, Bloomberg, G, Fisher, E & Strunk, R. 2003; 'Predictors of Repeat Hospitalisations in Children with Asthma: The Role of Psychosocial and Environmental Factors', *Health Psychology*, 22 (1), 12–18.

Finesilver, CA. 2001; 'Perfecting Your Skills: Respiratory Assessment', *Travel Nursing Today*, (April), (supplement), 17–20, 22, 24, 26, 28.

Howell, M. 2002; Pulse Oximetry: An Audit of Nursing and Medical Staff Understanding', *British Journal of Nursing*, 11 (3), 191–197.

Hunter, M & King, D. 2001; 'COPD: Management of Acute Exacerbations and Chronic Stable Disease', *American Family Physician*, 64 (4), 603–612, 621–622.

Kirksey, KM, Holt-Ashley, M & Goodroad, BK. 2001; 'An Easy Method for Interpreting the Results of Arterial Blood Gas Analysis', *Critical Care Nurse*, 21 (5), 49–54.

References

1. Thibodeau, G & Patton, K. 2004; *Structure and Function of the Body* (12th ed.), Mosby, St Louis.
2. Huether, S & McCance, K. 2004; *Understanding Pathophysiology* (3rd ed.), Mosby, St Louis.
3. Wilkins, RL, Stoller, JK & Scanlan, CL. 2003; *Egan's Fundamentals of Respiratory Care*, Mosby, St Louis.
4. Urden, LD, Stacy, KM & Lough, ME. 2002; *Thelan's Critical Care Nursing: Diagnosis and Management*, Mosby, St Louis.
5. Lowton, K. 1999; 'Pulse Oximeters for the Detection of Hypoxaemia', *Professional Nurse*, 14 (5), 243–350.
6. Horne, C & Derrico, D. 1999; 'Mastering ABGs: The Art of Arterial Blood Gas Measurement. *American Journal of Nursing*, 99 (8), 26–32.
7. Sheldon, LK. 2001; *Nursing Concepts: Oxygenation*, Slack, New Jersey.

8. Fuller, J & Schaller, J. 2000; *Health Assessment: A Nursing Approach*, Lippincott Williams and Wilkins, Philadelphia.

9. Stevens, A & Lowe, J. 2000; *Pathology* (2nd ed.), Mosby, London.

10. Price, S & Wilson, L. 2003; *Pathophysiology - Clinical Concepts of Disease Processes* (6th ed.), Mosby, St Louis.

11. Groer, M. 2001; *Advanced Pathophysiology: Application to Clinical Practice*, Lippincott, Philadelphia.

12. Finesilver, CA. 2001; 'Perfecting Your Skills: Respiratory Assessment', *RN*, (supplement: 'Travel Nursing Today'), 16–28.

13. Wong, FWH. 1999; 'A New Approach to ABG Interpretation', *American Journal of Nursing*, 99 (8), 34–36.

14. Berry, BF & Pinard, AE. 2002; 'Assessing Tissue Oxygenation', *Critical Care Nurse*, 22 (3), 22–40.

15. Place, B. 2000; 'Pulse Oximetry: Benefits and Limitations', *Nursing Times*, 95 (26), 42.

16. Siela, D. 2002; 'Using Chest Radiograph in the Intensive Care Unit', *Critical Care Nurse*, 22 (4), 18–27.

17. Connelly, MA. 2001; 'Chest X-Rays: Completing the Picture', *RN*, 64 (6), 57–62.

18. Corne, J. *et al.* 2002; *Chest X-Ray Made Easy*, Churchill-Livingston, Edinburgh.

19. Brown, AF. 2001; *Emergency Medicine: Diagnosis and Management*, Butterworth Heinemann, Port Melbourne.

20. Trott, AT. 2003; *Chest Trauma in Emergency Medicine: An Approach to Clinical Problem Solving*, Hamilton, *et al.* (eds.), W.B. Saunders, Philadelphia, 758–773.

21. Baumann, EA. 2001; 'Management of Spontaneous Pneumothorax: An American College of Chest Physicians Delphi Consensus Statement', *Chest*, 119, 590.

22. Sahn, S & Hefner, J. 2000; 'Spontaneous Pneumothorax', *New England Journal of Medicine*, 342, 868–873.

23. Crowley, LV. 1997; *Introduction to Human Disease* (4th ed.), Jones & Bartlett, London.

24. Kirchner, JT. 2000; 'Diagnosis and Management of Spontaneous Pneumothorax', *American Family Physician*, 62 (6), 1398–1400.

25. Ross, RT & Burnett, CM. 2001; 'Talc Pleurodesis: A New Technique', *The American Surgeon*, 67 (5), 467–468.

26. O'Reilly, M. 2003; 'Major Trauma Management', in G Jones, R Endacott & R Crouch (eds.), *Emergency Nursing Care*, Greenwich Medical Media, London.

27. Hudak, C, Gallo, B & Morton, P. 1998; *Critical Care Nursing: A Holistic Approach*, Lippincott, Philadelphia.

28. Lewis, S, Heitkemper, M & Dirksen, S. 2000; *Medical Surgical Nursing*, Mosby, St Louis.

29. Hockenberry, M. 2000; *Wong's Nursing Care of Infants and Children*, Mosby, St Louis.

30. Hagler, D. 2004; 'Nursing Management: Upper Respiratory Problems', in M Heitkemper, S Dirksen & S Lewis (eds.), *Medical Surgical Nursing: Assessment and Management of Clinical Problems*, Mosby, St. Louis, 566–591.

31. Crimlisk, JT. 2004; 'Nursing Management: Lower Respiratory Problems', in M Heitkemper, S Dirksen & S Lewis (eds.), *Medical Surgical Nursing: Assessment And Management Of Clinical Problems*, Mosby, St Louis, 592–636.

32. Tiziani, A. 2002; *Harvard's Nursing Guide to Drugs* (6th ed.), Mosby, Marrickville, New South Wales.

33. Drosten, C, Gunther, S, Preiser, W, vander Werf, S, Brodt, H, Becker, S, *et al.* 'Identification of a Novel Coronavirus in Patients with Severe Acute Respiratory Syndrome', *New England Journal of Medicine*, 348, 1967–1976.

34. World Health Organization (WHO). 2003; 'The Management of Severe Acute Respiratory Syndrome (SARS)', Available at http://www.who.int/csr/sars/management/en/.

35. World Health Organization (WHO). 2003; 'Consensus Document on the Epidemiology of Severe Acute Respiratory Syndrome (SARS)', Available at http://www.who.int/csr/sars/en/WHOconsensus.pdf.

36. American Thoracic Society. 2000; 'Diagnostic Standards and Classification of Tuberculosis in Adults and Children', *American Journal of Respiratory and Critical Care Medicine*, 161, 1376.

37. Bryant, B, Knights, K & Salerno, E. 2003; *Pharmacology for Health Professionals*, Mosby, Sydney.

38. Lubkin, I & Larsen, P. 2002; *Chronic Illness: Impact and Interventions* (5th ed.), Jones & Bartlett, London.

39. Hunter, M. 2001; 'COPD: Management of Acute Exacerbations and Chronic Stable Disease', *American Family Physician*, 64 (4), 603–612.

40. Ladebauche, P. 1997; 'Managing Asthma: A Growth and Development Approach', *Pediatric Nursing*, 23 (1), 37–44.

41. Guthrie, C & Tingen, M. 2002; 'Asthma: A Case Study, Review Of Pathophysiology And Management Strategies', *Journal of the American Academy of Nurse Practitioners*, 14 (10), 457–61.

42. Kerstjens, H. 1999; 'Stable Chronic Obstructive Pulmonary Disease', *Clinical Evidence*, 1 (1).

43. Snow, V, Lascher, S & Mottur-Pilson, C. 2001; 'Evidence Base for Management of Acute Exacerbations of Chronic Obstructive Pulmonary Disease: Position Paper', *Annals of Internal Medicine*, 134 (7), 595–99.

44. Kerstjens, H. 1999; 'Stable Chronic Obstructive Pulmonary Disease', *Clinical Evidence*, 1 (1).

45. McKenzie, D, Frith, P, Burdon, J & Town, G. 2003; 'The COPDX Plan: Australian and New Zealand Guidelines for the Management of Chronic Obstructive Pulmonary Disease', *Medical Journal of Australia*, 178 (supplement 17 March), S1–S40.

46. Snow, V, Lascher, S & Mottur-Pilson, C. 2001; 'Evidence Base for Management of Acute Exacerbations of Chronic Obstructive Pulmonary Disease: Position Paper', *Annals of Internal Medicine*, 134 (7), 595–599.

47. Younf, PD, Fergusson, M, Colb, J. 1999; 'Improvement in Outcomes for Chronic Obstructive Pulmonary Disease (COPD) Attributable to a Hospital-based Respiratory Rehabilitation Program', *Australian New Zealand Journal of Medicine*, 29, 59–65.

7 | Renal Health Breakdown

AUTHORS

KATHLEEN KILSTOFF

ANN BONNER

LEARNING OBJECTIVES

When you have completed this chapter you will be able to

- Recognise the important anatomical and physiological features of the renal and genitourinary systems;
- Describe the pathophysiological changes associated with renal health breakdown;
- Understand the use of diagnostic and therapeutic techniques associated with caring for a person with renal health breakdown;
- Identify the common pharmacological agents used in managing renal health breakdown; and
- Consider nursing interventions required for people with renal health breakdown.

INTRODUCTION

More than one million Australians are currently experiencing a renal health breakdown with most of these due to urinary tract disorders. While health breakdown of the kidneys and urinary system can be due to a number of causes, the content of this chapter will focus on four distinct disorders. This chapter commences with a review of the anatomy and physiology of the renal and urinary system. Then case studies will be employed to facilitate discussion of acute renal failure, chronic renal failure, prostatic hyperplasia, and renal calculi.

WHAT MAKES UP THE RENAL AND URINARY SYSTEM?

The main organs of the renal system are the kidneys, through which blood plasma is processed and waste products are eliminated as urine via the urinary (accessory) organs, which include the ureters, urinary bladder and urethra (as shown in Figure 7.1). Waste products are formed from the metabolism of nitrogen (food protein) and muscle breakdown (body protein). Nitrogenous waste products, such as urea and creatinine, can be detected in blood and other fluids[1]. Other major functions of the kidneys include the maintenance of fluid and electrolyte balance (particularly sodium and potassium), acid–base balance, regulation of blood pressure and the production of hormones and enzymes.

The kidneys are located outside the peritoneum on either side of the vertebral column (level of T12 to L3). In each kidney there are approximately one million microscopic functioning units called the nephrons (see Figure 7.2), which are named according to their location in the kidney. Approximately 85% of nephrons are found in the outer cortex region (cortical nephrons) and 15% of nephrons arise in the inner medullary region (juxtamedullary nephrons)[2]. A network of peritubular capillaries that assist in reabsorption and excretion surrounds each nephron.

REGULATORY FUNCTIONS

There are discrete processes that occur in the cortex and medulla of the nephron that maintain the complex functioning of the kidney. These processes are involved in *glomerular filtration, tubular reabsorption, tubular secretion* of the blood plasma, and *excretion of urine*. The mechanisms by which these three processes occur are by diffusion, active transport, osmosis and filtration.

GLOMERULAR FILTRATION

The cortex contains the renal corpuscle, which consists of the glomerulus and the surrounding Bowman's capsule (see Figure 7.2). The glomerulus is composed of a coil of capillaries that are supplied by the afferent arterioles and drained by the efferent arterioles. Each minute approximately 1–1.5 L of blood (a quarter of cardiac output) is passed through the two million glomeruli where ultrafiltration takes place[3]. The speed and pressure of blood flow is determined by hydrostatic pressure (blood pressure). This process of *filtration* prevents larger molecules such as red blood cells and plasma protein from entering the

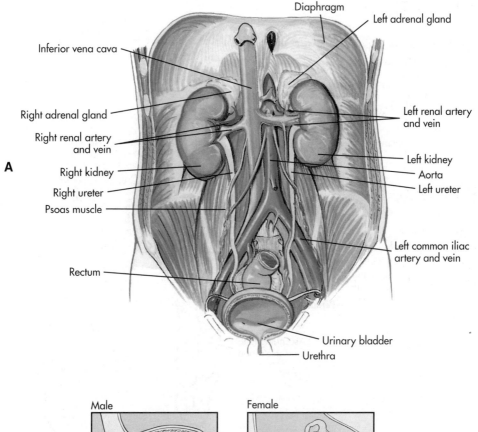

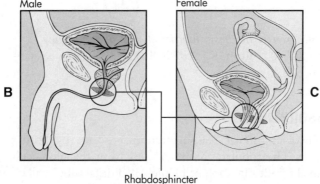

FIGURE 7.1 *Organs of the urinary system:* **A,** *upper urinary tract in relation to other anatomical structures;* **B,** *male urethra in relation to other pelvic structures; and* **C,** *female urethra*
Source: A, Thibodeau, GA & Patton, KT. 1999; *Anatomy and Physiology* (4th ed.), Mosby, St Louis, Fig. 28-1A, p. 824. B, C, Lewis, SM, *et al.* 2004; *Medical-Surgical Nursing* (6th ed.), Mosby, St Louis, Fig. 43.1, p. 1153.

glomerular filtrate but does include solutes (creatinine, urea, nitrogen and glucose), water and electrolytes[1]. Each day about 180 L of glomerular filtrate is formed and a normal glomerular filtration rate (GFR) averages about 120–125 mL/min in adults in normal conditions. The next part of the process involved in urine formation is reabsorption and occurs in the tubular system, where more than 99% of all filtered water is reabsorbed into the body again by the tubules.

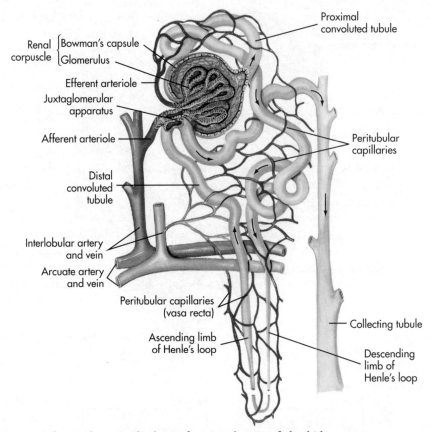

FIGURE 7.2   *The nephron is the basic functional unit of the kidney*
Source: Thibodeau, GA & Patton, KT. 1999; *Anatomy and Physiology* (4th ed.), Mosby, St Louis, Fig. 28.4A, p. 826.

TUBULAR REABSORPTION

Urine formation involves tubular reabsorption that occurs by both active and passive transport mechanisms. The tubular system extends from the glomerulus and consists of three parts: a proximal tubule, the loop of Henle and a distal tubule, all of which are critical to kidney function. The proximal convoluted tubule descends from the renal corpuscle down into the medulla of the kidney and is responsible for increasing the surface area available for *reabsorption* of almost 70% of the sodium, potassium and water contained in the glomerular filtrate and approximately 50% of urea[4]. Other substances that are reabsorbed include chloride, glucose, amino acids, phosphate and bicarbonate[5]. The reabsorbed filtrate is transported by either active or passive mechanisms into the peritubular capillary network. The proximal tubular system leads on to the first section of the Henle's loop in the medulla.

Henle's loop consists of a descending and an ascending limb and is an important part of the renal tubule because of its role in the production of either concentrated or dilute urine. This process occurs because of the kidney's countercurrent mechanism that is caused by the contents in the descending limb flowing in an opposite direction to the contents in the ascending limb. The main functions of the Henle's loop have to do with the reabsorption of water that occurs in the thicker portion of the descending loop. The active reabsorption of sodium and chloride occurs in the thinner portion of the ascending loop[2]. This reabsorption of sodium makes the tubule fluid more dilute. Urea is removed by diffusion in the descending loop. Henle's loop joins into the distal tubule that is situated in the renal cortex, where further concentration of the filtrate occurs[5].

The cells in the distal tubule and their collecting ducts, allow some sodium to be removed by active transport with the assistance of aldosterone (a hormone of the adrenal cortex), but not water[6]. If this were allowed to continue the urine would become too dilute (hypotonic) and lead to dehydration. In order to prevent this from occurring the body's regulatory mechanism produces antidiuretic hormone (ADH) that causes these cells to become more permeable to water. This means that the water is able to pass into the interstitial fluid and so maintain equilibrium.

TUBULAR SECRETION

A third mechanism involved in the formation of urine is tubular secretion, which is the opposite process to reabsorption. During this process substances (ammonium ions, hydrogen, and potassium ions) move from the peritubular capillaries through the cells that line the tubule wall into the tubular fluid. Potassium or hydrogen is actively transported from the blood to the tubular fluid in exchange for sodium that diffuses back into the blood. The secretion of potassium increases when the concentration of aldosterone, in the blood increases, which is an important process in the removal of excessive levels of potassium. Aldosterone, is the only hormone involved in the regulation of potassium[4]. A high level of aldosterone in the plasma causes the tubules to increase their reabsorption of sodium and water, which then means that less sodium and water is eliminated in the urine. If the aldosterone level in the plasma is low then the excretion of sodium and water is increased. Certain drugs, such as penicillin, are also secreted from the tubular cells[6]. The distal tubules then combine to form collecting ducts.

EXCRETION OF URINE

The collecting ducts are important for emptying urine into the pelvis of the kidney, which extends into the ureters. The ureters are composed of three layers of tissue: a mucousal inner lining, a smooth muscle middle layer and a fibrous outer layer. The muscular layer propels the urine, via peristalsis, to the bladder. The ends of the ureters act like valves and prevent the reflux or backflow of urine when the bladder is full. The urinary bladder is situated behind the symphysis pubis. It is formed of a smooth muscle wall called the detrusor muscle with an inner folded lining of mucous membrane that allows it to enlarge when full with urine. The function of the bladder is to store urine and excrete it via the urethra to the urinary meatus. The female urethra is about 3–4 cm long and the male urethra is about 20 cm long. The prostate gland surrounds the upper part of the male urethra.

FURTHER FUNCTIONS OF THE KIDNEYS

Aside from removing toxins from the blood, eliminating waste products and regulating fluid and electrolyte balance, the kidneys also have an important role in the regulation of blood pressure, vitamin D and calcium and the production of red blood cells.

REGULATION OF BLOOD PRESSURE

Blood pressure is controlled through the production and secretion of an enzyme called renin by the kidneys. The kidneys respond to either a decrease in blood pressure or low serum sodium in the circulatory system. Renin stimulates the conversion of angiotensinogen to angiotensin I (in the liver). Angiotensin I is converted to angiotensin II in the lungs by the angiotensin–converting enzyme (ACE). Angiotensin II produces a powerful vasoconstriction, the release of aldosterone and stimulation of the thirst centre in the brain that results in an increase in sodium and water in the body thereby increasing the blood pressure. This corrects the fluid deficit thereby increasing blood pressure.

REGULATION OF VITAMIN D AND CALCIUM

The kidneys regulate calcium and phosphate balance by converting the inactive form of vitamin D to an active form. Activated vitamin D regulates the secretion of parathyroid hormone and calcium concentration. Parathyroid hormone increases calcium absorption and decreases phosphate[3].

PRODUCTION OF RED BLOOD CELLS

The kidneys produce over 80% of erythropoietin (EPO) a glycoprotein hormone, which has a major role in red blood cell production and the prevention of anaemia. In a hypoxic state, the kidneys secrete EPO, which then directs the bone marrow to produce proerythroblasts, which then develop into erythrocytes[7]. The production of EPO is decreased when the oxygen supply to the tissues is corrected.

SUMMARY OF KEY CONCEPTS

- Kidneys are the primary organs responsible for fluid and electrolyte balance and removal of waste products such as urea and creatinine.
- Four processes are involved in the production of urine; namely, glomerular filtration, tubular reabsorption, tubular secretion and excretion of urine.
- Other functions of the kidneys include: regulation of blood pressure, acid–base balance, activation of vitamin D, and the production of erythropoietin.

ACUTE RENAL FAILURE

WHAT DOES IT MEAN?

Acute renal failure (ARF) is a rapid and sudden deterioration of renal function and results in the retention of metabolic wastes (azotaemia) and impaired fluid and electrolyte balance[5]. It usually develops over hours or days and usually follows severe, prolonged hypotension or hypovolaemia or exposure to a nephrotoxic agent. ARF is usually accompanied by oliguria (urine output less than 400 mL in 24 hours), although some people have nonoliguric ARF and maintain urine output of greater than 400 mL in 24 hours. Rarely does anuria (urine output less than 100 mL in 24 hours) occur. Unlike chronic renal failure, ARF is potentially reversible if the precipitating factors can be removed or corrected before permanent kidney damage has occurred. Despite advances in renal replacement therapies, ARF continues to have a mortality rate of approximately 50%[8].

> ● Case study
>
> Sandra Henderson, 65, lives at home with her husband. Mrs Henderson has been diagnosed with cancer of the transverse colon and has undergone a total colectomy and formation of ileostomy two days ago. Post-operatively she developed a paralytic ileus and had a nasogastric tube (NGT) inserted, which is connected to continuous low suction. At midnight, the fluid balance chart revealed the following: input 2.5 L (all intravenous fluids) and output 3.2 L (1.8 L via NGT and 0.5 L urine). By 0900 h the next morning, Mrs Henderson's observations were: BP 105/55, P 104, T 38.8°C, and she had not voided overnight. Mrs Henderson was reviewed by the medical staff and was commenced on regular ampicillin 1 g QID and a stat dose of gentamycin 240 mg. At 1600 h, her blood pressure was 95/55 and she had voided a total of 200 mL. Her most recent biochemistry revealed the following abnormalities: K^+ 4.5 mmol/L, urea 10.9 mmol/L, and creatinine 280 μmol/L. Medical staff then reviewed Mrs Henderson and suspected acute renal failure.

WHAT IS THE PATHOPHYSIOLOGY?

Acute renal failure can be caused by many types of conditions, including a reduction in blood flow to the kidney; toxic injury within the kidney; and obstruction of urine outflow from the kidney. The causes of ARF are commonly categorised as prerenal (55–60%), intrarenal (35–40%), and postrenal (<5%)[8].

PRE-RENAL FAILURE

Prerenal ARF results from any external factors that cause a sudden and severe reduction in blood flow to the kidneys and subsequent reduction in glomerular perfusion and filtration rate. The causes of prerenal failure can be broadly classified as conditions causing hypovolaemia, reduction in cardiac output, vasodilation, and obstruction of renal blood vessels. Table 7.1 summarises the causes of prerenal ARF.

Normally the kidneys receive approximately 20% of the cardiac output, and this is required to efficiently remove metabolic waste products and to regulate body fluids and electrolytes. Several protective mechanisms are in place to minimise the effect of reduced renal blood flow on renal tissue. These include the kidney's ability to: 1) autoregulate blood flow to preserve renal perfusion; 2) activate the renin-angiotensin-aldosterone mechanism to promote sodium retention; and 3) stimulate the secretion of anti-diuretic hormone from the pituitary gland to encourage the distal convoluted tubules and collecting ducts to conserve water. It is the ability of the kidney to retain sodium and water that allows prerenal failure to be separated from intrarenal and post-renal ARF[9].

In prerenal ARF, the reduction in renal blood flow is so profound it renders these protective mechanisms as ineffective, and severely diminishes the ability of the glomeruli to filter these wastes. Prolonged renal hypoperfusion also decreases the availability of nutrients and oxygen needed for basic cellular function and this can lead to tubular ischaemia (see acute tubular necrosis).

TABLE 7.1: CAUSES OF PRERENAL ACUTE RENAL FAILURE
Hypovolaemia/Fluid Volume Loss
• Haemorrhage (trauma, surgery, postpartum period)
• Dehydration (GIT loss – vomiting, diarrhoea, nasogastric suctioning)
• Renal loss (diuretics, osmotic diuresis, diabetes insipidus)
• Third spacing/volume shift (burns, ascites, pancreatitis, ileus)
Inadequate Cardiac Output
• Congestive heart failure
• Myocardial infarction
• Cardiogenic shock
• Pulmonary embolus
• Pericardial tamponade
Vasodilatation
• Septic shock
• Anaphylactic shock
• Drugs (antihypertensives)
Obstruction of Renal Blood Vessels
• Renal artery stenosis
• Renal artery thrombosis
• Renal vein thrombosis

INTRA-RENAL FAILURE

Conditions that directly injure functional renal tissue (glomerulus, tubules and interstitium) are classified as intrarenal causes of ARF (see Table 7.2). The most common cause of intrarenal ARF is acute tubular necrosis[8]. Less common causes are acute types of glomerulonephritis (i.e., Goodpasture's syndrome), vasculitis, systemic lupus erythematosus and haemolytic uraemic syndrome. Acute pyelonephritis can also be responsible for the development of intrarenal ARF.

ACUTE TUBULAR NECROSIS

Acute tubular necrosis (ATN) is a type of intrarenal ARF caused by ischaemia, nephrotoxic effects of drugs, intratubular obstruction (e.g., myoglobin pigments) or toxins released from severe sepsis[5,10]. Ischaemic and nephrotoxic ATN are responsible for 90% of intrarenal ARF cases[9]. Those at greatest risk of developing ATN include the elderly, diabetics, and patients who have a history of renal insufficiency[11]. ATN typically develops following prolonged ischaemia when perfusion to the kidney is considerably reduced. In some patients, ATN can eventuate after only a few hours of hypovolaemia or hypotension. The ischaemia associated with ATN predominantly damages the proximal tubule. The kidney is also susceptible to toxic injury because of its high blood flow, its mechanism for concentrating drugs and toxins, and its cellular structure[5]. Nephrotoxic agents may cause approximately 20% of all cases of ARF[10].

TABLE 7.2: CAUSES OF INTRA-RENAL FAILURE
Acute Tubular Necrosis
• Any of the prerenal causes above
• Prolonged hypotension
• Obstetric complications (abruptio placentae, placenta previa)
Glomerular or Vascular Dysfunction
• Acute glomerulonephritis (post-streptococcal, Goodpasture's syndrome)
• Vasculitis
• Malignant hypertension
• Systemic lupus erythematosus
• Haemolytic uraemic syndrome
• Disseminated intravascular coagulation
• Pregnancy induced hypertension/pre-eclampsia
• Thrombosis of renal artery or vein
Nephrotoxic Substances
• Drugs (aminoglycosides, amphotericin B, vancomycin, rifampicin, cisplatin, cyclosporin, frusemide, methotrexate, non-steroidal anti-inflammatory agents)
• Radiocontrast dye (particularly used during intravenous pyelogram and vessel angiography)
• Blood transfusion reactions
• Rhabdomyolysis (trauma, crush injury, alcohol or drug abuse, heat stroke)
• Chemical exposure (pesticides & fungicides)
Miscellaneous
• Heavy metals (mercury, arsenic, gold)
• Snake and/or spider bites
• Organic solvents (ethylene glycol)
• Pesticides

The renal protective mechanisms of autoregulation of renal blood vessels and activation of the renin-angiotensin-aldosterone system are able to increase renal perfusion during the early stages of ARF[8]. If, however, the blood flow is reduced for longer than one hour, these protective mechanisms begin to weaken, triggering a variety of factors that result in the development of ATN. These factors include: 1) decreased glomerular filtration rate and permeability, 2) medullary tissue hypoxia and cellular oedema, 3) intratubular obstruction, and 4) backleak of filtrate into the interstitium[8]. All of these factors cause a decrease in urine output.

POST-RENAL FAILURE

Post-renal ARF results from an obstruction of urine outflow from the kidneys (see Table 7.3). The obstruction can occur in the kidneys (e.g., renal cell carcinoma), ureter

TABLE 7.3: CAUSES OF POST-RENAL FAILURE
• Renal calculi/nephrolithiasis
• Tumours (bladder or kidney)
• Benign prostatic hypertrophy
• Obstruction of indwelling catheter
• Ligation of ureter during surgery (e.g., hysterectomy)
• Urethral strictures

(e.g., renal calculi), bladder (e.g., cancer), or urethra (e.g., prostatic hypertrophy)[12]. Obstruction can also result from iatrogenic causes such as blocked or kinked indwelling urinary catheters or from inadvertent surgical ligation of ureters. Prostatic hypertrophy is the most common underlying problem[12].

Urinary tract obstruction causes an increase in pressure proximal to the obstruction that often leads to dilation of the proximal collecting system (i.e., hydroureter and hydronephrosis). The elevated pressure in the collecting system is transmitted back into the tubular network and eventually stops glomerular filtration. The extent of damage depends on the degree, duration, and location of the obstruction as well as the presence and severity of infection[9]. Postrenal ARF is a urological emergency, and if the obstruction is not relieved, permanent renal damage can occur.

WHAT ARE THE CLINICAL MANIFESTATIONS?

Prerenal and postrenal ARF resolve relatively easily when they are identified early and treatment is commenced quickly[10]. Intrarenal failure and ATN have a prolonged course of recovery because actual parenchymal damage has occurred. Clinically, ARF usually progresses through four phases: initiating, oliguric, diuretic, and recovery. In some situations, the patient does not recover from ARF, and chronic kidney disease results.

INITIATING PHASE

This begins at the time of the insult and continues until the signs and symptoms become apparent. It can last for several hours to days. ARF is potentially reversible during the initiation phase.

OLIGURIC PHASE

The most common initial feature of ARF is the development of oliguria (<400 mL of urine in 24 hours). Oliguria usually occurs within 1 to 7 days of the causative event. If the cause is ischaemia, oliguria may occur within 24 hours. When nephrotoxic drugs are involved, the onset may be delayed for up to a week. About 50% of patients will not demonstrate oliguria, making the initial diagnosis more difficult. The oliguric phase lasts for approximately 10 to 14 days but can last months in some cases. The longer the oliguric phase persists, the poorer the prognosis for recovery of complete renal function[9].

It is important to distinguish prerenal oliguria from the oliguria of intrarenal ARF during this phase. Measurements of serum urea and creatinine levels are essential in patients who have ARF. If the ratio of urea:creatinine is more than 20:1, a prerenal cause of ARF is most likely[13]. In addition, urine with a high specific gravity (>1.015) and a low sodium concentration (<20 mmol/L) is characteristic of prerenal ARF[14]. This reflects the protective mechanisms of salt and water retention described earlier. In contrast, oliguria due to intrarenal failure is characterised by urine with a normal or fixed specific gravity (1.010) and a high sodium concentration (>40 mmol/L), indicating that the injured tubules cannot respond to protective mechanisms and lose sodium. Similarly, the oliguria of intrarenal failure caused by ATN is characterised by the presence of casts in the urine. These casts are formed from necrotic renal tubular epithelial cells, which detach or slough off into the tubules. The presence of protein on dipstick urinalysis may also be suggestive of intrarenal ARF due to glomerular damage[15]. It is during this phase that the clinical manifestations of significant renal impairment become apparent. These are described in more detail later in this chapter (see chronic renal failure).

DIURETIC PHASE

Over the next one to three weeks, there is a gradual repair and regeneration of renal tissue[9]. The diuretic phase begins with a gradual increase in daily urine output from 1 L to 3 L per day, and the urine volume may reach 3 L to 5 L or more per day. Although urine output is increasing, the nephrons are still not fully functional. An osmotic diuresis occurs due to salt and water accumulation in extracellular spaces as well as from high urea concentration in glomerular filtrate. The inability of the tubules to concentrate urine results in an increased urine volume. Hypovolaemia and hypotension can occur from massive fluid losses. Large losses of electrolytes, such as sodium, potassium also occur during this phase[14]. The kidneys have recovered their ability to excrete wastes, but not to concentrate urine. Near the end of this phase the patient's acid-base, electrolyte, and waste product (urea, creatinine) values begin to normalise.

RECOVERY PHASE

The recovery phase begins when GFR increases, allowing serum urea and creatinine levels to plateau and then decrease. Although major improvements occur in the first 1 to 2 weeks of this phase, renal function may take up to 12 months to stabilise.

WHAT SHOULD YOU BE LOOKING AT IN THE LABORATORY AND OTHER TESTS?

A thorough history is essential for diagnosing ARF. Prerenal causes should be considered when there is a history of dehydration, blood loss, or severe heart disease. Intrarenal causes may be suspected if the patient has been taking potentially nephrotoxic drugs[5] or has a recent history of prolonged hypotension or hypovolaemia. Postrenal ARF is suggested by a history of changes in urinary stream, stones or benign prostatic hypertrophy.

Urinalysis is an important diagnostic test; particularly urine osmolality, specific gravity and sodium content help to differentiate between the three types of ARF. To establish a diagnosis of ARF, other testing may be required. These include

• Renal ultrasound;
• Computed tomography (CT) scan and magnetic resonance imaging (MRI); and
• Renal scan.

WHAT IS THE TREATMENT?

ARF is potentially reversible if detected early. The primary goals of treatment are to eliminate the cause, manage the signs and symptoms, and prevent complications while the kidneys recover[14]. The first step is to determine if there is adequate intravascular volume and cardiac output to ensure adequate perfusion of the kidneys. This is assessed by the administration of volume expanders (Gelofusin®) or bolus amounts of crystalloids along with diuretic therapy, e.g., frusemide. If ARF is already established, forcing fluids and diuretics will not be effective and may, in fact, result in life-threatening fluid overload and pulmonary oedema. Conservative therapy involving dietary (e.g., sodium, potassium and protein) and fluid restrictions (i.e., 500 mL plus previous day's urine output), and medications (e.g., resonium, antihypertensive agents, phosphate binders, sodium bicarbonate supplements) may be all that is necessary to control the multi-systemic effects of ARF until renal function improves[8].

Hyperkalaemia, severe uraemia, pulmonary oedema and uraemic pericarditis all indicate that conservative measures are no longer able to control the symptoms of ARF and there is now a need for urgent renal replacement therapy (RRT)[16]. If RRT is required, three options are available: haemodialysis (HD), continuous venovenous haemodiafiltration (CVVH) and peritoneal dialysis (PD)[16]. HD is preferred for the hypercatabolic patient and for the individual who has had abdominal or thoracic trauma or surgery. HD is the method of choice when rapid changes are required in a short time especially if life-threatening symptoms have arisen (e.g., hyperkalaemia >6.5 mmol/L, pulmonary oedema). HD is technically more complicated because specialised staff, equipment and vascular access are required. In the haemodynamically unstable patient, CVVH provides gradual removal of excess fluid and solutes, and is, therefore, better tolerated by patients with ARF. It is technically similar to HD and is frequently used in the intensive care setting. PD is much simpler than HD, but it carries the risk of peritonitis, is less efficient, requires longer treatment times, and is not commonly used for ARF.

The patient's overall health, the severity of renal failure, and the number and type of complications influence the outcome of ARF. The majority of patients with ARF have potentially recoverable renal function. At least 60% of patients have full recovery of renal function, approximately 30% have mild to moderate renal impairment and only 6–10% progress to end-stage renal failure and require permanent RRT[8]. In addition, the older adult patient is less likely to recover full kidney function than the younger patient.

APPLIED PHARMACOLOGY

Pharmacological treatment is similar to chronic renal failure and is required to control: fluid overload (diuretics); hypertension (antihypertensive agents); and electrolyte imbalances, particularly hyperkalaemia (Resonium), and hypocalcaemia (Caltrate).

NURSING IMPLICATIONS

Monitoring fluid volume status is the most important nursing intervention of all patients at risk for the development of ARF or during the course of ARF. Accurate measurements of blood pressure, pulse, body weight, urine output, and jugular or central venous pressure as well as assessment of lung fields, skin turgor, mucous membranes and presence of oedema are all vital in determining the patient's fluid volume status. Monitoring the use of as well as careful administration of potentially nephrotoxic agents is also an important nursing responsibility.

> ## LEARNING EXERCISES
> 1. Outline the common causes of acute renal failure.
> 2. Describe the pathophysiology associated with the development of acute tubular necrosis.
> 3. Explain the different phases of acute renal failure.
> 4. When is renal replacement therapy required in acute renal failure?
> 5. Why is the monitoring of fluid status an important nursing consideration in acute renal failure?

In this case study, Mrs Henderson was becoming hypovolaemic (dehydrated) due to excessive gastric losses as a result of her paralytic ileus. This would have been evident on her fluid balance chart throughout the day. Nursing staff should have observed this and requested a review by the medical staff (i.e., increase of IV fluids). This should have occurred prior to midnight, but certainly Mrs Henderson's fluid imbalance, particularly her poor urine output, should have triggered this review.

Mrs Henderson was then anuric for at least nine hours prior to the medical staff review in the morning. Both medical and nursing staff should have been alerted to this. Mrs Henderson was exhibiting clear signs of hypovolaemia (i.e., hypotension and tachycardia). Her hypovolaemia would have also worsened as a consequence of being febrile; further signs of impending prerenal ARF. The prescription for gentamycin, while quite reasonable for a post-operative febrile patient, would have exacerbated this situation.

Unfortunately Mrs Henderson's deterioration was allowed to continue as evidenced by her reduced urine output (200 mL in at least 16 hours), and it is not until abnormal biochemistries are noted that interventions take place.

Mrs Henderson has developed ARF due to ATN. The ATN is a consequence of her prolonged hypovolaemia, hypotension and concomitant administration of a highly nephrotoxic medication. In essence, Mrs Henderson's ARF could have been avoided by careful and accurate monitoring of her fluid status by the nursing staff. This would have ensured timely medical intervention.

CHRONIC RENAL FAILURE

WHAT DOES IT MEAN?

Chronic renal failure (CRF) is characterised by a progressive and irreversible destruction of renal function that occurs over varying periods of time ranging from a few months to decades[5,14]. CRF results from a number of conditions that cause permanent loss of nephron function, and a decrease in glomerular filtration rate (GFR). A five-stage classification system for kidney disease progression, in which GFR is used to identify those at risk of developing CRF, exists (Table 7.4)[17]. The stages broadly indicate normal renal function (stage 1), diminished renal function (stage 2), renal insufficiency (stage 3), renal failure (stage 4) and end stage renal failure (stage 5). Stages 1 and 2 require close monitoring to preserve

TABLE 7.4: DEFINITIONS AND STAGES OF CHRONIC KIDNEY DISEASE		
Stage	Description	GFR (mL/min/1.73 m²)
1	Kidney damage with normal or increased GFR	≥90
2	Kidney damage with mild decreased GFR	60–89
3	Moderate decreased GFR	30–59
4	Severe decreased GFR	15–29
5	Kidney failure	<15 (or dialysis)

renal function; stage 3 requires aggressive treatment to slow the progression; and stages 4 and 5 require specialist management by a nephrologist to avoid the long-term complications of CRF[18].

● Case study

Peter Jones, 68, is a married man who has had type 2 diabetes mellitus for 23 years. Mr Jones was referred, by his local doctor, to a nephrologist for assessment and ongoing management of his renal function three years ago when he developed proteinuria. Today the nephrologist reviewed Mr Jones and his renal function has deteriorated significantly. His most recent blood tests revealed the following abnormalities: K^+ 5.9 mmol/L, urea 28.9 mmol/L, creatinine 870 μmol/L and Hb 8.8 g/dL. The nephrologist arranged for his admission to the renal ward for insertion of a peritoneal dialysis catheter tomorrow.

On admission to the ward, Mr Jones' observations were BP 165/95; P 86, T 37.0°C; BSL 14.7 mmol/L. Mr Jones advised that his normal medications are Actrapid 24 units TDS; Protophane 36 units daily; ramipril 2.5 mg daily, atenolol 50 mg BD; Caltrate 1500 mg TDS, sodium bicarbonate 840 mg TDS, and Lasix 250 mg BD. On arrival to the renal unit, Mr Jones had an ECG taken which revealed normal sinus rhythm. He was also prescribed Resonium 30 g STAT.

WHAT IS THE PATHOPHYSIOLOGY?

The major causes of CRF in Australia are glomerulonephritis (30%), diabetes mellitus (22%) and hypertension (14%)[19]. Other significant causes include polycystic kidney disease, analgesic nephropathy and reflux nephropathy, which are beyond the scope of this book. The indigenous populations of both Australia and New Zealand are over-represented in the number of people with renal failure with Aborigines accounting for 8% and Māori 31% of all patients with end-stage renal failure[19].

GLOMERULONEPHRITIS

Glomerulonephritis (GN) is an inflammatory process that affects the structures within the glomeruli, and it is the leading cause of chronic renal failure (CRF) in Australia[19]. There are numerous causes of GN which can be broadly labelled as either nephritic or nephrotic[14]. In addition, GN can be as a result of either primary conditions in which the glomerular abnormality is the only disease process involved or as secondary condition resulting from another disease such as diabetes mellitus, hypertension or systemic lupus erythematosus (SLE)[5,20]. A renal biopsy is commonly performed to identify the type of GN causing renal dysfunction.

NEPHRITIC SYNDROME

Nephritic syndrome is a collection of clinical features (haematuria, hypertension, fluid overload and oliguria) which are common to particular forms of GN[5]. Nephritic syndrome is also known as nephritis. The more common forms of GN which present as nephritic syndrome are: IgA nephropathy, acute proliferative GN and rapidly progressive GN.

IMMUNOGLOBULIN A (IGA) GLOMERULONEPHRITIS

This is the most frequently found type of GN in Australia[19] in which there is an increase in mesangial cells within the glomeruli due to deposits of immunoglobulin A (IgA). Its cause is not well understood, but it is believed that the immune response is triggered following ingested or inhaled pathogens[21]. There is no proven effective therapy for IgA GN and the goal of treatment is to control the decline in renal function.

ACUTE PROLIFERATIVE (POST-INFECTIOUS) GLOMERULONEPHRITIS

This form of GN frequently follows throat or skin infections due to certain strains of Group A beta-haemolytic streptococci, and is more common in children and young adults[22]. The exact mechanism causing the GN is not well understood but the immune response is dependent on host factors and organism characteristics. In all situations, however, there is activation of the complement cascade via the alternate pathway that causes the inflammatory process to occur in the glomeruli[5]. Laboratory findings reveal elevated antistreptolysin O levels along with reduced C3 complement. Treatment is mostly symptomatic with approximately 95% of children recovering spontaneously but in adults up to 40% develop permanent kidney damage[22].

RAPIDLY PROGRESSIVE GLOMERULONEPHRITIS

Rapidly progressive glomerulonephritis (RPGN) is not a common renal disease but causes a rapid decline in renal function. RPGN does not have a specific cause although it is often associated with an immune disorder called Goodpasture's syndrome. Goodpasture's syndrome develops due to the development of antibodies to the glomerular and alveolar basement membranes[23]. Its clinical features are haematuria, haemoptysis and severe (and often acute) renal failure. Treatment includes plasmapheresis to remove the circulating anti–glomerular basement membrane antibodies and immunosuppressive therapy (corticosteroids and cyclophosphamide) to inhibit antibody production[23].

NEPHROTIC SYNDROME

Nephrotic syndrome is another collection of particular clinical features that are more common to different forms of GN in comparison to nephritic syndrome[24]. The classic features of nephrotic syndrome are massive proteinuria, hypoalbuminaemia, oedema, hyperlipidaemia and altered coagulopathy[5]. The more common forms of GN which present as nephrotic syndrome are: minimal change GN and membranous GN.

MINIMAL CHANGE GLOMERULONEPHRITIS

Minimal change glomerulonephritis (MCGN) occurs suddenly and is more common in young children (2–6 years of age). Its name indicates that minimal changes occur in the glomeruli but there is damage to the epithelial layer of the glomerular membrane, which allows large quantities of plasma proteins to leak into the glomerular filtrate[14]. This form of GN is responsive to corticosteroids and there is usually a complete return of renal function[5].

MEMBRANOUS GLOMERULONEPHRITIS

Typically 60–70 year olds develop membranous GN and this causes the classic features of nephrotic syndrome[14]. Membranous GN can also be associated with systemic lupus erythematosus, diabetes mellitus and the use of drugs such as gold, penicillamine and captopril[5]. Although it can often be treated with corticosteroids, up to 50% of people will experience a slow but steady decline in renal function.

DIABETIC NEPHROSCLEROSIS

Nephropathy is a major complication of both type 1 (IDDM) and type 2 (NDDM) diabetes mellitus (see Chapter 4). People with type 1 of 15–30 years duration will have a 20% chance of developing CRF[25]. Type 2 accounts for the remaining 80% of diabetes with renal failure. In Australia, diabetic nephropathy is the second most frequent reason people need dialysis or a kidney transplant[19]. Structural changes occur in the nephrons due to diabetes mellitus[5]. Early indications of renal impairment are associated with the development of microalbuminuria, and it is recommended that all diabetics have yearly measurements of urinary proteins[26]. Strategies to minimise or slow the progression of diabetic nephrosclerosis include careful control of blood glucose levels, aggressive management of hypertension and the introduction of angiotensin converting enzyme inhibitors such as captopril[25].

HYPERTENSIVE NEPHROSCLEROSIS

Hypertension can cause renal failure and it is also a symptom once renal failure is established[5]. Hypertension results from damage to the small arterioles in the kidney. High pressure in these blood vessels causes them to become weak and to haemorrhage inside the kidney. Good control of hypertension is required to prevent or slow the progression of renal damage.

WHAT ARE THE CLINICAL MANIFESTATIONS?

Regardless of the cause of CRF, the clinical manifestations become increasingly more apparent due to the progressive deterioration in glomerular filtration rate[18]. Early symptoms of renal insufficiency begin during stage 3 when at least 50% of nephron function has been destroyed. Hypertension, elevated urea and creatinine levels, and anaemia develop. In later stages, oedema, electrolyte imbalances, metabolic acidosis and multi-systemic effects

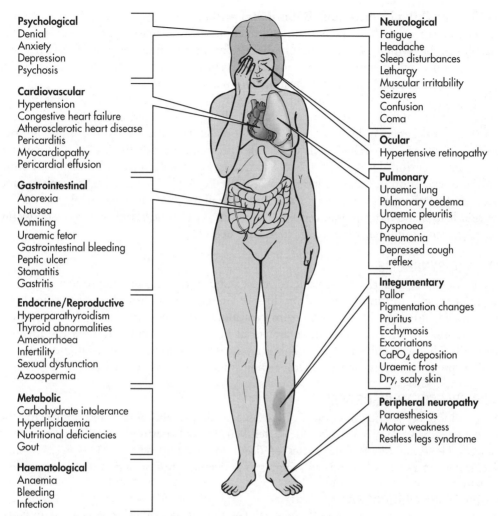

Psychological
Denial
Anxiety
Depression
Psychosis

Cardiovascular
Hypertension
Congestive heart failure
Atherosclerotic heart disease
Pericarditis
Myocardiopathy
Pericardial effusion

Gastrointestinal
Anorexia
Nausea
Vomiting
Uraemic fetor
Gastrointestinal bleeding
Peptic ulcer
Stomatitis
Gastritis

Endocrine/Reproductive
Hyperparathyroidism
Thyroid abnormalities
Amenorrhoea
Infertility
Sexual dysfunction
Azoospermia

Metabolic
Carbohydrate intolerance
Hyperlipidaemia
Nutritional deficiencies
Gout

Haematological
Anaemia
Bleeding
Infection

Neurological
Fatigue
Headache
Sleep disturbances
Lethargy
Muscular irritability
Seizures
Confusion
Coma

Ocular
Hypertensive retinopathy

Pulmonary
Uraemic lung
Pulmonary oedema
Uraemic pleuritis
Dyspnoea
Pneumonia
Depressed cough
  reflex

Integumentary
Pallor
Pigmentation changes
Pruritus
Ecchymosis
Excoriations
$CaPO_4$ deposition
Uraemic frost
Dry, scaly skin

Peripheral neuropathy
Paraesthesias
Motor weakness
Restless legs syndrome

DIAGRAM 7.1 *Clinical manifestations of chronic uraemia*
Source: Lewis, SM, *et al.* 2004; *Medical-Surgical Nursing* (6th ed.), Mosby, St Louis, Fig. 45.3, p. 1218.

of uraemia develop (see Diagram 7.1). Common clinical manifestations are described below, and eventually many of them become life-threatening.

URINARY CHANGES

In the early stages of renal failure, polyuria and nocturia are apparent as the kidneys are unable to concentrate urine, particularly overnight. The specific gravity of urine gradually becomes fixed at around 1.010 (the osmolar concentration of plasma) reflecting the kidneys' inability to dilute or concentrate urine. As CRF worsens, oliguria develops (urine output <400 mL per 24 hours). If the patient is still producing urine, haematuria, proteinuria and casts could be present depending on the cause of the kidney disease.

FLUID, ELECTROLYTE AND ACID-BASE IMBALANCES

There is a corresponding increase in fluid retention as urinary output decreases. The severity of the symptoms depends on the extent of the fluid overload. Oedema and hypertension may develop. Fluid overload can eventually lead to congestive heart failure (CHF), pulmonary oedema, and pericardial and pleural effusions.

There are also numerous abnormalities in electrolyte balance due to kidney dysfunction. Sodium excretion is impaired and is retained along with water. Sodium retention can contribute to oedema, hypertension, and CHF. Hyperkalaemia is the most serious electrolyte disorder associated with CRF. Life-threatening dysrhythmias can occur when the serum potassium level reaches 7 to 8 mmol/L. Hyperkalaemia results primarily from decreased excretion by the kidneys and metabolic acidosis. Calcium, phosphate and magnesium abnormalities also exist. Lastly, in renal failure, the kidneys are unable to excrete the acid load that builds up due to cellular function. As a result, plasma bicarbonate usually falls to 16 to 20 mmol/L resulting in metabolic acidosis.

URAEMIC SYNDROME

The kidneys are primarily responsible for the excretion of urea, an end product of protein metabolism, and creatinine, an end product of muscle metabolism. In renal failure these are elevated, although an elevated serum creatinine is the best indicator of renal failure. The retention of urea and creatinine affects all body systems and is termed the uraemic syndrome. The main clinical manifestations are nausea, vomiting, lethargy, fatigue, impaired thought processes, and headaches. Other clinical features are described below.

CARDIOVASCULAR DISORDERS

Hypertension is the most common cardiovascular abnormality and is responsible for the accelerated atherosclerotic vascular disease, left ventricular hypertrophy and congestive heart failure[27]. These are the leading causes of death for patients with CRF. Rarely, uraemic pericarditis can also develop and can progress to pericardial effusion and cardiac tamponade[28].

RESPIRATORY DISORDERS

Dyspnoea from fluid overload, pulmonary oedema, uraemic pleuritis (pleurisy) and pleural effusion are common in people with renal failure.

NEUROLOGICAL DISORDERS

Neurologic changes can range from fatigue and difficulty concentrating to seizures, stupor, and coma. Peripheral neuropathy is also apparent and patients complain of a restless leg syndrome and paraesthesias (burning sensations) in the feet.

METABOLIC AND ENDOCRINE DISTURBANCES

Renal failure is associated with several metabolic and endocrine disturbances. These include: hyperglycaemia, hyperinsulinaemia, abnormal glucose tolerance tests and hyperlipidaemia. Other metabolic and endocrine disturbances are linked to musculoskeletal abnormalities and are described below.

HAEMATOLOGICAL AND IMMUNOLOGICAL DYSFUNCTION

Anaemia is a common clinical manifestation because renal failure results in impaired erythropoietin production and is compounded by platelet abnormalities[29,30]. It has debilitating consequences and is the primary cause of left ventricular hypertrophy in

CRF[31]. White blood cells are also altered due to the retention of urea and this leads to some immunodeficiency making the patient more susceptible to infections[32]. While platelet count is normal, their function is abnormal due to uraemia, which cause bleeding tendencies.

GASTROINTESTINAL DISORDERS

Anorexia, nausea, and vomiting are associated with renal failure and this contributes to the weight loss and malnutrition seen in many patients. Every part of the gastrointestinal system is affected as a result of inflammation of the mucosa caused by excessive urea[14]. Stomatitis, oral ulcerations, a metallic taste in the mouth, and uraemic fetor (a uraemic, fruity odour of the breath) are commonly found. In addition, gastrointestinal bleeding, diarrhoea and/or constipation may also develop due to retained uraemic products.

MUSCULOSKELETAL DISORDERS

Renal failure impairs the activation of vitamin D. Activated vitamin D is required in the gastrointestinal tract to assist with the absorption of calcium. In CRF, this results in the development of hypocalcaemia. Parathyroid hormone (PTH) is secreted in order to compensate, and this stimulates bone demineralisation, thereby releasing calcium from the bones to increase serum calcium. Phosphate is also released from the bone, which exacerbates the already existing hyperphosphataemia. The action of PTH on bone results in renal osteodystrophy, a syndrome of skeletal changes found in chronic kidney disease[5,33].

INTEGUMENTARY DISORDERS

The most noticeable change in people with decreased renal function is the yellow-grey discolouration of the skin, which occurs due to the absorption and retention of urinary pigments. The skin is also pale (due to anaemia), and dry and scaly (due to decreased oil and sweat gland activity). Pruritis occurs due to the elevation in urea and the calcium-phosphate deposits in the skin[34]. The itching may be so intense that it can lead to bleeding or infections secondary to scratching. Hair is dry and brittle, and nails are thin and ridged. Lastly, petechiae and ecchymoses may be present and are due to platelet abnormalities.

REPRODUCTIVE DYSFUNCTION

Normal reproductive function is also altered in renal failure. Male and female hormones are decreased, and both sexes have a lowered libido and develop infertility problems[5,35,36].

WHAT SHOULD YOU BE LOOKING AT IN THE LABORATORY AND OTHER TESTS?

Important diagnostic interventions include measuring serum creatinine to estimate GFR, monitoring electrolyte and full blood count profiles, urinalysis will assist in detecting red and white blood cells, protein, and glucose. Other investigations include renal biopsy, ultrasound and renal scans.

WHAT IS THE TREATMENT?

Initially conservative methods of dietary and pharmacological treatment are needed to control and slow the progression of renal failure. When these methods fail to control the clinical manifestations of CRF, then long-term renal replacement therapy (RRT) are required to sustain life.

DIETARY MANAGEMENT

The aim is to maintain good nutrition whilst restricting protein, potassium, salt and phosphate in the diet[37]. Protein restriction must be used cautiously to avoid malnutrition (especially in ESRF), but it has been shown to slow the decline in GFR[38]. Diets should have adequate calories from carbohydrates and fat to minimise catabolism of body protein and to maintain body weight. Fluid intake is usually restricted to 500 mL plus an amount equal to the previous days' urine output. Sodium and potassium restriction depends on the amount of renal function available to excrete these electrolytes. Generally, sodium is restricted to avoid oedema and hypertension, and high potassium contain foods (e.g., some fruits and vegetables, chocolate) must be avoided. Lastly, foods high in phosphate such as dairy products (e.g., milk, ice-cream, cheese, yoghurt) are also restricted.

RENAL REPLACEMENT THERAPY

When renal function deteriorates to the point of end stage renal failure (ESRF) and conservative methods can no longer manage the symptoms, RRT is required. These treatments include haemodialysis, peritoneal dialysis and renal transplantation. Briefly haemodialysis (HD) involves access to the vascular system (usually an arteriovenous fistula is formed and cannulated), an extracorporeal circuit, dialyser and technological equipment. Typically, a patient with ESRF will receive a minimum of four hours of treatment on three occasions each week[19].

Peritoneal dialysis (PD) is performed by introducing 1 L to 3 L of a sterile dextrose-containing solution (dialysate) into the peritoneal cavity. Although there are several different techniques for PD, the most common is Continuous Ambulatory Peritoneal Dialysis (CAPD). CAPD requires the individual to manually change the dialysate in the peritoneal cavity 4 or 5 times each day, every day of the year[39].

The last type of RRT is renal transplantation, and is an option for most patients with ESRF, either before or after the initiation of dialysis. The donor kidney is placed in the iliac fossa and native kidneys are not removed[40]. Immunosuppression (e.g., prednisone, mycophenolate and cyclosporin) is required to avoid rejection.

APPLIED PHARMACOLOGY

The person with CRF requires numerous medications to control the symptoms associated with renal dysfunction. These medications include: antihypertensive agents; calcium-based phosphate binders such as calcium carbonate (e.g., Caltrate); erythropoietin (Eprex); sodium bicarbonate; sodium (or calcium) polystyrene sulfonate (Resonium), a cation-exchange resin; and vitamin D (Calcitriol).

In renal failure there can be a delayed or decreased elimination of drugs which can lead to an accumulation of drugs in the body[41]. Adjustments in drug doses and frequency of administration are required. Drugs of particular concern include digoxin, gentamicin, vancomycin and opiates[5]. Pethidine should never be administered to a person with CRF because it can accumulate and cause seizures.

NURSING IMPLICATIONS

Nursing implications are similar to ARF but with the added complexity of a chronic illness that requires specialist nursing care in the dialysis or transplant unit. This includes:

monitoring for life-threatening alterations in biochemistry and complications of uraemic syndrome; maintaining dialysis access (e.g., fistula and PD catheter patency); prevention of infection; monitoring for rejection; and psychosocial support[18,42]. A major goal in nursing care is education and empowerment of the patient to manage their illness themselves.

LEARNING EXERCISES

1. Outline the major causes of chronic renal failure in Australia.
2. Describe the pathophysiology associated with glomerulonephritis.
3. What is the difference between nephritic and nephrotic syndromes?
4. How does diabetes mellitus cause chronic renal failure?
5. Describe the major systemic effects of uraemia.
6. Why is it necessary to restrict dietary intake of sodium, potassium and protein in people with chronic renal failure?
7. Explain the differences between haemodialysis and peritoneal dialysis.

In this case study, Mr Jones has now reached end-stage renal failure secondary to his non-insulin dependent diabetes mellitus. Diabetes mellitus (DM) is the second leading cause of ESRF in Australia, and will shortly be the leading cause, due to the increasing incidence of DM. Patients with CRF should be referred early to a nephrologist in order to aggressively control and slow the progression of renal failure. Mr Jones has extremely elevated urea and creatinine levels that indicate his kidneys have now reached ESRF. He is also experiencing electrolyte abnormalities (hyperkalaemia and hypocalcaemia), anaemia and acidosis; some of these are being treated with medications (Caltrate and sodium bicarbonate). Ideally, Mr Jones should be on erythropoietin to correct his anaemia and may require Resonium from time to time to control his hyperkalaemia. Eventually, however, these strategies will fail and, like Mr Jones, patients will now require preparation for RRT, which, in his case, involves formation of an arteriovenous fistula and insertion of a PD catheter. His nursing care focuses on management of and education for his ESRF and RRT.

PROSTATIC HYPERPLASIA

WHAT DOES IT MEAN?

Hyperplasia is an abnormal increase in the number of cells that results in enlargement (prostatic hypertrophy) of the prostate gland[43]. The prostate goes through two stages of growth, the first occurring early in puberty and the second around 25 years of age. Although the prostate continues to grow it does not cause problems for many men until later in life, around 60 years or older. Hyperplasia of the prostate can occur from either benign prostatic hyperplasia (BPH) or from adenocarcinoma.

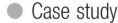 Case study

Alfred Talford, 75, was admitted to the ward for a radical retropubic prostatectomy. His medical history identified that three years ago he was diagnosed with lower urinary tract symptoms (LUTS), which included dysuria, a weak, hesitant and intermittent stream on voiding followed by some dribbling. Following a digital rectal examination (DRE) and a prostatic-specific antigen (PSA) test that showed a level 12.5 ng/mL, a formal diagnosis of benign prostatic hyperplasia (BPH) was made. Symptom control was initially by a treatment choice of 'watchful waiting' and the use of Minipress. Mr Talford found it increasingly difficult to cope with his symptoms and subsequently had a transurethral resection of his prostate (TURP). At this present time, his PSA was increased (27.5 ng/mL) and his prostatic biopsies revealed adenocarcinoma, necessitating his admission.

During his admission procedure, the nurse provided information about the purpose of the surgery, its effects on urinary elimination and sexual functioning. The nurse caring for Mr Talford in the early postoperative period was surprised when he explained to her that he 'was not sure about what to expect'.

WHAT IS THE PATHOPHYSIOLOGY?

The prostate gland lies just below the neck of the bladder and surrounds the urethra (see Figure 7.3). When abnormal enlargement or cell multiplication occurs from either benign or cancerous cells it causes pressure on the prostatic urethra, which can then lead to impeded urinary outflow. During this process the detrusor muscle begins to thicken and eventually the bladder becomes so irritable that contraction occurs even when there is only a little amount of urine. If pressure in the bladder is not relieved then it will result in the backward flow of urine into the ureters, called vesicoureteral reflux. Although it is not a frequent occurrence generally, it is still one of the more common causes of renal failure in old age for men[43]. This reflux can eventually end with hydroureter, hydronephrosis and impaired renal function[2]. Over time, urinary retention with the added strain on the bladder can impair function of the urinary tract resulting in infection.

Although an enlargement of tissue occurs in both BPH and prostate cancer, the site of tissue growth is different for each condition. Benign prostatic cells replicate in the central

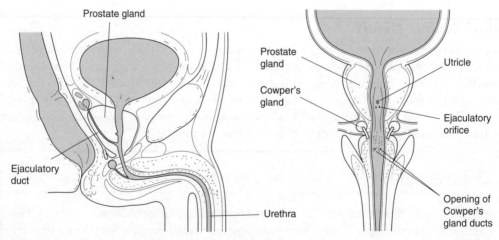

FIGURE 7.3 *Structure of male lower urinary tract*

or transition zone that surrounds the urethra whereas, cancerous cells tend to develop in the periphery or outer zone of the prostate[2,44]. As most of the prostate is composed of glandular epithelial cells all cancers that occur are mainly adenocarcinomas. These metastatic cells are slow growing and invade surrounding tissues in an expected pattern that involves the lymph nodes, bone marrow and bones of the pelvis, sacrum and lumbar spine[45]. Metastatic spread to other parts of the body occurs later in the disease via the lymph and venous bloodstream. The causes of prostatic hyperplasia are not fully known but it is believed that it may have something to do with testosterone being converted by the prostate into an androgen called dihydrotestosterone (DHT). DHT then stimulates the ageing cells in the prostatic glandular epithelium tissue to enlarge[2]. The proliferation of cells caused by DHT is a major concern for the spread of prostatic cancer. Another suggestion is that an increase in the level of oestrogen in association with ageing, may also contribute to the growth of cells in the prostate. Other causes proposed for prostatic cancer aside from hormonal changes, include genetic and environmental factors.

WHAT ARE THE CLINICAL MANIFESTATIONS?

The symptoms of prostatic hyperplasia are caused by outlet obstruction and irritation of the bladder often referred to as prostatism or more recently LUTS (lower urinary tract symptoms)[46]. As the enlargement of prostatic tissue is slow many symptoms are often tolerated until acute urinary retention occurs. Initially, clinical manifestations would include: frequency, hesitancy, diminished stream and force on micturition and dribbling or post-void overflow incontinence. Irritation of the bladder may lead to urgency, nocturia and incomplete emptying of the bladder, which then can result in residual urine and infection[47]. Haematuria occurs from the enlarged prostate and blood vessels that tear on straining. Complaints of pain may assist with differentiating between BPH and prostate cancer. With BPH pain may be lower in the abdomen, back or side with a slow onset and in comparison, pain from prostate cancer may characteristically be sudden and quickly increase in severity. If the cancer has metastasised then pain may be felt in other areas of the body (usually the spine) along with weight loss, bowel and bladder dysfunction and fatigue[2]. The time from the initial development of metastases and death is about five years[48].

WHAT SHOULD YOU BE LOOKING AT IN THE LABORATORY AND OTHER TESTS?

Diagnostic tests for prostatic hyperplasia include those for assessment of renal function. A urinalysis and urine culture would be required for both BPH and prostatic cancer in order to detect infection or any abnormality in the urine. If infection is present then the results from a urinalysis may show white blood cells, high pH (alkaline) and or red blood cells, which are more common with BPH than with prostate cancer. Problems with renal function may be detected from analysis of protein, specific gravity and glucose. A urine culture would demonstrate any abnormality in the urine or presence of infection.

Haematology could reveal anaemia or infection and biochemistry results for blood urea and creatinine would determine impaired renal function. A prostate-specific antigen (PSA) test and a serum acid phosphatase measurement are undertaken for suspected prostate cancer[43,49]. If the cancer has invaded the bone then serum alkaline phosphatase levels will most likely be elevated[2]. Other tests include X-rays of the kidneys, ureters, and bladder

(KUB) to reveal their outline. An intravenous pyelogram (IVP) would assist in evaluating the structure and function of the urinary tract (bladder filling and emptying, residual urine, hydronephrosis or tumours). Urodynamic flow rate analysis assesses bladder function during the emptying stage of micturition. Cystoscopy is used to visualise the bladder and urethra. Digital rectal examination is used to palpate the gland in order to assess its size and whether it is smooth, pliable and not tender as is usually the case in BPH or if it is a hard nodule as is found in prostate cancer.

WHAT IS THE TREATMENT?

There are several treatments available to relieve bladder outflow obstruction but their choice depends on the severity of symptoms. Non-surgical procedures include transurethral microwave thermotherapy (TUMT) and laser therapy that use heat at high temperatures to destroy the prostatic tissue adjacent to the urethra, thereby improving urine flow. Complications such as overheating, trauma, bleeding and swelling can occur. Electrical vaporisation, high intensity ultrasound waves and radio frequency energy can also be used to destroy the glandular tissue. Delayed haematuria and urinary retention can occur within days to weeks following electrovaporisation of the prostate[50]. Stents and balloon dilation that open the lumen of the prostatic urethra may be more suitable for high-risk patients. These procedures are not as effective in the long term as surgery.

There are four surgical procedures for removal of the prostate tissue. The most commonly used is *transurethral resection of the prostate* (TURP) that uses an endoscope via the urethra through which pieces of the obstructive prostate tissue can be cut away. Cauterisation is used to reduce bleeding and the insertion of a three-way urethral catheter assists the removal of clots and urine and allows for either intermittent or constant bladder irrigation. For mild to moderate enlargement of the prostate, early removal of the catheter following a brief irrigation period has not been found to increase post-operative complications[51]. Untoward effects of the procedure can lead to retrograde ejaculation, erectile dysfunction or urinary incontinence. There are three other surgical techniques that are used if the prostate is too large for transurethral removal. *Suprapubic prostatectomy* removes tissue through an abdominal incision into the bladder and is used to explore the abdomen. *Perineal prostatectomy* uses an incision through the perineum between the anus and the scrotum and is preferred for treating prostatic cancer. *Retropubic prostatectomy* bypasses the bladder and approaches the enlarged gland between the pubis and the bladder and is used when the enlarged gland is located high in the pelvic area. For prostatic cancer a radical retropubic prostatectomy is often preferred because it allows for improved visualisation of the prostate and bladder neck and access to the lymph nodes in the pelvic region as well as assisting with a greater control of bleeding[52].

APPLIED PHARMACOLOGY

Non-surgical treatment consists of using a medication (finasteride), which inhibits the enzyme that converts testosterone to dihydrotesterone (DHT)[53]. This medication reduces the size of the prostate and relieves urine flow through the urethra. Aside from some adverse effects (impotence and ejaculation disorder) finasteride can also lower PSA levels by around 50%, which can be problematic if screening for prostatic cancer. Alpha-adrenergic blockers (minipress) relax the smooth muscle in the prostate and the neck of the bladder, which then allows for the passage of urine through the urethra.

NURSING IMPLICATIONS

Preoperative education for the patient undergoing a surgical operation for prostatic enlargement is vital for recovery. It should involve information about immediate post-surgical care that includes continuous bladder irrigation and assessment for haemorrhage as well as the possibility of bladder spasm. Patients should also be assessed for water intoxication that occurs from the large amounts of irrigating solutions used during surgery. This complication is known as transurethral resection (TUR) syndrome and the early symptoms include confusion and agitation from cerebral oedema[47]. Coping with events after surgery is extremely stressful for most men and does affect their quality of life[54]. Problems such as incontinence and dribbling can be relieved with the use of pelvic floor exercises. It is important to include fibre in the diet and increase fluid intake in order to prevent constipation and straining as this increases pressure on the surgical site.

LEARNING EXERCISES

1. Outline possible causes for prostatic hyperplasia.
2. Describe the pathophysiology that occurs following an abnormal enlargement of the prostate gland.
3. What is the difference between benign prostatic cell and cancerous cell development?
4. Provide a rationale for the tests that may be undertaken for prostatic hyperplasia, including those for suspected prostate cancer.

In this case study, it is important to remember that in the early phase of his prostatic hyperplasia, Mr Talford was able to choose a more conservative approach for treatment. Although this was an appropriate decision at this time, he nevertheless was not coping with the lower urinary tract symptoms (LUTS) caused by his enlarged prostate. Living with LUTS symptoms affected his physical, social and emotional well-being, eventually resulting in his request for a TURP. At this stage his biopsies were still negative and it was not until two years later following his TURP, that his PSA level had nearly doubled to 27.5 ng/ml along with positive biopsies for adenocarcinoma. This progressive rise in his PSA level indicated that there could be the likelihood of prostatic cancer.

The significance of cancer and the overwhelming anxiety about the prognosis often affects the amount of information that is processed during patient education. The nurse in the case study needed to be aware that, even with such teaching, often there are gaps in understanding about the postoperative nursing care and the complications of the surgery which, for Mr Talford, included his catheter care, post-operative pain, possible incontinence and erectile dysfunction. Discharge planning is important for this man in order to improve his coping and quality of life in the recovery period. The first year following his surgery would be the most difficult for him in terms of living with possible dribbling or incontinence and sexual problems. Many men report that these symptoms leave them feeling that life is a burden because of physical deterioration and fear of ridicule. Nurses need to legitimise these fears and show that they are worthy of discussion and include partners and other family members in finding solutions for these problems.

RENAL CALCULI

WHAT DOES IT MEAN?

Renal calculi, or *urolithiasis*, is the formation of stone-like masses of crystals that, combined with proteins, can form at any level within the urinary tract (see Diagram 7.2)[2]. If formed within the kidneys these calculi are referred to as *nephrolithiasis* and can either remain in the kidney or move down the urinary tract, where they can cause an obstruction.

● Case study

John Hendricks, 45, presented to the emergency department complaining of fever, chills, haematuria and extreme, intermittent pain in his left groin that started yesterday as a nagging pain, higher up in his side and back. His right kidney was ballottable and very tender. For over three weeks he had been having difficulty passing urine. Five days ago, he saw his general practitioner who prescribed Augmentin Duo Forte 250 mg 8/24.

He was febrile with a temperature of 38.4°C, sweating and pale. His observations and the remainder of his physical examination were normal. The results from his urinalysis found large blood and leucocytes, positive nitrite, pH 7.5 and specific gravity was 1.025. The urine culture found *Escherichia coli* bacteria and Mr Hendrick was commenced on cephalexin, and naproxen. He was admitted to the ward for an endoscopic extraction of the stone under general anaesthetic the following day.

WHAT IS THE PATHOPHYSIOLOGY?

It is not clearly understood how renal calculi develop, but a primary function of the kidneys is to remove the by-products of metabolism that include, calcium, oxalate and uric acid. These minerals and other urinary organic matter are generally eliminated from the urinary tract, but when the urine volume is low they supersaturate the urine and crystals can form[55]. Crystal forming salts develop around a nucleus that continues to enlarge until it becomes a stone. The presence or absence of urinary inhibitors, such as magnesium, pyrophosphate, citrate and other substances, are also factors in stone formation.

Although different substances can form stones, the most commonly occurring is either *calcium oxalate (60%) or phosphate*

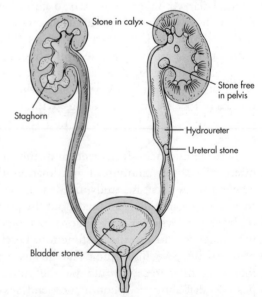

DIAGRAM 7.2 *Location of calculi in the urinary tract* Source: Lewis, SM, *et al.* 2004; *Medical-Surgical Nursing* (6th ed.), Mosby, St Louis, Fig. 44.5, p. 1187.

(10%) or a mixture of both (10%)[56]. These stones are associated with high levels of calcium in the urine or blood or from dehydration[1]. Calcium phosphate calculi are more likely to develop in infected urine[57]. *Struvite stone* (15–20%) is formed from magnesium, calcium and ammonium phosphate but can also develop from a bacterial infection (usually *Proteus mirabilis*), long-time use of antibiotics, alkaline urine, obstruction or following invasive procedures[52]. *Uric acid* (10%) calculi are found when there is an increased excretion of urate, acid urine (<pH of 5.5) or fluid deficit[56]. The least occurring stone is the *cystine*, (1–5%) which can form from a genetic defect and acid urine[55]. Aside from supersaturation, the development of stones can also occur from a history of previous calculi or stasis from immobility[56].

WHAT ARE THE CLINICAL MANIFESTATIONS?

The main symptom of renal calculi is an acute onset of severe pain that changes according to the size and location of the stone in the urinary tract. Some stones, if small enough, can be eliminated without any symptoms but if large in size they can cause an obstruction and trauma. When stones block the flow of urine they cause an increase in hydrostatic pressure and distension of the renal pelvis (hydronephrosis) and proximal ureter (hydroureter). The pain caused by either a partial or complete obstruction to the flow of urine in the renal pelvis is referred to as *renal colic*. This type of pain is associated with a constant, gnawing ache in the costovertebral (the point on the back corresponding to the 12th rib and the lateral border of sacrospinal muscle) region. A stone in the proximal ureter may cause pain that radiates anteriorly down to the testicle in the male and to the bladder in the female. The symptoms of renal colic can be so severe that it can cause a sympathetic response of nausea, vomiting, pallor and cool, clammy skin.

Characteristically, the pain that occurs from calculi in the ureter is known as *ureteric colic*, and can radiate lower in the abdomen to the genitalia and upper thigh. This pain is excruciating and intermittent in nature because of the spasms that occur in the ureter as it attempts to move the stone. The continuous inflammation caused by the rough surface of a stone can result in infection of the kidney (pyelonephritis) or the bladder (cystitis) leading to fever, chills, frequency, haematuria, burning and pain on voiding.

WHAT SHOULD YOU BE LOOKING AT IN THE LABORATORY AND OTHER TESTS?

The diagnosis of renal calculi can be confirmed by an X-ray of the abdomen (kidneys, ureter and bladder (KUB), an intravenous pyelogram (IVP) or a computed tomographic (CT) scan[57]. An IVP is used to identify structural damage, abnormalities or an obstruction from the calculi. If there is a risk with the contrast dye, other tests can be used such as an ultrasound, which can detect non radio-opaque stones and the presence of an obstruction. A CT scan provides a more definitive image of both the size and location of a stone than an ultrasound. Changes in biochemistry would assist in identifying a possible causative agent for stone formation (calcium, phosphorous, magnesium, albumin) or renal damage (blood urea and creatinine). Other tests would include a full blood count and a urine culture that would reveal the presence of red blood cells if there has been trauma and or white blood cells from a bacterial infection. Urinalysis is undertaken to identify whether there is an infection (increase in leucocytes), trauma (haematuria) or bacteriuria (nitrite). In addition, the urine is tested for its pH level as cystine and uric acid stones may form when the pH is less than 6.0 and both calcium phosphate and struvite stones favour a pH of more than 7.2.

WHAT IS THE TREATMENT?

Smaller stones, (less than 5–10 mm in diameter) might be passed without medical intervention but if not then there are four treatment options that are available. Extracorporeal shock wave lithotripsy (ESWL), is a frequently used non-invasive treatment where external shock waves are sent through the body to fragment the stone[6]. ESWL can reduce the need for using an invasive procedure and has been found to decrease hospital stay[58]. An X-ray or ultrasound is used to detect these particles that can then be removed by an endoscope or passed spontaneously with the urine. A uretheric stent is often inserted after the procedure to prevent obstruction and assist the passage of the broken calculi. If the stone is in the kidney, a percutaneous nephrolithotomy (PCN) can be used whereby a needle is passed into the renal pelvis and the stone can then broken up by ultrasound[46]. A nephrostomy tube is then inserted and sutured to the skin. A ureteroscopy procedure is used to remove stones that are in the ureter. A basket catheter is passed via the ureteroscope to remove the stone with or without the use of a laser[59]. When these techniques are not suitable to remove the stone then open surgical interventions are chosen.

APPLIED PHARMACOLOGY

Initially, analgesia may be prescribed to relieve the pain and allow time for the stone to be passed. Depending on the severity of the pain, either opioids (morphine sulphate injection; pethidine hydrochloride) or non-steroidal anti-inflammatory drugs (e.g., ketorolac and naproxen) can be used[3]. Propantheline can be used for ureteric spasm. Antibiotic cover should be given if there is a urinary tract infection present or for stone removal to prevent secondary infection.

On removal of the renal calculi it can then be analysed for its composition and certain medications can be prescribed which will either prevent or inhibit the formation of further stones. A thiazide diuretic decreases calcium content in the urine by reducing urinary calcium excretion in the renal tubules. The production of uric acid can be decreased by the use of allopurinal[55]. Acid urine may need to be alkalinised by citrate preparations.

NURSING IMPLICATIONS

For stones to be passed spontaneously, patients should be advised to increase their fluid intake to 3 L per day. Increased urine volume is one of the most important inhibitors of calculi development[56]. During this process it is important to strain all urine in order to observe when the calculi have been excreted[2]. Patients should be ambulated or, if immobile, repositioned every two hours in order to avoid urinary stasis. Following medical intervention, the urine should be observed for haematuria and crystallised material. Information about dietary modification can be made after the composition of the calculi has been analysed. For example, foods that contain dairy products, oxalate (dark green foods) and sodium that can affect calcium levels should be avoided.

LEARNING EXERCISES

1. How do renal calculi develop?
2. Describe the pain that is characteristically felt from renal and ureteric colic.
3. Which type of renal calculi is more likely to develop from a bacterial infection?
4. What is one of the most important inhibitors of calculi development?

In this case study, it was important, in triaging Mr Hendrick's lower abdominal pain (when he presented to the accident and emergency department) that the nurse took a thorough patient history because this is vital in understanding the probable diagnosis as well as the stone location. During the assessment process, the nurse was able to collect data from Mr Hendrick about his abdominal pain in relation to what had provoked the pain, its quality, radiation, severity, the time he had had it, and any treatment he had used to alleviate it. At the time he was assessed, Mr Hendrick had told the nurse that he had initially experienced sudden, severe pain high in his left flank, about the region of his kidney, which changed character as the stone migrated to his left groin. This aspect of the history may possibly have indicated that the stone was lodged in the ureter. The intermittent pain was suggestive of the distension and increased peristasis of the uterine contractions. The symptoms Mr Hendrick was experiencing, such as sweating and pale skin, were related to the severity of the pain. His fever, chills, dysuria and haematuria also supported the results from his urine culture that suggested an *Escherichia coli* infection of the urinary tract. Part of the assessment process would also include the measurement of vital signs, especially the temperature which, if elevated, would provide further cues for his urinary tract infection.

CONCLUSION

This chapter has reviewed the important anatomical and physiological features of the renal and urinary systems. This was followed by a discussion of four distinct health breakdowns associated with these systems. These were: acute renal failure, chronic renal failure, prostatic hyperplasia, and renal calculi. Case studies were utilised to examine specific pathophysiological, pharmacological and key nursing issues. Finally reflective questions have been prepared to stimulate student learning.

Recommended Readings

Andrews, L & Gibbs, M. 2002; 'Antihypertensive Medications and Renal Disease', *Nephrology Nursing Journal*, 29 (4), 379–382, 388.

Campbell, D. 2003; 'How Acute Renal Failure Puts the Brakes on Kidney Function', *Nursing*, 33 (1), 59–63.

Echlin, KN & Rees, CE. 2002; 'Information Needs and Information-Seeking Behaviours of Men with Prostate Cancer and Their Partners: A Review of the Literature', *Cancer Nursing*, 25 (1), 35–41.

Seaton-Mills, D. 1999; 'Acute Renal Failure: Causes and Considerations in the Critically Ill Patient', *Nursing in Critical Care*, 4 (6), 293–297.

Zimmerman, PG. 2002; 'Triaging Lower Abdominal Pain', *RN*, 65 (12), 52–58.

References

1. Baker, L. 1998; *Nephology*, Cavendish Publishing Ltd, London.

2. Datta, S. 2003; *Renal and Urinary Systems* (2nd ed.), Mosby, St Louis.
3. Phipps, W, Monahan, F, Sands, J, Marek, J, Neighbors, M. 2003; *Medical-Surgical Nursing*, Mosby, St Louis.
4. Chalmers, C. 2002; 'Applied Anatomy and Physiology and the Renal Disease Process', in N Thomas (ed.), *Renal Nursing* (2nd ed.), Baillière Tindall, London. 27–74.
5. Field, M, Pollock, C & Harris, D. 2001; *The Renal System*, Churchill Livingstone, St Louis.
6. Thibodeau, G & Patton, K. 2003; *Anatomy & Pysiology* (5th ed.), Mosby, St Louis.
7. Thomas, N. 2002; *Renal Nursing* (2nd ed.), Baillière Tindall, London.
8. Brady, HR, Brenner, BM, Clarkson, MR & Liebman, W. 2000; 'Acute Renal Failure', in BM Brenner (ed.), *Brenner and Rector's The Kidney* (6th ed.), Saunders, Philadelphia, 1201–1247.
9. Anderson, RJ & Schrier, RW. 2001; 'Acute Renal Failure', in RW Schrier (ed.), *Diseases of the Kidney and Urinary Tract* (7th ed.), 1093–1136, Lippincott Williams and Wilkins, Philadelphia.
10. Johnson, DC & Anderson, RJ. 2002a; 'Acute Renal Failure, Part 1: Seeking Cause', *Journal of Critical Illness*, 17 (7), 251–256.
11. Zellner, KM. 1999; 'Acute Tubular Necrosis', *RN*, 62 (10), 42–46.
12. Palmieri, PA. 2002; 'Obstructive Nephropathy: Pathophysiology, Diagnosis and Collaborative Management', *Nephrology Nursing Journal*, 29 (1), 15–21, 96.
13. Johnson, DC & Anderson, RJ. 2002b; 'Acute Renal Failure, Part 2: Zeroing In on the Diagnosis', *Journal of Critical Illness*, 17 (8), 301–305.
14. Parker, KP. 1998; 'Acute and Chronic Renal Failure', in J Parker (ed.), *Contemporary Nephology Nursing*, Janetti Inc, Pitman, New Jersey.
15. Al-Khafaji, A & Corwin, HL. 2002; 'Acute Renal Failure in the ICU: Balancing Diagnosis and Treatment', *Journal of Critical Illness*, 17 (10), 389–396.
16. Kalra, PA. 2002; 'Early Management and Prevention of Acute Renal Failure', *European Dialysis and Transplant Nurses Association/European Renal Care Association [EDTNA/ERCA]*, (supplement 2), 34–38, 42.
17. National Kidney Foundation. 2002; 'Kidney Disease Outcomes Quality Initiative', *American Journal of Kidney Diseases*, 39 (supplement 1), S17–S31.
18. Szromba, C, Thies, MA & Smith Ossman, S. 2002; 'Advancing Chronic Kidney Disease Care: New Imperatives for Recognition And Intervention', *Nephrology Nursing Journal*, 29 (6), 547–559.
19. McDonald, S & Russ, G. 2002; 'New Patients Commencing in 2001', in SP McDonald & G Russ (eds.), *ANZDATA Registry Report 2002*, Australia and New Zealand Dialysis and Transplant Registry: Adelaide, 7–13.
20. Couser, WO. 1999; 'Glomerulonephritis', *Lancet*, 35, 1509–1515.
21. Erikson, P. 1993; 'Idiopathic Glomerulonephritis: Is It IgA Nephropathy?', *American Nephrology Nurses' Association Journal*, 20 (2), 469–476, 504.
22. Lang, MM & Towers, C. 2001; 'Identifying Poststreptococcal Glomerulonephritis', *The Nurse Practitioner*, 26 (8), 34, 37–38, 40–42, 44, 47.
23. Fox, HL & Swann, D. 2001; 'Goodpasture's Syndrome: Pathophysiology, Diagnosis and Management', *Nephrology Nursing Journal*, 28 (3), 305–310.
24. Wiseman, KC. 1991; 'Nephrotic Syndrome: Pathophysiology and Treatment', *American Nephrology Nurses' Association Journal*, 18 (5), 469–476, 504.
25. Harvey, JN. 2002; 'Diabetic Nephropathy', *British Medical Journal*, 325, 59–60.
26. American Diabetes Association. 2002; 'Clinical Practice Recommendations: Diabetes Nephropathy', *Diabetes Care*, 25 (supplement I), S85–S90.
27. Levin, A & Foley, RN. 2000; 'Cardiovascular Disease in Chronic Renal Failure', *American Journal of Kidney Disease*, 36, (6 supplement 3), S24–S30.
28. Smith, SH. 1993; 'Uremic Pericarditis in Chronic Renal Failure: Nursing Implications', *American Nephrology Nurses' Association Journal*, 21 (2), 147–153.
29. Foret, JP. 2002; 'Diagnosing and Treating Anemia and Iron Deficiency in Patients', *Nephrology Nursing Journal*, 29 (3), 292–296.
30. Tong, EM. 2001; 'Erythropoietin and Anemia', *Seminars in Nephrology*, 21, 190–203.
31. Kammerer, J, Ratican, M, Elzein, H & Mapes, D. 2002; 'Anemia in CKD: Prevalence, Diagnosis, and Treatment', *Nephrology Nursing Journal*, 29 (4), 371–374.
32. Lewis, SL. 1990; 'Alterations of Host Defense Mechanisms in Chronic Dialysis Patients', *American Nephrology Nurses' Association Journal*, 17 (2), 170–182.
33. Pei, Y & Hercz, G. 1996; 'Low Turnover Bone Disease in Dialysis Patients', *Seminars in Dialysis*, 9 (4), 327–331.
34. Shoop, KL. 1994; 'Pruritis in End Stage Renal Disease', *American Nephrology Nurses' Association Journal*, 20 (4), 432–436.
35. Foulks, CJ & Cushner, HM. 1986; 'Sexual Dysfunction in the Male Dialysis Patient: Pathogenesis, Evaluation, and Therapy', *American Journal of Kidney Diseases*, 8, 211–212.
36. Rickus, MA. 1987; Sexual Dysfunction in the Female ESRD Patient', *American Nephrology Nurses' Association Journal*, 14, 185–186.

37. Hartley, GH. 2001; 'Nutritional Status, Delaying Progression and Risks Associated with Protein Restriction', *EDTNA/ERCA Journal*, 27, 101–104.

38. Levery, AS, Adler, S, Caggiula, AW, England, BK, Greene, T, Hunisker, HG, *et al.* 1996; 'Effects of Dietary Protein Restriction on the Progression of Advanced Renal Disease in the Modification of Diet in Renal Disease Study', *American Journal of Kidney Disease*, 27 (5), 652–663.

39. Burrows, L & Prowant, BF. 1998; 'Peritoneal Dialysis', in Parker, J (ed.), *Contemporary Nephrology Nursing*, Janetti Inc, Pitman, New Jersey, 603–660.

40. Allen, RDM & Chapman, JR. 1994; *A Manual of Renal Transplantation*, Edward Arnold, Melbourne.

41. Matzke, GR & Frye, RF. 1997; 'Drug Administration in Patients with Renal Insufficiency: Minimising Renal and Extrarenal Toxicity', *Drug Safety*, 16 (3), 205–231.

42. Yürügen, B. 2002; 'Chronic Renal Failure, Nursing Diagnoses and Intervention', *EDTNA/ERCA Journal*, 28 (1), 13–15, 20.

43. Cameron, S. 1999; *Kidney Failure*, Oxford University Press, Oxford.

44. Gallagher, R & Fleshner, N. 1998; *'Prostate Cancer: 3 Individual Risk Factors'*, *Canadian Medical Association Journal*, 159, 807–813.

45. Davis, D. 1998; 'Prostate Cancer Treatment with Radioactive Seed Implantation', *Association of Perioperative Registered Nurses Online*, 68 (1), 15–48.

46. Smith, P. 2001; *Urology*, Cavendish Publishing Ltd, London.

47. Chambers, A. 2002; 'Transurethral Resection Syndrome: It Does Not Have To Be a Mystery', *AORN Online*, 75 (1), 155–178.

48. Jewett, M, Fleshner, N, Klotz, L, Nam, R, Trachtenberg, J. 2003; 'Radical Prostatectomy as Treatment for Prostate Cancer', *Canadian Medial Association Journal*, 168 (1), 44–45.

49. Balk, S, Ko, Y & Bubley, G. 2003; 'Biology of Prostate-Specific Antigen', *Journal of Clinical Oncology*, 21 (2), 383–391.

50. Gray, M & Allensworth, D. 1999; 'Electrovaporization of the Prostate: Initial Experiences and Nursing Management', *Urologic Nursing*, 19 (1), 25–31.

51. Perera, N & Nandasena, A. 2002; 'Early Catheter Removal after Transurethral Resection of the Prostate', *Ceylon Medical Journal*, 47 (1), 11–12.

52. LeMone, P & Burke, K. 2000; *Medical-Surgical Nursing*, Prentice Hall Health, New Jersey.

53. Sullivan, M & Geller, J. 2002; 'The Effectiveness of Reducing the Daily Dose of Finasteride in Men with Benign Prostatic Hyperplasia', *BioMed Central Urology*, 2, 2.

54. Moore, K & Estey, A. 1999; 'The Early Post-Operative Concerns of Men after Radical Prostatectomy', *Journal of Advanced Nursing*, 29 (5), 1121–1129.

55. Ellsworth, P & Rous, SN. 2001; *Urology*, Blackwell Science, Massachusetts.

56. Morton, A, Iliescu, E & Wilson, J. 2002; 'Nephrology: 1. Investigation and Treatment of Recurrent Kidney Stones', *Canadian Medical Association Journal*, 166 (2), 213–218.

57. Ellis, H, Calne, S, Watson, C. 2002; *General Surgery*, Blackwell Publishing, Oxford.

58. Holman, C, Wisniewski, Z, Semmens, J & Bass, A. 2002; 'Changing Treatments for Primary Urolithiasis: Impact on Services and Renal Preservation in 16,679 Patients in Western Australia', *British Journal of Urology International*, 90 (1), 7–15.

59. Dawson, C & Whitfield, H. 1996; 'ABC of Urology: Urinary Stone Disease', *British Medical Journal*, 312 (7040), 1219–1221.

8 | Neurologic Health Breakdown

AUTHOR

JENNIFER BLUNDELL

LEARNING OBJECTIVES

When you have completed this chapter you will be able to
- Identify the major anatomical and physiological features of the neurological system;
- Describe the pathophysiological changes associated with neurologic health breakdown related to sensorimotor disorders, cerebrovascular disease, meningitis and epilepsy;
- Understand laboratory and diagnostic techniques used to form the diagnosis for these problems;
- Describe the management strategies associated with caring for a person with a neurologic health breakdown;
- Identify the common pharmacologic agents used in managing neurologic health breakdown; and
- Consider nursing interventions required in caring for people with neurologic health breakdown.

INTRODUCTION

This chapter includes a review of the anatomy and physiology of the central and peripheral nervous system. Using a case study approach, distinct common health breakdowns are presented. These are: Guillain–Barré syndrome, multiple sclerosis, myasthenia gravis and Parkinson's disease, cerebrovascular disease, meningitis, and epilepsy.

WHAT MAKES UP THE NERVOUS SYSTEM: KEY ASPECTS OF ANATOMY AND PHYSIOLOGY

There are two major components of the nervous system: the central nervous system comprising the brain and spinal cord that acts as the control centre for the body, and the peripheral nervous system consisting of the cranial and peripheral nerves. The peripheral nervous system acts as the information pathway, transmitting information between the central nervous system and the sensory receptors, muscles and organs of the body. Through this process, the nervous system organises and coordinates functions of all body systems, as well as consciousness and cognition[1,2].

THE NEURONE

The functional unit of the nervous system is the neurone or nerve cell, a specialised cell with the ability to receive and transmit electrochemical nerve impulses. Each neurone is composed of a cell body, an axon or nerve fibre carrying impulses away from the cell body, and processes called dendrites that carry impulses to the cell body (see Figure 8.1). This basic structure is similar for all neurones, but variations occur depending upon the site of the neurone and its specific function. For example, a motor neurone may have a long axon, or fibre, in order to transmit impulses from the central nervous system over a long distance in the body, whereas a sensory nerve may have a shorter axon[1,2].

The majority of axons have a fatty (lipoprotein) myelin sheath wrapped around them, with regular constrictions at approximately 1 mm intervals called the nodes of Ranvier. Outside the central nervous system, myelin is produced by Schwann cells that lie alongside the nerve, while in the central nervous system, myelin is produced by cells called oligodendrocytes. Unmyelinated nerve fibres are found in the autonomic nervous system, a division of the peripheral nervous system[1–3].

NERVE IMPULSE TRANSMISSION

At rest, the cell membrane of the neurone is relatively resistant to sodium ions (Na^+), but permeable to potassium ions (K^+) and has a negative electrical potential difference across its membrane; that is, the inside of the cell is negative to its external environment. This charge (resting potential) is maintained by the cell membrane pumping out any sodium ions that seep in.

When the axon receives a stimulus, its membrane becomes more permeable and sodium rapidly diffuses into the cell, causing a positive electrical charge. This is the first stage of the action potential and sets up a chain reaction along the axon (depolarisation).

Potassium leaves the cell as it fills with sodium, until the membrane becomes impermeable to sodium ions again and the sodium pump restarts. Three sodium ions then

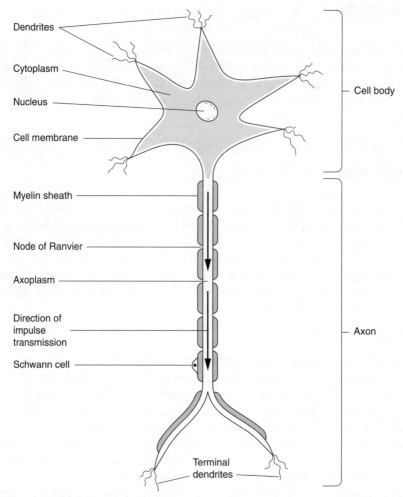

Dendrites

Cytoplasm

Nucleus

Cell membrane

Cell body

Myelin sheath

Node of Ranvier

Axoplasm

Direction of impulse transmission

Schwann cell

Axon

Terminal dendrites

FIGURE 8.1 *Structure of the neurone*

leave the cell, the resting potential of the axon is restored (repolarisation), and two potassium ions passively re-enter the axon. This whole process takes about 2 milliseconds[4]. A short period of time when another impulse cannot be transmitted (the refractory period) occurs, limiting the frequency of impulses. The transmission of an impulse is an 'all or nothing' event, that is, in a healthy neurone the impulse is the same size and speed for a given nerve, and if initiated is always transmitted[4]. However, the frequency of impulses can vary, with more frequent impulses occurring along the more important pathways of the central nervous system[1,4–6].

The speed at which a nerve impulse is transmitted depends on the diameter of the axon, with wider axons transmitting impulses more quickly. If the axon is myelinated, the impulse travels at greater speed, as depolarisation and repolarisation occurs at the nodes of Ranvier as the nerve impulse action potential travels down the axon from one node to the next (saltatory conduction)[1–6].

NERVE IMPULSES AND THE SYNAPSE

The area where nerves connect with each other, with muscles or other organs is called the synapse. This is where impulses are transmitted from the nerve cell to the target organ

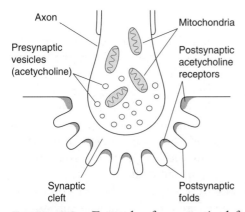

FIGURE 8.2 *Example of a synaptic cleft in a neuromuscular junction*

through the release of chemical transmitters from the presynaptic neurone to stimulate the postsynaptic neurone/s or organ (see Figure 8.2). There are a number of different chemical transmitters, but the most common one is acetylcholine (ACh). Acetylcholine diffuses across the synaptic cleft and binds to the postsynaptic membrane of a neurone, causing depolarisation of that nerve fibre. In turn, the postsynaptic membrane releases cholinesterase, an enzyme that inactivates the acetylcholine. In the brain, release of neurotransmitter substances is more complex, as is the arrangement of nerve fibres[1,4].

CENTRAL NERVOUS SYSTEM

The central nervous system receives, interprets and stores messages from the internal and external environment and transmits messages in return. The brain, a soft mass of tissue, is composed of a collection of nerve cells, white matter and supportive tissue connected to the spinal cord, which has a similar structure. The brain is subdivided into the cerebrum, cerebellum and brainstem (see Figure 8.3).

The skull and the vertebrae provide protection for the brain and spinal cord, along with three membranes called the meninges, and cerebrospinal fluid. These three dural membranes, the dura mater, arachnoid mater and pia mater, cover and support the brain. Cerebrospinal fluid (CSF) circulates through the ventricles of the brain, the central canal of the spinal cord, and the subarachnoid space between the arachnoid and pia mater, bathing and cushioning the brain and spinal cord.

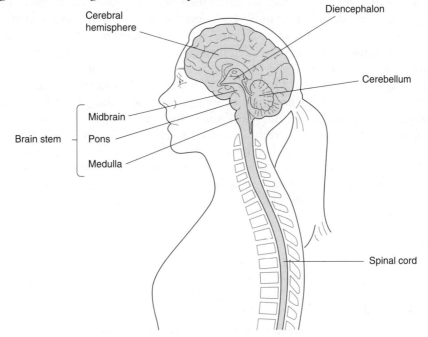

FIGURE 8.3 *Major divisions of the central nervous system*

CEREBRUM

The cerebrum, the largest part of the brain, consists of a right and left hemisphere, each of which is subdivided into four lobes. The hemispheres are connected by the corpus callosum. The outer layer or cortex of the cerebrum primarily consists of neuronal cell bodies or grey matter, while the inner part of the cerebrum is made up of the axons or white matter. The internal capsule carrying sensory impulses to the cortex, and motor impulses from the cortex to the body, is situated within the white matter in each hemisphere. Sensation and motor function for the left side of the body are controlled by the right cerebrum and on the right side of the body by the left cerebrum, as ascending and descending impulses cross at the medulla oblongata in the brain stem[3,4].

The frontal, parietal, temporal and occipital lobes are each responsible for controlling specific bodily functions. The frontal lobes are involved in voluntary movement, speech, intelligence, personality, thought, memory, emotion, and understanding, linking sensory and motor information, and coordinating sensory and motor function. The temporal lobes are responsible for interpretation of hearing, smell and taste, with the dominant temporal lobe responsible for understanding speech. The parietal lobes receive sensory impulses, interpreting information such as shape, size, texture and the sense of body position, and the occipital lobes are the primary area for vision. Cranial nerves 1 and 2 responsible for sight and smell have their origins within the cerebrum[1-4].

Deep within the cerebrum surrounding the third ventricle is the thalamus, a structure that acts as a relay centre with connections to the brain and spinal cord, the autonomic nervous system and pituitary gland. The thalamus also plays a role in control of primitive emotions, including fear and distinguishing noxious from pleasant stimuli. Another structure within each hemisphere is the basal ganglia, a mass of nerve cells responsible for mediating motor coordination and regulating muscle tone and force.

The hypothalamus, a structure situated at the base of the optic chiasm, acts as an autonomic centre with connections to the brain, spinal cord, autonomic nervous system and the pituitary gland. It is responsible for control of body temperature, appetite, blood pressure, breathing, sleep patterns, behavioural and emotional expression, pituitary secretions, and is partially involved in regulating the stress reaction. The pituitary gland, consisting of an anterior and posterior lobe, is attached to and gets messages from the hypothalamus which regulates production of hormone-stimulating substances that are involved in regulating the functions of other body systems, as well as prolactin, corticotropin, growth hormone, and anti-diuretic hormone[1-4].

Within the cerebrum are four ventricles or connected cavities consisting of two lateral ventricles, one in each cerebral hemisphere, the third ventricle, which surrounds the thalamus and the fourth, an expansion of the central canal in the medulla oblongata. About 500 mL of cerebrospinal fluid (CSF) is produced in the lateral ventricles every 24 hours. CSF is clear and contains water, glucose, protein and lymphocytes[2,3].

CEREBELLUM

The cerebellum, mirrors the structure of the cerebrum having two hemispheres, with an outer cortex of grey matter and an inner core of white nerve fibres, connecting the cerebellum to the cerebrum and brain stem. The cerebellar hemispheres receive sensory input from muscles, joints and the vestibular canals of the inner ear, and control muscle coordination, posture, equilibrium and balance on the same side of the body.

BRAIN STEM

The brain stem, where two-way transmission of nerve impulses from the spinal cord to the brain occurs, connects the cerebrum to the spinal cord and is composed of the midbrain, pons and medulla oblongata. The midbrain contains the cell bodies for cranial nerves 3 and 4 that mediate pupil reaction and eye movements. The origins of cranial nerves 5, 6, 7 and 8, responsible for chewing, saliva production, hearing and maintaining balance, are found in the pons. Cranial nerves 9, 10, 11 and 12, responsible for taste, gag reflexes, swallowing and tongue movement, arise from the medulla oblongata, which houses the cardiac, respiratory, vasomotor and vomiting centres.

The reticular formation, a network of nerves involved in arousal and the sleep-wake cycle is situated in the brainstem with connections to the thalamus and cerebral cortex. The reticular formation screens and mediates sensory information so that the cerebral cortex is not overwhelmed.

Voluntary muscle control occurs as impulses from the motor cortex of the brain, travelling via the descending motor pathways, receive input from the cerebellum and basal ganglia before crossing over (decussation) at the medullary pyramids to travel down the spinal cord. The pyramidal tracts from the cortex exert voluntary control of motor function, while the extrapyramidal tracts from the other areas of the central nervous system have an inhibitory influence and control involuntary movement[1,2,4].

SPINAL CORD

The spinal cord is continuous with the medulla oblongata to the level of the twelfth lumbar vertebra and consists of an inner mass of grey matter divided into horns containing the neuronal cell bodies which relay impulses related to reflex or voluntary motor activity. The surrounding white matter consists of myelinated nerve fibres grouped into columns called tracts that carry sensory or ascending impulses to the brain and descending or motor impulses to the nerve cells to refine voluntary muscle action. These messages travel from the spinal cord to the body via the 31 pairs of spinal nerves that are part of the peripheral nervous system (see Figure 8.4).

PERIPHERAL NERVOUS SYSTEM

The peripheral nervous system consists of 31 pairs of spinal nerves and their motor and sensory branches plus the 12 pairs of cranial nerves. The system has two divisions, the somatic and autonomic. The somatic division is involved with sensation and movement, while the autonomic nervous system (ANS) helps regulate the internal environment of the body through its effect on involuntary tissues in the lungs, and endocrine, cardiovascular and gastrointestinal systems. The autonomic nervous system includes the nerve cells and fibres that act upon these particular organs. It is subdivided into the sympathetic and the parasympathetic nervous system, each having antagonistic or opposing influences that help maintain homeostasis. The neurotransmitter of the sympathetic nervous system is noradrenaline and of the parasympathetic nervous system, acetylcholine. Control of the ANS is complex, involving the hypothalamus and brainstem structures[4].

The 31 pairs of spinal nerves connect to the spinal cord by two roots. Sensory information is transmitted from receptors in the body to the dorsal nerve root of the nerve cell, and motor information is transmitted to the muscles via the ventral nerve root. Each spinal nerve separates into branches that supply a specific area, with a degree of overlap between the areas of the body each nerve supplies.

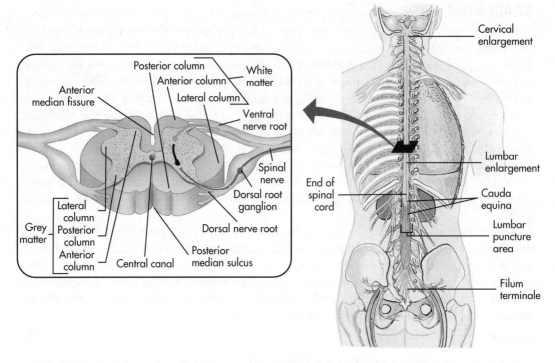

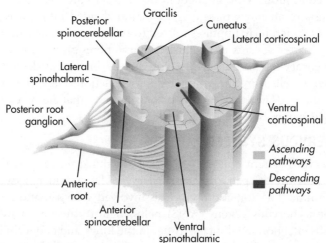

FIGURE 8.4 *Spinal cord*
Source: Adapted from Thibodeau, GA & Patton, KT. 1999; *Anatomy and Physiology* (4th ed.), Mosby, St Louis Fig. 13.6, p. 381.

CEREBRAL BLOOD SUPPLY

The brain requires a blood flow of approximately 750 mL/min for it to be able to function fully. The arteries and their branches in the brain receive blood supply from the right and left internal carotid arteries. These enter the skull anteriorly on each side through the base, and then branch to form the anterior and middle cerebral arteries that feed the anterior and middle part of the cerebral hemispheres. The posterior part of the cerebral hemispheres, including the occipital lobes, brain stem and cerebellum, receive their supply from the two vertebral arteries that enter at the foramen magnum to form the basilar artery, then this divides to form the two posterior cerebral arteries. The anterior and posterior communicating arteries join these two circulations to form a vascular ring called the circle of Willis. This potentially allows collateral circulation to develop if occlusion of a cerebral blood vessel occurs. Autoregulation in cerebral arterioles allows precise distribution of regional blood flow in the different areas of the brain[3].

Venous drainage occurs directly from cerebral tissue through veins into the venous sinuses found between the two layers of the dura mater, that in turn drain into the external jugular veins.

THE BLOOD BRAIN BARRIER

The blood brain barrier (BBB) maintains constancy in the intracerebral environment through controlling the passage of substances from the vascular system by a series of passive and selective active transport mechanisms. Substances such as oxygen, glucose, and essential nutrients enter the brain easily, while other substances are prevented from entering. This means that drugs require certain properties to allow them to cross the BBB if they are to act on the nervous system. For example, nicotine and alcohol enter easily while levodopa, the precursor of dopamine, is used to treat Parkinson's disease because it can reach the brain from the vascular system, while dopamine is unable to enter. The protective effect of the BBB is diminished in the presence of cerebral disease, inflammation or trauma and certain organisms appear to be able to breakdown the barrier and cross into the nervous system[4,5].

SUMMARY OF KEY CONCEPTS

- The neurone is the functional unit of the nervous system.
- The central nervous system is responsible for controlling intelligence, consciousness, sensation, movement and all other functions of the body.
- Impulses are transmitted to and from the structures in the cerebrum via a relay centre, the thalamus.
- The cerebellum assists coordination of movement and posture.
- Impulses related to sensory and motor function are relayed to and from the cerebrum via the spinal cord.
- The peripheral nervous system relays sensory information to the spinal cord and initiates voluntary muscle activity.
- The autonomic nervous system is involved in regulating the internal environment.

GUILLAIN-BARRÉ SYNDROME

WHAT DOES IT MEAN?

Guillain-Barré syndrome (GBS) was named after two French doctors who first described a number of cases of acute ascending muscular weakness[6]. It is an acute immune-mediated disorder associated with inflammation and demyelination of the cranial and spinal nerves, characterised by a rapid progressive ascending muscle weakness resulting in varying degrees of motor dysfunction[4,6,7]. The syndrome occurs in children and adults, and is the most common cause of acute neuromuscular paralysis in developed countries[8,9]. There appear to be two major peaks of occurrence, in young adults and in persons aged over 55 years[10,11]. Although it can be fatal, prompt diagnosis and good management of symptoms leads to recovery of 80–90% of patients, with few or no remaining disabilities[7,8].

● Case study

Sandra Probona, 23, presented complaining of a three-day history of mild weakness in her lower limbs, 'feeling funny' in her legs, and a recent tendency to trip when walking. She said that about two weeks ago, she had had the 'flu' with a runny nose and a cough and had felt cold. As it was the weekend, she had not seen a doctor, and had treated it with over-the-counter medication and rest, and had felt able to go to work by the Monday.

On examination, she had abnormal gait with loss of plantar flexion, and a marked decrease in her ability to dorsiflex, invert and evert her feet. She had loss of sensation to deep pressure in her feet and decreased deep tendon reflexes at the ankle and knee. The strength in her quadriceps was reduced with a score of 3/5. Further examination demonstrated loss of position sense below mid-calf, and slight reduction in her ability to discriminate between temperature extremes and between sharp and blunt objects. Sensation, movement and strength were normal in her trunk and arms. No speech or swallowing deficits, breathing difficulties or cardiac arrythmias were present at this time. A diagnosis of Guillain-Barré syndrome was made following diagnostic tests that excluded other possible diagnoses.

Following admission, Sandra was monitored for progression of the paralysis, cardiac irregularities and respiratory function. Progression of her symptoms continued with loss of quadriceps strength and tendon reflexes. Cardiac monitoring showed sinus rhythm; her respiratory rate and depth, vital capacity and pulse oximetry remained within normal limits. Treatment with intravenous immunoglobulin was commenced and the physiotherapist consulted for assessment for splinting of her paralysed legs. Nerve conduction studies performed 10 days after admission showed reduced response in the peroneal and tibial nerves.

WHAT IS THE PATHOPHYSIOLOGY?

GBS is believed to be caused by a cell-mediated autoimmune attack on the myelin surrounding the cranial and spinal nerves in response to a virus. Of patients with GBS, 50% have reported a viral-like illness 10–14 days prior to onset of symptoms[7,12]. *Haemophilus influenzae*, *Mycoplasma pneumonia*, Epstein-Barr virus, HIV and *Camyplobacter jejuni* infection have all been linked to GBS, as have patients who are immunocompromised, such as those who have AIDS or are post-organ transplant[12–14].

In GBS, it is believed that an immunologic reaction results in inflammation and oedema of the myelin sheath of the nerve axon and the anterior and posterior nerve roots of the spinal nerve. In response, lymphocytes and macrophages move in to the area, which results in patchy loss of myelin (demyelination) from the affected peripheral nerves and wider spaces between the nodes of Ranvier. The more highly myelinated motor, and some cranial, nerves are affected more than those responsible for cutaneous pain, touch and temperature. In some cases, there may be injury to the axon itself[4,6,11].

Demyelination causes impaired transmission of electrical impulses along the affected nerves due to the inability of the action potential to travel down the neuron and reach the target organ (loss of saltatory conduction). The result is a decrease in or loss of function in the organs the affected nerves innervate. The degree of dysfunction the patient experiences depends upon the degree of demyelination in the affected nerves. In motor nerves, muscle weakness and a flaccid paralysis (areflexia) can occur. Similarly, disruption of the posterior sensory nerve roots results in paresthesia, numbness, tingling and burning sensations, while the consequence of disruption to the autonomic nervous system may be a labile blood pressure and cardiac arrythmias[4,6,11].

There is a range of variants of GBS based on the degree of peripheral nerve involvement or the site of inflammation, but ascending GBS or acute motor-sensory axonal neuropathy is the most common type, with symmetrical weakness and numbness starting in the legs and progressing to the trunk, arms and cranial nerves. Respiratory function is affected in 50% of cases[8]. Other variants are descending GBS, pure motor GBS or acute motor axonal neuropathy in which there is no sensory loss; and Miller-Fisher, a rare type, more common in China, Japan, Africa, and South America, which results in ophthalmoplegia, areflexia and ataxia[8].

WHAT ARE THE CLINICAL MANIFESTATIONS?

The presenting signs and symptoms depend upon the degree of peripheral nerve involvement and the severity of the demyelination. Characteristically, the person will present with a progressive symmetrical ascending weakness of skeletal muscles. The weakness usually starts in the legs and may then affect the trunk, arms, and cranial nerves, with reduction in or loss of tendon reflexes[8-14]. In severe cases, respiratory failure may occur if the nerves supplying the intercostal muscles and diaphragm or the 10th cranial (vagus) nerve are affected. If the cranial nerves are involved, clinical signs will depend upon the nerve affected. For example, if the facial nerve is affected, there will be difficulty in smiling, frowning, or drinking with a straw. Dysphagia and paralysis of the larynx can occur due to involvement of the 9th, 10th, 11th and 12th cranial nerves[8].

If there is sensory involvement, then paresthesia, sensations of tingling, altered sensation to touch and numbness in the extremities, reduced proprioception and sensory loss in a 'stocking and glove' distribution may be present. Pain and muscle stiffness in the limbs and back are also reported in about 25% of patients, and may become severe[8].

Rapid shallow breathing with the use of the accessory muscles of respiration (abdominal, intercostal muscles, shoulder girdle) is present as the intercostal muscles and diaphragm become weaker. If vital capacity falls below 15 mL/kg, there is a risk of respiratory failure and mechanical ventilation is indicated as alveolar hypoventilation and respiratory acidosis develop[8,15]. The most serious complication, respiratory failure requiring admission to ICU and mechanical ventilation, occurs in approximately 20–35% of cases[16].

Autonomic dysfunction results in hypotension, hypertension or a labile blood pressure, and tachycardia, bradycardia or cardiac arrhythmias. Paralytic ileus, urinary retention, and inappropriate antidiuretic hormone secretion can also occur[8,9].

GBS has three phases: acute, plateau and recovery. Symptoms usually occur 10–14 days following a viral infection and reach their peak in the third or fourth week. However in some cases, respiratory failure occurs within 48 hours of the onset of symptoms[10,15]. The acute phase lasts 1–3 weeks and begins when the first obvious symptoms develop, ending when no further symptoms appear or deterioration has ceased. The plateau phase, during which no change or improvement occurs, lasts from days to two weeks, while recovery time when remyelination and regrowth of axons occur can last from four months to three years. Approximately 80% of people recover from most effects by one year, although a 3% relapse rate has been reported after complete or near recovery[9,15].

WHAT SHOULD YOU BE LOOKING AT IN LABORATORY AND OTHER TESTS?

The diagnosis is based on medical history and assessment of the level of motor, sensory or autonomic involvement. A full assessment of motor and sensory (touch, proprioception, temperature) function, deep tendon and plantar reflexes, cranial nerves, respiratory effort and spirometry is required. Although a number of laboratory tests can be carried out, most will not show any change in the initial stages of the disease.

Lumbar puncture and examination of the CSF will demonstrate an increase in protein over several days, peaking 4–6 weeks after onset of the disease, normal white cell count and some increase in CSF pressure. Blood tests may show an elevated erythrocyte sedimentation rate (ESR) and raised levels of immunoglobulin can be measured in the serum. Electromyography (EMG) and nerve conduction studies will demonstrate a slowing of the velocity of nerve conduction to voluntary muscle as demyelination occurs[8,13].

WHAT IS THE TREATMENT?

GBS is potentially reversible in the majority of cases if it is detected early. The primary goals of treatment are to modify the course of the disease, provide supportive management related to the signs and symptoms, and prevent complications; and this requires a multidisciplinary team approach.

Immunomodulation therapy has been found to prevent further progression of the disease and reduce recovery time if instigated within the first two weeks of the disease[9]. Indications for immunomodulation therapy are rapid progression of the disease, bulbar involvement, respiratory dysfunction, and/or loss of mobility. Intravenous immunoglobulin (IVIg) is the most commonly used treatment, as it is less invasive than plasmapheresis and is usually given over 2–5 days for a total dose based on body weight[8]. Plasmapheresis aims to remove circulating antimyelin antibodies, and a daily exchange of plasma is performed over 4–5 days[17]. However, it has been reported as less useful for the treatment of children, a proportion of who may have poorer long-term outcomes[18–20].

APPLIED PHARMACOLOGY

Pharmacological management is based on immunomodulation therapy, prevention of complications and treatment of signs and symptoms. Anticoagulant therapy (heparin)[21] is administered to prevent deep venous thrombosis and pulmonary embolus, both complications related to reduced venous return due to the flaccid paralysis and loss of normal muscle pump activity. Analgesia will be required if muscle pain is present and may include narcotics. Autonomic system manifestations, such as cardiac arrhythmias, bradycardia, and hypotension, may require appropriate medication to treat these symptoms. Neuromuscular blocking agents are to be avoided due to the risk of prolonging muscle paralysis.

NURSING IMPLICATIONS

Monitoring to detect signs of ascending paralysis and sensory loss are paramount. In particular, observing for poor airway clearance, respiratory failure, poor swallowing, and autonomic complications is essential to provide early treatment. Further, in determining the progress of the disease and preventing complications, assessment of motor and sensory function, pain, respiratory patterns, vital capacity, swallowing, cardiac rate and rhythm, blood pressure and urinary output are all important. Nursing interventions to prevent secondary complications, such as superimposed respiratory and urinary infection, limb contractures, bowel and bladder dysfunction, pressure ulcers, muscle atrophy, thrombo-embolic episodes and inadequate nutrition, are essential if the patient is to recover with minimal side effects. Psychological support, communication and education for both patients and their families are important to reduce anxiety and fear of the possible outcome.

LEARNING EXERCISES

1. Describe the pathophysiology associated with demyelination of peripheral nerves.
2. Why are cardiac monitoring, assessment of motor and sensory function, vital capacity, speech and swallowing important nursing considerations in Guillain-Barré syndrome?
3. When are intubation and ventilatory support indicated?
4. What nursing interventions are essential to prevent secondary complications?

In any patient diagnosed with Guillain-Barré syndrome, it is important that frequent and accurate monitoring of motor and sensory, respiratory and autonomic function is carried out to evaluate the progression of the disease and the need for prompt intervention of supportive therapy if respiratory failure or cardiac involvement occurs. In this case study, the disease progression following admission affected the motor function in Sandra's lower limbs and did not progress further to involve her trunk muscles or arms. This, in conjunction with prompt diagnosis and commencement of a five-day course of immunomodulation therapy, meant that she was transferred to a rehabilitation unit 17 days following admission. Electromyography confirmed that demyelination was present. She received intensive inpatient rehabilitation for a period of 4 months and continued to receive physiotherapy on an outpatient basis for a further 7 months. At this time she appeared to have made a full recovery, with no residual motor or sensory deficits.

MULTIPLE SCLEROSIS

WHAT DOES IT MEAN?

Multiple sclerosis (MS) is unpredictable inflammation, demyelination and scarring of the myelin in the brain, spinal cord and cranial nerves, resulting in widespread neurologic dysfunction. It is characterised by remissions and exacerbations of varying severity, with some patients having a rapidly progressive disease; however the majority (70%) have prolonged remissions[22].

The incidence of disease is more common in people of northern European descent, in women born in the northern hemisphere from urban and high socioeconomic backgrounds, and there is often a family history[8]. Multiple sclerosis is a major cause of disability in people between 18–40 years, with average age at onset being 30 years[8].

There is no one identified cause of MS and environmental agents, a slow acting virus, autoimmune response, allergic response, anoxia, toxins, and nutritional, traumatic and genetic factors have all been considered. The risk of developing the disease decreases in people who migrate from a high-risk area before adolescence, leading to a hypothesis that an environmental agent may trigger an autoimmune response in genetically susceptible people. An increase in humoral and cell-mediated T and B cells has been identified in the plaque[22].

● Case study

Gilda Swensson, 32, an accountant, presented to her general practitioner four months ago complaining of 'fuzzy' vision. This resolved with no further problems until recently, when the fuzziness returned, accompanied by double vision. At the last visit she complained of weakness in her legs and a tendency for her right foot 'to trip her up'. Her general practitioner referred her to a neurologist for further investigation.

During her assessment, she said she had migrated from northern Europe with her family when she was 18 years of age. On examination, she had 75% of normal muscle strength in her right lower leg and 60% in her left leg. Examination of her gait showed mild right foot drop and slight knee hyperextension. A visual evoked potential test demonstrated a decrease in her visual sensory conduction time. An appointment for an MRI was to be made, and she was referred to physiotherapy for assessment.

WHAT IS THE PATHOPHYSIOLOGY?

There is sporadic patchy demyelination of the white matter of the central nervous system in brain, spinal cord and cranial nerves, with a preference for the optic nerves, brain stem, cerebellum and spinal cord white matter secondary to inflammation[4]. Scarring from proliferation of the glial cells (gliosis) of the myelin sheath occurs in the affected areas with hard yellow plaques replacing the myelin. This scar tissue damages the axon fibre and causes disruption of the conduction of nerve impulses, usually in the brain, spinal cord or optic nerves. Nerve impulses may be slowed, blocked or be abnormal or ectopic, and this disruption accounts for the variation in symptoms with which patients present[8].

Remission, with an improvement in symptoms, is thought to occur when the inflammation ceases or the lesions heal, with impulse transmission returning as remyelination by the oligodendrocytes occurs. Residual disability may be due to only part remyelination of lesions occurring. Symptoms become irreversible if further lesions develop, with permanent myelin loss and axonal loss if the disease progresses[6,23].

Classification of multiple sclerosis is based upon the timing of exacerbations and disease progression, with remissions varying from months to years and relapses lasting days to months[23,24] (see Table 8.1).

WHAT ARE THE CLINICAL MANIFESTATIONS?

Clinical manifestations vary depending on the extent and location of demyelination, and therefore the varying presentations and unpredictable progress of the disease can make diagnosis difficult. The most common initial manifestations are visual and sensory alterations. Blurred vision and pain in the eye (optic neuritis), diplopia (double vision)

TABLE 8.1: TYPES AND CHARACTERISTICS OF VARIANTS OF MULTIPLE SCLEROSIS	
Type	**Characteristics**
Relapsing-remitting MS (RRMS) Most common	Recurrent episodes of neurological dysfunction with full, incomplete or no recovery. No progression of symptoms between attacks. 80% of cases are stable between attacks
Secondary progressive MS (SPMS)	Begins as RRMS but the number of attacks reduces and is replaced by a steady deterioration unrelated to attacks after twenty years or more
Primary progressive MS (PPMS) 10–15%	Older age onset. Characterised by a progressive course from the beginning signs and symptoms with no acute attack
Progressive relapsing MS (PRMS) 5%	Progressive deterioration from first symptoms, with an occasional acute attack

and/or sensory disturbances, such as paresthesia, numbness and tingling, loss of balance, decreased ability to distinguish temperature and proprioception, are most commonly reported[24].

Other signs and symptoms include emotional lability due to involvement of white matter in the frontal lobes. Gait ataxia, problems with balance and coordination, tremor, slurred speech and nystagmus occurs due to involvement of the cerebellum. Brain stem lesions affect swallowing and speech, while muscle weakness and spasticity are related to spinal cord tract involvement, as are bladder, bowel and sexual dysfunction[24].

Approximately 65% of patients will have some form of cognitive impairment affecting functions such as memory, attention, information processing, executive function and visual spatial skills[25]. These are independent of disease progression and are often undiagnosed or mistaken for depression.

The onset of an attack may be preceded by stress or an upper respiratory tract infection, and as the disease progresses, heat sensitivity and fatigue exacerbate the symptoms.

WHAT SHOULD YOU BE LOOKING AT IN LABORATORY AND OTHER TESTS?

There is no single test that diagnoses MS and initially, testing may not demonstrate any specific findings consistent with the disease. A negative test result does not rule out the diagnosis of multiple sclerosis, as it is based on the total picture rather than a single test[23]. Diagnosis is based on past and present patient history, full neurological examination including cranial nerves, motor, sensory and cerebellar function, and mental status. Magnetic resonance imaging (MRI) is the most sensitive test for multiple sclerosis, although CT scanning may show lesions in the white matter. MRI shows the size, number and location of lesions in the white matter brain or spinal cord in about 95% of cases. Evoked potential testing demonstrates slowed absent or abnormal conduction pathways of visual, auditory, sensory or motor nerve impulses in 85% of people[23].

Components of the breakdown of myelin are released into the CSF as demyelination occurs and these components can be measured by three tests. The CSF IgG (immunoglobulin G) Index test detects IgG synthesis if the ratio of IgG: albumen is greater than the serum ratio. The normal IgG index is 0.77 or less, and the normal ratios of IgG: albumin in CSF is 0.15–0.38 and 0.15–0.41 in serum. The oligoclonal band test is used to examine if synthesis of immunoglobulin G (IgG) has occurred and is positive in more than 90% of patients with multiple sclerosis[8]. The third test, the CSF myelin basic protein test, is positive if elevated above 4 ng/mL. However, as elevated levels occur in other demyelinating disorders, CNS trauma or infection, it cannot be used as the only test[26].

Diagnosis is based on age, signs and symptoms of disease of the brain or spinal cord following neurological examination, evidence of 2 or more lesions on an MRI scan and a history of two or more episodes lasting at least 24 hours and occurring at least one month apart, or progressive development of signs and symptoms over at least 6 months with no other cause or explanation[8,26].

WHAT IS THE TREATMENT?

There is no standard treatment to prevent or cure multiple sclerosis. The aims of treatment are to shorten the length of an attack, decrease demyelination, enhance recovery from an acute attack, and reduce the rate of relapse, as well as to slow disability and development of new lesions. This is achieved through pharmacological means and a multidisciplinary approach. The pharmacological approach includes the use of drugs that modify the immune processes (immunomodulators). Corticosteroids are used to reduce the severity and length of an acute attack or relapse by reducing oedema, and relieving symptoms. Interferons reduce the rate of relapse in relapsing–remitting MS (RRMS) and secondary progressive MS (SPMS) versions of the disease. Other drugs may be prescribed if the patient has a poor response or develops adverse reactions including chemotherapeutic agents, and humoral therapy through IVIG and plasmapheresis[27–29].

Other management is focussed on managing the symptoms by supporting altered body functions, maintaining muscle tone and strength, improving function and preventing complications such as falls, constipation, urinary tract infection, joint contractures, pressure sores, and pneumonia through a multidisciplinary approach. Reduction of stress and prevention of fatigue are important components of management[30,31]. Physiotherapy for muscle strengthening and balancing exercises, spasticity reduction and development of a daily exercise routine plays a major role in management. Pain management may be required. Procedures to reduce severe spasticity include botulinum toxin injection, implantation of an intrathecal pump to administer the antispasmodic drug baclofen, or in extreme cases, surgical interventions such as adductor tendonotomy and dorsal rhizotomy. Deep brain stimulation has been used in cases where a disabling tremor is present[26–27].

Once MS has been definitely diagnosed, patient education about the disease, current management, and complementary or alternative medical treatments and their effect are required, supplemented with appropriate counselling.

APPLIED PHARMACOLOGY

Pharmacological management is used to reduce the course of attacks and manage other signs and symptoms, such as tremor, spasticity, fatigue, pain, bladder and bowel dysfunction, depression and mood alterations.

Corticosteroids are used to reduce the severity and length of an acute attack by reducing oedema, relieving symptoms, and shortening the length of an acute attack or relapse. A short course of intravenous (IV) methylprednisone (3–7 days) and an oral prednisone taper is the most commonly used approach.

A daily subcutaneous (SC) injection of glatiramer acetate (Caponex) is used for initial treatment of relapsing-remitting multiple sclerosis. Interferon–beta 1a (Avonex) via intramuscular injection (IMI) weekly, or interferon–beta 1b (Betaferon) SC every second day, is thought to increase protein synthesis, and decrease the frequency of acute attacks[28]. However, approximately 24–35% of patients will develop neutralising antibodies to these medications, therefore a decision about when to commence this treatment and close monitoring of its effect needs to be given serious consideration[28,29].

Chemotherapeutic agents such as cyclosporin and methotrexate have been used in the treatment of progressive multiple sclerosis to disrupt immune function and alter the process of demyelination.

Depending upon the signs and symptoms, a number of other medications may be prescribed. These include: antispasmodics for muscle spasticity (baclofen, diazepam or dantrolene sodium); anticholinergics for detrusor muscle spasm or urinary frequency and urgency (propantheline bromide); stool softeners, stimulants and bulking agents for bowel dysfunction; anticonvulsants (carbamazepine, gabapentin) for neuropathic pain; antidepressants; beta blockers or central nervous system depressants for tremor (propranolol, clonazepam); and amantadine which has been found to reduce fatigue[27–31].

NURSING IMPLICATIONS

The majority of care for a person with multiple sclerosis occurs outside the acute hospital setting, except for hospitalisation for severe attacks or other health problems. Patient education is an important component of care. Patient teaching should include expected action of any drug therapy, as the patient may be on multiple drugs and, if receiving immunomodulation therapy, they should be aware of adverse reactions that may occur.

Signs and symptoms of multiple sclerosis are exacerbated by fatigue, heat, infection, fever, stress and pregnancy. Decreased mobility may result in weight gain over time. Pain and depression are often masked by mood alterations. In the progressive forms of multiple sclerosis, severe muscle weakness puts the patient at risk of aspiration pneumonia and respiratory failure. The patient's problems should be adequately assessed as they occur and appropriate management interventions planned, as all body functions can be affected.

LEARNING EXERCISES

1. Describe how the effect of demyelination of central nervous system white matter differs from demyelination in peripheral nerves.
2. Why does spasticity occur in multiple sclerosis but not in Guillain-Barré syndrome?
3. Differentiate between cognitive alterations and depression.
4. Why is it necessary to limit activity and control the temperature of the environment in people with multiple sclerosis?
5. Access the web site for your national Multiple Sclerosis Society and read about the current research into Multiple Sclerosis.

In this case study, following further investigations including an MRI, a diagnosis of relapsing–remitting multiple sclerosis was made. Gilda had migrated to Australia from northern Europe in her late teens, thereby being at the same risk for multiple sclerosis as people from her point of origin, whereas migration in the pre-teen years confers the same risk as the country to which the person migrates. The 'fuzzy' vision she complained of was optic neuritis, confirmed by visual evoked response studies. She met the criteria for diagnosis of multiple sclerosis based on her age, signs and symptoms, and her neurological examination. There was evidence of three lesions characteristic of plaque in the motor region of the cerebral cortex on an MRI scan, and she had a history of two episodes of neurological dysfunction lasting at least 24 hours and occurring at least one month apart with no other cause or explanation.

Corticosteroids were prescribed, and the more obvious aspects of her limb weakness and foot drop resolved over three weeks. The physiotherapist assessed her and she received muscle strengthening exercises and gait training. Her foot drop resolved and no orthosis was required. Patient teaching included avoidance of overexertion, control of environment and stress.

MYASTHENIA GRAVIS

WHAT DOES IT MEAN?

Myasthenia gravis (MG) means 'grave muscle weakness' from the Greek words for muscle and weakness and the Latin word *gravis* for severe[32]. It is an autoimmune disease affecting the neuromuscular junction, causing unpredictable alterations in transmission of electrical impulses, leading to generalised or specific muscular weakness that can be debilitating or life-threatening[27].

● **Case study**

John Smithson, 65, a retired welder, was admitted for management of myasthenia gravis. He was first diagnosed with the disease six years ago when he noticed that his ability to hold and use his welding equipment became more difficult as the day progressed due to his arm and shoulder muscles feeling 'tired'. He also noticed that he was having some visual problems and finding it difficult to 'keep his eyes open'. He had thought at first that it was 'old age coming on' as he usually felt better after resting and in the mornings. Following investigation, a diagnosis of myasthenia gravis was made at that time and he was prescribed Mestinon.

One year ago, neostigmine was added to his drug regime as he had developed a generalised weakness and complained of muscle weakness in the morning. One week ago, he developed a 'flu-like' illness and has been admitted to hospital with respiratory difficulties and acute exacerbation of his myasthenia gravis. On examination, he sits on the side of the bed, supporting his jaw with his hand, as he is unable to hold his head up. His speech is weak and he is having difficulty swallowing his saliva. He is to start on plasmapheresis.

WHAT IS THE PATHOPHYSIOLOGY?

In MG, there is a defect in impulse transmission between the nerve and muscle fibre at the neuromuscular junction. Normally, the nerve impulse travels down the neurone to the motor nerve terminal, stimulating the release of the neurotransmitter acetylcholine (ACh). ACh diffuses across the synapse to acetylcholine receptor (AChR) sites in the muscle fibre membrane, triggering depolarisation of the muscle fibre. Calcium is then released and the muscle stimulated to contract. This cycle ends when acetylcholinesterase (AChE) hydrolyses the ACh, thus terminating the action[4].

In MG, the ACh receptor sites on the postsynaptic membrane of the muscle cell are weakened, blocked and destroyed by antibodies (Anti AChR). The reduced number of AChR sites limits normal conduction and speed of impulses across the synaptic cleft, causing an inability to initiate muscle contraction. This results in progressive mild to severe weakness and abnormal fatigue of voluntary skeletal muscle, both exacerbated with activity and repeated muscle movement, and alleviated by rest. The muscles most commonly affected are those of the face, lips, tongue, neck and throat, but any group of muscles can be affected. The degree of muscle weakness is associated with the number of receptor sites affected[27,33]. Eventually, degeneration of the muscle fibres occurs and the weakness may become irreversible.

Myasthenia gravis occurs at any age, with the highest incidence in women between 18–25 years and men between 50–60 years[33–34]. It is more common in women than men, with a 3:1 ratio until 40 years of age, when it equalises. As well, 20% of children born to women with myasthenia gravis will have signs of the disease, however, for most this will be transient[33–34].

Myasthenia gravis can be classified according to clinical manifestations or disability level. In the ocular form, there is weakness of the eyes and eyelids. The second form, the bulbar type, affects the muscles for breathing, swallowing, and speech due to the motor cranial nerves 11 and 12 being affected. The third type, classified as generalised, ranges from mild to severe, affects the proximal muscles of the neck and limbs, and usually includes symptoms of the ocular or bulbar types[27,33,34].

WHAT ARE THE CLINICAL MANIFESTATIONS?

The onset of myasthenia gravis may develop insidiously and the disease progresses gradually over 5–7 years, although a more rapid onset occurs for some people. The severity of the disease varies from patient to patient, and may vary from hour to hour in the same patient. The most common complaint is of generalised muscle weakness and fatigability that worsens throughout the day, improving with rest. Fatigability is associated with repeated muscle use and is different from tiredness[27,33–35].

The most common presentation (90%) is the ocular type[33] with the patient complaining of inability to move their eyes and eyelids, or close their eyes properly, causing diplopia and ptosis. This gets worse over the day and improves with rest. As the day progresses, the patient has to tilt their head back to see properly. Patients with the second or bulbar type will have difficulty chewing and swallowing[33].

Involvement of the facial and neck muscles affects expression, speech and eating. Due to the weakness of the facial muscles, patients have a lack of facial expression and attempts to smile result in a snarl. They appear to have a mask-like sleepy look with a drooping jaw, and to overcome this, they may bob their head or support jaw their jaw with their hand.

Speech quality may become nasal and weak and chewing, swallowing and managing saliva difficult, with regurgitation of food and drooling[33,34].

Eighty-five per cent of patients develop a generalised weakness[27]. Most affected are the proximal muscle groups, neck extensors and the diaphragm. Weakness of the neck extensor muscles results in changes in posture with the head falling forward, while diaphragmatic involvement results in respiratory difficulties and the need for assisted ventilation. Complications of myasthenia include respiratory distress, pneumonia, difficulty in chewing and swallowing that can cause choking, and aspiration of food. Weakness may be reported as worse during menses, infection, or in extremes of temperature[26,33].

WHAT SHOULD YOU BE LOOKING AT IN LABORATORY AND OTHER TESTS?

Diagnosis is based upon patient history, clinical manifestations, assessment for muscle weakness, anticholinesterase testing, screening for presence of antibody titre for AChR, electrophysiological testing and stimulation of ACh receptors, screening of thymus gland[8].

Assessment of proximal muscles will show decreased ability to climb stairs, bend the knees or lift the arms over the head. Anticholinesterase testing involves intravenous injection of an anticholinergic drug, edrophonium (Tensilon). The test is positive if there is improvement in muscle strength for a period of 5–10 minutes following administration of the drug. The antibody titre of AChR is elevated in 80–90% of people with generalised myasthenia gravis[8]. A panel of four tests can detect the antibodies to acetylcholine receptors in blood. The four tests performed are to detect above-normal levels of AchR binding antibodies, AchR modulating antibodies, AChR blocking antibodies and Striational antibodies[8,34].

Electrophysiological testing demonstrates a decreased response to repeated nerve stimulation and delay at the neuromuscular junction in single-fibre studies[4,33]. A chest X-ray or MRI of the mediastinum may show an enlarged thymus or thymoma. The thymus gland, situated behind the sternum, is involved in the development of cell-mediated immunity and the maturation of T cells[5]. In the adult, this gland normally shrinks and is replaced with fat[33]. However, hyperplasia of the thymus is common in people with myasthenia gravis[33], and approximately 15% of people diagnosed with myasthenia gravis have a thymoma[8,34].

WHAT IS THE TREATMENT?

Treatment is planned on an individual basis, the aim being to assist the person to have quality of life with minimal symptoms. Four alternative management approaches can be used: anticholinesterase, immunosuppressive therapy, plasmapheresis or IVIG, and thymectomy.

Anticholinesterase drugs are used to inhibit ACh destruction by cholinesterase, thus boosting the amount of ACh available and causing improved impulse transmission. However, these drugs become less effective over time. Immunosuppressive agents are used if response to anticholinesterase drugs is poor. Plasmapheresis to remove the anti-AchR antibodies and IVIg temporarily reduces symptoms and is used to stabilise the condition of people during an acute exacerbation of the disease. Plasmapheresis may also be used to treat people having their thymus removed[8,33].

Thymectomy is performed when a thymoma is present and results in improvement for 85% of people who undergo the surgery, with 35–40% experiencing a remission with cessation of drug treatment[8,26,27]. Due to the disease process, patients are at risk of variable responses to drugs used during anaesthesia, and surgery is planned carefully due to the risk of respiratory failure.

Intensive care and assisted ventilation are required if myasthenic or cholinergic crisis occurs, as both put the patient at risk of respiratory failure. Myasthenic crisis occurs in patients with moderate, severe or generalised myasthenia who have a sudden relapse, commonly due to infection, temperature extremes, stress and when anticholinergic therapy is ineffective. However, many drugs can affect neuromuscular transmission and any other medications need to be monitored[8]. A cholinergic crisis develops slowly and is caused by the adverse effects of anticholinesterase therapy.

Strategies to increase muscle tone and strength and improve fatigue are planned with the patient. Psychosocial support is needed to assist the patient to deal with their disease, body changes when an acute exacerbation, myasthenic or cholinergic crisis occurs, or steroid therapy is prescribed[8,35].

APPLIED PHARMACOLOGY

The anticholinesterase pyridostigmine (Mestinon) is the most commonly prescribed drug, and amount and frequency of dosage is calculated on an individual basis to provide maximal muscle strength with the least side effects. It is important that the drug is taken on time or muscle weakness may interfere with swallowing the medication[8]. Adverse cholinergic effects of increased acetylcholine at receptors in skeletal and smooth muscle and glands can occur if drug toxicity develops[4]. Neostigmine (Prostigmine), another drug in this group, can be given in combination if patients have weakness during the night or on awakening. There is a narrow therapeutic range between effectiveness and side effects which occur due to the drug's action on smooth muscle and glands in the gastrointestinal, genitourinary, cardiovascular and respiratory systems, as well as pupillary muscles and sweat glands. These side effects are generalised muscle weakness, impaired respiratory function, abdominal pain and diarrhoea, excess pulmonary and salivary secretions, twitching and spasms in skeletal muscle[8,33]. If there is a poor response to anticholinesterase therapy, immunosuppressive therapy including corticosteroids (Prednisone), azathioprine (Imuran) and cyclosporin can be used.

Medications that impair neuromuscular transmission should be avoided. Examples include neuromuscular blocking agents (succinylcholine, vercuronium), anti-arrhythmics (quinine, quinidine, procainamide), aminoglycoside antibiotics (gentamycin, neomycin, streptomycin, kanamycin) and ciprofloxacin, beta-blockers, calcium channel blockers and iodine-based contrast agents[36].

NURSING IMPLICATIONS

The patient is usually managed in the community and presents to hospital for management of a crisis situation or because of another medical or surgical condition. Differentiating between myasthenic and cholinergic crisis is important, as both result in the patient requiring respiratory support, but have different precipitating events and management. The patient should be monitored for deterioration in their symptoms after commencing any new medication, and anaesthesia should be carefully planned if surgery is needed. Respiratory function, muscle strength and movement, voice quality should be assessed. During a crisis, the patient may need assistance with nutritional support including enteral feeding, and all activities including skin and eye care. During the Tensilon test, a cardiac monitor should be in situ.

Patient education about the disease, treatment and drugs is very important. To maintain a good quality of life with minimal weakness and reduce the risks of exacerbations, strategies to reduce or manage the following should be discussed with the patient: fatigue, nutritional needs, prevention of infection and environmental control. Strategies to reduce falls and the risk of other injury due to muscle weakness should be included.

LEARNING EXERCISES

1. How does myasthenia gravis cause muscle weakness?
2. What is the difference between muscle weakness due to demyelination and impaired neuromuscular transmission?
3. Differentiate between myasthenic and cholinergic crisis.
4. What specific interventions are required to care for the skin of a person in myasthenic crisis?

In this case study, Mr Smithson is exhibiting signs and symptoms of a myasthenic crisis related to an exacerbation of his disease due to an infection. He will require close monitoring of arterial blood gases, pulse oximetry and respiratory function tests (spirometry) and cranial nerve function for difficulty in swallowing and loss of gag reflex, peripheral muscle strength and diplopia as signs of further deterioration and the need for mechanical ventilation to assist his breathing.

He received a five-course regimen of plasmapheresis every other day, as well as IVIg daily for five days. Fortunately, the myasthenic crisis resolved without the need for mechanical ventilation. However, his disease has progressed and he now has the generalised form of myasthenia gravis.

During this period of acute exacerbation, Mr Smithson required assistance with all activities of daily living, chest physiotherapy and suctioning of secretions, eye and skin care, and nutritional support via a nasogastric tube.

PARKINSON'S DISEASE

WHAT DOES IT MEAN?

Parkinson's disease is named after the physician who first described it in 1817[4]. It is a progressive degenerative disorder of the central nervous system caused by loss of dopaminergic neurons in the substantia nigra of the basal ganglia. It is distinguished by muscle rigidity, difficulty in initiating movement and an involuntary tremor at rest.

Parkinson's disease affects men slightly more than women, and the mean age of onset is 58–62 years of age, with an incidence of 1:100 over 60 years[36]. The disease occurs worldwide, affecting quality of life[36,37].

Case study

Keith Gordon, 77, is attending the Parkinson's disease clinic. His wife, who accompanies him, tells the nurse running the clinic that he is becoming more incapacitated and less able to look after himself, with his tremor spreading to both arms and increasing difficulty in moving independently. On examination, he has a blank inexpressive face and oily-looking skin and speaks with some difficulty in a monotone voice. He has a rhythmical resting tremor of both hands, the right more pronounced than the left. When his mobility is assessed, he stands with a stooped posture with semi-flexed arms, and shuffles when asked to walk. He is unsteady when asked to turn around and walk back, and demonstrates loss of ability to balance.

His medications include Sinemet 25/100 q.i.d., which he was prescribed when his disease moved to stage II.

WHAT IS THE PATHOPHYSIOLOGY?

Parkinson's disease is due to the destruction of dopaminergic nerve cells in the substantia nigra. Normally, input from the cerebral cortex, midbrain and thalamus go to the basal ganglia comprised of the caudate nucleus, putamen, globus pallidus (corpus striatum) and other nuclei. Together with nuclei in the thalamus and midbrain, the interconnections and related neurotransmitters form the extrapyramidal system that controls muscle tone, posture and coordinates movement[1,4]. The loss of the dopaminergic cells in the substantia nigra and other structures of the basal ganglia and the formation of Lewy bodies cause an imbalance between the inhibitory effect and excitatory effects of the neurotransmitters within the basal ganglia and its connections[4,8].

The effect is a decrease in voluntary movement due to reduced activity in the motor cortex. Reduction of normal inhibitory functions of the basal ganglia influences initiation, modulation and completion of movement. The result of these changes is rigidity due to muscle contraction causing resistance of the muscle to movement, bradykinesia (slow or decreased movement), and resting tremor due to unopposed neuronal activity. Up to 75–80% of cells can die before the classic signs and symptoms of Parkinson's disease appear[4,8,36].

Toxins, pesticides, environmental agents and genetic factors have been suggested as possible causes of primary or idiopathic Parkinson's disease, the most common type[37]. Secondary causes include encephalitis, drugs that block dopamine receptors such as haloperidol, prochlorperazine, lithium, and pyridostigmine. Other causes include substances that destroy dopamine pathways, such as carbon monoxide and methylphenyltetrahydropyridine (MPTP), vascular changes, trauma, neoplasm[27,37].

WHAT ARE THE CLINICAL MANIFESTATIONS?

In the early stages, not all the signs and symptoms are present and as they develop, slowly may not be recognised or are thought to be due to ageing. The characteristic signs and symptoms are tremor, muscle rigidity and bradykinesia (slowness of movement). The tremor initially occurs unilaterally in the distal parts of a limb, particularly the hands, where it is described as having a pill rolling action, in later stages it becomes bilateral and may also occur in the foot, lips, tongue or jaw. It is present at rest (resting tremor), decreasing with purposeful movement and during sleep, and may increase with stress and anxiety.

Muscle rigidity, an increase in resistance to passive stretch, may be jerky, rhythmic muscle contractions (cogwheel) or uniform (lead pipe). Bradykinesia may progress to akinesia and temporary freezing of movement for several seconds. This results in difficulties with activities of daily living and movements, such as rising from a chair. A characteristic stooped-over posture with semi-flexed arms and flexed fingers develops. Gait becomes affected with short shuffling steps, and once movement is initiated rapid acceleration (festination) occurs. Balance becomes affected and the person needs a broad base to turn around, and the potential for falls increases as their centre of gravity alters.

Secondary signs include difficulty with fine movement. For example, handwriting deteriorates and there is difficulty with manipulating buttons. There is generalised weakness and muscle fatigue. The facial muscles become mask-like and blinking decreases. If dysarthria develops, speech may become slurred, monotonous and whisper quiet (hypophonia). In time, cognitive changes affect memory, executive function and dementia may occur, and more than 50% of patients develop depression[8]. Autonomic dysfunction results in oily skin, increased perspiration, orthostatic hypotension, constipation, and urinary hesitancy and frequency[8,36–38].

As the disease progresses, patients develop bilateral signs and are at risk of falls, aspiration pneumonia and urinary tract infections. Postural changes become severe and by the latter stages, the patient is confined to a chair or bed.

WHAT SHOULD YOU BE LOOKING AT IN LABORATORY AND OTHER TESTS?

There is no one test available to verify Parkinson's disease, and diagnosis is based on clinical signs and symptoms and full neurological examination. For the diagnosis to be confirmed, the patient must demonstrate two or more of the principal features, that is, tremor, rigidity, bradykinesia and postural instability, and have secondary causes excluded[8,37,38]. Positron emission tomography (PET) and single proton emission therapy (SPECT) imaging may show a decrease in dopamine activity, but is not widely available or used. However, CT or MRI can help rule out other possible neurological conditions or causes, such as vascular disease or atrophy[36–38].

WHAT IS THE TREATMENT?

The aims of treatment are to relieve symptoms, maintain function and quality of life, and protect from injury, and this is achieved through pharmacological and non-pharmacological means, as progression of the disease cannot be slowed. Patient and family education is an important component of any treatment regime as patients are managed in their home. There are six types of drugs used in managing Parkinson's disease aiming to relieve symptoms while minimising the side effects of medication. Anticholinergic agents are commonly used in the early stages of the disease when tremor is the most prominent manifestation. An antiviral agent (amantadine) may be used if the disease is mild or as an adjunct. A dopaminergic agent such as carbidopa/levodopa, a precursor of dopamine, is the most effective drug but has limitations in relation to the period for which it is effective and side effects. Other medications used singly, or as adjuncts, include dopamine agonists, monoamine oxidase B inhibitors (MAOI-B) and catechol-O-methyltransferase (COMT) inhibitors, such as entacapone[36–39]. Strategies to manage the side effects of medication such as dry mouth and constipation are necessary.

Physiotherapy and an exercise program to maintain muscle tone, function, strength, balance, flexibility and joint mobility help maintain quality of life and prevent injury. Assessment of the patient's abilities and living environment for modifications will assist independent living and prevent injury as the disease progresses. Referral to a speech therapist for assessment of swallowing may be indicated if the patient is having difficulty drinking or eating due to choking and coughing, or for teaching of vocal techniques if hypophonia has developed.

Maintenance of nutritional status, mouth and dental care and management of urinary problems and constipation are also required.

Surgical intervention through the use of stereotactic neurosurgery may be performed if drug therapy is not controlling the symptoms. Pallidotomy is used for motor complications not completely controlled by levodopa or dopamine agonists. Tremor can be relieved by thalamotomy, but in some patients may result in worsening of gait and speech problems[37]. The procedures are not a cure and are best performed if the patient is young or there is severe unilateral muscle rigidity, bradykinesia or tremor. Deep brain stimulation can be used to treat tremor or the symptoms of advanced Parkinson's disease by blocking neuronal activity with implanted electrodes in the thalamus[36-38].

Implantation of dopamine-rich tissue obtained from the adrenal medulla into the caudate nucleus has been performed, but long-term outcomes need to be assessed[8]. Stem cell therapy has also been proposed, but the ethical implications of both these procedures will need to be explored further and resolved[8].

APPLIED PHARMACOLOGY

Pharmacological management of Parkinson's disease is complex. There are six classes of drugs available, each with different mechanisms of action that require use of the right drug with the least side effects for the stage and signs and symptoms of the disease. Anticholinergics (benzotropine, orphenadrine, trihexyphenidyl) correct central cholinergic overactivity by antagonising the cholinergic neurones that become disinhibited with reduced dopaminergic neurones. This class of drugs is often used in the early stages and relieve tremor more than rigidity. Caution is required in use with elderly patients, as confusional states and general muscarinic effects may occur[8,37,39].

Amantadine (symmetrel) is an antiviral agent that promotes synthesis and release of dopamine and is used singly for rigidity, tremor and bradykinesia in early stages of the disease or as an adjunct to carbidopa/levodopa where it appears to decrease side effects of dyskinesia[39].

Dopamine receptor agonists (bromocriptine, pergolide) are ergot derivatives that stimulate the dopamine receptors. They can be used singly in early treatment, thus delaying the side effects that occur when carbidopa is introduced[8,37,39], or in conjunction with dopaminergics. However, due to widespread stimulation of dopamine receptors, side effects are more common with this group of drugs.

Levodopa, the precursor of dopamine, is the standard for treatment. However, when given on its own, only 1% crosses the blood brain barrier for use in the brain, the rest being converted to dopamine in the peripheries[38,39]. Therefore, levodopa is combined with carbidopa (Sinemet), a substance that inhibits peripheral conversion, thereby increasing brain uptake, reducing the dosage of levodopa needed, and reducing adverse effects. The aim is to prescribe a dose that relieves symptoms without causing side effects. However, the effectiveness of the drug decreases over time. Complications that develop with long-term use include abnormal movements (dyskinesia) that can be disabling and embarrassing, occurring at peak dose or as the dose is wearing off. Management may be a reduction in dosage or addition of a dopamine agonist. Another complication is the return of symptoms despite taking the medication. This is due to a waning of peripheral levels of dopamine over time. Reducing time between doses, using a controlled-release form of the drug, or adding a dopamine agonist or a COMT inhibitor are methods that may be used to treat this problem[8,36–39].

Monoamine oxidase B inhibitors (selegiline) block metabolism of central dopamine and delay the need for levodopa, and are best prescribed in the early stages for patients below 65 years of age[37]. COMT inhibitors (comtan) inhibit the breakdown of levodopa, thus prolonging the action of levodopa and reducing the required dose[39].

NURSING IMPLICATIONS

Patients with Parkinson's disease are managed in the community, although they may require placement in long-term care in the last stages of the disease due to dementia and the need for total care. Admission to hospital is usually due to other diseases, injury due to falls or surgery. An understanding of the progress of the disease and the side effects of medication are essential. Monitoring of nutritional and fluid status is necessary, as the patient's ability to eat can be affected. Medication side effects include reduction of saliva, nausea and constipation. Therefore, mouth and dental care, strategies to decrease nausea and constipation are important interventions. Psychological support and communication skills are required as the disease progresses and physical signs become more pronounced.

LEARNING EXERCISES

1. What are the functions of the basal ganglia?
2. Name the neurotransmitter deficient in Parkinson's disease.
3. Identify the four primary signs of Parkinson's disease.
4. Differentiate the difference between the actions of levodopa and anticholinergic drugs.
5. What is the reason for the generalised side effects of anticholinergic drugs?

In this case study, Keith Gordon's disease has progressed to stage III as he has bilateral signs of the disease and impaired postural reflexes, as well as some autonomic manifestations, but is still able to move independently, although requiring some assistance. He has progressed from stage I where he had tremor of one arm, and stage II where there are bilateral signs but intact postural reflexes. Over time, he will progress to stage IV and V as his signs and symptoms worsen and he requires more assistance[8]. At this time, his medications will be reviewed and adjusted to decrease his signs and symptoms. He will also be referred to a physiotherapist, occupational therapist and speech therapist for assessment and planning of a program to assist with his mobility, activities of daily living and vocal abilities. If his wife is having difficulties with his care, due to his disease or her own health and abilities, then assessment for home support and care will be arranged.

EPILEPSY

WHAT DOES IT MEAN?

Epilepsy is the term used for recurrent transitory disturbances of electrical activity in the nerve cells of the brain, affecting one or more of the following: movement, sensation, emotions, behaviour or consciousness[40]. A seizure or fit is the term used to describe the outward signs of the electrical disturbance. For the diagnosis of epilepsy, the seizures need to be recurrent, as seizures can occur as a once-only event in a range of neurological and other conditions.

Epilepsy is classified as primary or secondary depending upon the cause of the seizure. In primary epilepsy, also called idiopathic or cryptogenic, there is no identifiable cause and 60–70% of cases fall into this group[8]. In secondary epilepsy, known as symptomatic or organic epilepsy, there is an identifiable intracranial cause such as a brain tumour, infection, injury or developmental abnormality. Chemical, electrolyte or metabolic imbalances, hyperthermia, drug and alcohol abuse, fatigue, hypoxia or flashing lights can trigger seizures in some people.

● Case study

Sandra O'Connor, 28, arrives by ambulance to the emergency department, accompanied by her sister Tara, visiting from interstate. Tara says that they were out shopping when Sandra 'got a funny look on her face and 'wasn't there' when she spoke to her. Sandra then cried out and went stiff and fell to the ground, where her arms and body started jerking and she made grunting sounds. Tara is not sure how long this lasted, but says that gradually the jerking became less, and the colour of her sister's face became more normal and she 'woke up'. Tara says that, as far as she knows, this has never happened before.

On assessment, Sandra is drowsy with slurred speech and says she wants to be 'left alone'. Her blood pressure and pulse are within normal limits and she is afebrile with no neurological deficits. There are signs that she has been incontinent of urine. A provisional diagnosis of an epileptic seizure is made and a CT scan arranged.

WHAT IS THE PATHOPHYSIOLOGY?

A number of areas are being explored to explain the cause and sequence of events that take place in epilepsy. A seizure is thought to occur because there is an imbalance between excitatory and inhibitory neurotransmitter activity in neurons in the brain, either within a localised area of the cerebral cortex (focal seizure) or over the entire cerebral cortex (generalised seizure). This imbalance is thought to be due to abnormally low levels of inhibitory transmitters, such as GABA (gamma-aminobutyric acid), or high levels of excitatory transmitters, such as glutamate[8]. Excessive excitation of the neurons may also be caused by a disorder of the ion or calcium channels of the cells[8,41]. Epilepsy following brain injury, infection, stroke or after birth may occur because of the development of abnormal neuronal connections following injury or during brain development.

During a seizure, the membrane potential of the neurons alters in response to environmental changes, such as an alteration in intracellular sodium concentration, and this causes hypersensitive or hyperactive neurones to fire excessively. This burst of activity forms the focus of the seizure that then extends to related brain areas or the opposite hemisphere by connecting pathways[8]. Eventually, the electrical discharge decreases and the seizure stops due to inhibitory processes[4].

WHAT ARE THE CLINICAL MANIFESTATIONS?

Seizures have a range of clinical manifestations that include hallucinations, motor, sensory, psychic or autonomic disturbances, involuntary movement and altered consciousness. Some seizures have three clear stages, first an aura where the person has a forewarning sensation, second a period of altered consciousness and/or seizure activity (ictus), followed by the third or postictal stage (recovery).

Epileptic seizures are classified as partial or generalised, according to the type of brain activation that occurs during a seizure[8].

Partial or focal seizures involve a group of neurones in one area of a cerebral hemisphere and clinical manifestations reflect the location of seizure activity. Generalised seizures involve neurones in both cerebral hemispheres. These two classifications are further divided into types of seizures based on their clinical presentation. A third – unclassified seizures – refers to activity that does not fit into either of the other groups[8]. Partial seizures are classified according to the following categories.

SIMPLE PARTIAL SEIZURES

Consciousness remains intact and the person will demonstrate seizure activity related to the area of involvement. Examples include

- Motor activity if the motor cortex is the source;
- Sensory activity, such as visual and auditory hallucinations from parietal or occipital lobe involvement;
- Autonomic manifestations, such as epigastric sensation and skin pallor; or
- Psychic activity (disturbed cerebral function).

COMPLEX PARTIAL SEIZURES

Consciousness is impaired with the person appearing to be in a trance-like state; and automatisms, involuntary repetitive motor activity such as lip smacking, chewing, pacing in a repetitive pattern, may occur.

PARTIAL SEIZURES EVOLVING TO GENERALISED SEIZURES

Partial seizure activity spreads into a generalised seizure.

GENERALISED SEIZURES

Generalised seizures may involve loss of consciousness and are subdivided into six categories based upon their clinical presentation and electrical activity:

1. Absence seizures (formerly called petit mal seizures) common in childhood, and their incidence decreases with age. These are brief seizures characterised by decreased awareness of the environment or ability to respond to stimuli, with episodes of staring into space for 30–60

seconds, followed by resumption of activity. Some people may exhibit purposeless movements, such as blinking of the eyelids.

2. Myoclonic seizures are more common in childhood and consist of sudden, rapid involuntary contractions of one or more muscle groups.
3. Tonic seizures are characterised by episodes of stiffening due to long muscle contraction.
4. Clonic seizures where there are episodes of muscle contraction alternating with periods of relaxation causing repeated jerking movements.
5. Tonic-clonic seizures (formerly called grand mal), is the most common generalised seizure with loss of consciousness. There is a tonic phase where there is contraction of large muscle groups, and there may be a cry as air is forced through the vocal cords. This is followed by a clonic phase with alternating spasm and relaxation of muscles. There may be an aura and the postictal phase is of variable length.
6. Atonic seizure. There is sudden loss of normal muscle tone, leading to 'drop attacks' which may be precipitated by auditory, photic, touch stimuli, stress or fever.

STATUS EPILEPTICUS
Status epilepticus is the term for persistent and recurrent seizures without a return to usual functional level or consciousness. These may last 30 minutes or longer, can occur for any type of seizure, and they are life-threatening.

WHAT SHOULD YOU BE LOOKING FOR IN LABORATORY AND OTHER TESTS?
Diagnosis is based upon a detailed past and current patient history including antenatal and developmental history. Information about drug use, previous brain trauma or infection, and possible exposure to environmental toxins, assist in diagnosis and exclusion of other causes. A complete description of any seizures is obtained from the patient and any witness and includes onset of seizure, precipitating factors, presence or absence of an aura, loss or impairment of consciousness, behaviour before, during or following the seizure. A description of any abnormal movement or sensation, the parts of the body affected, skin colour changes, cyanosis, or eye deviation, incontinence and the length and frequency of the seizure is also important information to be collected[40].

The diagnosis of epilepsy is based upon electroencephalograph (EEG) findings together with the clinical manifestations of the seizure. An EEG records superficial electrical activity or brain waves through electrodes placed on the scalp and detects changes in the wave pattern associated with epilepsy. However, abnormal electrical activity may be undetected if it is occurring deeper within the brain, and approximately 50% of people diagnosed with epilepsy have a normal wave pattern if the recording is taken between seizure activity[8]. Triggers such as repeated hyperventilation, light stimulation, rapid eye movement, or sleep deprivation may be used as an adjunct during the recording to stimulate abnormal wave activity. Characteristic findings include asymmetrical alpha and beta waves, focal spike and wave discharges with differences in frequency and amplitude[8]. Continuous EEG monitoring during sleep or video-EEG monitoring using superficial or intracranial electrodes may be used to assist diagnosis and locate epileptic foci.

Other diagnostic tests that may be ordered include MRI scanning if lesions such as tumours and structural abnormalities are thought to be the cause of seizures. Positron emission tomography (PET scan) and functional MRI are able to identify changes in glucose uptake and metabolism and single photon emission computed tomography (SPECT) can detect changes in blood flow. During a seizure, increased metabolism and blood flow occur at the focus of the seizure, with decreased metabolism and perfusion between seizures. Magnetic resonance spectroscopy (MRS) and magnetoencephalogram (MEG) are other diagnostic techniques being developed to monitor brain activity and assist in diagnosis.

WHAT IS THE TREATMENT?

Treatment of epilepsy is primarily achieved by an individual program of drug therapy, with the aim of treatment to reach a balance between control of seizures, lifestyle and side effects of drugs. In 78% of patients, a single drug controls seizure activity[8]. The addition of a second drug may occur if the seizures are not controlled. However, there is an increased risk of side effects as the number of drugs increases. Patients need to be monitored so that they receive the optimum dose with minimal side effects for control of their seizures. Monitoring of blood levels of the drug is important to ensure that a therapeutic dose is being received[4,40]. Treatment also includes patient education in relation to avoidance of precipitating factors, drug therapy, seizure management, and psychological support.

Surgical intervention is used to treat severe or intractable epilepsy when there is an underlying condition such as a brain tumour or an identified focus for the seizures and there is no risk of a major neurological deficit. Prior to any procedure, extensive diagnostic testing and psychological assessment will be carried out. Removal of the focal lesion or a lobectomy is performed for partial epilepsy. Other surgical procedures are severing of the neural connections between the cerebral hemispheres (corpus callosotomy) to prevent the spread of seizure activity from one hemisphere to the other such as occurs in tonic and atonic seizures. However, seizures will still occur in the hemisphere where the focus is situated. A modified hemispherectomy may be performed for severe epilepsy in infants or young children. Anticonvulsant therapy is continued postoperatively after all types of surgery, and discontinuation at a later date is based on the electroencephalogram[8].

Vagal nerve stimulation via an implanted battery-powered device delivering bursts of electrical activity to the brain via the vagus nerve has been found to reduce partial seizures by 50%, and has less adverse effects than a corpus callosotomy[42]. This treatment requires the patient to continue anticonvulsant therapy, but a reduced dosage in conjunction with the device may be sufficient for seizure control.

A high-fat, low-carbohydrate diet (ketogenic diet) has been found to reduce seizures in some children whose epilepsy was poorly controlled by medications[43]. However, it can result in nutritional deficiency and must be supervised by medical and nutritional specialists.

Status epilepticus requires intravenous administration of an anticonvulsant, usually a benzodiazepine, with airway support, oxygen therapy, cardiac monitoring and ventilatory support. A loading dose of phenytoin is also administered[40].

APPLIED PHARMACOLOGY

There are a varying number of mechanisms by which antiepileptic drugs exert their effect, but most act to achieve a balance between inhibitory and excitatory activity in the brain. Some are effective for only a specific type of epilepsy, such as ethosuximide, which acts on calcium channels and is only used for absence seizures, or carbamazepine, a sodium channel blocker that inhibits the firing of neurons and is useful for partial seizures but aggravates absence seizures[8].

Other sodium channel blockers, such as phenytoin and lamotrigine, have a wide spectrum of activity and are prescribed as first-line drugs for a wider range of seizure types. Sodium valproate affects calcium and sodium channels and is a first-line drug for most types of epilepsy, especially as it has little sedative effect. Benzodiazepines, vigabatrin, gabapentin and phenobarbitone act on GABA mediated inhibition[8]. Withdrawal or cessation of anticonvulsant therapy can result in status epilepticus. To prevent this, when an anticonvulsant drug is introduced to replace another drug, the dosage of the initial drug should be reduced gradually once the second drug dosage has reached the desired level[8, 39].

Adverse effects, such as liver toxicity (sodium valproate), tolerance or sedation (phenobarbitone, benzodiazepines) or hypertrophy of gums, skin problems (phenytoin), mean that serum levels of the drug should be measured to ensure a therapeutic level without toxic effects. Women with epilepsy should seek advice about pregnancy, as many of the drugs are potentially teratogenic[8].

NURSING IMPLICATIONS

The ability to recognise, fully assess and accurately record a seizure is essential in assisting diagnosis. During a seizure, the nurse should stay with the person, protect them from injury and maintain their airway. During a generalised tonic-clonic seizure, the patient's limbs should not be forcibly restrained nor articles forced between clenched teeth. Tight clothing should be loosened, dangerous objects removed and the person turned onto their side if possible to maintain the airway. Once the seizure is over, assess airway, breathing and circulation, neurologic status and injury, record sequence of events and duration of seizure. Allow the person privacy to recover.

Because drugs bind to plasma proteins, the dosage might need adjustment to maintain therapeutic blood levels in cases where patients are being tube fed or have diseases that affect protein levels such as chronic renal failure, liver disease or burns. To best assist people with epilepsy the nurse needs to be aware of potential effects and interaction/effects of antiepileptic drugs, as well as understand the effect of epilepsy on people's social interaction.

> ### LEARNING EXERCISES
> 1. Differentiate between partial and generalised seizures.
> 2. Identify the clinical manifestations of a complex partial seizure originating from the temporal lobe.
> 3. List all the factors you should observe and record when witnessing a seizure.
> 4. What monitoring tests should be undertaken for patients prescribed phenytoin or sodium valproate?
> 5. Describe the effect the diagnosis of epilepsy and drug management has for lifestyle and social interactions.

In this case study, Sandra presented with a description of a generalised tonic-clonic seizure. Because this was her first seizure for investigation, a CT scan was arranged to exclude an intracranial lesion as the cause. No lesion was detected. However, Sandra had a second seizure five days after the initial one, and during a full neurological assessment and evaluation, it emerged that 20 years previously, Sandra had been diagnosed with encephalitis (inflammation of the brain tissue). She had recovered without any complications at the time. Further testing with EEG was ordered and a diagnosis of epilepsy made. Sandra was commenced on sodium valproate at that time.

MENINGITIS

WHAT DOES IT MEAN?

Meningitis is inflammation of the meninges of the brain and spinal cord and is caused by pathogenic organisms gaining entry to the central nervous system. Organisms gain entry via the blood from a pre-existing infection (bacteraemia, pneumonia) or viral infections (echo virus, mumps, measles, and less commonly herpes simplex) or through extension of infection from an extracranial source. Extracranial sources include the sinuses, middle ear, mastoid process, skull or facial bones. Infection can also occur by a direct route, such as through a penetrating head injury, fracture of the base of skull or a neurosurgical procedure[8,27].

Meningitis can occur at any age, but is most serious in infants, children, young adults and the elderly, with people who are malnourished or immunosuppressed being most at risk. Meningitis is commonly caused by bacteria and viruses, but may also be due to fungi or protozoa. The most common types of bacterial meningitis are caused by the organisms *Streptococcus pneumoniae*, *Haemophilus influenzae*, or *Neisseria meningitidis*[44]. The latter organism is responsible for meningococcal meningitis in infants and young children, although outbreaks occur in young adults or adults living in close proximity. *Haemophilus influenzae* is the organism commonly responsible for meningitis in infants[44], while *Cryptoccoccus neoformans* is the most common cause of fungal infection, and people who are immunocompromised are susceptible to infection by it[45].

● Case study

John Harbin, 19, presents to the emergency department feeling unwell and complaining of a headache, vomiting, stiff neck and backache. He thinks he has the 'flu', as he has had a 'runny nose and stuffed up feeling' for the last week. He looks flushed and his skin is hot and dry. His observations are: BP 102/60, P 96, R24 and T 38.3C.

On examination, he has neck rigidity and on passive flexion of his neck, his hips and knees are observed to flex involuntarily and he cries out with pain. John is unable to straighten his knee when it is flexed onto his abdomen. When his pupil reaction is tested, John screws up his eyes and complains that 'the light hurts', He is irritable, wanting to be 'left alone'.

Nose and throat swabs, full blood count, blood and urine cultures are ordered and a lumbar puncture is performed. Lumbar puncture results are: CSF pressure 240 mm H_2O and the CSF is turbid looking. Laboratory results are: CSF protein 70 mg/dL, CSF glucose 20 mg/100 mL, and CSF WBC 35000/mm^3, with many polymorphs. A diagnosis of meningitis is made, and a broad-spectrum IV antibiotic commenced until microbiology results are available.

WHAT IS THE PATHOPHYSIOLOGY?

In bacterial meningitis, inflammation may involve all three layers of the meninges and can involve the underlying cortex. There is rapid multiplication of bacteria in the subarachnoid space and lysis of these bacteria releases substances from their cell walls that stimulates an inflammatory response by macrophages and some brain cells (microglia and astrocytes). The permeability of the blood brain barrier alters, and leucocytes and neutrophils proliferate. This results in an increase in purulent exudate and obstruction of the flow of cerebrospinal fluid. There is also an increase in intracranial pressure due to brain oedema. The exudate can also affect cranial nerve function if there is inflammation at the point where the nerves leave the meninges[8,27].

Fibrotic changes and scarring of the arachnoid layer can occur, resulting in adhesion and effusions and obstruction of normal CSF circulation, leading to hydrocephalus. Other complications include seizures, visual and hearing deficits, and cranial nerve palsies[8].

Waterhouse-Friderichsen syndrome may develop in meningococcal meningitis due to the release of endotoxins from the organism into the circulation damaging the vascular system. This results in endothelial necrosis, inflammation, thrombosis and perivascular haemorrhage with the development of disseminated intravascular coagulation (DIC) causing signs and symptoms of septic shock and hypolvolaemia[8]. The vascular complications may result in the need for limb amputation.

Viral meningitis, also known as aseptic meningitis as there is no exudate present, is usually mild and self-limiting, with complete recovery occurring[8,45].

WHAT ARE THE CLINICAL MANIFESTATIONS?

Classical clinical manifestations include headache due to irritation of the dura mater, nuchal (neck) rigidity, and a positive Kernig's and Brudzinski sign due to meningeal irritation. Photophobia and fever are also present, especially with bacterial meningitis. Alterations in consciousness including lethargy, irritability, confusion and a decrease in conscious level may occur rapidly with accompanying seizures. In infants, clinical manifestations may be less specific and complicate the diagnosis. Such manifestations include fever, anorexia, lethargy, vomiting and diarrhoea, seizures, a high-pitched cry and bulging fontanelles[44].

The occurrence of petechiae or a rash that spreads rapidly is indicative of meningococcal meningitis[46]. Seizures occur in forty to fifty per cent of patients with a bacterial infection, and some develop a syndrome of inappropriate secretion of antidiuretic hormone (SIADH)[8].

In viral or aseptic meningitis, there is usually fever, drowsiness, stiff neck, and headache and a history of a recent viral infection.

WHAT SHOULD YOU BE LOOKING AT IN LABORATORY AND OTHER TESTS?

Diagnosis is based on clinical history, including respiratory, sinus, and middle ear infection or recent head trauma, physical assessment and examination of cerebrospinal fluid.

Kernig's sign is pain and hamstring muscle spasm when passive extension of the knee is attempted while the patient's hip is at a 90° angle from the abdomen. Flexion of the hip and knee in response to passive flexion of the neck onto the chest is Brudzinski's sign. Both signs indicate inflammation of the meninges and spinal nerve roots, which are irritated when stretched during these tests[8].

Unless there is evidence of increased intracranial pressure, cerebrospinal fluid (CSF) is obtained from a lumbar puncture. Findings indicative of bacterial meningitis are an elevated CSF pressure (above 180mmH$_2$O), cloudy or milky CSF, decreased CSF glucose level, increased protein and white blood cells. A culture and Gram stain of the CSF will identify the causative organism, providing antibiotic therapy is not established at the time of collection. In viral meningitis, the CSF is clear, glucose and protein levels normal or elevated and no bacterial organisms are seen on culture.

A virus can sometimes be isolated from blood, CSF or throat swab, but these results are not available immediately[44]. Nose and throat swabs are taken, as well as blood, urine and sputum culture if a primary infection is suspected as being the cause of the meningitis. An elevated white cell count is indicative of infection. In meningococcal meningitis, blood tests show the presence of neutropenia and a low platelet count, and the organism may be cultured from the skin lesions. X-ray of the chest, skull and sinuses may identify pre-existing infection.

WHAT IS THE TREATMENT?

If the disease is recognised early and treatment instigated, then the prognosis is good. Untreated, there is a high mortality rate in bacterial meningitis[47], particularly in infants and the elderly. Treatment is pharmacological, with intravenous administration of the appropriate antimicrobial agent for the infective organism. A broad-spectrum antibiotic, or an antifungal or viral agent if indicated, is used while waiting for results of culture of the CSF. If meningococcal meningitis is suspected, treatment must be instigated immediately[44-46].

Care to avoid direct contact with nasopharyngeal secretions to prevent transmission of the organism should be taken, especially if meningococcus is suspected, until cultures are negative[8,44,46]. Any co-existing disease is also treated and measures to relieve fever and headache are taken. Other treatment may be instigated for management of sepsis, respiratory distress, myocardial dysfunction, seizures, raised intracranial pressure, electrolyte imbalance or adrenal insufficiency if these occur. Treatment for such problems includes fluid replacement, airway management, drugs to improve myocardial contractility, anticonvulsant therapy, and monitoring of electrolyte and acid-base balance.

In aseptic meningitis, the symptoms are treated and most patients do not require hospitalisation and recover completely[44].

APPLIED PHARMACOLOGY

Large doses of intravenous antibiotics specific to the identified organism are prescribed, with intravenous penicillin the treatment of choice, with third-generation cephalosporines (cefotaxine, ceftriaxone) if sensitivity to penicillin is present. These drugs are able to enter the CSF circulation, and are active against most meningitis-causing bacteria. The antiviral agent aciclovir is prescribed if the herpesvirus is thought to be the cause of meningitis and for cryptoccocus. Oral rifampicin is given to people who have been in close contact with a patient diagnosed with meningococcal meningitis. Vaccine for serogroups A, C, W-135 and Y is also available[45-46].

Analgesia and antipyretics are prescribed for headache and fever. Corticosteroids (dexamethasone) have been found to be beneficial in treating adults with bacterial meningitis due to their effect on the inflammatory process[47].

NURSING IMPLICATIONS

The primary aspect is to be aware of the potential outcomes of meningitis, and be alert for signs of disease progression, deterioration and complications. Accurate assessment of baseline neurological, respiratory and cardiovascular status, monitoring of fluid balance, any seizure activity, prompt recognition and reporting of change and timely administration of antimicrobial therapy is essential, especially if meningococcus is suspected.

Positioning to assist comfort and reduce intracranial pressure, maintenance of a restful environment and reduced lighting assist to reduce the discomfort of photophobia and meningeal irritation.

LEARNING EXERCISES

1. Identify the common routes for CNS infection.
2. Describe the rationale for signs and symptoms of meningitis.
3. Differentiate between CSF findings in viral and bacterial meningitis.
4. Describe nursing measures that are used to reduce the discomfort associated with the signs and symptoms of meningeal irritation.

BRAIN ATTACK OR STROKE

WHAT DOES IT MEAN?

Brain attack is the contemporary term for stroke or cerebral vascular accident (CVA), and refers to a sudden interference to the brain's blood supply due to a partial or complete occlusion, or rupture of a cerebral blood vessel. This disruption to blood flow reduces the supply of oxygen, glucose and other nutrients to the part of the brain the affected blood vessel supplies and results in a range of impaired brain functions. Stroke occurs in all ages, but predominantly over the age of 75 years[48].

WHAT IS THE PATHOPHYSIOLOGY?

Most strokes (85%)[8] are ischaemic and occur due to an occlusion of a cerebral artery by a thrombosis or embolism related to atherosclerosis. Thrombosis, the most common cause of stroke, usually occurs in older adults. Risk factors include hypertension, heart disease, diabetes mellitus, hyperlipidaemia and history of transient ischaemic attack (TIA)[8,48–50]. A transient ischaemic attack (TIA) may last from minutes to 24 hours, and usually resolves without permanent damage. It is caused by microemboli temporarily interrupting small distal branches of cerebral blood vessels followed by return to normal function, and is a warning sign of impending thrombosis. Embolism can occur at any age, especially in people with cardiac disease, atrial fibrillation, heart valve disease or following open-heart surgery[8,48–49].

Initially in atherosclerosis, yellow, fatty areas form on the intimal surface of the arteries. Over time, fibrous plaques (atheroma) form at localised sites, such as where arteries branch and opposite bifurcations of extracerebral arteries. Platelets then adhere to the surface of the plaque (aggregation) and along with fibrin, slowly enlarge the size of the plaque to form a thrombus. In smaller arteries, a hyaline-lipid membrane forms on the walls of the vessels. In both cases, the lumen of a cerebral or extracerebral blood vessel, such as the carotid artery, are narrowed. In an embolus, a portion of thrombus or other material such as tumour, fat or bacteria breaks off and travels until it lodges in a distal blood vessel. A septic embolus may lead to formation of a cerebral aneurysm (mycotic), with subsequent rupture and haemorrhage[8,49].

The narrowing or occlusion of a cerebral artery results in reduced cerebral blood flow (CBF) to the region normally supplied by the affected blood vessel, and this reduction in blood flow governs the severity of the injury to the brain. Focal ischaemia and irreversible infarction of the area of brain tissue supplied by the affected artery occurs unless blood flow is restored. A zone called the ischaemic penumbra surrounds a core of infarcted tissue and although non-functioning, the neurons in this area are viable, and can recover if blood flow can be re-established and subsequent ischaemia and infarction prevented[8,50].

A lack of oxygen and the breakdown of glucose cause the neurons to become acidotic. Their electrical activity is disrupted as sodium, chloride and water enter and potassium leaves the cell, and local cerebral oedema occurs. An influx of calcium triggers a cascade of cellular reactions producing free radicals that cause lipid perioxidation and destruction of cell membranes. The neuron shrinks and dies and an inflammatory response is triggered. Phagocytes remove the necrotic tissue and it is replaced by scar tissue over time[8,50].

Haemorrhage from a ruptured cerebral artery, although less common (11%), is the most common cause of stroke-related death and can occur at any age, although 50% occur in people over 75 years[50]. Hypertension or rupture of a cerebral aneurysm are the most common causes of this type of stroke. Others causes include bleeding from an arteriovenous malformation, brain tumour and drug induced hypertension, such as can occur with some types of amphetamine[8,48,49].

Haemorrhagic stroke causes a reduced blood supply to the area of brain fed by the affected artery. Blood is forced into the surrounding brain tissue forming a haematoma that causes displacement and compression of adjoining tissues (parenchyma). This results in local ischaemia, a zone of cerebral oedema around the haematoma, and an increase in intracranial pressure and possible herniation of the brain. This type of haemorrhage has a mortality rate of 30–35% in the first 30 days[8].

When a cerebral aneurysm has ruptured, blood enters the subarachnoid space causing signs and symptoms of meningeal irritation as previously discussed in meningitis. Further cerebral ischaemia may occur 4–7 days following the initial haemorrhage due to spasm of the cerebral arteries.

● Case study

Mr Spooner found his wife, Vivian, 76 years, lying on the bedroom floor when he arrived home in the evening. He was unable to rouse her fully or get her to move, and called the ambulance service.

On arrival in the emergency department Mrs Spooner responded to loud verbal command with unintelligible sounds. She moved her left arm and leg purposefully to painful stimuli, but her right limbs were flaccid and the reflexes reduced. Her pupils were equal and reacting to light sluggishly.

Mrs Spooner showed P 90, BP 170/100, R 18, T 36.7°C, her skin was pale and swallowing and coughing reflexes were reduced. Oxygen therapy was continued, an intravenous infusion and nasogastric tube inserted. A provisional diagnosis of stroke was made and Mrs Spooner was sent for a CT scan. A diagnosis of ischaemic stroke due to a thrombosis of the left middle cerebral artery was made following the CT scan.

WHAT ARE THE CLINICAL MANIFESTATIONS?

Clinical manifestations depend upon the cerebral artery involved, the functions controlled or mediated by the affected part of the brain, the severity of the damage and size of the affected area, as well as the degree of collateral circulation.[1,3,8] (see Table 8.2). Clinical signs and symptoms include one or more of the following: alterations in level of consciousness, mobility, sensation, language, swallowing, sensory perception, cognitive function, concentration, and continence. There is a variation in clinical manifestations related to the side of the brain involved (see Table 8.3)[3,8].

Bleeding into the subarachnoid space causes meningeal irritation due to the presence of blood and the products of blood cell breakdown. The patient will present with history of an explosive headache, photophobia, nuchal (neck) rigidity, and positive Kernig's and Brudzinski sign due to meningeal irritation as well as clinical manifestations related to the affected blood vessel. Patients with intracerebral haemorrhage demonstrate an altered level of consciousness, headache, nausea and vomiting. Signs and symptoms of increased intracranial pressure (ICP) are often present in haemorrhagic stroke[8].

WHAT SHOULD YOU BE LOOKING AT IN LABORATORY AND OTHER TESTS?

Diagnosis is based upon a comprehensive history and neurological examination including consciousness, blood pressure, heart rate, temperature, and respiratory patterns. There are a number of diagnostic tests that can be performed, depending upon the suspected type of stroke. A computerised tomogram (CT) is the standard diagnostic test[51] and is able to distinguish cerebral haemorrhage from infarction, and differentiate between stroke and disorders that may present with the same clinical manifestations, such as cerebral tumour or traumatic haemorrhage. This test will show any distortion of cerebral structures caused by haemorrhage or cerebral oedema, and, if a contrast medium is used, may show if a large cerebral aneurysm or arteriovenous malformation is present. A negative result is expected in the early hours of an acute ischaemic stroke or a transient ischaemic attack. Subsequent scans show infarction and later cavitation as the necrotic tissue breaks down.

A full blood picture, 12-lead ECG, electrolytes, renal function, glucose, lipids, cholesterol and triglycerides are performed to assist in diagnosis. For example, a 12-lead ECG can assist in identifying a cardiac cause if an embolic stroke is suspected. An elevated haematocrit with a high blood viscosity is a predisposition for thrombosis[51].

Other tests that can be performed include magnetic resonance imaging (MRI) to show lesions such as a haematoma, and distinguish between ischaemia and infarction. Magnetic

TABLE 8.2: CLINICAL PRESENTATION RELATED TO INVOLVED ARTERY	
Artery Involved	**Clinical Presentation**
Internal carotid artery	• Contralateral weakness (hemiparesis) or paralysis of face, arm and leg • Contralateral sensory deficit of face, arm and leg • Aphasia or dysphasia if dominant hemisphere • Apraxia, agnosia and unilateral neglect if non-dominant hemisphere • Visual disturbances
Anterior cerebral artery	• Contralateral paralysis of the foot and leg • Contralateral sensory loss of foot and leg • Impaired gait and coordination • Slowed voluntary actions • Decreased spontaneity, distractible, interest • Cognitive impairment (confusion) • Urinary incontinence
Middle cerebral artery	• Contralateral hemiparesis (arm more than leg) • Contralateral sensory impairment (arm more than leg) • Visual field deficits (homonymous hemianopia) • Aphasia or dysphasia (if dominant hemisphere) • Language problems related to ability to read and write
Vertebral artery	• Dizziness • Nystagmus • Dysarthria • Dysphagia • Sensory loss and weakness of face on side of lesion • Ataxia and impaired coordination
Basilar artery	• Quadriplegia • Pharyngeal, tongue and facial muscle weakness
Cerebellar arteries	• Ataxia, vertigo, dizziness and nystagmus • Nausea and vomiting • Impaired pain and temperature sensation of trunk and limbs on the contralateral side • Paralysis of gaze • Small pupil and ptosis of eyelid-affected side

TABLE 8.3: CLINICAL MANIFESTATIONS RELATED TO AFFECTED SIDE OF BRAIN	
Right side of the brain (dominant for spatial and visual perception and creativity)	**Left side of the brain** (dominant for speech; analytical capabilities; and auditory and verbal memory)
Left-sided hemiplegia	Right-sided hemiplegia
Impaired judgement	Expressive, receptive or global aphasia
Loss of non-verbal memory	Impaired-thought processes
Left visual field defects	Right visual field defects
Decreased awareness of the left side of body	Cautious behaviour
Note: lesions affecting the cerebellum produce ipsilateral signs and in the brain stem there is cranial nerve involvement.	

resonance angiography (MRA) is a non-invasive method of visualising the carotid and cerebral circulation and can show the presence of an occlusion.

Carotid ultrasound and transcranial Doppler measure cerebral blood flow and detect reduced blood flow and stenosis in the carotid and vertebrobasilar arteries, as well as the extent of collateral circulation. It can be used to assess the progression of vascular disease and evaluate effects of therapy for vasospasm, such as occurs with a subarachnoid haemorrhage. Cerebral angiography is an invasive procedure using a contrast medium to show the cerebral blood vessels, patency, and the site of stenosis, occlusion or aneurysm. Cerebral blood flow studies assist in determining the degree of vasospasm[8].

In subarachnoid haemorrhage (SAH), a lumbar puncture will demonstrate bloody CSF and elevated CSF pressure. However, this test will only be performed if an intracerebral lesion has been excluded and there is no risk of increased intracranial pressure.

WHAT IS THE TREATMENT?

Treatment is determined by the cause of the stroke and may be pharmaceutical, interventional radiology or surgical. Early recognition and accurate diagnosis is essential so that appropriate treatment can be instigated as soon as possible to restore circulation and prevent secondary injury, thereby improving the chances for recovery and reduced disability. For ischaemic stroke, treatment aims are to increase perfusion to the brain, assist lysis of the clot and prevent further thrombosis, protect viable brain tissue and prevent other secondary injury. In haemorrhagic stroke, the aim is to prevent secondary damage by controlling intracranial pressure and vasospasm, and preventing further bleeding[50].

Thrombolytic therapy can be used to restore blood flow by causing lysis of a clot, but needs to commence within three hours of clinical manifestations appearing, and only after exclusion of haemorrhage or other causes[50,51]. Anticoagulant therapy is controversial, and the latest evidence-based guidelines do not recommend routine use of this treatment following ischaemic stroke unless there is a high risk of a recurrent embolism due to valvular heart disease, recent myocardial infarction or atrial fibrillation[51]. In acute ischaemic stroke aspirin, unless contraindicated, can be given once haemorrhage is excluded[50,51].

Supportive therapy to prevent extension of a stroke and increase cerebral perfusion includes management of airway and oxygenation, blood pressure monitoring and control to prevent further haemorrhage, analgesia for headache, and management of fever and anticonvulsant therapy if seizures occur. Control of hyperglycaemia in patients with diabetes is important, as deviations from the norm increases the area of infarction[8]. In cases of severe hypertension, if antihypertensive therapy is used, close monitoring of blood pressure is important as a sudden decrease may cause lowered cerebral perfusion[50,52].

Surgical intervention may be required to clip a ruptured cerebral aneurysm to prevent further haemorrhage, although interventional radiology and embolisation of the aneurysm are becoming more common in some centres[53]. Management of the person with a haemorrhagic stroke and cerebral aneurysm includes the use of hypervolaemic haemodilution to prevent vasospasm, and calcium channel blockers to prevent contraction of the walls of the blood vessels.

In cases of carotid artery atheroma, carotid endarterectomy and removal of plaque is performed when the patient has symptoms of reduced blood flow and a stenosis of more than 70%, or if asymptomatic, with a stenosis of greater than 50%[8,51]. Removal of intracerebral haematoma may occur in cases where the lesion is accessible and well defined.

Prevention of further stroke is managed through reduction of modifiable risk factors, such as hypertension, smoking, weight and cholesterol, and glucose control in those with diabetes. Antiplatelet medication may be prescribed to prevent further blood clot formation and improve blood flow[50].

The management of the person following stroke involves a collaborative approach involving the health care team, the patient and their family, with the aim of assisting the patient to regain their ability to carry out their normal activities of daily living. A multidisciplinary assessment is carried out within the first 48 hours of admission. This includes the speech pathologist's assessment of swallowing ability to reduce the risk of aspiration, and assessment for communication problems. The physiotherapist and occupational therapist assess mobility and the ability of the patient to perform cognitive and functional activities. They provide therapy to assist mobility and strategies to help regain the ability to perform activities of daily living.

APPLIED PHARMACOLOGY

Thrombolytic therapy using recombinant tissue plasminogen activator (rTPA) alteplase can restore blood flow in acute ischaemic stroke by dissolving the blood clot. This drug is administered intravenously and needs to start within three hours of the onset of symptoms following exclusion of cerebral haemorrhage as the cause. It is recommended that it only be administered in acute stroke units where staff members are experienced in its use, and in conjunction with the guidelines[51]. It is contraindicated if the patient has a history of recent surgery, gastric ulceration, bleeding, or a prolonged clotting time.

Antiplatelet therapy, such as aspirin, dipyridamole or clopidogrel, may be prescribed to reduce thrombus formation and prolong clotting time. Anticoagulant therapy with warfarin places the patient at risk of haemorrhage and is not advised until seven days following a stroke, and then only for ischaemic stroke of cardiac origin[50,51].

NURSING IMPLICATIONS

Regular assessment of airway, breathing, and circulation, as well as neurological status, is necessary to monitor changes in condition and responses to treatment. Raised intracranial pressure due to cerebral oedema or further haemorrhage may occur, especially if the original stroke was extensive. Severe hypertension increases the risk of haemorrhage, which can occur up to four days following infarction, but any treatment to lower the blood pressure must be carefully monitored[8]. If thrombolytic therapy is administered, monitor bleeding by testing urine and faeces for blood, check skin mucous membranes and avoid IM and SC injections.

Bleeding tendencies, fluid imbalance, poor nutrition, and safety problems related to the type of cerebral damage, systemic complications, anxiety and depression are other potential problems. Other complications that pose a risk and require assessment and preventive care include aspiration pneumonia, pulmonary embolus, cardiac arrhythmias, decreased gastrointestinal motility and incontinence. Joint contractures, shoulder pain, falls and pressure sores can also be prevented by risk assessment and correct positioning techniques.

As part of the multidisciplinary team, nurses also play a role in maintaining and reinforcing management aimed at reducing disability and maximising function and the ability to carry out activities of daily life, as well as education in risk reduction to prevent further stroke.

LEARNING EXERCISES

1. Describe the two main causes of stroke.
2. Explain how ischaemia is caused by the two main causes of stroke.
3. Identify the clinical manifestations when there is an occlusion of the left middle cerebral artery.
4. What strategies and nursing interventions are directed at reducing injury to the brain?
5. Identify the three major areas that have implications for the nurse in caring for patients with stroke.

In this case study, it was not possible to estimate the time when Mrs Spooner experienced her stroke and therefore, thrombolytic therapy could not be administered. She was admitted to a high dependency area within the neurosciences unit where her neurological status continued to be monitored using the Glasgow coma scale. An indwelling urinary catheter was inserted and intravenous therapy continued. Positioning to maintain her airway, assist cerebral venous return and minimise changes to intracranial pressure, as well as prevent joint and limb contractures was carried out two hourly. Nursing care related to maintaining all body functions and preventing complications was commenced. Intragastric feeding was commenced on day two.

On day three, Mrs Spooner started to open her eyes and exhibit spontaneous movement of her left limbs. The reflexes in her right limbs were brisk, and there was evidence of increased muscle tone, particularly in her right arm, but there was no spontaneous movement. Her left facial paralysis remained and although she focused on objects, she did not speak and appeared agitated at times. On day four, she was attempting to remove her nasogastric tube, but her swallowing remained impaired and enteral feeding continued until day seven, when oral diet was commenced after further testing demonstrated an improvement in her swallowing reflex, although the weakness of her facial muscles continued. However, she remained aphasic.

Transfer to a rehabilitation facility was planned for further mobilisation, gait and balance training, speech therapy and programs to enable her to carry out activities of personal care and daily living.

Recommended Reading

Calne, SM & Kumar, A. 2003; 'Nursing Care of Patients with Late-Stage Parkinson's Disease', *Journal of Neuroscience Nursing*, 35 (5), 242–251.

Cunning, S. 2000; 'When the Dx is Myasthenia Gravis', *RN*, 63 (4), 26, 28–31.

Costello, K. & Harris, C. 2003; 'Differential Diagnosis and Management of Fatigue in MS: Considerations for the Nurse', *Journal of Neuroscience Nursing*, 35 (3), 139–148.

Fischer, D. 2004; 'Help Your Patient Manage Myasthenia Gravis', *Nursing Made Incredibly Easy!* 2 (1), 28–33.

Penna, C. 2003; 'Seizure: A Calm Response and Careful Observation Are Crucial', *American Journal of Nursing*, 103 (1), 73–81.

Schretzman, D. 2001; 'Acute Ischemic Stroke', *Dimensions of Critical Care Nursing*, 20 (2), 14–21.

References

1. Waxman, SG & de Groote, J. 1996; *Correlative Neuroanatomy* (23rd ed.), Prentice Hall International, Stanford.
2. Nolte, J. 2002; *The Human Brain: An Introduction to Its Functional Anatomy* (5th ed.), Mosby, St Louis.
3. Thibodeau, GG & Patton, K. 2003; *Anatomy & Physiology* (5th ed.), Mosby, St Louis.
4. Barker, RA, Barasi, S & Neal, MJ. 1999; *Neuroscience at a Glance*. Blackwell Science, Oxford.
5. McCance, KL & Huether, SE. 2002; *Pathophysiology: The Biologic Basis For Disease in Adults and Children* (4th ed.), Mosby, St Louis.
6. Bonduelle, M. 1998; 'Guillain-Barré Syndrome', *Archives of Neurology*, 55, 1483–1484.
7. Hund, E, O'Borel, C, Cornblath, D, Hanley, D & McKhann, G. 1993; 'ICU Management of

Guillain-Barré', *Critical Care Medicine*, 21 (3), 433–446.

8. Hickey, J. 2003; *The Clinical Practice of Neurological and Neurosurgical Nursing* (5th ed.), Lippincott Williams & Wilkins, Philadelphia.

9. Van der Meche, FGA & van Doorn, PA. 1995; 'Guillain-Barré Syndrome and Chronic Inflammatory Demyelinating Polyneuropathy: Immune Mechanisms and Update on Current Therapies', *Annals of Neurology*, 37 (supplement 5), 14S–31S.

10. McMahon-Parkes, K & Cornock, MA. 1997; 'Guillain-Barré Syndrome: Biological Basis, Treatment and Care', *Intensive and Critical Care Nursing*, 13, 42–48.

11. Worsham, TL. 2000; 'Easing the Course of Guillain-Barré Syndrome', *RN*, 63, 46–50.

12. Mishu, B & Blaser, M. 1993; 'Role of Infection Due to *Campylobacter jejuni* in the Initiation of Guillain-Barré Syndrome', *Clinical Infectious Diseases*, 17, 104–108.

13. Waldock, E. 1995; 'The Pathophysiology of Guillain-Barré Syndrome', *British Journal of Nursing*, 4, 818–821.

14. Allos, BM. 1998; '*Campylobacter jejuni*: Infection as a Cause of Guillain-Barré Syndrome', *Infectious Disease Clinics of North America*, 12 (1), 173–184.

15. Pascuzzi, RM & Fleck, JD. 1997; 'Acute Peripheral Neuropathy in Adults', *Neurology Clinics*, 15 (3), 529–545.

16. Sharshar, T, Chevret, S, Bourdain, F & Raphael, J. 2003; 'Early Predictors of Mechanical Ventilation in Guillain-Barré Syndrome', *Critical Care Medicine*, 31 (1), 278–283.

17. Sharief, MK, Ingram, DA, Swash, M & Thompson, FJ. 1999; 'IV Immunoglobulin Reduces Circulating Proinflammatory Cytokinines in Guillain-Barré Syndrome', *Neurology*, 52 (9), 1833–1888.

18. Vajsar, J, Fehlings, D & Stephens, D. 2003; 'Long-Term Outcome in Children with Guillain-Barré Syndrome', *The Journal of Pediatrics*, 142 (3), 305–309.

19. Raphael, JC, Chevret, S, Hughes, RAC & Annane, D. 2003; *Plasma Exchange for Guillain-Barré Syndrome*, The Cochrane Library, Oxford, 2 (CD001798).

20. Graf, WD, Katz, JS, Eder, DN, Smith, AJ & Chun, MR 1999; 'Outcome in Severe Pediatric Guillain-Barré Syndrome After Immunotherapy or Supportive Care', *Neurology*, 52 (7), 1494–1497.

21. Gaber, TAK, Kirker, SGB & Jenner, JR. 2002; 'Current Practice of Prophylactic Anticoagulation in Guillain-Barré Syndrome', *Clinical Rehabilitation*, 16 (2) 190–193.

22. Weinshenker, BG. 1996; 'The Epidemiology of MS', *Neurology Clinic*, 14, 291–308.

23. Lublin, FD & Reingold, SC 1996; 'Defining the Clinical Course of MS', *Neurology*, 46, 907–911.

24. Burks, JS & Johnson, KP (eds.). 2000; *Multiple Sclerosis: Diagnosis, Medical Management, and Rehabilitation*, Demos, New York.

25. Halper, J, Kennedy, P, Miller, CM, Morgante, L, Namey, M & Rioss, AP. 2003; 'Rethinking Cognitive Function in Multiple Sclerosis: A Nursing Perspective', *Journal Neuroscience Nursing*, 35 (2), 70–81.

26. Ross, AP & Crabbe, RA 2003; *Neurologic Problems*. Springhouse, Philadelphia.

27. Stewart-Amidei, C & Kunkel, JA. (eds.), 2001; *AANN's Neuroscience Nursing: Human Responses To Neurologic Dysfunction* (2nd ed.), W.B. Saunders Company, Philadelphia.

28. Tullman, MJ, Lublin, FD & Miller, AE. 2002; 'Immunotherapy of Multiple Sclerosis: Current Practice and Future Directions,' *Journal of Rehabilitation, Research and Development*, 39 (2), 273–286.

29. Goodin, DS, Frohman, EM, Garmany, GP, Halper, J, Likoskey, WH, Lublin, FD, *et al.* 2002; 'Disease Modifying Therapies in Multiple Sclerosis: Report of the Therapeutics and Technology Assessment Subcommittee of the American Academy of Neurology and the MS Council for Clinical Practice Guidelines', *Neurology*, 58, 169–178.

30. Bakshi, R. 2003; 'Fatigue Associated with Multiple Sclerosis: Diagnosis, impact and management', *Multiple Sclerosis*, 9, 219–227.

31. Costello, K & Harris, C 2003; 'Differential Diagnosis and Management of Fatigue in Multiple Sclerosis: Consideration for the Nurse', *Journal Neuroscience Nursing*, 35 (3), 139–148.

32. Pascuzzi, R. 1994; 'The History of Myasthenia Gravis', *Neurology Clinics*, 12 (2), 231–242.

33. Kernich, CA & Kaminski, HJ. 1995; 'Myasthenia Gravis: Pathophysiology, Diagnosis and Collaborative Care', *Journal of Neuroscience Nursing*, 27 (1), 207–217.

34. Cunning, S. 2000. 'When the Dx is Myasthenia Gravis.' *RN*, 63 (4), 26, 28–31, 37.

35. Kittiwatanapaisan, W, Gauthier, DK, Williams, AM & Oh, SJ. 2003. 'Fatigue in Myasthenia Gravis Patients', *Journal of Neuroscience Nursing*, 35 (2), 87.

36. Calne, D & Calne, SM (eds.). 2001; *Parkinson's Disease*. Lippincott Williams & Wilkins, Philadelphia.

37. Smolowitz, J & Waters, C. 2001; 'Clinical Management of the Adult with Parkinson's Disease', *The American Journal for Nurse Practitioners*, 5 (7), 9–10, 15–17, 21–22.

38. Duvoisin, RC. 1996; '*Parkinson's Disease: A Guide for Patient and Family.*' Lippincott-Raven, Philadelphia.

39. Bryant, B, Knights, K & Salerno, E. 2003; *Pharmacology for Health Professionals.* Elsevier (Australia) Pty. Limited, Marrickville.

40. Penna, C. 2003; 'Seizure: A Calm Response and Careful Observation Are Crucial', *American Journal of Nursing*, 103 (1), 73–81.

41. Celesia, GG. 2003. 'Are the Epilepsies Disorders of Ion Channels?', *The Lancet*, 361, 1238–1239.

42. Buchhalter, JR & Jarrar, RG. 2003; 'Symposium On Seizures: Therapeutics in Pediatric Epilepsy, Part 2: Epilepsy Surgery and Vagus Nerve Stimulation', *Mayo Clinic Proceedings*, 78 (3), 371–378.

43. Freeman JM, Vining EPG, Pillas DJ, Pysik PL, Casey JC & Kelly MT. 1998; 'The Efficacy of the Ketogenic Diet-1998: a Prospective Evaluation of Intervention in 150 Children', *Pediatrics*, 102, 1358–1363.

44. Parini, SM. 2002; 'The Meningitis Mind-bender', *Nursing Management*, 33 (8), 21–25.

45. Leaver, M. 1998; 'Meningococcal Disease in Australia', *Collegian*, 5 (1), 44–45.

46. Communicable Diseases Network Australia 2001. *Guidelines for the Early Clinical and Public Health Management of Meningococcal Disease in Australia.* Public Affairs, Parliamentary and Access Branch, Commonwealth Department of Health and Aged Care, Canberra.

47. De Gans, J & van de Beek, D. 2002; 'Dexamethasone in Adults with Bacterial Meningitis', *The New England Journal of Medicine*, 347 (20), 1549–1556.

48. Australian Institute of Health and Welfare, 2001. *Heart, stroke and vascular diseases, Australian facts.* AIHW, Heart Foundation and National Stroke Foundation of Australia, Canberra.

49. Schretzman, D. 2001; 'Acute Ischaemic Stroke', *Dimensions of Critical Care Nursing*, 20 (2), 14–21.

50. Cadilhac, D. 1998; 'The Changing Face of Stroke: Medical Management Revolution', *Australian Nursing Journal*, 5 (11), 18–21.

51. National Stroke Unit Program Steering Committee Expert Working Group of National Stroke Foundation 2003; *National Clinical Guidelines for Acute Stroke Management.* National Stroke Foundation, Melbourne.

52. International Society of Hypertension Writing Group 2003; 'International Society of Hypertension (ISH): Statement on the Management of Blood Pressure in Acute Stroke', *Journal of Hypertension*, 21 (4), 665–672.

53. Bader, MK. 1998; 'Case Presentations of Neuroradiologic Interventions for Acute Cerebrovascular Disease', *Journal of Cardiovascular Nursing*, 13 (1), 1–16.

9 | Gastrointestinal Health Breakdown

AUTHORS

JOHN SIBBALD

MALCOLM ELLIOTT

VICKI BAKER

LEARNING OBJECTIVES

When you have completed this chapter you will be able to

- Identify the important anatomical and physiological features of the gastrointestinal system;
- Describe the common pathophysiological changes associated with gastrointestinal health breakdown;
- Identify the common pharmacological agents used in managing gastrointestinal health breakdown and the associated nursing implications; and
- Consider nursing interventions required for people with gastrointestinal health breakdown.

INTRODUCTION

This chapter includes an overview of the anatomy and physiology of the gastrointestinal tract. Using a case study approach, the following common health breakdowns are presented: cholecystitis, cirrhosis of the liver, pancreatitis, hepatitis, appendicitis, peptic ulcer disease, Crohn's disease, and ulcerative colitis.

The gastrointestinal (GI) tract is essentially a tube running through the body with its lumen open to the outside (see Figure 9.1). The GI tract is the only (normal) input channel to the body for water and nutrients. Four major functions are associated with the GI tract: ingestion, digestion, absorption and defaecation[1]. Ingestion refers to the taking in of food and water and is a voluntary action. Digestion is the breakdown of food into absorbable particles. There are two main ways in which this happens:

1. Mechanical breakdown, which involves muscular movement of the GI tract; and
2. Chemical breakdown, which involves the secretion of various enzymes and solutions.

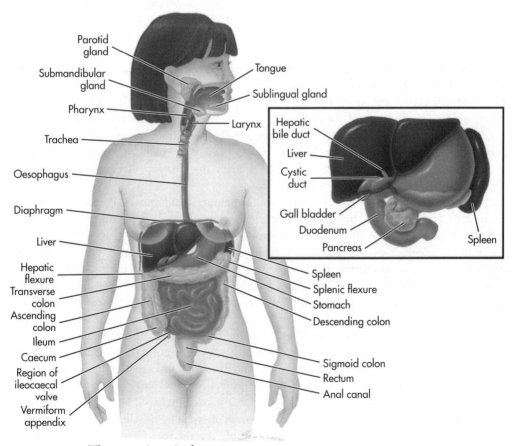

FIGURE 9.1 *The gastrointestinal system*
Source: Adapted from Thibodeau, GA & Patton, KT. 2003; *Anatomy and Physiology* (5th ed.), Mosby, St Louis, Fig. 25.1, p. 740.

Gut movements also help to mix food with the secreted solutions and so hasten digestion. Absorption is the process by which nutrients cross the gut lining and enter the body proper. Defaecation involves the excretion of unwanted or unusable ingested material together with shed epithelial cells from the gut lining plus some substances secreted into the gut, bile pigments for example, for excretion by this route[2].

The GI tract or tube has the same basic structure throughout. It consists of layers of tissue, some with sub layers[1]. The innermost layer, forming a barrier between the outside and inside of the body is the mucosa, in most parts a single layer of epithelium rich in mucus-secreting goblet cells and in many parts also enzyme and hormone secreting cells. Immediately underlying the mucosa is a thin layer of smooth muscle, the muscularis interna, contraction and relaxation of which brings about movement of the mucosa. Beneath the mucosa is a layer of connective tissue containing blood vessels, lymphatics, and autonomic submucosal nerve plexuses. The muscularis externa, a layer of smooth muscle lies underneath this and forms the bulk of the GI tract wall. Generally it consists of two layers of muscle, an inner circular layer and an outer longitudinal layer. In some parts of the tract there is an additional oblique layer, and in some places there are thickenings of the circular layer forming sphincters, which prevent backflow and control the passage of food. There are autonomic myenteric nerve plexuses between the two muscle layers. The serosa forms a protective outer layer. In most parts of the GI tract within the abdomen, the outer layer is a double-layered serous membrane, the peritoneum[1].

Put simply, the peritoneum may be regarded as a single continuous membrane. It lines the walls of the abdomino-pelvic cavity (as the parietal peritoneum) and also extends into the abdominal cavity and covers the external surfaces of most of the GI tract (as the visceral peritoneum). The peritoneal cavity is the area contained within the peritoneum and contains serous fluid, which acts as a lubricant. To provide a route for blood vessels, lymphatics and nerves supplying the GI, viscera two layers of peritoneum are fused, to form mesenteries. Most GI tract organs lie within the peritoneal cavity but some are retroperitoneal, for example the pancreas[1].

Apart from movements involving the mouth, pharynx, and anus, GI tract movement is involuntary and mediated by smooth muscle[1]. Although not requiring a motor nerve stimulus for the initiation of contraction smooth muscle still contracts in a fairly ordered way and the gut has several pacemaker regions in the more proximal parts of the gut, which initiate waves of contraction (very similar to the pacemaker region in the heart)[3]. Smooth muscle contracts more slowly and sustains contraction longer than skeletal muscle. Its contraction is modified by autonomic nerves (hence the myenteric nerve plexuses) and by hormonal action. Parasympathetic (cholinergic) nerves increase contraction strength, duration and frequency, while sympathetic (adrenergic) nerves inhibit activity[2].

Food is moved along the GI tract by peristalsis[3], a wave of contraction passing along the gut from proximal to distal. This wave of contraction may involve the whole gut or just a segment, and contributes to mixing of the gut contents. Other types of contraction contribute to the breakdown of food into smaller particles as well as helping to mix the contents of the gut[3]. Segmentation is a movement in which muscle in different parts of the gut contract simultaneously, making the gut look like a string of sausages. On relaxation, this movement may be repeated by contraction of different areas of muscle.

Once food has been ingested the digestive process begins. Mechanical digestion begins in the mouth with chewing and movement of the food with the tongue[1]. This starts the breakdown process and mixes food with saliva, which begins the process of chemical digestion. Salivary secretion is a parasympathetic reflex and involves cerebral as well as local stimuli. The sight, smell, taste or even thought of food will cause secretion of saliva as will the presence of food in the mouth[3]. Saliva contains water (97–99%), ions, mucus, an enzyme (salivary amylase), antibodies, and the antibacterial compound lysozyme. Salivary amylase begins the breakdown of starches (polysaccharides) to smaller molecules (oligosaccharides).

Swallowing (deglutition) is a complex process involving the tongue, soft palate, pharynx and oesophagus[2]. Food is first compacted into a bolus by the tongue. It is then 'tipped' back into the oropharynx by the tongue. The tip of the tongue is raised against the hard palate. This is the voluntary or buccal phase of swallowing. After this point food is out of our voluntary control.

The pharyngeal-oesophageal phase of swallowing is controlled by the swallowing centre in the medulla oblongata[2]. The bolus is gripped by the muscles of the wall and 'squeezed' downwards. All routes except the correct one, the oesophagus, being blocked off. The tongue blocks off the mouth; the soft palate rises to block off the nasopharynx; and the larynx rises so that the epiglottis blocks off the respiratory passages. The bolus of food then passes down the oesophagus into the stomach by peristaltic action.

Once in the stomach the bolus comes into contact with gastric juice, secreted by various cells in the gastric glands[1]. Mucous neck cells (found at the necks of gastric pits) secrete special mucus, which protects the stomach lining from the effects of its acid secretions. Parietal (oxyntic) cells found among the mucous cells of the neck secrete hydrochloric acid, which keeps the pH of the stomach at approximately 2.0. Zymogenic (chief) cells located at the base of the glands secrete pepsinogen (an inactive form of a proteolytic enzyme). When food enters the stomach, at first the pH rises because the protein content buffers H^+ but as the pH falls salivary amylase ceases to act. The acid pH converts pepsinogen to pepsin – an enzyme which breaks proteins into large polypeptides. The acid continues the further breakdown of the food and effectively kills most microorganisms present.

Gastric juice is secreted in three phases[3]. The sight, smell, taste or thought of food cause gastric secretions to occur. This is mediated via a branch of the vagus nerve and begins before food enters the stomach. Distension of the stomach by food initiates local gut reflexes and 'long loop' reflexes, involving the central nervous system, which result in the secretion of more gastric juice. The presence in the stomach of partially digested protein, a high pH, or caffeine, stimulate the secretion of gastrin, a hormone secreted by the enteroendocrine cells of the gastric mucosa. Gastrin is secreted into the systemic circulation. However, it only affects the secretory cells of the gastric glands causing them to release both HCl and pepsinogen. HCl secretion is also increased by histamine, released by the enteroendocrine cells of the gastric mucosa in response to the presence of food in the stomach.

When food first enters the duodenum there is a release of intestinal gastrin, from enteroendocrine cells in the duodenum[1]. Gastrin circulates systemically and brings about a further increase in gastric secretion. Later as larger amounts of H^+ and fats enter the duodenum there is inhibition of gastric secretion via both nervous and hormonal factors (secretin, cholecystokinin [CCK] and gastric inhibitory peptide [GIP]). Gastric secretion is also inhibited by a fall in pH in the stomach.

The stomach continually compresses, kneads and twists to mix the contents, producing chyme[1]. Muscular activity is also enhanced by the same hormonal and nervous reflexes that enhance gastric secretion (and is similarly inhibited by the same inhibiting factors). There are receptors for the hormones on the gastric smooth muscle.

Peristaltic activity in the pylorus causes release of small amounts (3–5 mL) of chyme into the duodenum up to 2 to 3 times each minute[2]. Gastric emptying is inhibited by chyme rich in fats. Liquids pass through the stomach fairly rapidly – generally the stomach empties within 4 hours of a meal – but a fatty meal may delay this by a further 2 hours or so[3].

Only a few fat-soluble substances are absorbed in the stomach (e.g., aspirin, alcohol, some drugs)[1]. The oxyntic cells also secrete intrinsic factor – a glycoprotein essential for the absorption of vitamin B_{12}. These two substances combine in the stomach and are absorbed in the small intestine[2]. The glands in the duodenum secrete an alkaline-rich juice, which neutralises the acid chyme coming from the stomach[1]. In the duodenum chyme also mixes with pancreatic juice and bile.

The exocrine cells of the pancreas secrete from 1200 to 1500 mL/day[1]. Pancreatic juice contains water, enzymes and ions, especially HCO_3^- which further contributes to the neutralisation of the acid chyme. The pancreatic enzymes are concerned with the digestion of all food types. A major component of pancreatic juice is a series of proteases or protein splitting enzymes – trypsinogen, chymotrypsinogen and procarboxypeptidase. These are all initially inactive. Trypsinogen is activated by enterokinase, normally bound to the surface of the duodenal lining cells, to form trypsin. Once present trypsin in turn activates chymotrypsinogen to form chymotrypsin, then chymotrypsin in turn activates procarboxypeptidase to form carboxypeptidase. The pancreas also secretes amylases, to digest carbohydrates; lipases, to digest fats; and nucleases, to digest nucleic acids.

Stimulation of the vagus nerve, brought about by eating and by the presence of food in the stomach, also causes some pancreatic secretion[3]. The presence of HCl in the duodenum brings about secretion of two hormones: secretin, which causes the secretion of pancreatic HCO_3^-; and cholecystokinin (CCK), which causes secretion of pancreatic digestive enzymes.

Bile is secreted by the liver and stored and concentrated in the gall bladder[1]. It is released in small quantities in response to vagal stimulation and in large quantities in response to CCK. Five hundred to 1000 mL of bile is secreted each day[1]. Bile is a yellow-green, alkaline fluid containing bile salts, which are cholesterol derivatives and the bile pigments, bilirubin and biliverdin. The latter are waste products from the breakdown of haemoglobin. Bile salts emulsify fats and so make their digestion easier. They are also important in fat absorption. Bile salts are not excreted but are reabsorbed in the small intestine and recycled. Bile pigments colour and deodorise faeces and so are excreted.

Chyme is moved further on into first the jejunum and then the ileum[1]. The intestinal glands here secrete 1 to 2 L of juice per day[3]. The intestinal juice is mainly water but also contains a great deal of mucus as well as digestive enzymes. Intestinal digestive enzymes are bound to the microvilli on the surfaces of the intestinal epithelial cells, and, for that reason are often called 'brush border' enzymes. These are found mainly in the duodenum and are most active here.

Digestive processes are essentially completed in the small intestine[3]. Proteins are finally broken down to amino acids (or often pairs of amino acids). Carbohydrates are broken down to monosaccharides, while fats are broken down to fatty acids and glycerol.

Daily we ingest up to 10 L of food and drink, but only about 500 mL to 1 L reaches the large intestine[1]. The rest is absorbed in the small intestine. Absorption occurs all along the small intestine but is mostly completed by the time chyme reaches the ileum. At the end of the ileum all that remains is water, indigestible food material (e.g., cellulose) and millions of bacteria. This all passes into the large intestine or colon.

Most nutrients are absorbed through the mucosa of the villi[3]. Water-soluble products, such as amino acids and monosaccharides are transported into and across the lining cells of the intestine and then enter capillary blood in the villus. Lipids, however, diffuse passively across the mucosa and are taken up by the lacteal (lymph vessel) and carried to the blood via the lymph system. The veins draining the stomach and small intestine empty into the hepatic portal vein and the blood passes through the liver before returning to the systemic circulation[1]. The liver is able to extract and process absorbed nutrients from the blood as required.

Chyme entering the colon contains few nutrients[3]. The colon absorbs water, ions and some vitamins. The terminal ileum and colon contain large quantities of bacteria. Some bacteria enter the GI tract via the anus, while others survive passage through the stomach and small intestine. The more neutral pH of the ileum and colon may encourage their growth. These bacteria present in the colon play important roles in body metabolism. They digest some of the remaining carbohydrates in chyme, in the process producing some irritating acids and gases. The human body produces about 500 mL of gas each day. These gases are eventually passed as flatus. Bacteria in the colon also synthesise some B-complex vitamins and most of the vitamin K required by the body[3].

Two main types of muscular activity are observed in the colon[3]. Haustral contractions are slow segmenting movements. Distension of a haustrum causes a contraction, which moves the contents along the colon into the next haustrum. This type of movement also mixes the contents and aids in water absorption. Mass movements are long, slow moving, contractile waves, which move over the entire length of the colon 3 or 4 times a day[1]. These mass movements usually occur during or just after eating (the gastrocolic reflex).

Material that reaches the anus is semi-solid[1]. Most of the water still present when chyme enters the caecum, has been absorbed by the colon and the material present is now called faeces. Faeces are forced into the rectum by mass movements. The rectum is usually empty and when faeces enter, the rectal wall becomes stretched, which initiates the defaecation reflex.

This is a spinal cord mediated parasympathetic reflex[3]. It involves contraction of the walls of the sigmoid colon and rectum and relaxation of the internal anal sphincter (smooth muscle). The external sphincter can be controlled since it is composed of skeletal muscle and so defaecation can be delayed for a time. Expulsion of faeces is aided by contraction of the levator ani muscle and raising the intra-abdominal pressure. The latter is achieved by the valsalva manoeuvre, essentially exhaling against a closed glottis[2].

CHOLECYSTITIS

● Case study

Leslie Wynne, 42, presented to the hospital with acute abdominal pain. The pain radiated into her right shoulder, and was worse on inspiration and movement. She had nausea and had vomited. Her blood pressure was normal. Her heart rate was 94 beats/min and her temperature was 38.2°C. Her abdomen was distended and bowel sounds were absent. She was mildly jaundiced.

WHAT IS THE PATHOPHYSIOLOGY?

Cholecystitis is inflammation of the gallbladder, most commonly caused by a build up of bile in the gallbladder when the cystic duct is obstructed by gallstones[1]. The common (though not exclusive) risk factors for the disease are known as the four Fs: female, forties, fat, and fertile[2].

The gallbladder holds bile that has been produced by the liver, before it is used by the gut. Bile is made from cholesterol and becomes more concentrated in the gallbladder. Sometimes the cholesterol precipitates, forming crystals and gallstones. This can occur if the bile becomes too concentrated, or if there is an oversupply of cholesterol[3]. Stone formation is a slow process. It is approximately eight years from the beginning of stone development to the onset of symptoms, and another four years to cholecystectomy[4].

WHAT ARE THE CLINICAL MANIFESTATIONS?

Commonly intense sudden pain in the right upper quadrant is experienced. The pain is recurrent in nature, occurring after fatty meals and classically, the pain increases on deep inspiration[2]. The abdominal pain typically radiates to the right shoulder and scapula. Murphy's sign is also frequently seen in cholecystitis. It is characterised by the patient holding their breath, in response to pain, when their abdomen is palpated in the right subcostal region[5].

DIAGNOSTIC TESTS

In the patient's blood results, a raised bilirubin level and raised liver function tests (LFT) will be present. The white blood cell count may be increased[2]. Ultrasound, computerised tomography (CT) and cholangiography (dye and X-rays) may be used to diagnose the disease. An ultrasound of the abdomen is the least invasive of these procedures and is able to be done at the bedside[6].

WHAT IS THE TREATMENT?

Initially, intravenous fluids to correct or prevent dehydration are commenced, and analgesia is given, usually morphine[2]. The patient is made nil by mouth. Surgical intervention is the normal treatment involving the removal of the gall bladder. This is called a cholecystectomy and is done either laparoscopically or through a laparotomy. Laparoscopic techniques are safer, cause the patient less pain and are the preferred method of cholecystectomy[4]. Traditionally surgery was delayed for several weeks, however early surgery is now advocated by most clinicians[7].

APPLIED PHARMACOLOGY

Antibiotics are given if peritonitis or sepsis is suspected. This may occur if infective organisms or bile leaks from gallbladder rupture into the sterile peritoneal cavity. But in an uncomplicated case of acute cholecystitis antibiotics are usually not given[2].

NURSING IMPLICATIONS

The main nursing considerations are analgesia and hydration. The analgesics used are typically opioids, such as morphine, given via the intravenous or intramuscular route. The intravenous route is favoured as smaller doses can be given at frequent intervals. Giving smaller doses of morphine at close intervals maintains a steadier therapeutic blood level, and thus better pain relief. 'An order for intramuscular morphine every four hours is unlikely to provide satisfactory analgesia for more than 20% of that interval'[8]. Antiemetic cover should also be given.

LEARNING EXERCISES

1. What are the four risk factors for cholecystitis?
2. What are the benefits of intravenous over intramuscular morphine?
3. Describe Murphy's sign.

CIRRHOSIS

 ## Case study

Frank Sloane, 55, presented to the emergency department suffering a large (greater than 500 mL) haematemesis. He was a frail, thin man and had a large distended abdomen. He was resuscitated with intravenous fluids and blood products. An endoscope was used to visualise his oesophageal varices, and they were injected with adrenaline and banded to reduce the bleeding. Mr Sloane experienced multiple episodes of variceal bleeding. He had a long history of heavy alcohol consumption.

WHAT IS THE PATHOPHYSIOLOGY?

Cirrhosis is damage to the liver by the formation of small nodules that are surrounded by fibrotic tissue. This occurs throughout the entire liver. The nodules and the fibrotic tissue cause irreversible deterioration in liver function. Chronic alcohol abuse is the most common cause of cirrhosis.

The changing of the microscopic architecture of the liver in cirrhosis causes many complications. All functions of the liver, including filtering of blood draining from the small intestine, and the production of albumin and blood clotting products are decreased[9]. The small nodules and recurring strips of connective tissue toughen the normally spongy liver. If the liver is too solid for blood to flow through it, back pressure will occur. This will cause distension of the veins that flow to the liver from the gut[10]. This distension is called portal hypertension and leads to the creation of varices and collateral blood flow. Oesophageal varices are prone to massive bleeding,[11] which often presents as haematemesis.

WHAT ARE THE CLINICAL MANIFESTATIONS?

The disease has a long latent period as the liver becomes slowly less efficient. Ascites (accumulation of protein-rich fluid in the peritoneum due to obstruction of the portal circulation) and jaundice (yellow-green discolouration of the skin and sclerae due to rising bilirubin levels, reflecting deteriorating liver function) are common manifestations. Dramatic haematemesis can also occur. Generalised weakness and weight loss are frequently observed. Eventually complete liver failure can ensue, leading to coma and death[12]. This is believed to be caused by high levels of ammonia in the blood. As the liver normally breaks down ammonia, the high blood levels seen with this disease precipitate hepatic encephalopathy.

DIAGNOSTIC TESTS

Initially liver function tests may be normal. Decreased albumin and increased prothrombin time indicate worsening liver function. Prothrombin is a blood–clotting factor produced by the liver. Anaemia is common as alcohol directly suppresses red blood cell production in the bone marrow[13].

WHAT IS THE TREATMENT?

The only definitive treatment for cirrhosis is liver transplantation[9]. The majority of interventions in cirrhosis management are supportive, as donor livers for transplantation are scarce. Good nutrition and abstinence from alcohol are imperative. Ascites can usually be controlled with diuretics and a diet that is salt restricted[9]. Oesophageal varices, visualised with an endoscope, may be injected with adrenaline, or banded with small rubber bands, in order to achieve haemostasis. This technique in combination with intravenous pharmacotherapy is most effective. Intravenous shunts are infrequently used as they carry a mortality rate between 40 and 100%[10]. A shunt is inserted from the liver to the inferior vena cava, to reduce the pressure from the distended veins. Occasionally a balloon tamponade device (a special nasogastric tube which has balloon inflation components) is inserted. The balloons put direct pressure on the bleeding varices. This type of nasogastric tube is called by one of three names: a Sengstaken Blakemore tube, Linton tube, or a Minnesota tube. This is typically a bridging procedure to more definitive medical care[14].

APPLIED PHARMACOLOGY

Pharmacotherapy is a first-line approach to controlling variceal bleeding. Vasopressin, a potent vasoconstrictor, may be used to try to control bleeding. It reduces blood flow to the abdominal organs[11]. Its use is controversial and not recommended in the elderly as it can cause cardiac and bowel ischaemia[9]. Terlipressin is a synthetic form of vasopressin, with much longer half-life but less potent vasoconstriction effects than vasopressin. It is an effective treatment for variceal bleeding, and it has a lower mortality rate[15].

Somatostatin and octreotide are two intravenously administered peptides that can also reduce bleeding from oesophageal varices. Although these two drugs reduce blood loss, they have not been found to reduce overall mortality[16]. The mechanism of action is not known, however they may reduce portal pressure by having an effect on vasoactive peptides, such as glucagon[11]. There is some evidence that milk thistle (*Silybum marianum*) may exert a protective effect on the cirrhotic liver; however the mechanism of action is not understood[17].

NURSING IMPLICATIONS

Sudden abstinence from alcohol can cause severe withdraw symptoms (delirium tremens). This can make nursing care of the patient with cirrhosis challenging. Symptoms include tremor, hallucinations and agitation. Gross ascites can cause respiratory distress by increasing upward pressure on the diaphragm which compromises lung expansion. The patient may require oxygenation and ventilatory support. Haematemesis can be remarkable and difficult to control. It is common for the patient to be haemodynamically unstable[11]. Timely resuscitation and administration of blood products is important.

LEARNING EXERCISES
1. What is portal hypertension?
2. What treatment options are most successful in treating bleeding oesophageal varices?

PANCREATITIS

 Case study

Paul Kelley, 52, presented to the emergency department with acute, penetrating upper abdominal pain. He had a two-day history of nausea and vomiting. He was thin, had poor skin turgor and dry oral mucosa. His blood pressure was 90/55 mmHg and his temperature was 38.2°C. His pulse rate was 125 beats/min, and his respirations were rapid and shallow. On examination, his abdomen was tender and rigid and there were no bowel sounds. He reported drinking twelve cans of beer a day.

WHAT IS THE PATHOPHYSIOLOGY?

Pancreatitis is an acute or chronic inflammation of the pancreas. Cases can range from mild to severe. In a severe case, necrosis and haemorrhage of the pancreas can cause hypovolaemic shock and death of the patient.

Acute pancreatitis is believed to result from the autodigestion of the pancreas by its own enzymes[18]. The pancreas is usually protected from autodigestion because it produces inactive digestive enzymes. The enzymes are activated when they reach the small intestine. In pancreatitis the organ may produce active enzymes, thus damaging itself. There are multiple theories about how the process of pancreatic irritation begins, most revolving around the blocking of the bile duct or the premature activation of pancreatic enzymes[19]. The main causes of pancreatitis are alcoholism and gallstones, which account for about 70% of cases[20]. Other causes include drugs, toxins, abdominal trauma, infections and surgery on or close to the pancreas[21].

WHAT ARE THE CLINICAL MANIFESTATIONS?

Classically patients have persistent, severe abdominal pain[22]. Nausea and vomiting that does not provide relief is common. This may be severe enough to cause dehydration. Other symptoms include fever, respiratory distress and tachycardia.

DIAGNOSTIC TESTS

Raised serum amylase levels are normally present. Serum calcium is frequently low. Radiological testing, such as ultrasound, CT scanning and MRI, will define the pancreas and give some evidence of the severity of disease by showing oedema, gallstones, necrosis or haemorrhage[2].

WHAT IS THE TREATMENT?

Treatment is mainly supportive and includes analgesia, hydration, nutrition, and suppression of pancreatic secretions[23]. A nasogastric tube may be inserted if vomiting is severe and the patient is kept strictly nil by mouth. Total parenteral nutrition should be initiated as fasting may continue for two to three weeks. Fasting is an attempt to rest the pancreas by decreasing the workload of the gut[18]. Use of antibiotic therapy has not been supported by research, unless a specific infection has been confirmed by blood culture. Surgery may be considered if the damage to the pancreas is extensive.

APPLIED PHARMACOLOGY

Severe pain in pancreatitis is most commonly treated with intravenous pethidine or intravenous or transdermal fentanyl. Morphine should be avoided as it causes biliary tract spasm and further pain[24].

A common pharmacological therapy for pancreatitis is to reduce acid secretion from the gut by giving antisecretory medication. By reducing acid secretion from the gut, stimulation of the pancreas is believed to be decreased[25]. The medication often used is octreotide; however there is little evidence to support therapy of this kind[26]. Pancreatic enzymes may be administered to the patient who is taking food orally. A combination of enzymes is taken with each meal to improve digestion[23]. This is done in an attempt to advance the patient's nutritional status.

NURSING IMPLICATIONS

The assessment and treatment of severe pain typically experienced by these patients is a challenge for clinicians[25]. Pain should be documented in intensity, duration and character. Good documentation and knowledge of the patient will lead to better levels of analgesia. It is important to monitor clinical parameters closely including: oxygenation, blood pressure, temperature, and blood glucose level. As insulin is produced in the pancreas, there may be a decrease in insulin production and so the patient's blood glucose level may rise. The patient is usually kept nil by mouth (includes no ice) in order to rest the gut completely. Frequent mouth care will improve the patient's level of comfort. The monitoring of hydration is important as fluid loss may be great. Supportive measures such as education in relation to reducing alcohol intake should be provided.

HEPATITIS

 Case study

Luke Straub, 28, presented to his GP with decreased appetite, nausea, fever, general malaise, muscle aches and jaundice. He had been sick for three weeks. He is normally healthy, and told the doctor that he occasionally used recreational drugs, such as heroin and cocaine. Blood tests were taken and Luke returned in three days for results. He was overwhelmed when he was told that he had hepatitis C.

WHAT IS THE PATHOPHYSIOLOGY?

Hepatitis or an inflammation of the liver has many viral and non-viral causes. The non-viral causes include drugs and chemicals, as well as immune and metabolic causes[27]. The majority of cases, however, are caused by viruses, including hepatitis A, B, C, D, E, and G.

The viral invasion of the liver cells causes inflammation. The virus damages but does not kill the liver cells. The injury causes swelling, and a decrease in liver function. If the damage is ongoing (chronic) then scarring or fibrosis occurs. Fibrosis is caused by the formation of collagen fibres as the liver tries to repair itself. When fibrosis is extensive it is called cirrhosis. Fibrosis, and thus the damage, is permanent[28]. Hepatitis B, C, D and G are transmitted through blood-to-blood contact, whereas hepatitis A and E are spread by ingesting food and water that have been contaminated by the virus[29].

WHAT ARE THE CLINICAL MANIFESTATIONS?

All viral hepatitis infections have similar symptoms, but the difference is in the severity of symptoms and whether the infection leads on to chronic liver injury[29]. Signs and symptoms include anorexia, nausea, vomiting, fever, jaundice, malaise, and muscle aches.

Hepatitis B, C, and D have more severe, longer lasting symptoms. Hepatitis B is the most commonly occurring form. Most people recover fully from hepatitis B, with only 5–10% progressing to chronic liver failure. In those with hepatitis C, only 30–40% of people infected show any symptoms. The majority of these people however, will go on to have some degree of chronic liver disease[29]. Hepatitis D is unusual in its mode of transmission. A person must first be infected with hepatitis B, and then be exposed to hepatitis D. This is a more serious form of the disease. Little is known about hepatitis G, except that it is believed to be blood-borne.

Symptoms of hepatitis A and E are similar to a case of mild influenza, often lasting less than two weeks[29]. Infection is mainly through contaminated food and water. Hepatitis E however affects pregnant women in a more serious way, with death in one in five cases[30].

DIAGNOSTIC TESTS

Blood test will be positive for the specific IgM antibody for each kind of hepatitis.

WHAT IS THE TREATMENT?

In acute hepatitis the treatment is mainly supportive, with some pharmacotherapy available for hepatitis B and C. There is no specific treatment available for hepatitis A, E D or G. There is some evidence for a herbal medication called milk thistle (*Silybum marianum*). Research is not strong but suggests it has 'hepatoprotective, anti-inflammatory, and regenerative properties producing a beneficial effect for some types of hepatitis'[31]. Chronic liver disease, such as hepatitis, is the most common cause of hepatocellular carcinoma. In this group of patients, ongoing treatment should include regular screening (CT scan) for liver tumours[32].

APPLIED PHARMACOLOGY

The main medications used are antiviral drugs. The aim of treatment is to slow or stop chronic inflammation of the liver. There is no specific pharmacological therapy for hepatitis A, D, E or G. For hepatitis B, a choice of interferon alpha or lamivudine is the standard treatment[33]. Interferons are glycoproteins that occur naturally in the body and are produced by all cells to fight viral infection. Interferons have been manufactured commercially for several years. They offer protection by preventing viruses from entering cells, and stimulate the destruction of infected cells by macrophages[34]. Interferons must be injected, either daily or weekly. The many side effects include malaise, depression, hair loss, thyroid dysfunction and a decrease in both red blood cell, and platelet counts[28]. Lamivudine is available in oral form and is usually taken for 6 to 12 months. It prevents viral replication, hence the virus is not killed, and viral load will increase when the medication is stopped[28]. Interferon alpha with ribavirin is the treatment for hepatitis C,[35] and has been shown to improve outcomes and decrease viral load[36]. This combination, however is effective in less than half of patients, and has multiple side effects[37]. It is generally well tolerated; however it will cause a fall in haemoglobin as it destroys older red blood cells[28].

WHAT ARE THE NURSING IMPLICATIONS?

The difficulty of daily self injections and strict adherence to oral medication regimes should be taken into consideration, when assessing patient compliance. The side effects can greatly affect the quality of life of the patient. Supportive measures such as antiemetic medications are useful. A clear liquid, low-fat diet may also help to reduce nausea. The patient needs to be aware to avoid agents that are toxic to the liver, such as morphine, paracetamol and alcohol[29].

LEARNING EXERCISES
1. Which forms of hepatitis are spread by the faecal-oral route?
2. What are the side effects from prescribed interferon use?

APPENDICITIS

 Case study

Lorick Pembury, 23, presented to the emergency department with gradual onset of lower right quadrant pain. The pain had woken him in his sleep, at which stage the pain was located in the epigastric region. He also had nausea, vomiting and was anorexic. Despite having a bowel movement that morning, the patient felt constipated. Other symptoms included abdominal guarding, rigidity and rebound tenderness. Pain was also present in the lower right quadrant when the lower left quadrant was deeply palpated then suddenly released ('Rovsing's sign').

WHAT IS THE PATHOPHYSIOLOGY?

Appendicitis, by definition, is inflammation of the vermiform appendix. Because of its twisted structure, the appendix provides an ideal location for bacteria to accumulate and multiply[38]. Appendicitis can occur at any age though it is more common in adolescents and young adults[39].

Potential causes of appendicitis include obstruction of the lumen by a faecalith (a hard mass of faeces), calculus, foreign body, tumour or oedema; kinking of the appendix; swelling of the bowel wall; and external occlusion of the bowel by adhesions[39,40,41]. Regardless of the cause, when the appendix becomes obstructed, the pressure within its lumen increases. This impairs its blood supply resulting in inflammation, oedema, necrosis, gangrene or perforation.

DIAGNOSTIC TESTS

Diagnosis of appendicitis is based strongly on the patient's history and physical examination. However laboratory tests aid in making the correct diagnosis. Abnormal results include elevations in white blood cell count and C-reactive protein[42] although these are not unique to appendicitis. Abdominal X-rays and ultrasound may reveal a right lower quadrant density or localized distension of the bowel[41] though a negative abdominal X-ray should never exclude the diagnosis of appendicitis[42].

APPLIED PHARMACOLOGY

There is no specific pharmacological management for appendicitis. Treatment primarily consists of surgical removal of the appendix. Preoperative care involves intravenous fluids and antibiotics[40]. Because perforation may occur less than 24 hours after the onset of symptoms, laparotomy is the only safe procedure when appendicitis is the provisional diagnosis[43]. Many trials have demonstrated the efficacy of preoperative antibiotics in lowering infectious complications, but if simple acute appendicitis is encountered, there is no benefit in extending antibiotic coverage beyond 24h[44].

Due to the presence of Gram-negative organisms in the gut, antibiotic therapy involves the use of a third-generation cephalosporin effective against many Gram-negative bacteria[39,43]. Examples of third-generation cephalosporins include cefotaxime, ceftriaxone and ceftazidime. These agents destroy bacteria by inhibiting synthesis of their cell walls[45].

NURSING IMPLICATIONS

Cephalosporins should be used cautiously in patients with known allergies or sensitivity to penicillins. Cross-sensitivity between the drugs in the penicillin, cephalosporin and carbapenem groups occurs in 5–10% of individuals[34]. Caution should also be taken if the patient has renal impairment and dosage adjustment may be necessary[46]. Cephalosporins may also interact with anticoagulants further prolonging clotting time, so the nurse should observe for signs of increased bleeding[47,48].

In order to maintain therapeutic serum levels, antibiotics should be administered at the prescribed intervals. Ceftriaxone should not be administered in fluids containing calcium, such as Hartmann's solution[46].

LEARNING EXERCISES
1. What are the differential diagnoses for a person with acute abdominal pain?
2. What is the typical presentation of a patient with appendicitis?
3. What are the most reliable ways of diagnosing appendicitis?

PEPTIC ULCER DISEASE

 Case study

William Rubin, 52, presented to his general practitioner complaining of burning pain between his xiphisternum and umbilicus. He had had the pain intermittently for the past three months; it usually lasted from a few minutes to hours and was relieved by eating. He had been a tobacco smoker for five pack/years, and consumed four standard glasses of alcohol and five cups of coffee a day. The patient believed the pain to be due to indigestion, even though it was relieved by food consumption. He therefore had not sought medical attention. On questioning, he denied taking aspirin or other non-steroidal anti-inflammatory drugs (NSAIDS).

WHAT IS THE PATHOPHYSIOLOGY?

Peptic ulcer disease refers to ulceration either of the stomach, pylorus, duodenum or oesophagus. Risk factors for the development of peptic ulceration that are suspected though unproven, include stress, family history and people with blood type O^{41}.

The Gram-negative bacteria *Helicobacter pylori* (*H. pylori*), however, is the primary causal factor in the majority of peptic ulcers. It is present in 70% of patients with gastric ulcers and 95% of patients with duodenal ulcers[41]. Peptic ulcers mainly occur in the gastroduodenal mucosa because this tissue cannot withstand the digestive action of gastric acid and pepsin[41]. Ulceration occurs either due to increased acid secretion, breakdown of the protective epithelial lining or inadequate mucus secretion[39].

DIAGNOSTIC TESTS

As the organism *H. pylori* is the common causative agent for peptic ulcer disease, patients should be tested for its presence. This can be achieved through breath tests, antibody assays, biopsy or the direct identification of the organism by culture[41,49]. Other tests that may prove useful for diagnosing peptic ulcer disease include barium studies of the upper gastrointestinal tract and endoscopy. Gastroscopy allows tissue to be sampled for biopsy[39]. A full blood count may reveal anaemia secondary to a bleeding ulcer.

APPLIED PHARMACOLOGY

The drugs used most commonly to treat peptic ulcer disease include antibiotics, antacids, H_2 (histamine) receptor antagonists, proton pump inhibitors and mucosal protective agents[50].

ANTACIDS

Common examples of these include aluminium hydroxide, calcium carbonate and sodium bicarbonate, all of which may be given in a variety of combinations. Antacids have a number of important actions that provide relief for the person with a peptic ulcer. The most significant actions are the neutralising of gastric acidity and reducing pepsin activity[51].

As described above, a number of compounds such as magnesium hydroxide and magnesium carbonate make up most antacids[51]. The nurse therefore must be aware of the risk of metabolic and electrolyte disturbances associated with the use of antacids. These disturbances may occur if a person takes excessive amounts of antacids in a short period. They may do so because they are not obtaining relief from symptoms. The electrolyte disturbances include hypophosphataemia, hypercalcaemia, hypermagnesaemia and alkalosis. Antacids can also alter or reduce the absorption of various other drugs including cimetidine, ranitidine, chlorpromazine, digoxin, phenytoin and tetracyclines[51].

H_2 RECEPTOR ANTAGONISTS

Common examples of these available in Australia include ranitidine, cimetidine, famotidine and nizatidine. This group of drugs reduce gastric acid secretion by reversibly competing with histamine for binding to H_2 receptors on the basolateral membrane of parietal cells[52]. H_2 receptors are located primarily in gastric parietal cells but also in the central nervous system and in cardiac muscle[34]. Stimulation of these receptors normally results in the release of hydrochloric acid[38].

The nursing implications are that because H_2 receptor antagonists can impair renal and hepatic function, this should be monitored carefully. The common side effects of H_2 receptor antagonists include headaches, blurred vision, confusion, bradycardia, hypotension and arrhythmias. A number of drugs can interact with H_2 receptor antagonists, particularly cimetidine, leading to toxic levels of these agents. Other drugs include warfarin, phenytoin, beta-adrenergic blockers, quinidine, theophylline, nifedipine, carbamazepine and tricyclic antidepressants[47].

PROTON PUMP INHIBITORS

These drugs decrease gastric acid secretion by inhibiting the hydrogen-potassium adenosine triphosphatase gastric enzyme system, which catalyses the final stage of acid production[47].

Common examples of these available in Australia include omeprazole, pantoprazole, lansoprazole, esomeprazole and rabeprazole.

Proton pump inhibitors may slow the absorption of a number of drugs, such as iron, digoxin and ampicillin[47]. Their use has also been associated with upper respiratory tract infections presumably via the migration of organisms up the oesophagus. This is an issue for patients with a nasogastric tube[34].

MUCOSAL PROTECTIVE AGENTS

The two main drugs in this group include sucralfate and misoprostol. These drugs complement the protection offered by the gastric mucosa by providing a physical gel barrier over the ulcer[53]. Misoprostol also has antisecretory properties[54].

The nursing implication is that administration of other oral medications should occur two hours before or after sucralfate as it can cause reduced absorption and bioavailability of these drugs[47]. Due to the aluminium content, sucralfate should be administered cautiously to patients with chronic renal failure because of the risk of aluminium toxicity. Other agents containing aluminium, such as some antacids, should also therefore be avoided[55]. The main side affects of misoprostol are diarrhoea, abdominal pain and menorrhagia[34].

ANTIBIOTICS

Peptic ulcer disease caused by the bacterium H. pylori is best treated with antibiotics[49]. 'With the exception of patients with gastrinoma and those taking non–steroidal anti-inflammatory drugs, more than 95% of patients with duodenal ulcers and more than 80% of patients with gastric ulcers are infected with H. pylori'[56]. Patients with H. pylori develop peptic ulcer disease at a rate of about 1% per year, which is about three times the rate of the H. pylori-negative population[57].

Usual treatment involves one of the following triple regimens: proton pump inhibitor, clarithromycin and amoxicillin; proton pump inhibitor, clarithromycin and metronidazole; ranitidine bismuth citrate, clarithromycin and amoxicillin[53]. Metronidazole resistant strains of H. pylori are now common so it is not recommended as a first-line agent[58].

The nursing implications are that, as with all antibiotic treatments, patients must be aware of the need to take the full course of treatment. This is particularly important because H. Pylori is difficult to eradicate partly because it is protected by the stomach lining[59]. Poor compliance may be an issue if the treatment is to be taken over 10 days or more. Patients must therefore be educated about the importance of adhering to the medication regime. To encourage compliance, some manufacturers have produced the three drugs packaged together. For example, Losec Helipak contains omeprazole, amoxicillin and metronidazole.

Patients should be warned that amoxicillin may reduce the effectiveness of oral contraceptive pills and that administration may also result in a black 'hairy' tongue[46]. Metronidazole can enhance the activity of warfarin so signs of bleeding should be observed for in patients who are concomitantly taking this drug. Similarly, metronidazole may also increase serum digoxin levels so the patient should be monitored for signs of digoxin toxicity[46] such as nausea, vomiting, abdominal pain, diarrhoea, arrhythmias and visual disturbances. Patients should be warned that metronidazole may cause the urine to become a harmless dark colour and to avoid alcohol during treatment to prevent a disulfiram–like reaction (chest pain, confusion, vomiting, vertigo, respiratory difficulties)[34,51].

LEARNING EXERCISES
1. What are the risk factors for developing peptic ulcer disease?
2. How common is the organism *H. pylori* in the general population?
3. Differentiate between the effects produced by the stimulation of H_1 versus H_2 receptors.

CROHN'S DISEASE

 Case study

Anna Pelloso, 24, presented to her GP with a recent history of persistent diarrhoea, crampy, intermittent abdominal pain, fatigue, and weight loss. A diagnosis of food allergy was considered and Anna was told to keep a record of what she ate and to try excluding dairy products from her diet. The symptoms continued for a number of months but she also developed rectal bleeding. The GP ordered a colonoscopy, which showed ulceration and inflammation of the bowel. A diagnosis of Crohn's disease was made.

WHAT IS THE PATHOPHYSIOLOGY?

Crohn's disease, also known as regional enteritis, is a chronic, relapsing inflammatory disorder of the bowel[39]. Crohn's disease is one of the two diseases that constitute 'inflammatory bowel disease', the other being ulcerative colitis. The disease can occur at any age though presents most commonly between the ages of 15 and 30. Any part of the intestinal tract from the mouth to the anus can be affected, with the most common location being the terminal ileum. The specific cause of the disease is unknown.

Crohn's disease begins with small inflammatory lesions, which may regress or progress to involvement of all layers of the bowel wall[39]. Thickening of the bowel wall occurs as well as narrowing of the lumen with stricture development[48]. Local complications of the disease include malabsorption, obstruction, fistulas, abscesses and anal fissure[40,48].

DIAGNOSTIC TESTS

The diagnosis of inflammatory bowel disease depends on the clinical history, physical findings, and endoscopic, radiologic, and histologic features, as well as routine laboratory tests[60]. Although laboratory tests are not definitive tools for diagnosing Crohn's disease, there are a number of abnormalities to look for. These include raised white cell count, erythrocyte sedimentation rate and C-reactive protein; and decreased serum albumin, ferritin, calcium, zinc and magnesium levels[61,62]. Anaemia may also be present due to deficiencies of iron, vitamin B$_{12}$ or folate[63].

APPLIED PHARMACOLOGY

Two main groups of drugs are used to treat Crohn's disease – oral or parenteral steroids and drugs related to sulphonamides[34]. Antibiotics are also beneficial when treating mild to moderate disease and they help maintain disease remission[64]. Crohn's disease is not curable by surgical or medical intervention[65].

AMINOSALICYLATES

Examples of drugs in this class include sulphasalazine, mesalazine and olsalazine. They decrease inflammation by inhibiting prostaglandin synthesis[34]. Aminosalicylates result in remission in 30 to 40% of patients and have fewer side effects than steroids[58].

The nursing implication is that sulphasalazine can interact with numerous drugs including antibiotics, digoxin, folic acid, iron, oral anticoagulants and oral hypoglycaemic agents[46]. The interaction involves either reduced absorption of the drug or increased effect. Patients should be monitored for signs of these interactions.

If mesalazine is administered with oral hypoglycaemics or anticoagulants, increased effects of these drugs may occur. Their concomitant use should therefore either be avoided or these effects monitored closely[46]. Sulphasalazine, mesalazine and olsalazine should be administered cautiously to patients with pre-existing renal disease as deterioration in renal function may occur.

CORTICOSTEROIDS

This group of drugs are highly effective in inducing remission in people with Crohn's disease[66]. Examples include prednisone and prednisolone. Corticosteroids can be a challenging group of drugs to understand as they have a wide variety of actions and thus uses. Actions include: increasing gluconeogenesis; decreasing peripheral glucose utilisation; decreasing anabolism; depressing inflammatory and allergic responses; delaying healing; increasing fat deposition; and sodium retention[51]. These drugs are used in the treatment of Crohn's disease primarily for their anti-inflammatory action.

There are a number of issues nurses must be aware of when administering corticosteroids. Due to the variety of actions of corticosteroids, numerous adverse effects may be experienced such as raised blood glucose levels, muscle atrophy, increased susceptibility to infection, increased blood pressure, hypernatraemia and hypokalaemia[34]. Nurses must also teach patients that they must be slowly weaned from steroid therapy and to never suddenly stop taking these medications. This is to allow time for the hypothalamic-pituitary mechanisms to resume normal hormone production thus avoiding adrenal insufficiency[51,55].

ANTIBIOTICS

Two antibiotics commonly used are metronidazole and ciprofloxacin[67]. Metronidazole is as effective as sulfasalazine and whilst ciprofloxacin may also be used, no trials have established its efficacy[58].

Ciprofloxacin may increase the anticoagulant effect of warfarin and elevate plasma theophylline levels, whilst antacids and sucralfate can decrease the absorption and bioavailablility of ciprofloxacin[53]. Patients should be instructed to avoid milk products, antacids, iron and sucralfate as these can reduce the effectiveness of ciprofloxacin[47]. Oral fluid intake should also be encouraged to avoid crystalluria[46].

LEARNING EXERCISES
1. What are the common signs and symptoms of Crohn's disease?
2. When is surgical intervention indicated for the management of Crohn's disease?
3. Describe the extra-intestinal manifestations of Crohn's disease.

ULCERATIVE COLITIS

● Case study

Diane Chen, 31, presented to her general practitioner with a 12-week history of abdominal cramps, diarrhoea and anorexia. On further questioning, it was revealed that some of her bowel motions were dark and watery and she said some were coated with blood. She had been a smoker for 10 years but had recently quit. She also described symptoms of tiredness, weight loss and malaise.

She had not travelled overseas recently and her GP excluded food poisoning. The GP ordered a sigmoidoscopy, which showed discontinuous areas of inflammation, erythema and superficial ulceration. This resulted in the diagnosis of ulcerative colitis.

WHAT IS THE PATHOPHYSIOLOGY?

Ulcerative colitis is a chronic inflammatory bowel disease involving only the mucosa and submucosa of the colon. The specific cause of the disease is unknown but numerous causative theories have been proposed. These theories include bacterial infection, allergic reaction, altered immunity or autoimmunity, environmental factors (e.g., smoking) and diet[39,40].

The affected mucosa becomes oedematous and hyperaemic, with multiple abscesses developing and eventually becoming ulcerated[48]. Inflammation, thickening and congestion of the bowel also occur. Ulcerations destroy the mucosal epithelium causing bleeding and diarrhoea[48]. Intestinal complications of the disease include haemorrhage, strictures, perforation, toxic megacolon, cancer and colonic dilatation[39,40,48]. Extra-intestinal complications include malabsorption, kidney stones, gallstones, liver disease and peptic ulcer disease[48].

	Crohn's Disease	Ulcerative Colitis
TABLE 9.1: COMPARISON OF CROHN'S DIEASE AND ULCERATIVE COLITIS[34,39,40,48,61–64,68]		
Cause	Unknown	Unknown
Person affected	Most commonly females, aged 15–30 or 50–80 years Twice as common in smokers	High incidence in Jewish and Caucasians Peak incidence 30–50 years of age
Anatomical location	Any part of the intestinal tract, most commonly the terminal ileum	Colon
Pathology	Small inflammatory lesions Thickening of the bowel wall Narrowing of the lumen	Oedematous and hyperaemic mucosa Ulceration Abscess formation
Manifestations	Crampy, abdominal pain Diarrhoea Weight loss Anaemia	Diarrhoea Rectal bleeding Abdominal pain Tenesmus Vomiting Anorexia
Local complications	Malabsorption Obstruction Fistulas Abscesses Anal fissures	Malabsorption Haemorrhage Strictures Perforation Toxic megacolon Dilatation
Systemic complications	Malnutrition Fluid and electrolyte imbalance Arthritis	Kidney stones Gallstones Liver disease Peptic ulcer disease
Treatment	Aminosalicyclates Corticosteroids Antibiotics	Aminosalicyclates Corticosteroids Immunomodulators Colectomy if indicated
Prognosis	Not curable	High mortality rate. 10–15% develop colon carcinoma Potentially curable by colectomy

DIAGNOSTIC TESTS

Diagnosis of ulcerative colitis is challenging given its similarity to Crohn's disease (see Table 9.1). There are no specific signs on clinical examination but inflammation of the rectal mucosa can be seen at endoscopy[68]. If the patient has diarrhoea, hypokalaemia would be expected. Hypoalbuminaemia may also be present from the loss of protein from damaged gastric mucosa or from malnutrition due to systemic inflammation[15].

APPLIED PHARMACOLOGY

The main aim of treatment is symptom relief[68]. Pharmacologic treatment typically includes aminosalicylates and corticosteroids. Colectomy is indicated if the disease is unresponsive to medical treatment or when it is fulminant and toxic megacolon or perforation is suspected[69]. Surgery is generally curative[70,71].

Apart from aminosalicylates and corticosteroids, the other group of drugs used in the treatment of ulcerative colitis include immunomodulatory agents, such as infliximab and azathioprine[70]. These drugs work by binding to tumour necrosis factor, which is a cytokine believed to mediate chronic inflammation[51].

WHAT ARE THE NURSING IMPLICATIONS?

As their name suggests, immunomodulators suppress the actions of the immune system. Administration of this group of drugs carries a risk of bacterial, viral and fungal infection and increases the risk of developing neoplasms[51].

When immunosuppressants are being administered, electrolytes, renal and hepatic function tests should be monitored closely. The patient should be instructed to report any signs of abnormal bleeding or signs of infection[47]. The nurse should also observe for these.

LEARNING EXERCISES

1. What are the primary differences between Crohn's disease and ulcerative colitis?
2. What are the side effects of corticosteroid use?
3. What is the role of surgery in the management of ulcerative colitis?

CONCLUSION

This chapter provided an overview of the anatomy and physiology and gastrointestinal health breakdown with applied pharmacology. It is important that the nurse understands the physiology, normal values as well as the pathophysiology of the condition in order to give the appropriate assessment, nursing care and treatment to the patient. Part of the role of the nurse is to monitor and evaluate the patient's condition. In order to provide care, the nurse also needs to understand the treatments and the side effects of medication administration. It is vital that the nurse is aware of the significant nursing implications associated with the condition and reflect on the care they give.

Recommended Readings

Achord, JL. 2002; *Understanding Hepatitis*, University Press of Mississippi, Mississippi.

Kefalides, P & Hanauer, S. 2001; 'Ulcerative Colitis: Diagnosis and Management', *Journal of Clinical Outcomes Management*, 8 (9), 40–48.

Knutson, D, Greenberg, G & Cronau, H. 2003; 'Management of Crohn's Disease: a Practical Approach.' *American Family Physician*, 68 (4), 707–714.

Meyers, RP, Regimbeau, C, Thevenot, T, Leroy, V, Mathurin, P, et al. 2003; 'Hepatitis C', *The Cochrane Database of Systematic Reviews*, Issue 3.

Smoot, D & Cryer, B. 2001. 'Peptic Ulcer Disease.' *Primary Care: Clinics in Office Practice*, 28 (3), 487–503.

References

1. Parmet, S. 2003; 'Acute Cholecystitis', *Journal of the American Medical Association*, 289 (1) 124.
2. Farrar, J & Kearney, K. 2001; 'Acute Cholecystitis', *American Journal of Nursing*, 10 (1), 35–36.
3. Guyton, AC. 2000; *Textbook of Medical Physiology* (10th ed.), Saunders, Philadelphia.
4. Fletcher, D. 1997; 'Gall Stones', in GJ Clunie, JJ Tjandra & DM Francis (eds.), *Textbook of Surgery*, Blackwell Science, Melbourne.
5. Urbano, FL & Carroll, M. 2000; 'Murphy's Sign of Cholecystitis', *Hospital Physician*, 36 (11), 51–52.
6. Rosen, CL, Brown, DF, Chang, Y, Moore, C, Averill, NJ, Arkoff, LJ, *et al.* 2001; 'Ultrasonography by Emergency Physicians in Patients with Suspected Cholecystitis', *American Journal of Emergency Medicine*, 19 (1), 32–36.
7. Trowbridge, RL, Rutkowski, NK & Shojania, KG. 2003; 'Does this Patient Have Acute Cholecystitis?' *Journal of the American Medical Association*, 289 (1), 80–86.
8. Blake, D. 1997; 'Anaesthesia and Pain Relief', in GJ Clunie, JJ Tjandra & DM Francis (eds.), *Textbook of Surgery*, Blackwell Science, Melbourne.
9. Anand, BS. 2001; 'Drug Treatment of the Complications of Cirrhosis in the Older Adult', *Drugs and Aging*, 18 (8), 575–585.
10. Bouley, G, Grimshaw, K, Lindenwall-Matto, D & Kiernan, L. 1996; 'Transjugular Intrahepatic Portosystemic Shunt: An Alternative', *Critical Care Nurse*, 16 (1), 23–29.
11. Sharara, AI & Rockey, DC. 2001; 'Medical Progress: Gastroesophageal Variceal Hemorrhage', *The New England Journal of Medicine*, 345 (9), 669–681.
12. Gerber, T & Schomerus, H. 2000; 'Hepatic Encephalopathy in Liver Cirrhosis: Pathogenesis, Diagnosis and Management', *Drugs*, 60 (6), 1353–1370.
13. Casagrande, G & Michot, F. 1989; 'Alcohol Induced Bone Marrow Damage', *Blut*, 59 (3), 231–236.
14. Cook, D & Laine, L. 1992; 'Indications, Technique and Complications of Balloon Tamponade for Variceal Gastrointestinal Bleeding', *Journal of Intensive Care Medicine*, 7 (4), 212–218.
15. Ioannou, GN, Doust, L & Rockey, DC. 2003; 'Systematic Review: Terlipressin in Acute Oesophageal Variceal Haemorrhage', *Alimentary Pharmacology & Therapeutics*, 17 (1), 53–64.
16. Gotzsche, PC. 2003; 'Somatostatin Analogues for Acute Bleeding Oesophageal Varices', *The Cochrane Database of Systematic Reviews*, Issue 3.
17. Boerth, J & Strong, KM. 2002; 'The Clinical Utility of Milk Thistle in Cirrhosis of the Liver', *Journal of Herbal Pharmacotherapy*, 2 (2), 11–17.
18. White, AH, 2001; 'Acute Pancreatitis', in SD Melander (ed.), *Case Studies in Critical Care Nursing*, Saunders, Philadelphia.
19. Hennessy, K. 1996; 'Patients with Acute Pancreatitis', in JM Clochesy, C Breu S Cardin AA Whittaker & EB Rudy (eds.), *Critical Care Nursing*, Saunders, Philadelphia, 1091–1104.
20. British Society of Gastroenterologists. 1998; 'United Kingdom Guidelines for the Management of Acute Pancreatitis', *Gut*, 42 (supplement 2), June, S1–S13.
21. McArdle, J. 2000; 'The Biological and Nursing Implications of Pancreatitis', *Nursing Standard*, 14 (48), 46–53.
22. Giuliano, K & Scott, S. 1999; 'Acute Pancreatitis', in L Bucher & S Melander (eds.), *Critical Care Nursing*, Saunders, Philadelphia, 764–778.
23. Trolli, PA, Conwell, DL & Zuccaro, G. 2001; 'Pancreatic Enzyme Therapy and Nutritional Status of Outpatients with Chronic Pancreatitis', *Gastroenterology Nursing*, 24 (2), 84–87.
24. Stevens, M, Esler, R & Asher G. 2002; 'Research Brief: Transdermal Fentanyl for the Management of Acute Pancreatic Pain', *Applied Nursing Research*, 15 (2), 102–110.
25. Khalid, A & Whitcomb DC. 2002; 'Conservative Treatment of Chronic Pancreatitis', *European Journal of Gastroenterology and Hepatology*, 14 (9), 943–949.
26. Uhl, W, Buchler, MW, Malfertheiner, P, Berger, HG, Adler, G & Gaus, W. 1999; 'A Randomized, Double Blind, Multicentre Trial of Octreotide in Moderate to Severe Pancreatitis', *Gut*, 45 (1), 97–104.
27. Marsano, LS. 2003; 'Hepatitis', *Primary Care*, 30 (1), 81–107.
28. Achord, JL. 2002; *Understanding Hepatitis*, University Press of Mississippi, Jackson.
29. Garza, A & Forshner, L. 1997; 'Hepatitis Update', *RN*, 60 (12), 39–44.
30. Krawczynski, K, Aggarwal, R & Kamili, S. 2000; 'Hepatitis E', *Infectious Disease Clinics of North America*, 14 (3), 699–687.
31. Giese, LA. 2002; 'Complementary Healthcare Practices: Milk Thistle and the Treatment of Hepatitis', *Gastroenterology Nursing*, 24 (2), 95–97.
32. Valls, C, Andia, E, Roca, Y, Cos, M & Figueras, J. 2002; 'CT in Hepatic Cirrhosis and Chronic Hepatitis', *Seminars in Ultrasound, CT and MRI*, 23 (1), 37–61.

33. Befeler, AS & Di Bisceglie, AM. 2000; 'Hepatitis B', *Infectious Disease Clinics of North America*, 14 (3), 617–632.

34. Galbraith, A, Bullock, S & Manias, E. 2004; *Fundamentals of Pharmacology* (4th ed.), Pearson Education Australia, Frenchs Forest.

35. Colgan, R, Michocki, R, Greisman, L & Moore, TA. 2003; 'Antiviral Drugs in the Immunocompetent Host, Part 1: Treatment of Hepatitis, Cytomegalovirus, and Herpes Infections', *American Family Physician*. 67 (4), 757–762.

36. Meyers, RP, Regimbeau, C, Thevenot, T, Leroy, V, Mathurin, P, Opolon, P, *et al.* 2003; 'Hepatitis C', *The Cochrane Database of Systematic Reviews*, Issue 4.

37. Burak, KW & Lee, SS. 2000; 'Treatment Options in Patients with Chronic Hepatitis C', *Canadian Journal of Public Health*. 91 (supplement 1), S22–S26.

38. Marieb, E. 2001; *Human Anatomy and Physiology* (5th ed.), Benjamin Cummings, San Francisco.

39. LeMone, P & Burke, K. 2000; *Medical-Surgical Nursing: Critical Thinking in Client Care* (2nd ed.), Prentice Hall, New Jersey.

40. Rogers, H. 2001; 'Management of Clients with Intestinal Disorders', in J Black, J Hawks & A Keene, *Medical-Surgical Nursing: Clinic Management for Positive Outcomes*, Saunders, Philadelphia, 765–800.

41. Smeltzer, S & Bare, B. 2004; *Brunner and Suddarth's Textbook of Medical-Surgical Nursing* (10th ed.), Lippincott, Philadelphia.

42. Pisarra, VH. 2001; 'Recognising the Various Presentations of Appendicitis', *Dimensions of Critical Care Nursing*, 20 (3), 24–27.

43. Beers, M & Berklow, R. 1999; *Merck Manual of Diagnosis and Therapy* (17th ed.), Merck Research Laboratory, New Jersey.

44. Schwartz, S, Shires, G, Spencer, F, Daly, J, Fischer, J & Galloway, A. 1999; *Principles of Surgery* (7th ed.), McGraw Hill, New York.

45. Carruthers, S, Hoffman, B, Melmon, K & Nierenberg, D. 2000; *Melmon and Morrelli's Clinical Pharmacology* (4th ed.), McGraw Hill, New York.

46. Comerford, K (ed.). 2003; *Australian and New Zealand Nursing Drug Handbook* (2nd ed.), Lippincott Williams & Wilkins, Philadelphia.

47. McGuistion, L & Gutierrez, K. 2002; *Real World Nursing Survival Guide: Pharmacology*, Saunders, Philadelphia.

48. Bliss, D & Sawchuk, L. 2004; 'Lower Gastrointestinal Problems', in S Lewis, M Heitkemper & S Dirksen, *Medical-Surgical Nursing: Assessment and Management of Clinical Problems* (6th ed.), Mosby, St Louis, 1052–1103.

49. Smoot, D & Cryer, B. 2001; 'Peptic Ulcer Disease', *Primary Care: Clinics in Office Practice*, 28 (3), 487–503.

50. Turkoski, BB. 2002; 'Orthopaedic Patients and the Risk for Peptic Ulcer Disease (PUD)', *Orthopaedic Nursing*, 21 (1), 70–74.

51. Tiziani, A. 2002; *Harvard's Nursing Guide to Drugs* (6th ed.), Mosby, Sydney.

52. Hoogerwerf, W & Pasricha, P. 2001; 'Agents Used for Control of Gastric Acidity and Treatment of Peptic Ulcers and Gastroesophageal Reflux Disease', in J Hardman & L Linbird (eds.), *Goodman & Gilman's Pharmacological Basis of Therapeutics* (10th ed.), McGraw Hill, New York, 1005–1020.

53. Bryant, B, Knights, K & Salerno, E. 2003; *Pharmacology for Health Professionals*, Mosby, Sydney.

54. Crozier, A. 2003; 'The Management of Dyspepsia', *Nursing Times*, 99 (38), 30–32.

55. Reiss, B & Evans, M. 2001; *Pharmacological Aspects of Nursing Care* (6th ed.), Delmar Thomson, Albany, New York.

56. Cummings Stegbauer, C. 1999; 'Understanding Peptic Ulcer Disease Pharmacokinetics', *The Nurse Practitioner*, 24 (3), 128–132.

57. Lara, L & Mishra, G. 2002; 'Peptic Ulcer Disease', *Emergency Medicine*, 19–22.

58. Therapeutic Guidelines Limited. 2002; *Therapeutic Guidelines: Gastrointestinal, Version 3*, Therapeutic Guidelines Limited, Melbourne.

59. Aranson, B. 1998; 'Update on Peptic Ulcer Drugs', *American Journal of Nursing*, 98 (1), 41–46.

60. Podolsky, D. 2002; 'Medical Progress: Inflammatory Bowel Disease', *New England Journal of Medicine*, 347 (6), 417–429.

61. Baron, M. 2002; 'Crohn Disease in Children', *American Journal of Nursing*, 102 (10), 26–34.

62. Klonowski, EI & Masoodi, J. 1999; 'The Patient with Crohn's Disease', *RN*, 62 (3), 32–37.

63. Metcalf, C. 2002; 'Crohn's Disease: An Overview', *Nursing Standard*, 16 (31), 45–52.

64. Knutson, D, Greenberg, G & Cronau, H. 2003; 'Management of Crohn's Disease: A Practical Approach', *American Family Physician*, 68 (4), 707–714.

65. Sercombe, J. 2001; 'Surgical Therapy for Inflammatory Bowel Disease', *Nursing Times*, 97 (10), 34–36.

66. Zaidel, O & Abreu, M. 2003; 'Crohn's Disease: An Evidence-based Approach to Medical Management', *Journal of Clinical Outcomes Management*, 10 (5), 279–286.

67. Hanauer, S & Sanborn, W. 2001; 'The Management of Crohn's Disease in Adults', *American Journal of Gastroenterology*, 96 (3), 635–643.

68. Ghosh, S, Shand, A & Ferguson, A. 2000; 'Ulcerative Colitis', *British Medical Journal*, 320 (7242), 1119–1123.

69. Kefalides, P & Hanauer, S. 2001; 'Ulcerative Colitis: Diagnosis and Management', *Journal of Clinical Outcomes Management*, 8 (9), 40–48.

70. Maltz, C. 2002; 'Ulcerative Colitis', *Emergency Medicine*, 34 (6), 43–48.

71. Thirlby, R, Sobrino, M & Randall, J. 2001; 'The Long-Term Benefit of Surgery on Health-related Quality of Life in Patients with Inflammatory Bowel Disease', *Archives of Surgery*, 136 (5), 521–527.

10 | Female Reproductive Health Breakdown

AUTHORS

LINDA JONES

KERRY CHOUZADJIAN

LEARNING OBJECTIVES

When you have completed this chapter, you will be able to
- Recognise the important anatomical and physiological features of the female reproductive system;
- Describe the pathophysiological changes associated with a cross section of female reproductive health breakdown;
- Outline the role of the nurse in caring for women experiencing reproductive health breakdown;
- Consider the diagnostic techniques and common pharmacological agents associated with caring for a woman with endometriosis; and
- Outline the nursing care of a woman experiencing a complex degree of endometriosis, including the psychosocial implications for the woman and her family.

INTRODUCTION

This chapter includes an overview of the anatomy and physiology of the female reproductive system, followed by a discussion of health breakdown of the female reproductive system using exemplars. These examples include benign conditions of menstruation, structural, inflammation, and ovarian disorders and cancer. It is not within the scope of this chapter to discuss all possible aspects of female reproductive system health breakdown. Finally, a case study of a woman with endometriosis will link the diagnostic procedures, common pharmacological agents and nursing interventions involved in the care of this woman.

It is important to remember in discussion that the female reproductive system inter-relates with other body systems, such as the urinary, neurologic and endocrine systems. Not so obvious is the inter-relationship between the female reproductive system and general physiology. The production of oestrogens, primarily from the ovaries, which influences bone density, is one such example. One function of the female reproductive system relates to sexual intercourse, and the complexity of psychosocial norms and cultural values. A second function is perpetuation of the species through fertilisation, implantation, pregnancy maintenance and subsequent birth of a baby. This chapter briefly examines issues related to these linked functions of reproduction.

STRUCTURE OF THE FEMALE REPRODUCTIVE SYSTEM

The female reproductive system consists of the internal and external genitalia. The internal genitalia comprise the ovaries, fallopian tubes, uterus, and vagina, with the external genitalia including the mons pubis, labia majora and minora, clitoris, introitus, and perineal body (see Figures 10.1 and 10.2). Even though the female urinary tract is separate anatomically from the reproductive structures, their close proximity is a means of potential cross contamination and shared symptomatology between the two structures.

INTERNAL GENITALIA
OVARIES

There is a pair of ovaries usually located on either side of the uterus below the fimbriated ends of the two fallopian tubes. The ovaries are attached to the posterior surface of the broad ligament and by the ovarian ligament to the uterus. Each ovary is a flat, almond-shaped structure and measures on average 1.5 cm wide, 3 cm long and 2 cm deep, weighing approximately 2–3 g.

The function of the ovaries is twofold in that they store the female germ cells, or oocytes, and produce the two major female reproductive hormones, oestrogen and progesterone. Structurally, the ovary is

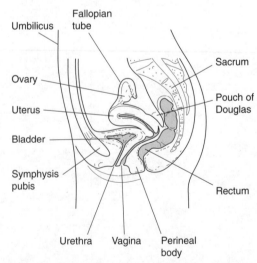

FIGURE 10.1 *Female reproductive organs mid-sagittal section*

composed of an inner medulla containing supportive connective tissue directly attached to the broad ligament. The cortex of the ovary consists of highly vascular tissue where the ovarian follicles are embedded. Each primordial follicle contains an immature egg or germ cell encased in a layer of squamous-like follicle cells. The primary follicle is then surrounded by two or more layers of granulosa cells. These cells protect and nourish the germ cells until the follicle matures and ovulation occurs. Thus the primary germ cell, under the influence of the pituitary and ovarian hormones, becomes a fully developed graafian follicle. During a woman's reproductive years, one germ cell usually matures each monthly cycle to be extruded from the ovary and engulfed by the fallopian tube fimbriae. This expulsion of the germ cell, or ovulation, occurs as a consequence of the stimulus of the gonadotrophic hormones, follicle stimulating and luteinizing hormones. After ovulation, the ruptured follicle transforms into a structure called the corpus luteum. In the absence of a pregnancy, the corpus luteum degenerates in approximately six months into a corpus albicans. If pregnancy occurs the corpus luteum is than maintained until the placenta is established, taking over the endocrine function[1,2].

Prior to birth, the fetal ovary contains over 2 million primordial follicles. By menarche (commencement of menstrual cycles), only approximately 200,000 remain, continuing then to decrease throughout a woman's reproductive years. Only 300 to 400 are actually released by ovulation during the woman's reproductive life. Of the remainder, a process termed atresia occurs in over 80%. This process involves the primordial and primary follicles becoming smaller and then being reabsorbed by the body[1].

FALLOPIAN TUBES

The fallopian tubes are also called uterine tubes or oviducts, of which there are two. Each tube is a slender, cylindrical and muscular structure approximately 10 cm long. The tube is an extension of the cornu of the uterus and travels to the side walls of the pelvis, turning downwards and backwards before reaching the ovaries. Both tubes communicate with the uterus at the medial end and the ovaries at the lateral end, being supported by the upper folds of the broad ligament. At the ovary end, the fallopian tubes form a funnel-shaped opening with fringed projections or fimbriae. These finger-like projections massage the ovaries at ovulation to help extract the mature ovum[1,2].

The primary function of the fallopian tubes is to provide a passageway for the ova and sperm to travel and possibly encounter, with fertilisation occurring. Most fertilisations occur within the outer one third of the fallopian tubes. This is assuming that sperm are present following recent coitus. Sperm are viable for 24–48 hours. An ovum can be fertilised up to 72 hours following ovulation.

Travel in the fallopian tubes occurs as a result of two factors:

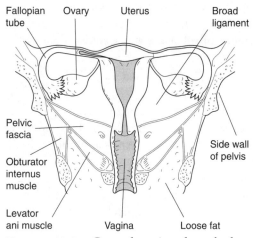

FIGURE 10.2 *Coronal section through the pelvis*

1. The fallopian tubes are formed of smooth muscle, which makes contractile movements; and
2. The tubes are lined with a ciliated mucus-producing epithelial layer. Together, the peristaltic movements of the muscle and the beating of the cilia propel the non-mobile ova to the uterus. This function of the fallopian tubes can be impaired through infection and inflammation, disrupting its patency.

Further, the fallopian tube provides a passageway through which tubal secretions can drain into the uterus. It should also be noted that the fallopian tube provides a direct passageway between the vagina and the peritoneal cavity. This is, therefore, a direct route for the entry of ascending infection into the peritoneal cavity[1,2].

UTERUS

The uterus is a thick-walled, muscular, pear-shaped, hollow structure located between the bladder and the rectum. In a woman that has never been pregnant (nulliparous), the uterus measures approximately 6 cm in length and 4 cm wide. Principally, the broad and round ligaments provide the uterus with support on both sides. The uterus is divided into three components, the fundus, the body or corpus and the cervix. Eighty percent of the uterus consists of the body, which is connected via the isthmus or neck to the cervix.

Most women have a forward-lying or anteverted uterus, with the uterine fundus and body resting on the bladder. It is possible, however, for the uterus to be in a number of other positions without causing any difficulties. These positions include anteflexion, retroflexion, or retroversion. This variation in position occurs in response to a variety of factors.

The wall of the uterus consists of three layers. The outer serosal layer, derived from the abdominal peritoneum, is the perimetrium. This layer merges with the peritoneum that covers the broad ligament. The perimetrium is reflected over the bladder wall anteriorly and forms the vesicouterine pouch. Posteriorly, the perimetrium extends to form the cul-de-sac or pouch of Douglas. The proximity of the perimetrium to the bladder means that a bladder infection often causes uterine symptoms, especially during pregnancy.

The major portion of the uterine wall is the middle layer or myometrium. This layer has the amazing ability to change in length during pregnancy and labour. The inner layer of the uterus is the endometrium and is continuous with the inner layer of the fallopian tubes and vagina. There are then two layers of the endometrium, a basal and superficial layer. The superficial layer is shed during menstruation, but is then regenerated by the cells of the basal layer. Ciliated cells promote movement of tubal-uterine secretions out of the uterine cavity into the vagina[1,2].

CERVIX

In the nulliparous female, the cervix constitutes about 15%–20% of the uterus and is the part that invaginates or projects into the anterior wall of the vaginal canal. It is the outer portion, or ectocervix, that protrudes into the vagina. This ectocervix has a smooth, pinkish appearance due to the squamous epithelial cell covering. The inner, opening canal of the cervix is called the endocervix, containing a lining of columnar epithelial cells, giving it a rough, reddened appearance. Under hormonal influence, the columnar epithelium provides enough elasticity during labour for the cervix to adequately stretch to allow passage of a fetus. The squamocolumnar junction is where the two types of epithelial cells meet. This junction contains the optimal type of cells needed for an accurate Papanicolaou (Pap) test for malignancy screening. If there are endocervical cells present in the Pap test sample, this ensures that the squamocolumnar junction, or transformational zone, has been sampled.

The cervical canal or os, approximately 2–4 cm long, is tightly closed. The vaginal opening is termed the external os, and the internal os, the uterine opening. The os does, however, allow the passage of sperm to enter and menses to be expelled from the uterus. A rich supply of protective mucus is produced by glandular tissue in the endocervix, which changes in character and quantity during the menstrual cycle and pregnancy. Under the influence of oestrogen, the cervix produces mucus, which facilitates the entrance of sperm. Normally, the cervical mucus at ovulation becomes watery, more abundant, and can stretch several centimetres (spinnbarkeit). These conditions then allow the sperm to easily enter the cervical canal into the uterus. In contrast, the mucus becomes thick under the influence of progesterone following ovulation, inhibiting the passage of sperm. These physiological changes form the basis of natural family planning. The endocervical secretions also protect the uterus from infection and form a mucoid plug or operculum during pregnancy.

The cervix is richly supplied by blood from the uterine artery. This, therefore, can be a site of significant blood loss during birth. The cervix consists of a connective tissue matrix of glands and muscular tissue. This forms a firm fibrous structure that becomes soft and pliable under the influence of the hormones of pregnancy[1,2].

VAGINA

The vagina connects the internal and external genitalia, and is located behind the urinary bladder anteriorly and posteriorly adjacent to the rectum. The shape of the vaginal opening may be oval, circular, or sleeve-like, and may be partially or completely occluded. This occlusion may occur as a consequence of the presence of an intact or partially intact hymen. The hymen is a thin membrane of connective tissue, which varies the size of the vaginal opening from that of a pinhole to an opening large enough to permit two fingers to enter. It is a commonly held belief that an intact hymen indicates virginity. The hymen may, however, become stretched without tearing or becomes torn due to childhood activity, tampon usage or accidents.

A vagina consists of a fibromuscular tube approximately 7.5–10 cm in length, lined with mucus–secreting squamous epithelial cells. Vaginal secretions include cervical mucus, desquamated epithelium, and, during sexual stimulation, a direct transudate. The purpose of these secretions is to protect the vagina from infection. Consequently, the vaginal tissue is usually moist, with a pH maintained at 4–6, considered a bacteriostatic level, as further protection against vaginal infection. The squamous epithelial cells of the vagina store glycogen under the influence of oestrogen. The oestrogen levels also influence both the pH and keratinisation of these cells.

The vaginal walls' muscular and erectile tissue allows enough dilatation and contraction to accommodate penetration of the penis during intercourse, as well as the passage of the fetus during birth. The membranous vaginal wall, which forms two longitudinal folds and several transverse folds or rugae, contributes to this dilatation[1,2].

EXTERNAL GENITALIA

The external genitalia, commonly referred to as vulva, are located at the base of the female pelvis in the perineal area. Structures that make up the vulva include the mons pubis, labia majora, labia minora, clitoris and perineal body (see Figure 10.3). Other structures usually considered as part of the vulva include the urethra and anus, although they are not considered to be part of the genital structures.

MONS PUBIS (VENERIS)

The rounded eminence located anteriorly to the symphysis pubis of the bony pelvis is the mons pubis. This consists of a fat pad covered with skin and coarse hair that lies in an upside-down triangular pattern. Under the hormonal influence of puberty, the amount of fat and hair increases and the colour deepens. The skin is abundant with sebaceous glands, which may become infected for a variety of reasons, including changes in diet, normal variations, or poor hygiene. This is also the site of pubic lice infestation[1,2].

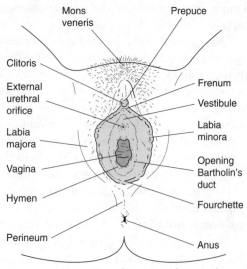

FIGURE 10.3 *Female external genital organs*

LABIA MAJORA

Beginning anteriorly at the base of the mons pubis and extending posteriorly to the anus are the outermost lips of the vulva called labia majora. This structure consists of folds of skin and fat, becoming covered with hair at the onset of puberty. The labia majora are rich in sebaceous glands and sweat glands and subject to the same types of problems as the mons pubis[1,2].

LABIA MINORA

Between the labia majora is the smaller delicate cutaneous structure of the labia minora, beginning anteriorly at the hood of the clitoris and ending posteriorly at the base of the vagina. This hairless structure consists of skin, fat and some erectile tissue, and is light pink in colour. The edges of the labia minora may be smooth or ragged and may protrude from the labia majora. During sexual arousal, the labia minora become distended with blood and enlarge, returning to normal following a period of labial throb. Sebaceous glands located in the labia minora secrete odoriferous fluid, both in the presence or absence of sexual arousal.

The vestibule is the area between the labia minora, extending anteriorly from the clitoris to the vagina posteriorly. This is a boat-shaped fossa that contains the ureteral and vaginal opening or introitus, and the Bartholin's lubricating glands. These glands are located at the posterior and lateral aspects of the vaginal orifice where the labia minora end. The purpose of the Bartholin's glands is to secrete a thin, mucoid material to lubricate the vestibular area. This is believed to contribute slightly to lubrication during sexual intercourse[1,2].

CLITORIS

Anteriorly, the two labia minora join, forming the clitoral hood or prepuce. Just below this structure, anterior to the urethral meatus, the clitoris is located. This structure consists of erectile tissue, rich in blood and nerve supply, which becomes distended during sexual stimulation. The clitoris is homologous to the male glans penis. Stimulation of the clitoris is an important part of sexual activity for women[1,2].

PERINEAL BODY

The perineal body or perineum is the tissue located posterior to the vagina and anterior to the anus. This area is composed of fibrous connective tissue and is the site of insertion of several perineal muscles. During childbirth, this area may be torn or incised (episiotomy) to facilitate birth of the baby[1,2].

FEMALE SEXUAL MATURITY

Physiological changes that occur during puberty include alterations in reproductive organs, the commencement of menstrual cycles and the development of secondary sex characteristics. The first change in the reproductive organs is the onset of breast budding, which usually occurs at around 10 years of age and may be accompanied by the first appearance of hair on the mons pubis[3].

The arrival of the first menstrual period is known as *menarche*, and usually occurs about two years after the start of breast budding. Just prior to the onset of the first menstrual period, a spurt in somatic growth is often experienced. The age at which menstrual cycles begin is influenced by nutritional status, weight, general health, genetic background, exercise and environmental factors; however, menarche generally occurs at approximately 12–13 years of age[4].

Other changes during puberty include development of the breasts and vulva, vagina, uterus and fallopian tubes. Vaginal secretions increase and become more acidic, pubic and axillary hair appears, the pelvis widens and fat is deposited on the breasts, hips and buttocks[4].

THE MENSTRUAL CYCLE AND THE CONTROL OF OVULATION

The menstrual cycle is a reflection of the cyclical release of hormones produced by the hypothalamus, pituitary and ovaries[1]. The hypothalamus controls the release of hormones from the anterior pituitary gland, which in turn regulates ovarian hormone production. Ovarian hormones control changes within the uterus and other parts of the reproductive tract[5,6]. During each cycle an oocyte is prepared for release at ovulation and, simultaneously, preparations begin within the woman's body for pregnancy and subsequent lactation[1].

The length of a menstrual cycle is the number of days between the first day of menstrual bleeding of one cycle to the onset of bleeding in the next cycle. The median duration of a menstrual cycle is 28 days (a lunar month) but most cycle lengths are between 25 and 30 days[4]. On the 14th day of a typical cycle ovulation occurs, during which an oocyte is released from the ovary. Menstrual cycles occur regularly throughout a woman's reproductive life except during pregnancy and lactation[5]. The menstrual cycle is characteristically most irregular around the extremes of reproductive life, at menarche and menopause[4].

THE OVARIAN CYCLE

At puberty, there are many thousands of primordial follicles embedded in the cortex of the ovary. Each of these primordial follicles consists of a primary oocyte (egg cell) surrounded by a single layer of follicle cells[1,4]. During each cycle a number of follicles will start to mature becoming known as Graafian follicles[1,5]. One of the follicles will mature at a faster rate than the others and this follicle will be the one that releases an oocyte at ovulation[1,4,5]. The Graafian follicle comprises the following (see Figure 10.4):

- Primary oocyte: the egg cell, which is undergoing first meiotic division. It is located at one end of the follicle;
- Perivitelline space: a narrow space surrounding the oocyte;
- Discus proligerus: a clump of cells surrounding the perivitteline space. These cells radiate outward to form the corona radiata;
- Zona pellucida: the innermost clear layer of the discus proligerus. This acts as a membrane around the oocyte;
- Granulosa cells: cells lining the follicle and enclosing the follicular fluid;
- External limiting membrane: the outer coat of the follicle; and
- Theca cells: compressed ovarian stroma cells surrounding the follicle.

The ovarian cycle can be considered in two phases, the follicular phase and the luteal phase[1,5,6]. During the follicular phase there is maturation of ovarian follicles and ovulation. The luteal phase involves the development of the corpus luteum from luteinization of the granulosa cells and theca interna cells[4]. The average ovarian cycle is 28 days with ovulation occurring on day 14. However, there is great variability between cycles both in the individual woman and between women. It is usually the length of the follicular phase that is variable. The length of the luteal phase is generally constant[1,4].

FOLLICULAR PHASE

The follicular phase begins with the first day of menstrual bleeding and continues until immediately before ovulation occurs. This phase is initiated by the release of gonadotrophin releasing hormone (GnRH) from the hypothalamus, which in turn stimulates the secretion of two gonadotrophins, follicle–stimulating hormone (FSH) and luteinising hormone (LH) from the anterior pituitary gland. Under the influence of FSH, a number of follicles will begin to mature but one will mature more quickly than the others[1,4].

The main hormones produced by the ovary are oestrogen, progesterone and androgens[4]. Oestrogen comprises a number of compounds including

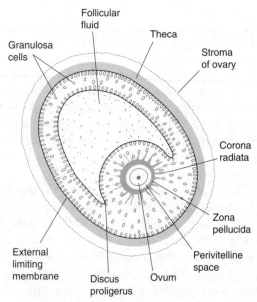

FIGURE 10.4 *A ripe Graafian follicle*

oestriol, oestradiol and oestrone[1,5]. LH stimulates the theca cells to produce androgens which are transported to the granulosa cells for conversion to oestrogen. FSH stimulates the granulosa cells to produce the enzymes that convert the androgens to oestrogen[1,4,6]. Proliferation of the granulosa and theca cells occurs and the follicle further increases in size[1]. The larger and more mature the Graafian follicle becomes, the greater the amount of oestrogen produced. As oestrogen levels rise, a negative feedback mechanism inhibits the production of FSH, ensuring that the growth and maturation of other follicles is controlled[1,4,5,6].

FSH and LH function synergistically to complete maturation of the dominant follicle. The follicle continues to grow and as it reaches maturity, there is a marked rise in oestrogen production. This rise initiates a surge in LH secretion approximately 36 hours before ovulation occurs[1,4,6]. Just prior to ovulation the primary oocyte completes its first meiotic division, becoming known as a secondary oocyte. The final stage of meiosis will take place on fertilization of the ovum[1].

The process of ovulation is assisted by the local secretion of prostaglandins and proteolytic enzymes which facilitate breakdown of collagen in the wall of the follicle[1]. The oocyte escapes from the follicle still surrounded by the zona pellucida, some follicular fluid and cells[6]. Some women experience pain at the time of ovulation, known as *mittelschmerz*. The ovum released at ovulation remains fertile for up to 72 hours[5].

LUTEAL PHASE

After ovulation has taken place, the walls of the follicle collapse inward. The remaining tissues become vascularised and change into the corpus luteum (yellow body)[4]. The function of the corpus luteum is to secrete the hormone progesterone, which has a profound influence on the preparation of the reproductive system for possible pregnancy. If pregnancy does occur, human chorionic gonadotrophin (HCG) maintains the corpus luteum and progesterone continues to rise. If pregnancy does not occur, the function of the corpus luteum declines by the end of the luteal phase and menstruation is triggered[5,6]. The corpus luteum then atrophies, becoming the corpus albicans (white body). During this regression, there is a rapid decline in the production of progesterone and oestrogen. When levels become low enough, the anterior pituitary is stimulated to produce FSH and LH and a new ovarian cycle begins[1,4].

THE MENSTRUAL (UTERINE) CYCLE

The changing patterns of gonadotrophins and ovarian hormones cause changes to occur within the endometrium of the uterus. This cycle can be considered in three phases, the menstrual phase, the proliferative phase and the secretory phase (see Figure 10.5).

MENSTRUAL PHASE

This phase is characterised by vaginal bleeding, known as menstruation or menses. Menstruation typically lasts 3 to 6 days[6]. Although the first day of bleeding is considered to be the first day of the cycle, physiologically it is the end point of the cycle as it involves the shedding of the endometrium down to the basal layer[5]. If pregnancy does not occur, the function of the corpus luteum declines and levels of ovarian hormones fall. The endometrium undergoes vasospasm, ischaemic necrosis and sloughing of tissue[4]. Endometrial tissue and accompanying blood are discarded through menstruation with the aid of uterine contractions stimulated by prostaglandins. These contractions may cause pain,

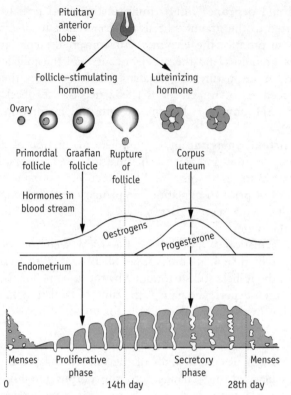

FIGURE 10.5 *Menstrual cycle*
Source: Henderson, C & Macdonald, S. 2004; *Mayes' Midwifery: A Textbook for Midwives* (13th ed.), Ballière Tindall, Edinburgh, Fig. 6.1, p. 89.

known as dysmenorrhoea. Normal blood loss during menstruation ranges from 30 to 80 mL[4]. The basal layer of the endometrium is not affected by the menstrual cycle and is, therefore, the foundation for endometrial regeneration[6].

PROLIFERATIVE PHASE

This phase begins once menstruation has ceased and ends at the time of ovulation. After menstruation, the inner lining of the uterus or endometrium is very thin. During the proliferative phase, under the influence of oestrogens being produced by the maturing Graafian follicle, the endometrium thickens from 1 mm to 3–6 mm[1]. The endometrium becomes more vascular and the endometrial glands proliferate. Increased levels of oestrogen also cause cyclical changes in the cervix, vagina and breasts[6].

SECRETORY PHASE

This phase corresponds with the luteal phase of the ovarian cycle, spanning from ovulation to the onset of menstruation. Changes occurring during this phase are largely stimulated by the secretion of progesterone from the corpus luteum[4]. The endometrium and its supporting stroma continue to thicken, blood vessels proliferate, dilate and become coiled. Endometrial glands continue to hypertrophy and begin to secrete fluid rich in glycogen[1]. Under the influence of oestrogen and progesterone, further changes to the reproductive system occur including to the alveolar system of the breasts, resulting in them feeling heavy and tender[4,6]. The purpose of these changes is to prepare the reproductive system for implantation of a fertilised ovum and to begin preparation for lactation.

PERIMENOPAUSE AND MENOPAUSE

Perimenopause is the phase during which a woman moves from reproductive life to non-reproductive life. The perimenopausal transition typically begins about four years before menstrual cycles finally cease. During the perimenopause, the ovaries become less responsive to the stimulatory effects of FSH and LH. During this phase, women may experience menstrual irregularity, changes in amount and length of menstrual flow, and reduced fertility[7]. Women may also suffer menopausal symptoms, such as changes in sexual function, vasomotor symptoms, psychological changes and insomnia[8].

Female reproductive life ends with the cessation of menstrual cycles at *menopause*, which usually occurs at around 47–55 years of age. Menopause is defined as 12 consecutive months of amenorrhoea sometimes accompanied by hot flushes and urogenital atrophy[8]. Symptoms can, however, be varied or absent.

ALTERATIONS IN STRUCTURE AND FUNCTION OF THE FEMALE REPRODUCTIVE SYSTEM

Disorders of the female reproductive system may have widespread effects on both physical and psychological functions of a woman. These conditions bear close relationships to sexuality and reproductive function, and for these reasons, have the potential to have a significant impact. There is a wide range of health breakdown of female reproductive system, all of which cannot be discussed in this chapter. For this reason the discussions in this section have been divided into benign and malignant conditions[9].

BENIGN CONDITIONS

Benign conditions of the female reproductive system are generally indicated by disturbances in function and structure. This section focuses on discussions on menstrual disorders, structural defects, inflammatory conditions, and benign ovarian disorders. Abnormal benign growth of uterine tissue will be discussed in detail in the case study that follows this section.

MENSTRUAL DISORDERS

Menstruation is a normal physiological process that starts from the time of menarche until menopause. Cultural and social norms influence women's perceptions of managing menstruation. Women may ignore changes in menstrual patterns and not seek treatment for menstrual disorders, even though they may represent more serious underlying problems[1,2,10].

DYSMENORRHOEA

Dysmenorrhoea is defined as abdominal cramping pain or discomfort associated with menstrual flow that restricts normal activity and requires medication, affecting approximately 50% of women[2,10]. This condition can be classified as either primary or secondary. Secondary dysmenorrhoea occurs when a pelvic disease or condition, such as endometriosis, is the underlying cause. This will be discussed in more detail in the case study at the end of this chapter.

Primary dysmenorrhoea occurs when there is no underlying pathological cause and is thought to be either the result of an excess of prostaglandin F2 alpha and/or an increased sensitivity to it. The endometrium is firstly stimulated by estrogen followed by progesterone, which results in a dramatic increase in prostaglandin production by the endometrium. Degeneration of the endometrium and the onset of menses release prostaglandins. At the local level, prostaglandins increase contractions of the myometrium and constriction of small endometrial blood vessels. This results in tissue ischaemia and increased sensitisation of the pain receptors, resulting in dysmenorrhoea. Absorption of prostaglandins into the circulation may in turn be responsible for headaches, diarrhoea and vomiting, other manifestations of dysmenorrhoea.

Characteristically, primary dysmenorrhoea starts 12–24 hours before the onset of menses. The first day of menses is usually when the pain is most severe, rarely lasting more than two days. The pain is lower abdominal and colicky in nature, radiating frequently to the lower back and upper thighs. Nausea, diarrhoea or loose stools, fatigue, headache and light-headedness may accompany this pain.

Treatment of primary dysmenorrhoea begins first with a thorough evaluation in order to find a cause and, therefore, distinguish it from secondary dysmenorrhoea. Management is then based on symptom control. Heat may be applied to the lower back or abdomen. Regular exercise is thought to be beneficial in reducing the endometrial hyperplasia and subsequently, reduce prostaglandin production[2,10].

Drug therapy includes non-steroidal anti-inflammatory drugs (NSAID) started at the first sign of menses and maintained every 4–8 hours, in order to inhibit prostaglandin synthesis. Oral contraceptives reduce the amount of endometrial growth and hence severity of symptoms. Diuretics may also be used to reduce oedema. Explanation and reassurance of the women is essential in providing individualised and holistic care[2,7,9].

DYSFUNCTIONAL UTERINE BLEEDING

A common disorder of the female reproductive system is irregular vaginal bleeding or dysfunctional uterine bleeding, which occurs in the absence of any pelvic pathology. This can be classified as one of the following:

- Oligomenorrhea: when there are long intervals between menses or infrequent menses;
- Secondary amenorrhea: cessation of menses for at least six months when the women has previously menstruated normally;
- Menorrhagia: excessive vaginal bleeding; and
- Metrorrhagia: irregular bleeding or bleeding between menses.

The causes of dysfunctional uterine bleeding vary from anovulatory menstrual cycles to more serious causes, such as blood dyscrasias, ectopic pregnancy, and miscarriage or endometrial cancer. Dysfunctional bleeding can originate as a primary disorder of the ovaries or as a secondary defect in ovarian function related to hypothalamic-pituitary stimulation. The latter can be initiated by emotional stress, marked variation in weight (sudden gain or loss), or by non-specific endocrine or metabolic disturbances[2,9].

Diagnosis occurs through a thorough history-taking, including the woman keeping a record of her bleeding pattern. This will often strongly suggest the cause. A complete physical examination is also necessary, including body mass index and gynaecological examination. Other means of diagnosis are laparoscopy and dilatation and curettage (D & C), with a laparoscopy providing a more precise diagnosis through visualisation and biopsy[7,10]. Management depends on the underlying cause.

PREMENSTRUAL SYNDROME

Premenstrual syndrome (PMS) is a condition where there is marked exaggeration in the physical, mental and emotional states that accompany the hormonal and metabolic changes associated with the premenstrual phase of the normal menstrual cycle. These symptoms are not present at any other time in the menstrual cycle. The symptoms usually occur from day 14 onwards, improve dramatically once menstruation starts and disappear after about 2–3 days. To be diagnosed with PMS, the symptoms must be severe enough to affect daily activities[11]. The symptoms include difficulty in concentrating, depression, irritability, emotional lability, anxiety, paranoia, low self-esteem, headaches, insomnia, breast discomfort and swelling, abdominal bloating, lethargy, acne and lack of libido.

Aetiology of PMS is not well understood and is thought to have a biological trigger with compounding psychological factors. It is not believed that this is an abnormality of hormones, even though some women may be affected by hormonal fluctuations[11]. There is increasing evidence to suggest that serotonin may be lower in women who suffer from PMS. It is speculated that there may be a genetically determined sensitivity to the neurotransmitter serotonin. This sensitivity results in heightened responses to the normal cyclic fluctuations of ovarian hormones. Other proposed causes are nutritional deficiencies of pyridoxine or magnesium[2,10].

Diagnosis is difficult and is based on eliminating other possible causes and completing a symptom diary for two months. Management strategies are based on relieving symptoms and enhancing the woman's sense of control. No simple treatment is available. To decrease autonomic nervous system arousal, women should avoid caffeine, reduce refined carbohydrates, exercise on a regular basis, and practise relaxation techniques. Increasing calcium intake may also help. Eating complex carbohydrates high in fibre, and foods rich in pyridoxine, are thought to promote serotonin production. Exercise results in release of endorphins, resulting in an elevation of mood and self-esteem. Other therapies that may be of assistance include hypnotherapy, acupuncture and relaxation therapy[2,11].

Informing the woman about PMS and its possible causes and treatment may help reassure the woman that her symptoms are real and she is not 'going crazy'. This education also involves discussions with the partner, as it assists in understanding PMS and how to support the woman during these times. Drug therapy may also be suggested. This includes oral contraceptives, diuretics, prostaglandin inhibitors, tranquillisers, and serotonin reuptake inhibitors[2,11].

STRUCTURAL DEFECTS

There are a number of ligaments that maintain the proper position of the uterus and pelvic structures, including

- Uterosacral ligaments which hold the uterus in a forward position;
- Round ligaments;
- Two cardinal ligaments which maintain the cervix at its normal level;
- A semirigid structure of the strong investing fascia encasing the vagina; and
- The muscular floor of the pelvis which supports the uterus and the vagina.

The main support for the pelvic viscera is the pelvic diaphragm, consisting of muscles and connective tissue that stretch across the bones of the pelvic outlet. These structures not only have to support the pelvic viscera against the force of gravity and increases in intra-abdominal pressure associated with coughing, sneezing, laughing, obesity and straining, but at the same time, permit urination, defaecation and normal reproductive tract function, specifically birth of a baby. This makes for an inherent weakness in the pelvic diaphragm because of the openings that must exist to make these functions possible. During pregnancy and childbirth, the muscles of the pelvic diaphragm become stretched and strained. Difficulties arising from this stretching may only appear in later life when there is further loss of muscle tone and elasticity. The combination of ageing and postmenopausal decreases in oestrogen levels may cause problems related to relaxation of pelvic support structures, even in women who have not borne children.

Pelvic floor disorders may affect up to half of the female population at some time during their lives, with many women not seeking any assistance. These disorders include pelvic organ prolapse and urinary and faecal incontinence. Approximately 20–35% of women over 40 years of age experience urinary incontinence, potentially undermining the quality of life for a number of women of all ages[10,12]. Urinary incontinence, usually referred to as stress incontinence, is the involuntary leaking of urine that occurs often with coughing, sneezing, walking, lifting or any other stressors. Other symptoms include urgency, urge incontinence, frequency and nocturia[9]. Although about half of older people have periods of incontinence, this is not a natural consequence of ageing, and not exclusively a problem of older women. Predisposing factors have been traditionally thought to be ageing, childbearing, obesity and menopause. The relative significance of each of these factors is unclear, specifically whether it is pregnancy or the actual birth that predisposes to pelvic dysfunction. However, a recent large study concluded that the effects of pregnancy more than birthing contributes to long-term pelvic floor dysfunction[9,12,13].

Diagnosis is through a thorough history-taking and physical examination, including mid-stream urinalysis (MSU) and a diary of urinary function. Management then depends on the diagnosis, but includes such measures as: lifestyle intervention (weight loss, caffeine reduction, avoidance of constipation); adjusting medications; pelvic floor muscle training; and use of devices to support the bladder[10].

INFLAMMATORY CONDITIONS

Inflammation, including infections in the lower genitourinary tract (vulva, vagina and cervix), are relatively common. This is due to the ready accessibility of the area to infectious organisms and because the warmth and moisture of these tissues provide an excellent environment for the growth of microorganisms. On the other hand, the upper genitourinary tract (uterus, fallopian tubes and ovaries) is less accessible to infectious organisms. The reason for this is that the mouth of the cervix acts as a natural barrier. Even though infections of the upper genitourinary tract are less common, the consequence of such infections is more severe because of the proximity to the peritoneal cavity. An example of an infection affecting the upper and lower genitourinary tract will be given in the next section.

Sexually transmissible infections (STIs) are infectious diseases that occur as a consequence of intimate sexual contact. Historically, these have been referred to as venereal diseases[2]. Usually these infections affect only the lower genitourinary tract and include gonorrhea, syphilis, genital herpes simplex virus (HSV) type 2, genital warts (human papilloma virus HPV), cytomegalovirus (CMV), hepatitis B virus, and human immunodeficiency virus (HIV)[10,11].

CHLAMYDIA

The most prevalent bacterial STI is caused by the Gram-negative bacterium *Chlamydia trachomatis*. To give an indication of the prevalence, between 1987 and 1996 in the United States, the reported cases of genital *Chlamydia* soared from 47.8 per 100,000 to 194.5 cases per 100,000[2]. In Australia, the incidence is reported to have risen by 80% from 1996 to 1999; most of the infections occurring in people aged 20–29, 60% being women[11].

Symptoms of a *Chlamydia* infection in women may be absent or minor in nature. Asymptomatic chlamydial infections can then be unknowingly transmitted during sexual intercourse. Typically, *Chlamydia* results in a superficial mucosal infection that can become more invasive. Women with a chlamydial infection may have cervicitis (mucopurulent discharge and hypertrophic ectopy [area that is edematous and bleeds easily]), urethritis (dysuria, frequent urination, and pyuria), and bartholinitis (purulent exudate). Chlamydial infections are a major contributor to pelvic inflammatory disease, ectopic pregnancy and infertility among women. Such complications develop from chlamydial infections that are undiagnosed, inaccurately diagnosed or poorly managed. There also appears to be a high incidence of recurrence, which may be a result of failure to treat the infected sexual partner/s of infected persons. The 1–3 weeks incubation period and the high prevalence of asymptomatic infections adds to the likelihood of recurrence. It has been suggested that all high-risk populations be screened to identify those infected[2]. Women deemed to be high risk include those less than 25 years, having multiple sexual partners, sex partners who themselves have had multiple partners, having a history of STIs, and who use non-barrier contraceptives. Transmission of chlymadial infection is also possible from a mother to her newborn, resulting in conjunctivitis or pneumonia[2,7,11].

Diagnosis is by endocervical swabs. Treatment of chlamydial infections occurs with a course of Vibramycin, azithromycin, or ofloxacin for seven days. The safety and efficacy of these medications in women under 15 years has not been established. These medications are contraindicated in pregnancy, with erythromycin or amoxicillin being the drugs of choice. The women should then be advised to return for further treatment if symptoms persist or recur; sexual partners also need to be treated. The use of condoms should be encouraged during all sexual encounters[7,9].

PELVIC INFLAMMATORY DISEASE

Pelvic inflammatory disease (PID) is an inflammation of the upper reproductive tract or pelvic cavity that may involve the uterus (endometritis), the fallopian tubes (salpingitis), the ovaries (oophoritis), and/or pelvic peritoneum. A woman may not perceive any symptoms, referred to as 'silent' PID, or be in acute distress. It is a disease of the reproductive years, with most women being young (75% under 25 years) and sexually active. The incidence of PID is increasing worldwide[7,10].

The most common causative organisms of PID are *Chlamydia* (60% of cases), which is increasing[9], or gonorrhoea, which is decreasing. Characteristically, the organisms ascend through the endocervical canal to the endometrial cavity and then to the fallopian tubes and ovaries. The endocervical canal is slightly dilated during menstruation, thus allowing the organism to enter the uterus and other pelvic structures. Organisms may gain entry during sexual intercourse or after pregnancy terminations, pelvic surgery or childbirth. Once inside the uterus, this provides an ideal environment for the organism to rapidly multiply in the favourable sloughing endometrium. It is important, however, to remember that not all PID is a result of STIs[7].

Typically, a woman with PID will seek medical assistance complaining of lower abdominal pain, which starts off gradually, and then becoming consistent. The intensity of the pain may vary from mild to severe, and increase with movements such as walking. There is also an exquisitely painful cervix, with pain increasing during sexual intercourse. Women may also complain of spotting following intercourse, have abnormal vaginal discharge, fever and chills and have an elevated white cell count. Women may have less acute symptoms, complaining of increased cramping pain with menses, irregular bleeding, and some pain with intercourse. In the case of mild PID, women may go untreated, either because they do not seek care or the complaint is misdiagnosed.

Diagnosis of PID may be difficult, and is based on signs and symptoms and information gained from the bimanual pelvic examination, STI screen, blood cultures, ultrasound and laparoscopy. Typically, women with PID have lower abdominal tenderness, bilateral adnexal tenderness, and tenderness when the cervix is moved. A culture of the abnormal vaginal discharge should be obtained from the endocervix.

Complications of PID included septic shock and *Fitz-Hugh–Curtis syndrome*, occurring when PID spreads to the liver causing acute perihepatitis. Women will complain of right upper quadrant pain but have normal liver functions test results. Another possible complication of PID is leaking, or rupture of pelvic, or tuboovarian abscesses, resulting in pelvic or generalised peritonitis. This may further result in toxic shock, as the general circulation is flooded with bacterial endotoxins from the infected area. It is also possible for embolic episodes to occur as a result of thrombophlebitis of the pelvic veins. Asymptomatic PID can cause irreversible damage.

Long term, women may experience further complications, such as ectopic pregnancy resulting from adhesions and strictures in the fallopian tubes. Partial obstruction of the tube results in the sperm being able to pass through the stricture but the fertilised ovum is unable to pass through to the uterus. In fact, one episode of PID increases a woman's chance of an ectopic pregnancy tenfold. PID is, therefore, a major cause of female infertility[9]. Another complication of PID is chronic pelvic pain.

Post termination of pregnancy or childbirth, PID can be more serious and life threatening. This is because the uterus following childbirth or termination is extremely susceptible to infection. Basically, the placental attachment site with its rich vascular channels offers little protection against bacterial invasion, affording direct tissue penetration. This may result in diffuse cellulitis (inflammation) and peritonitis. This PID is mostly a result of a mixed bacterial invasion, frequently by Gram–negative bacteria (e.g., *Escherichia coli, Pseudomonas, Proteus, Klebsiella*). These bacteria are highly virulent, liberating massive quantities of toxins. Absorption of these endotoxins results in generalised vasoconstriction causing pale, cold and clammy skin despite the fact that there is marked fever. Haemodynamic changes may eventually result in endotoxic shock with progressive renal, cardiac, hepatic and pulmonary failure and possibly death. Clinically, the woman appears extremely ill with a high fever, rapid pulse, shaking chills, purulent cervical discharge and extreme pelvic pain.

Treatment of PID is usually on an outpatient basis. A combination antibiotic therapy is used to provide a broad coverage against the causative organism. Women must be encouraged to rest and drink plenty of fluids. The woman's sexual partner must also be examined and treated. Couples should abstain from sexual intercourse for 3 weeks during treatment. Women should return to the clinic after 48–72 hours for reassessment of their condition.

Admission to hospital may be required if outpatient treatment is unsuccessful or the woman is acutely ill or in severe pain. In hospital, the woman is given maximum doses of intravenous antibiotics, with the possible addition of corticosteroids to reduce the inflammation. This allows for faster recovery and improvement in subsequent fertility. Women may be placed on bed rest in the semi-Fowler's position to facilitate pelvic drainage and help prevent abscess formation. Pain management is also part of the care of these women.

Prevention, early recognition, and prompt treatment of cervical and vaginal infections are crucial to prevent the development of PID and its complications[2,7,9,10].

BENIGN OVARIAN DISORDERS

Disorders of the ovaries frequently result in menstrual and fertility problems. These disorders include functioning ovarian tumours, benign ovarian cysts and polycystic ovary syndrome.

Ovarian cysts are the most common form of ovarian tumour, which are mostly benign (90%)[10]. Cysts are usually soft, surrounded by a thin capsule, and are seen mainly during the reproductive years. The most common ovarian cysts are corpus luteum and follicle cysts. Each month, several follicles begin to develop and become blighted at various stages of development. These follicles may form cavities that become filled with fluid, thus producing a cyst. Bleeding into the cyst may occur, resulting in considerable discomfort, manifesting as a dull ache on the affected side. A cyst may become twisted, or rupture into the abdominal cavity. Predominantly, cysts regress spontaneously.

Characteristically, ovarian cysts are often asymptomatic until they are large enough to cause pressure in the pelvis. This results in a sharp, stabbing pain on the affected side. Diagnosis is made from pelvic examination with or without a follow-up ultrasound. If the cyst is smaller than 8 cm, the woman is re-examined in 4–6 weeks. The cyst will be either smaller and need no action, or enlarged in size and best removed to avoid the risk of torsion and loss of the ovary. If the cyst is greater than 8 cm, laparoscopic surgery or laparotomy is performed. Immediate surgery is required if there is twisting of the ovary. The aim of surgical techniques to remove cysts is to save as much of the ovary as possible with the cyst being removed from the ovary. Management also involves excluding malignancy[7,9,10].

CANCER

Significant changes in the frequency of common gynaecological cancers have occurred in recent years. Malignant tumours of the female reproductive system include cancer of the vulva, vagina, cervix, endometrium, and ovaries.

CERVICAL CANCER

Cervical cancer is fortunately the most readily detected and the most easily curable of all of the female reproductive system cancers. If detected early, the cure rate is 80–90%[14]. Unfortunately, however, the screening is not universally followed, making the cure rate only about 60%[14]. Obviously, there is a need for more widespread screening. Cancer of the cervix is the eighth most common cancer in Australian women, with one in 101 women developing cancer of the cervix in their lifetime[14]. Worldwide, cervical cancer is the second most common malignancy after breast cancer[9]. The number of deaths attributed to cervical cancer has decreased in the past 40 years, attributed to better and earlier diagnosis through widespread use of the Pap test[14]. There is still a problem of the women being most at risk for cervical cancer not being screened[15].

An increased risk of cervical cancer is seen in women with low economic status, where there is early sexual activity (before 17 years of age), there are multiple sexual partners, infection with HPV and smoking (increases with longer duration, increased number smoked and use of unfiltered cigarettes). Cervical cancer has also been seen more frequently in women who have had several children and whose male sex partner is uncircumcised (the reasons for this are unclear)[7,10,14].

One of the most important developments in the early diagnosis and treatment of cervical cancer was the observation that this cancer arises from precursor cell changes. This begins with the development of atypical cervical cells, which progress to cancer in situ and finally to invasive cancer of the cervix. Atypical cells differ from normal cervical squamous epithelium in that there are changes in the nuclear and cytoplasmic parts of the cell, and more variation in cell size and shape (dysplasia). Cancer in situ is localised to the immediate area, whereas invasive cancer of the cervix spreads beyond the epithelial layer of the cervix. A system of grading and specific terminology has been devised to describe the dysplastic changes using the term cervical intraepithelial neoplasia (CIN). This system grades according to changes in the epithelial thickness of the cervix: grade I involves one third of the epithelial layer; grade II, one third to two thirds; grade III, two thirds to full thickness changes. The Pap test detects the atypical cells and cancer. The test obtains cells from the cervical canal for cytological examination. By treating the dysplasia, progression to cervical cancer can be prevented. It is recommended by the National Cervical Screening Program that women should have a Pap test every two years[14]. This is based on the premise that cervical cancers are mostly slow growing[7]. The Pap test should be obtained mid cycle for greater accuracy[7].

The progression from normal cervical cells to dysplasia and on to cervical cancer appears to be related to repeated injuries to the cervix[16]. The progression occurs slowly over many years, with a latent period of approximately 8–30 years. The peak incidence of CIN is in women in their early 30s, with the average age for women with invasive cancer being 50 years[10,14].

Precancerous changes are asymptomatic, as is early cancer, which highlights the importance of routine screening of women. Eventually, women will complain of leukorrhea and intermenstrual bleeding. Usually, the discharge starts as thin and watery, becoming dark and foul smelling as the disease advances. Initially, the vaginal bleeding is only spotting, becoming heavier and more frequent as the tumour enlarges. Late symptoms are pain, followed by weight loss, anaemia and cachexia.

Diagnosis is through Pap tests, colposcopy and biopsy. The initial diagnosis is made with a Pap test, with abnormal findings indicating the need for follow-up. On the finding of atypical cells, follow-up may be a repeat Pap test in 3–6 months, with the majority (80%) reverting to normal test results spontaneously[2,10]. Findings of abnormal cells consistent with dysplasia will receive additional procedures before a definitive diagnosis is made. Firstly, a colposcopy involving the examination of the cervix with a binocular microscope helps identify possible epithelial abnormalities. A punch biopsy may be performed on an outpatient basis using special punch biopsy forceps, and sent to pathology for examination[7,10].

Further investigation would involve taking of a cone biopsy or cone-shaped section of the cervix for diagnosis and treatment. Usually, this procedure is undertaken as an inpatient. Complications of this procedure include excessive bleeding and possible cervical stenosis following tissue healing. Women who have had a colposcopy and cone biopsy would then be followed up by 6-monthly Pap tests[7,10].

Treatment of cervical cancer depends on the stage of the tumour and the age, and general state of health of the woman. A cone biopsy may be sufficient if the excised tissue demonstrates that a wide area of normal tissue surrounds the biopsy. Treatment may also include laser, cautery and cryosurgery to destroy the dysplastic tissue. A dilatation and curettage may also be performed[9,10].

Treatment of invasive cancer involves surgery, radiation, or a combination of the two to remove or destroy the cancer and involved lymph nodes. Surgery usually involves hysterectomy, radical hysterectomy (involving adjacent structures), and rarely pelvic exenteration (uterus, ovaries, fallopian tubes, vagina, bladder, urethra and pelvic lymph nodes)[9,10].

● Case study

Julie began menstruating at 13 years of age. Some months after her menstrual cycles started, Julie began to experience cramping pain during her periods. Her mother reassured her that this was normal and that many women shared this experience. The cramping was so uncomfortable that Julie was missing a day of school each month.

By the time Julie was 16 years old, the pain at the time of each period had become so severe that she was missing two or three days of school each month, and she was also experiencing sharp pelvic pain in between her periods. Her menstrual bleeding was heavy, necessitating frequent sanitary pad changes, sometimes every two hours. The family doctor prescribed the combined oral contraceptive pill to help control Julie's unpleasant menstrual symptoms and he advised Julie to take ibuprofen to relieve her period pain.

Julie is experiencing the menstrual disorders of dysmenorrhoea and menorrhagia. Dysmenorrhoea is pain experienced during or immediately before menstruation. It is a common condition that can impact significantly on a woman's quality of life[17,18]. Many women do not seek medical assistance for dysmenorrhoea as they are conditioned to consider the pain as normal, even when it is severe enough to affect daily life[18]. Women who do seek help from their doctor may be discouraged by the tendency to dismiss their complaints as normal experience[17,18].

As discussed earlier in this chapter, dysmenorrhoea is categorised as primary or secondary. Secondary dysmenorrhoea has an underlying pelvic pathology, such as pelvic inflammatory disease, fibroid polyps and endometriosis[7]. Dysmenorrhoea that does not respond well to treatment should therefore be further investigated by ultrasound or laparoscopy to detect any underlying cause[19].

Heavy menstrual flow often accompanies dysmenorrhoea. Normal loss for a single menstrual period is considered to be about 70 mL, although there is great variation between women and in an individual woman at different times in her life[17]. A menstrual flow of greater than 80 mL is considered excessive. Menstrual flow is difficult to quantify, but the presence of clots is highly suggestive of a heavy flow[7].

Dysfunctional uterine bleeding occurs most commonly at extremes of reproductive age with 20% of cases occurring in adolescence[7]. Many causes of abnormal bleeding may be identified by history and self-observation alone but further diagnostic procedures such as endometrial sampling may be indicated[7]. The use of oral contraceptives may be effective in controlling heavy menstrual flow, however, other hormonal regimens or even surgery may be required in some cases[17].

APPLIED PHARMACOLOGY

Management choices for primary dysmenorrhoea include education regarding healthy lifestyle, use of non-steroidal anti-inflammatory drugs (NSAIDs), often combined with the oral contraceptive pill[10,18]. In the case of secondary dysmenorrhoea, treating the underlying cause should provide relief. The NSAIDs and combined oral contraceptives can be used alone or in combination. Use of oral contraceptives can also help to control the heavy blood flow that often accompanies painful menstrual periods[17]. There is increasing reluctance, however, to using the combined contraceptive pill in very young women because of the inherent long-term health risks[18]. Consequently, if a woman does not require concurrent contraception, NSAIDs such as ibuprofen may be the first drug of choice[7,17].

NON-STEROIDAL ANTI-INFLAMMATORY DRUGS

NSAIDs produce analgesic, anti-inflammatory effects and antipyretic effects. Its mechanism of action is not known but is thought to be related to prostaglandin inhibition[20]. Aspirin is a commonly used drug in this group as it can be easily bought over the counter. Aspirin may provide quite effective, analgesia, although it is quickly metabolised and so needs to be taken frequently[17].

Ibuprofen is a commonly recommended anti-inflammatory drug that provides effective pain relief for many women. It is also obtainable over the counter without prescription. Women should be advised to use it at the earliest onset of symptoms (pain or bleeding), as it is most effective when taken before pain becomes established[7]. The recommended dose is an initial 400–800 mg, followed by 400 mg every 4–6 hours, with a maximum dosage of 1200 mg per day. Side effects of NSAIDs are few but gastric irritation, such as dyspepsia and nausea have been reported[20]. It is recommended that ibuprofen be taken with food or milk.

COMBINED ORAL CONTRACEPTIVE PILL

Ethinyl oestradiol (synthetic oestrogen) in daily doses of 20–50 μg is combined with a variety of progestogens to provide a variety of brands[10]. The contraceptive pill is usually taken for 21 days of each cycle followed by a 7-day break during which time menstruation occurs. It may also be taken continuously so that no cycles occur[7]. There are three different types of formulation, monophasic, biphasic and triphasic:

- Monophasic: The dose of oestrogen and progestestogen does not vary through the cycle.
- Biphasic: The dose of oestrogen stays the same but the dose of progestogen is increased in the last 11 pills of the cycle.
- Triphasic: The dose of oestrogen is increased in the middle of the cycle to decrease the rate of breakthrough bleeding. The progestogen dose is initially low but increases stepwise as the cycle progresses[10].

The method of pain relief achieved with oral contraceptives is believed to be related to the absence of ovulation or endometrial changes, which results in reduced prostaglandin production. The combined oral contraceptive pill can be used in conjunction with ibuprofen to increase relief of dysmenorrhoea. Heavy or irregular menstrual bleeding may also be regulated by the use of the oral contraceptive pill[7].

Side effects of oral contraceptives include nausea, headaches, weight gain, and break through bleeding. Adverse reactions such as thrombosis development can occur with oral contraceptive use, although risks have now been significantly reduced by alterations in formulation. Women who are smokers, have a body mass index over 35 or are asthmatic are considered to be at greater risk[7].

In this case study, Julie experienced some relief from her symptoms for a number of years following commencement of the combined oral contraceptive pill and ibuprofen, but her menstrual problems returned when she ceased taking the pill two years after her marriage to Peter. She dreaded the days leading up to each period, during which she would experience intense fatigue, nausea, abdominal bloating, bowel disturbances and menstrual cramping that radiated into her lower back and rectum. Julie was also experiencing pain during sexual intercourse and was suffering pelvic pain and spotting intermittently throughout her cycle. Her symptoms were seriously affecting her quality of life. A year after ceasing the oral contraceptive pill, pregnancy had not occurred. Julie was subsequently referred to a gynaecologist for further investigation and assessment. Following collection of Julie's history, the gynaecologist advised an exploratory laparoscopy. Julie underwent an exploratory laparoscopy to investigate the cause of her menstrual symptoms and pelvic pain. The laparoscopy revealed that Julie had endometriosis with ovarian endometriomas. Adhesions of the fallopian tubes, ovaries and utero-sacral ligaments were also identified.

ENDOMETRIOSIS

WHAT IS THE PATHOPHYSIOLOGY?

Endometriosis is a progressive disorder where tissue resembling endometrium is found in locations other than the uterine lining[21]. These abnormal growths of endometrial tissue are referred to as endometrial implants or plaques. Implants can appear in a variety of areas, the most common being the ovaries, fallopian tubes, and utero-sacral ligaments. They may also appear on the outer surface of the uterus, pelvic cavity and rectum. Occasionally, implants may form blood-filled ovarian cysts known as endometriomas or chocolate cysts. In rare instances, implants have also been found in other parts of the body, such as the pleural cavity[22].

During the menstrual cycle, the endometrial lining of the uterus thickens in preparation for implantation of a fertilised egg. If fertilisation does not occur, the lining sloughs off in the form of menstrual blood. In the case of endometriosis, the endometrial implants respond in the same way as the endometrial lining of the uterus. During each menstrual cycle, the endometrial implants respond to hormone changes and bleeding occurs. The blood has nowhere to go, and so causes inflammation and scar tissue formation, which in most cases causes pain[23]. The size of implants varies widely from being microscopic to large invasive masses that cause extensive damage and adhesion formation[7].

The aetiology of endometriosis is not well understood, but is thought to be multifactorial in origin[7]. A popular theory has been that of retrograde menstruation, a condition in which menstrual flow backs up, leading to leakage of endometrial tissue through the fallopian tubes and into the abdominal cavity, where it implants[10]. However, the phenomenon of retrograde menstruation occurs in many if not most women and only a much smaller number of these women develop endometriosis. It is thought that immune alterations may also contribute to the development of the condition and to endometriosis-associated infertility. Another theory holds that peritoneal epithelium can undergo changes to become endometrial tissue, possibly as a result of chronic inflammation or chemical irritation from refluxed menstrual blood. A third theory suggests that müllerian remnants may be able to differentiate into endometrial tissue[7].

WHAT ARE THE CLINICAL MANIFESTATIONS?

Symptoms experienced are cyclical in nature and may include: dysmenorrhoea; ovulation pain; pelvic pain; lower back pain; dyspareunia (particularly with deep penetration);

premenstrual spotting; heavy menstrual bleeding; cyclical abdominal bloating; fatigue; bladder and bowel symptoms; and infertility[21,24,25]. However, there is wide variation in the experience of women with endometriosis, some being asymptomatic and others suffering severe disabling pain. It is possible for some women to have quite extensive endometriosis and not experience any symptoms. The severity of symptoms does not necessarily reflect the severity of the disease[23]. Women with endometriosis may experience some or all of the following symptoms:

- Ovulation pain: Pain is usually felt in one ovary at a time. The pain may begin 12–24 hours prior to ovulation and may last for some days. The pain is due to cyclical changes in the ovary which cause stretching of the implants and adhesions lying on the surface of the ovary[25].
- Dyspareunia: Painful sexual intercourse or dyspareunia can be divided into two types, superficial and deep. Superficial dyspareunia refers to pain in the vagina on entry and may be caused by a local inflammatory condition. Deep dyspareunia is associated with organic sources, such as pelvic inflammatory disease and endometriosis[10]. Deep dyspareunia is a common symptom of endometriosis, tending to occur particularly with deep penetration[7]. Pain may even be felt up to 48 hours after sexual intercourse[25].
- Pelvic pain: Gynaecological causes for acute pelvic pain may be related to such conditions as ovarian tumours or torsion, pelvic inflammatory disease and endometriosis[10]. Adhesions from endometriosis can cause discomfort at any time during the cycle[7].
- Intermenstrual bleeding: Lesions on or near the external surfaces of the cervix, vagina, vulva, rectum or urethra can cause post-coital bleeding at any time during the menstrual cycle. Premenstrual spotting may also occur[7].
- Urinary symptoms: There may be dysuria, urinary frequency or even haematuria in the perimenstrual period if implants involve the urinary tract[7,25].
- Gastrointestinal symptoms: Symptoms may include bouts of diarrhoea or constipation, painful bowel movements, bloating, nausea and vomiting[25].
- Fatigue: Fatigue is a common symptom experienced around the time of a period, though some women are unfortunate enough to experience it throughout the month[25].
- Infertility: The mechanism of infertility is not completely understood, although in some cases it may be due to damage of the fallopian tubes or ovaries, or distortion of the normal anatomy as a result of adhesion formation[22].

DIAGNOSIS

Endometriosis is notoriously difficult to diagnose, and women may suffer a great deal of discomfort for years before a diagnosis is made. Women may not initially seek help as they may have become accustomed to unpleasant menstrual symptoms from an early age and may not realise that what they are experiencing is abnormal[21]. Diagnosis depends heavily on the recognition of associated symptoms. A striking feature of endometriosis is that there is a cyclical pattern to the symptoms.

However, many women with endometriosis go unrecognised despite seeking help, and this leads to a delay in effective treatment[23]. Some women may be asymptomatic except for infertility, making a diagnosis of endometriosis less evident. Diagnosis can be confirmed by laparoscopy, during which the implants can be either directly visualised or confirmed by histology of a tissue sample[10].

In this case study, Julie discussed treatment options with her gynaecologist. She was not only seeking to gain relief from her symptoms, but also to maximise her chances of achieving pregnancy.

WHAT IS THE TREATMENT?

There are a number of treatment options available once a diagnosis of endometriosis has been made. Symptomatic endometriosis can be managed medically or surgically, or a combination of both approaches may be required[21,23].

MEDICAL APPROACH TO TREATMENT

Medical treatment of endometriosis has concentrated on altering the normal hormonal cycle to create a pseudo-pregnancy, pseudo-menopause, or chronic anovulation. The aim is to provide conditions that suppress endometrial growth and maintenance, thereby causing resolution of the endometrial implants[26].

APPLIED PHARMACOLOGY

In women who are strongly suspected to have endometriosis based on their symptomology alone, treatment usually begins with analgesia (usually NSAIDs) and combined oral contraceptives[23]. The aim is to create a hormonal pseudo-pregnancy[26]. Generally, monophasic products are selected and the woman is advised to take a pill daily continuously for 6–12 months. The aim is to effect changes in the endometrium and its glands[7]. A welcome adjunct to continuous administration is the control of dysmenorrhoea.

In the case of visually proven endometriosis, another medical pathway may be selected. A number of hormonal preparations are used in the treatment of endometriosis, including progestogens, androgens, GnRH agonists and antiprogestational steroids[26]. Treatments seem to be equally effective in managing endometriosis, but the range of side effects that may be experienced make some treatments more acceptable than others[23].

PROGESTATIONAL AGENTS

Progestogens cause decidualisation of endometrial tissue and eventual atrophy[7,26]. An example of a progestational agent used in the treatment of endometriosis is dydrogesterone (Duphaston). Side effects of progestogens include irritability, depression, fluid retention, breakthrough bleeding and breast tenderness[7,26].

ANDROGENS

Danazol is an example of an androgen given for the treatment of endometriosis. Danazol inhibits gonadotrophin release, thereby suppressing the mid-cycle surge of FSH and LH and subsequently, ovarian oestrogen production. The resulting hypoestrogenic environment and the androgenic effects of danazol suppress the growth of the endometrial implants[7]. When treatment is ceased, the pituitary suppressive action reverses, and ovulation recommences within a few weeks. Danazol is associated with unpleasant androgenic side effects, such acne, oily skin, hirsutism and voice deepening. It may cause serious adverse reactions including thrombosis and hepatic toxicity[20].

GONADOTROPHIN RELEASING HORMONE AGONISTS

The aim of this therapy is to suppress the secretion of gonadotrophins, thereby suppressing ovarian hormone production and subsequent control of endometrial implants. GnRH agonists can be administered intramuscularly, intranasally or subcutaneously. An example of a GnRH agonist is goserelin (Zoladex), which is in the form of a subcutaneous implant.

The use of these products is usually limited to 6 months because of possible adverse side effects. Side effects are related to suppression of oestrogen, and include loss of bone mineral density, vaginal dryness, mood changes and vasomotor symptoms[7].

ANTIPROGESTATIONAL STEROIDS

An example of an antiprogestational steroid is ethylnorgestrienone (Gestrinone). This drug acts to suppress the secretion of FSH and LH[7]. Most side effects are mild and transient, but some are irreversible, such as possible deepening of the voice, hirsutism and clitoral hypertrophy[26].

SURGICAL APPROACH TO TREATMENT

Surgical management may be conservative or radical. The aim of conservative surgery is to retain the woman's reproductive potential, and may include excision or destruction of the endometrial plaques, removal of adhesions and restoration of the pelvic anatomy as far as possible. The contemporary surgical approach to conservative surgery is by laparoscopy (use of a fiberoptic scope inserted through a small incision in the abdominal wall) as this approach is associated with shorter hospital stay and reduced recovery time, lower morbidity and cost effectiveness[7,23].

Excision or destruction of endometrial plaques and lysis of adhesions can be achieved through laparoscopic CO_2 laser vaporisation, electrosurgical cauterisation or ultrasonic scalpel use. The presence of extensive abdominal adhesions or widespread endometriosis may necessitate a laparotomy[21]. Sometimes, even conservative surgery may be relatively radical involving such procedures as dissection of the urinary tract, the bowel and the rectovaginal septum[23].

Additional surgical strategies may be aimed specifically at relieving the pain of endometriosis through procedures such as laparoscopic ablation or resection of the uterosacral sacral nerve or presacral neurectomy[26].

Radical surgery involves a total abdominal hysterectomy (removal of the uterus) and bilateral salpingo-oopherectomy (removal of both ovaries and fallopian tubes), with the aim of removing the endometrial tissue that has implanted outside the uterus. Unfortunately, this is not always successful and for some women, symptoms persist[23].

INFERTILITY

Infertility is usually defined as the inability of a couple to conceive within a certain period of time, commonly a year[7]. The term primary infertility refers to those who have never conceived. The term secondary infertility is applied to those who have conceived some time in the past. Approximately 90% of couples can be expected to conceive within one year[7]. Both partners, of course, contribute to the ability to conceive and both may be subfertile. A combination of male and female factors is found in 20–30% of cases, and a female factor alone is found in 40–50% of cases[7]. There are many factors that may be responsible for female infertility, including an underlying endocrine disorder, ovarian dysfunction and pelvic organs and structures that have been damaged by inflammatory conditions or endometriosis.

Endometriosis at all stages is associated with a reduction in conception rates[32]. The reported incidence of endometriosis found at laparoscopy in infertile women is 20–55%, in comparison with 5–10% in the general population[22]. Extensive endometriosis can alter normal pelvic anatomy rendering conception difficult, and the presence of endometriomas decreases ovarian responsiveness to gonadotrophins[27]. The process of infertility in the case of minimal and mild disease is less clear. For some women, infertility may be their only symptom of endometriosis. The condition may be revealed for the first time when the woman undergoes laparoscopic investigation for infertility. A number of possible causes has been proposed, including disturbances in ovulation, defective ovum capture and gamete transport, impaired implantation, luteal-phase dysfunction and toxic factors within peritoneal fluid[22,27].

The current treatment of choice for endometriosis-associated infertility, even in the case of minimal and mild disease, is laparoscopic ablation or resection of endometriotic tissue[22,26]. If conception still does not occur following surgical treatment, the woman may be counselled regarding appropriate assisted reproductive techniques, such as ovulation induction, intra-uterine insemination and in vitro fertilisation[22].

In the case study, a combination of surgical and medical management was considered the most appropriate approach for Julie. Laparascopic ablation for removal of endometrial plaques and lysis of adhesions was undertaken. Postoperatively, Julie was prescribed danazol for a period of six months. Nine months after ceasing danazol, Julie remained well, although not symptom free, but pregnancy had still not occurred. In light of her history of endometriomas, ovulation induction was considered to be an appropriate course of action, and Julie became pregnant three months later.

NURSING IMPLICATIONS

Nurses may encounter women who suffer from endometriosis in a range of clinical settings. Nurses working in school health, community health centres, clinics, medical practices and emergency departments will often see women and adolescent girls presenting with the many symptoms associated with this disease. They may also care for women in the hospital setting as they undergo diagnostic procedures and surgical treatments.

Skilled history-taking is an essential aspect of assessment, appropriate referral and ongoing management of symptoms for women with endometriosis. Women and young girls who present with specific symptoms may need to be guided to seek appropriate medical diagnosis and intervention. Nurses have an important role in helping women who have been diagnosed with endometriosis to understand their condition and the treatments they are undergoing. Sufferers of endometriosis who are well informed and well supported and who take an active role in their treatment will be able to manage their disease more successfully[28]. Nurses should also be aware of, and refer women to, local, national and international resources regarding endometriosis. In Australia and New Zealand, women and health care providers can obtain information from a variety of Internet resources, including:

- Endometriosis Association Victoria (Australia): www.endometriosis.com.au;
- The Jean Hailes Foundation: www.jeanhailes.org.au;
- New Zealand Endometriosis Foundation: http://www.nzendo.co.nz/;
- New Zealand consumer health site: http://conditions-diseases.nzpages.co.nz/health_and_fitness/conditions_and_diseases/Endometriosis/; and
- Women's Health Victoria: www.whv.org.au.

As can be seen, treatment of endometriosis focuses on reducing physical symptoms, instigating medical or surgical strategies, attending to physical health, modifying lifestyle, and coping with stressors that further aggravate symptoms. Pain is one of the most distressing symptoms experienced by women with endometriosis. It is also a symptom that is not always relieved in the long term by either medical or surgical treatments[29]. Nurses can help women to identify effective means of managing their pain, as well as other unpleasant symptoms that may be experienced. Dietary changes, such as avoiding caffeine, sugary and fatty foods, may be helpful to some women. The inclusion of certain vitamins and herbs, such as vitamin B complex and evening primrose oil, may be beneficial. The woman can be advised on the benefits of regular exercise, rest and relaxation and the use of pain relieving strategies, such as heat packs and massage. The woman can also be guided to other sources of assistance, such as alternative health practitioners, for example, acupuncturists and naturopaths[25].

Endometriosis is a chronic disease with an associated emotional impact[29]. In addition to providing understanding and emotional support, the nurse can guide the woman to other sources of support such as the Endometriosis Association and support groups. If appropriate, it may also be beneficial to assist the woman to raise the awareness of those close to her, so that they may better understand her experience and ways in which they can support her.

CONCLUSION

This chapter has provided an overview of the anatomy and physiology of the female reproductive system, followed by a discussion of health breakdown exemplars. These included the benign conditions of menstruation, structural, inflammation and ovarian disorders, and cancer. Finally, a case study of a women with endometriosis was used to link in the diagnostic procedures, common pharmacological agents and nursing interventions involved in the care of a woman experiencing a complex degree of reproductive health breakdown.

Recommended Readings

DeCherney, AH & Nathan, L (eds.). 2003; *Current Obstetric and Gynecologic Diagnosis and Treatment* (9th ed.), Lange Medical Books/McGraw Hill, Sydney.

Hart, D & Norman, J. 2000; *Gynaecology Illustrated* (5th ed.), Churchill Livingstone, Edinburgh.

Lee, C (ed.). 2001; *Women's Health Australia: Progress on the Australian Longitudinal Study on Women's Health, 1995–2000*, Australian Academic Press, Brisbane.

O'Connor, V & Kovacs, G. 2003; *Obstetrics, Gynaecology and Women's Health*, Cambridge University Press, Melbourne.

Stables, D & Rankin, J. 2004; *Physiology in Childbearing with Anatomy and Related Biosciences*, Baillière Tindall, Edinburgh.

References

1. Stables, D & Rankin, J. 2004; *Physiology in Childbearing with Anatomy and Related Biosciences*, Baillière Tindall, Edinburgh.

2. Brown, D & Edwards, H. 2004; *Lewis's Medical-Surgical Nursing: Assessment and Management of Clinical Problems* (6th ed.), Mosby, St Louis.

3. Reeder, S, Martin, L & Koniak-Griffin, D. 1997; *Maternity Nursing: Family, Newborn and Women's Health Care* (18th ed.), Lippincott, Philadelphia.

4. Blackburn, S. 2003; *Maternal Fetal and Neonatal Physiology: A Clinical Perspective* (2nd ed.), W.B. Saunders, Philadelphia.

5. Fraser, D & Cooper, M. 2003; *Myle's Textbook for Midwives* (14th ed.), Churchill Livingstone, Edinburgh.

6. Olds, S, London, M, Ladewig, P & Davidson, M. 2003; *Maternal-Newborn Nursing and Women's Health Care* (7th ed.), Prentice Hall, New Jersey.

7. DeCherney, AH & Nathan, L (eds.). 2003; *Current Obstetric and Gynecologic Diagnosis and Treatment* (9th ed.), Lange Medical Books/McGraw Hill, Sydney.

8. Stewart, D & Robinson, G (eds.). 1997; *A Clinician's Guide to Menopause*, Health Press International, Washington.

9. Pitkin, J, Peattie, AB & Magowan, BA. 2003; *Obstetrics and Gynaecology: An Illustrated Colour Text*, Churchill Livingstone, Sydney.

10. O'Connor, V & Kovacs, G. 2003; *Obstetrics, Gynaecology and Women's Health*, Cambridge University Press, Melbourne.

11. 'Family Planning Victoria. Sex Life! Choice not Chance'. Retrieved 2 June, 2003 from http://www.fpv.org.au.

12. Chiarelli, P, Brown, WJ & McElduff, P. 1999; 'Leaking Urine: Prevalence and Associated Factors in Australian Women', in C Lee (ed.). 2001; *Women's Health Australia: Progress on the Australian Longitudinal Study on Women's Health, 1995–2000*, Australian Academic Press, Brisbane.

13. MacLennan, AH, Taylor, AW, Wilson, DH & Wilson, D. 2000; 'The Prevalence of Pelvic Floor Disorders and their Relationship to Gender, Age, Parity and Mode of Delivery', *British Journal of Obstetrics and Gynaecology*, 107, 1460–1470.

14. 'National Cervical Screening Program'. Retrieved 3 June 2003 from http://www.health.gov.au/pubhlth/strateg/cancer/cervix.

15. Harris, MA, Byles, JE, Mishra, G & Brown, WJ. 1998; 'Screening for Cervical Cancer', in C Lee (ed.). 2001; *Women's Health Australia: Progress on the Australian Longitudinal Study on Women's Health, 1995–2000*, Australian Academic Press, Brisbane.

16. Moore, GJ. 1997; *Women and Cancer*, Jones and Bartlett, Boston.

17. Gould, D. 1998; 'Uterine Problems: The Menstrual Cycle', *Nursing Standard*, 12, 38–45.

18. Kennedy, S. 1997; 'Primary Dysmenorrhoea', *The Lancet*, 34, 116–117.

19. Edmonds, DK. 1999; 'Dysfunctional Uterine Bleeding in Adolescence', *Baillière's Best Practice Research Clinical Obstetrics and Gynaecology*, 13, 239–249.

20. 'MIMS Online'. Retrieved 20 August 2004 from http://mims.hcn.net.au.

21. Taylor, M. 2003; 'Endometriosis: A Missed Malady', *AORN Journal*, 77, 297–316.

22. Buyalos, R & Agarwal, S. 2000; 'Endometriosis: Associated Infertility', *Current Opinion in Obstetrics and Gynecology*, 12, 377–381.

23. Prentice, A. 2001; 'Endometriosis', *British Medical Journal*, 323, 93–95.

24. Colwell, H, Mathias, S, Pasta, D, Henning, J & Steege, J. 1998; 'A Health-related Quality-of-Life Instrument for Symptomatic Patients with Endometriosis: A Validation Study', *American Journal of Obstetrics and Gynecology*, 179 (1), 47–55.

25. Cagliarini, G & Woods, R. *Understanding and Managing Endometriosis*. The Epworth Hospital, Endometriosis Association (Vic) Inc and School of Nursing, Deakin University. Retrieved 30 November 2003 from http://www.endometriosis.org.au.

26. Olive, D & Pritts, E. 2001; 'Drug Therapy: Treatment of Endometriosis', *The New England Journal of Medicine*, 345, 266–275.

27. Mahutte, N & Arici, A. 2001; 'Endometriosis and Assisted Reproductive Technologies: Are Outcomes Affected?' *Current Opinion in Obstetrics and Gynecology*, 13, 275–277.

28. Miller, JF. 1992; *Coping with Chronic Illness: Overcoming Powerlessness* (2nd ed.), F.A. Davis, Philadelphia.

29. Lemaire, G. 2004; 'More Than Just Menstrual Cramps: Symptoms and Uncertainty Among Women with Endometriosis', *JOGNN*, 33, 71–79.

11 | Musculoskeletal Health Breakdown

AUTHORS

KIM VAN WISSEN

CHARLOTTE
  THOMPSON

LEARNING OBJECTIVES

When you have completed this chapter, you will be able to
- Describe the anatomy and physiology pertaining to the musculoskeletal system;
- Discuss a variety of musculoskeletal health breakdowns that occur with reference to skeletal muscle and joints;
- Discuss bone disease concerning anomalous calcium metabolism, infection and fracture;
- Explain the use of diagnostic tools and forms of treatment in managing musculoskeletal health breakdown;
- Identify pharmacotherapeutics used in treating musculoskeletal health breakdown; and
- Identify nursing interventions essential for people with musculoskeletal health breakdowns.

INTRODUCTION

This chapter first reviews the anatomy and physiology of the musculoskeletal system. A number of common clinical case studies are discussed demonstrating health breakdown of the musculoskeletal system. The case studies include: trauma (fractures), osteomyelitis, rickets, osteoporosis, fibromyalgia, gout, osteoarthritis and rheumatoid arthritis.

The musculoskeletal system includes the bones, muscles and joints with related tendons and ligaments that provide the framework for body support and movement. Bones provide a unique structure at a minimum weight and maximum support strength. This system is pivotal to mobility and maintaining activities of daily living (ADLs). In today's communities a person's independence is partially judged in terms of mobility and the ability to maintain ADLs and related social roles. Nurses can play a noteworthy part in rehabilitation where they are involved returning people back to a level of independent mobility. This chapter will assist students in becoming more familiar with the intricacies of the pathophysiology of bone and muscle and some of their associated treatments and nursing care.

THE MUSCULOSKELETAL SYSTEM

BONE: STRUCTURE AND FUNCTION

The four main functions of the skeletal system are

1. Internal organ protection;
2. Attachment for muscles and ligaments;
3. Allow functional movement; and
4. Storage of minerals and blood cell precursors.

Bone is highly vascular and remains active metabolically throughout the life span.

HEALTHY BONE

Collagen fibres make up 90–95% of the organic composition of bone. These fibres run the length of bones and give it tensile strength. The cellular components of bone include[1,2]

- Fibroblasts and fibrocytes, which are responsible for collagen production;
- Osteoblasts, which generate new osteoid (the organic matrix of bone), are responsible for synthesis of new bone and repair;
- Osteocytes, which are mature osteoblasts that have become surrounded by osteoid and have lost their ability to form bone matrix; and
- Osteoclasts, whose main activity is that of bone resorption.

To gain a clearer understanding of how these cells work together, see Figure 11.1.

The Haversian system is the basic structural unit within bone. Central to the system is the Haversian canal, which contains blood vessels and nerves. Around each Haversian canal are deposited the bony matrix as concentric rings (lamellae) where osteoblasts become osteocytes (see Figure 11.1). Extensions from the osteocytes, known as canaliculi, run as smaller canals linking lamellae to the Haversian canal. This system is important for transport of ions and nutrients to and from the blood to bone tissue.

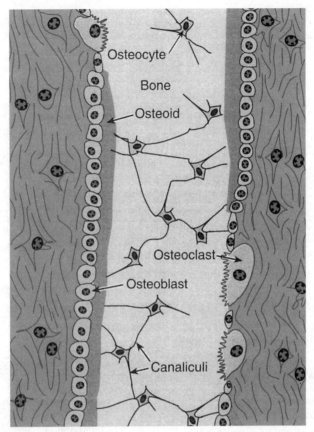

FIGURE 11.1 *Microscopic detail of principal bone cells: three principal cells important to bone metabolism*
Source: Rhoades, RA & Tanner, GA (eds.). 2003; *Medical Physiology 2E*, Lippincott Williams & Wilkins, Philadelphia, Fig. 36.3, p. 638.

BONE GROWTH

Major skeletal growth occurs in childhood. In a growing long bone, the epiphyses and the metaphysis are separated by a layer of cartilage (growth plate) where longitudinal growth takes place[3]. From infancy to adolescence, bones are actively growing in length, width, thickness and density (see Table 11.1). The epiphyseal plate gradually becomes less responsive to the hormones that stimulated them throughout childhood and adolescent growth. As hormones and tissues decline with age so too the status of the musculoskeletal system.

Cartilagenous thickening and continuing growth creates distance between the epiphyses and metaphysis[1]. Numerous hormones contributing to bone growth are summarised in Table 11.2.

Other factors affecting bone growth are

• Physical factors, such as weight bearing; and
• Absence of stress on bones (e.g., prolonged immobility) will cause bone demineralisation.

TABLE 11.1: SUMMARY OF BONE GROWTH	
	Bone Growth
Infancy	Rapid dimensional growth as calcium is added to cartilage-like bones. Calcium content in relation to body size increases faster than any other stage of life[3]
Childhood	Dimensional growth: skeletal height, length and width[4] in bone continue. Bone density and thickness increase. Bone deposition is greater than resorption
	Dimensional growth accelerates, bone growth peaks around ages 12–17 years in boys and 11–15 years in girls. Bone density and thickness increase while bone deposition outpaces resorption[4]
Middle adulthood	Bone mass loss after people reach 35 years[5] in both men and women
Later life	Loss of height due to osteoporosis and intervertebral disc thinning for both men and women. Metabolic changes (menopause) and reduced activity also contribute to osteoporosis. Bones lose their strength and alter in shape. Loss in size and number of muscle fibres due to myofibril atrophy due to increased inactivity and decline in neuromuscular stimulation[5]

TABLE 11.2: EFFECT OF HORMONES ON BONE GROWTH[2]	
Stimulation of Osteoblast Activity Parathyroid hormone Vitamin D_3 Thyroxine Growth hormone Testosterone	**Stimulation of Osteoclast Activity** Parathyroid hormone Vitamin D_3
Inhibition of Osteoblast Activity Glucocorticoids	**Inhibition of Osteoclast Activity** Oestrogen Prostaglandin E_2 Androgens

Bone is a specialised connective tissue that makes up 25% of the weight of a normal adult. Its major mineral components are calcium, phosphate and magnesium. Hormones (mainly parathyroid hormone) maintain this mineral homeostasis.

CALCIUM, PARATHYROID HORMONE AND VITAMIN D

The level of calcium in the blood must be maintained within a narrow range to perform the regulatory functions of this ion. When serum levels of calcium are low, parathyroid hormone (PTH) is released in greater amounts from the parathyroid gland[2], causing an increase in calcium absorption from the gastrointestinal tract, and further resorption by the kidneys into bone. When serum calcium levels are high, PTH secretion and activity are inhibited. PTH also regulates the synthesis of the active metabolites of vitamin D, which then increases gastrointestinal reabsorption. During infancy, bones grow rapidly as calcium is added to the cartilage-dominated bones and calcium content increases in relation to body size[3].

Vitamin D is necessary for normal bone mineralisation because of its role in calcium and phosphorous metabolism. The processes by which this vitamin reaches its final biological effects are summarised in Figure 11.2. Two sources of vitamin D contribute to serum calciferol: photochemically produced vitamin D from skin 7-dehydrocholesterol[6], known as cholecalciferol; and secondly, dietary vitamin D from plants and yeast. The second source, known as vitamin D_2 (ergocalciferol), is produced by ultraviolet ray exposure of plants[7], which we ingest.

CALCIUM HOMEOSTASIS AND REGULATION

Calcium homeostasis is regulated mainly by the effects of PTH and $1,25-(OH)_2-D_3$ (see Figure 11.2) on intestinal absorption, renal tubular absorption and bone resorption. Dietary calcium deficiency is rarely a major cause of bone disease in that absorption of calcium increases in states of calcium deficiency. Calcium fluxes between the gut plasma, bone and kidney. The circulating pool of calcium (approximately 12 mmol/L) is small when comparing the body reservoirs and daily fluxes of calcium levels[8,9].

LEARNING EXERCISES

1. What are the main functions of bone?
2. What are the principal ions deposited in bone matrix?
3. Why is it important to understand how the biochemical balance in bone is maintained?

NURSING IMPLICATIONS

The development of bone can be affected by numerous hormones and physiological processes (e.g., ageing or adolescent growth spurts). Therefore, it is important for nurses to be aware of the normal biochemical activities within bone, and be able to apply this knowledge when dealing with health breakdowns. For example, if an adolescent were not eating properly (e.g., anorexia nervosa) this would have a significant effect on their bone density for the rest of their life, hence a need to encourage good nutrition.

SKELETAL MUSCLE: STRUCTURE AND FUNCTION

Approximately 40% of body weight is attributable to skeletal muscle[10]. The four main functions of muscle are to

1. Enable movement of bones at the joint;
2. Provide strength and stability;
3. Protect the skeleton; and
4. Provide shock absorption.

SKELETAL MUSCLE CONTRACTION

A skeletal muscle is composed of many muscle fibres. Within each fibre are numerous muscle cells bundled together by a sarcolemma into fasciculi. Skeletal muscle is striated,

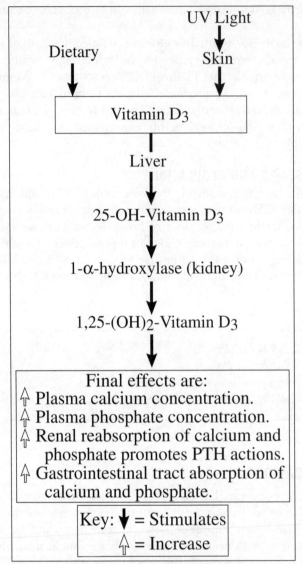

FIGURE 11.2   *Conversion of D3 and its final biological effects*

meaning it has a microscopic appearance of being striped. This is due to the specific organisation of contractile proteins, actin and myosin[10]. Myosin is the thick filament, the thinner filament being actin. Fasciculi that lie parallel to each other, as found in striated muscle, have the combined functions of strength and extensive range of motion at the associated joint.

Free intracellular calcium is essential to muscle contraction. The myosin heads have a high affinity to actin filaments, but they are prevented from interacting by tropomyosin protein attachment to actin. The position of the tropomyosin on actin is controlled by troponin[9,10]. When calcium ions are not available, the actin binding sites are covered by tropomyosin (which is stimulated by troponin). When calcium ions do become available through their release from the sarcoplasmic reticulum (a large storage for calcium ions) or extracellular space, the actin binding sites also become available as tropomyosin moves to another position. This allows actin and myosin to quickly interact to form a cross-bridge, the essential activity of muscle contraction[9].

ELECTROMECHANICAL COUPLING

To initiate contraction, a nerve impulse travels along the axon from the nerve cell body to muscle. The distal axon will divide many times, and these divisions will end on numerous motor end-plates. This nerve ending is positioned close to the sarcolemma. Acetylcholine is released to ensure depolarisation of the sarcolemma, which then spreads to the sarcoplasmic reticulum. When the action potential reaches the sarcoplasmic reticulum, calcium is released into the myofibril. This free calcium then stimulates chemical contraction, as the actin binding sites become available to bind with myosin. As a state of repolarisation is reached, the calcium ions return to the sarcoplasmic reticulum, and actin and myosin binding is reversed[9,10].

Muscle temperature increases with activity, and so too does the speed increase at which an action potential moves across the sarcolemma. As athletes warm up, muscle capability also increases. Accessibility to ATP sets a limit to contractile function. Prolonged muscle contraction and relaxation is sustainable while ATP and oxygen are available. As these two substrates become less available, muscle tension weakens and fatigue sets in.

Muscle is attached by tendons (fibrous tissue) or aponeuroses (flat sheets of connective tissue) to muscle and bone[2]. Ligaments (also fibrous connective tissue) bind bone to bone and are responsible for joint stability.

LEARNING EXERCISES
1. What are the main functions of skeletal muscle?
2. What is the main function of calcium in contraction?

NURSING IMPLICATIONS

Knowledge of muscle physiology is important to nurses because of close synergy with the skeletal system. Consequently dealing with issues such as good nutrition is important for muscle as well as bone function. Understanding and assessment of muscle groups for their 'range of movement' and alterations in muscle activity is also an important nursing skill.

JOINTS: STRUCTURE AND FUNCTION

Synarthroses are joints that are very inflexible or fused joints[2] such as skull bones or innominate bones (ileum or ischium) due to the presence of cartilage and fibrous tissue between bones. The symphysis pubis joint is an amphiarthrosis meaning the fibrous cartilage joining of the two pubic bones of the pelvis becomes flexible at specific times, for example, during the hormonal conditions of late pregnancy[4]. Diarthroses are those joints possessing a synovial sheath or joint capsule (examples are the hip or knee joint).

Movement of our body is only made possible through the coordinated movement of muscles and bone attached to joints. Joints or articulations are designed for a particular purpose and therefore have particular structures and surfaces.

Most significant joints of the body are synovial joints. Articular cartilage covers the points at which bone may articulate with bone. The synovial membrane secretes synovial fluid into the joint cavity to lubricate and cushion activity. Synovial fluid also acts as a medium for nutrient/waste movement in and out of the joint[1]. Articular cartilage at the ends of bones that articulate with each other, are smooth, shiny and able to cope with stress induced by body movement. The larger surface of the bone functions to

- Distribute weight or joint stress work load over a greater surface area;
- Cope with joint compression; and
- Cope with joint movement with articulation but likely deterioration as a person gets older.

Articular (hyaline) cartilage has no blood vessels, lymph or innervation. As a consequence, any defect in the cartilage will result in limited recuperation and disturbance to joint activity. Hyaline cartilage is 70% water and inorganic salts, lipids and glycoproteins[1]. The chondrocytes (cartilage secreting cells) produce the organic matrix of cartilage. During any health breakdown of the joint, the maintenance of articular cartilage can be severely altered, reducing its capacity to buffer against pressure and shearing forces. Uncharacteristic joint movement potentially disrupts natural joint activity. Therefore, a complex joint such as the knee, presenting with numerous articulations with complex ligament and tendon attachment, can potentially present with various joint health breakdowns.

LEARNING EXERCISES
1. What are the main structures of human joints?
2. What is the function of articular cartilage?
3. Why is it important to understand how joints function?

NURSING IMPLICATIONS

Understanding the mineral requirements of bones, muscles and joints gives nurses a greater appreciation of how the electrical and chemical environments of these structures work. For example, the balance of calcium (and other associated ions, such as phosphate) is necessary for conditions of growth and regeneration. Nurses need to assist patients to optimise these chemical microenvironments. Therefore a musculoskeletal health breakdown requires nursing consideration of the following potential issues: pain, sleep disturbances, fatigue, changes in mobility (with associated risk for disuse syndrome) and linked to changes in ability to attend to ADLs[5]. To assist regeneration and repair of bone and muscle, adequate nutrition is required. These broad nursing implications will assist in refining specific implications for each case study.

A number of common clinical cases of musculoskeletal breakdown are discussed below. The cases are: trauma, osteomyelitis, rickets, osteoporosis, fibromyalgia, gout, osteoarthritis and rheumatoid arthritis.

TRAUMA

The musculoskeletal system is open to trauma both mechanically and from infection. As bone and muscle are both highly vascular, infection within these tissues can be common. If bone is fractured, the capacity for repair is immense as bone is metabolically highly active. Hence bone is highly adapted to the mechanical and metabolic demands of the body.

FRACTURES

A fracture is defined as morphologic damage to bone continuity or part of the bone, such as the epiphyseal plate or cartilage. An estimated 66% of all injuries affect the musculoskeletal system[11] as a range of outcomes such as fractures and soft tissue injury. When fractures occur, tremendous reparation needs to be made to regenerate bone to original status. When a bone fracture occurs, the physical force causing the fracture will also cause damage to adjacent tissues/structures.

Fractures can be described by their anatomical position and arrangement of fragments. A classification of most fractures is described in Table 11.3.

The five main stages of bone healing are outlined in Table 11.4, differing in their time frame according to age and state of health.

The above table simplifies the various activities that may be occurring at the site of a fracture at any one time. Healing is a dynamic process, therefore as a fractures heal, some of the above processes will occur simultaneously, (e.g., remodelling will occur while other parts of the fracture are still being ossified).

● Case study

Enid Burrows, 77, lost her balance in the bathroom one night, fell and sustained a painful left hip. The ambulance officer noted her left leg was slightly externally rotated and shortened, and that she was hypotensive. Enid takes antihypertensive medication. Because she is hypotensive and is normally slightly hypertensive even on her medication, the ambulance officers commenced intravenous fluids. She was probably hypotensive because of local bleeding at the site of the fracture, causing hypovolaemia. In the emergency department, her X-ray showed a non-displaced (the bone pieces are in correct alignment for bone healing) left fractured neck of femur.

DIAGNOSTIC TESTS

Enid had lost blood into the site of the fracture, and because she needed surgery for her fracture, the following investigations were conducted: haemoglobin, white blood cell count,

TABLE 11.3: TYPOLOGY OF FRACTURES[5]	
Avulsion	Fracture wherein a fragment of bone is pulled from a main bone by a ligament/tendon
Comminuted	Fracture has fragmented into many small pieces
Compound/open	Fracture includes tissue damage such as skin or mucous membranes e.g., compound comminuted fracture is a common combination
Compression	Fracture in which bone is compressed or squashed
Epiphyseal	Fracture through the epiphyseal plate
Greenstick	Incomplete fracture common in children where in the bone is bent and not completely fractured through the bone
Impacted	Fracture in which bone fragments are driven into each other
Oblique	Fracture line lies angular to the bone shaft, making the fracture less stable
Pathological	Fracture may occur with trauma or spontaneously but affects diseased bone such as osteoporotic bone, bone cancer or renal failure (see Chapter 7)
Simple	Fracture does not break skin or mucous membrane
Spiral	Fracture spirals through the bone shaft, caused by a twisting action
Stress	Fracture caused by repeated activity 'stressing' the bone and associated muscles e.g., seen in athletes during repetitive training
Transverse	Fracture line is straight across the affected bone(s)

TABLE 11.4: STAGES OF BONE HEALING	
Haematoma formation	Inflammation: 1–3 days • Haematoma gives fracture site stability and seals bone ends to potential infection • Due to lack of circulation, bone distal to the fracture will become necrotic, and be replaced via bone resorption and deposition[11]
Fibrocartilage formation	Reparative: up to the first 2 weeks • Granular tissue with blood vessels, fibroblasts and osteoblasts
Callus formation	Reparative: 2–6 week (may start earlier) • Callus formation after granulation matures • Initially, new bone forms at the edges of periosteum where vascularity is greater
Ossification	Reparative: up to 6 months • Bone ends unite by ossification • Callus is resorbed • Bone stress lines have trabecular bone laid down
Remodelling	Up to a year after injury • Remodelling is constant while bone is resorbed and redeposited along stress lines according to activity[11]

creatinine, and electrolytes, such as sodium and potassium. These blood tests provide baseline data for comparison intraoperatively and after surgery. Also before anyone goes to theatre it is expedient to check that they have the capacity to oxygenate themselves (haemaglobin), have normal kidney function so they can excrete the anaesthetic (creatinine), do not have an infection (white blood cell count), and don't have electrolyte derangement. Enid's results showed a slightly lowered haematocrit, probably due to her blood loss, coupled with having intravenous fluids, which had diluted out the red blood cells she still had in her vascular compartment.

PHYSIOLOGY OF THE HIP JOINT

The hip joint is supplied by branches of the deep femoral artery. Most of the vessels traveling to the femoral head need to pass through the neck of the femur, the origin arising from a vascular ring at the neck base. The hip joint is a ball and socket synovial joint that allows movement in a variety of planes. The head of the femur articulates with the acetabulum of the pelvis. This particular joint has a tough, fibrous capsule maintaining femoral head and acetabulum articulation[1].

WHAT IS THE PATHOPHYSIOLOGY?

This type of fracture occurs more frequently in females than males, with frequency increased in the postmenopausal period of life. Osteoporosis is the most significant predisposing factor to fracture. As in Enid's case, this type of fracture occurs frequently by a simple fall at home. Diagnosis can be made observing for all the signs and symptoms that Enid demonstrated: shortening and external rotation of the affected leg as the gluteal muscle exerts an unopposed pull on bone. People with this sort of injury will not be able to weight-bear. They will experience tenderness over the affected groin as blood accumulates at the fracture site. Diagnosis is confirmed by X-ray: anterior-posterior (AP) view of the pelvis and a lateral view of the affected hip.

Treatment for people in the older age group, such as Enid, is to surgically replace the joint with a hemiarthroplasty (replacement of fractured bone by a titanium prothesis) determined by the severity and configuration of the fracture[11]. Avascular necrosis of the head of the femur can occur if the vascular supply to the femoral head is disrupted. Secondary osteoarthritis is also a common complication.

WHAT IS THE TREATMENT?

Enid's fracture was not displaced, so her fracture was immobilised by internal screwing of her two fractured bone surfaces to each other; hence, she did not need a hemiarthroplasty. The main aim of surgery is to facilitate swiftness of bone healing (see Table 11.3). As Enid has hypertension and therefore is at risk of perioperative myocardial infarction, a femoral nerve catheter was inserted by the anaesthetist, so the screws could be inserted under a regional anaesthetic.

Any procedure such as this, where artificial means are instigated to assist bone healing and a surgical incision is made, calls for prophylactic antibiotics. Enid was treated with an intravenous cephalosporin (cefuroxime, 750 mg eight hourly for two days) and consequently, did not acquire an infection.

Enid did have an episode of high blood pressure prior to surgery. After her femoral vein catheter was inserted, she was given an injection of bupivacaine (15 mL). Some time later that same day, her blood pressure was found to be 210/105 mmHg, and later decreased to 158/85 mmHg. The possible reason why her blood pressure was up was due to a lack of analgesia. Her antihypertensive medication (enalapril 15 mg once daily) was increased to preclude any cardiac incident, and she was given regular bupivacaine via the femoral nerve catheter and oral analgesia as necessary. It is worth mentioning here that throughout the hypertensive episode, she continued to receive intravenous fluids (normal saline eight hourly) for two reasons: she was 'nil per mouth' until surgery could proceed; secondly, as a precaution, some anaesthetists give intravenous fluids because the regional block may cause systemic hypotension.

The death rate within one year of a fractured neck of femur is between 20–35%[12,13]. In each case, these are reported as in-hospital mortality, not as deaths in the community.

APPLIED PHARMACOLOGY

As part of the nursing assessment the question needs to be posed, 'Was Enid on any medications that would cause her to fall?' For example, was she taking sleeping tablets or other medications that would make her drowsy or impair her balance? Another assessment consideration is to detail possible pharmacological reasons why Enid would have osteoporosis. Had Enid been taking steroids for some time? Over time steroids will generate a negative nitrogen balance hence causing a reduction in growth[14].

NURSING IMPLICATIONS

Determining why an older person has fractured their hip is as crucial as understanding treatments and management of fractures. Even though trauma as presented by this case is relatively common, it becomes vital for nurses to assess the patient thoroughly and consider the effect that co-morbidities (such as cardiac or respiratory conditions) will have on the recovery rate. Issues to consider for this case are: pain, immobility due to fracture and/or surgery, prevention of deep vein thrombosis during the postoperative period and preventing infection and how these specifically relate to the older person with a fracture.

LEARNING EXERCISES
1. Why do fractures occur more frequently in women in later life?
2. What would be considered the major nursing implications for the person with a fractured neck of femur?

BONE PATHOPHYSIOLOGY

Health breakdown of bone structure and mass occurs both in children and adults. The following three cases are presented to highlight how breakdown of skeletal health occurs and how nurses contribute to the management of osteomyelitis; rickets; osteoporosis.

OSTEOMYELITIS

Osteomyelitis is an acute or chronic inflammation of the bone and associated structures secondary to bacterial infection[15].

● Case study

Joey Jenkins, 6, presented with a painful left knee, which he knocked on a soccer goal post. He continued to play all day, but his parents noticed he was limping at home that night. The next day he awoke unwell, anorexic, lethargic and febrile. Taken to the family doctor, he was given antibiotics for otitis media (as he often gets this,) and his painful knee was explained as bruising/soft tissue injury. The next day, his knee was still very painful and he was taken back to the family doctor, who referred him to the emergency department. At the hospital, X-ray showed no changes, but there was also no evidence of otitis media.

WHAT SHOULD YOU BE LOOKING AT IN THE LABORATORY AND OTHER TESTS?

Joey's blood tests showed

- Neutrophils = 10.3×10^9/L (normal = 2.2–7.5 10^9/L);
- Erythrocyte sedimentation rate (ESR) = 62 mm/h (normal = 1–10 mm/h); and
- Complement reactive protein (CRP) = 30 mg/L (normal = <5 mg/L)

    Note the high CRP and ESR, which are commonly raised during the initial infection[16].

All three test results are indicative of a new acute infection and are standard tests used to identify acute infectious states. Four days later, diagnosis was confirmed by magnetic resonance imaging, showing osteomyelitis of the proximal tibial metaphysis.

WHAT IS THE PATHOPHYSIOLOGY?

Osteomyelitis is an acute infectious bone process, occurring through exogenous or endogenous (haematogenous) sources[15,17]. Exogenous infections can arise from open fractures or other external routes, such as wounds. Haematogenous osteomyelitis is the most common and occurs as an existing infection spreads from its local focus. Common examples are chest infections, otitis media, or common skin conditions, such as impetigo or abcesses. Osteomyelitis usually occurs in children aged 5–16 years[18], and can be caused by any organism, but age seems to be related to organism type[19], as summarised in Table 11.5.

TABLE 11.5: HAEMATOGENOUS ORGANISMS CAUSING OSTEOMYELITIS[19]	
Newborn	Gram-Negative Infections Group B Streptococcus
Younger children	*Haemophilus influenzae*
Older children	*Staphylococcus aureus*

Predominantly, osteomyelitis is a bacterial infection in otherwise healthy infants and children, occurring twice as frequently in boys[20]. An infective bolus leaves the point of the initial infection and travels to the small arterioles in the bone metaphysis, where a new infective focus commences[18,21,22]. Depending on whether the epiphyseal plate has closed or not, the metaphysis of rapidly growing long bone is most often involved. If the epiphysial plate has not closed yet, the infective bolus can travel into the epiphysis and set up an infective focus there[23]. Children such as Joey can appear well, but present with severe pain, fever, and toxaemia[24,25]. Once antibiotics are commenced, infection is usually quickly curtailed.

WHAT IS THE TREATMENT?

Intravenous antibiotics that penetrate bone and joint cavities are important to initiate as soon as possible. Joey was also referred to an orthopaedic surgeon and a microbiologist, to check that there would be no recurrence of his infection and that his infection was localised.

Selecting the appropriate antibiotics can best be achieved by direct culture from the infected site[26]. Surgical management can involve removal of the infection core and implantation of antibiotic beads.

Joey did not require surgical intervention, but was admitted for intravenous antibiotics: flucloxacillin and benzylpenicillin (both 100–200 mg/kg/day up to 12 g/day divided as 4–6 hourly doses). Some children will experience pain and are febrile, so an appropriate dose of paracetamol is also advised.

NURSING IMPLICATIONS

Assessment of infection is imperative to avoid incorrect diagnosis and commence appropriate treatment as soon as possible. Checking for raised neutrophil and CRP levels is an expedient way to find an indication of acute infection. CRP levels now supercede the ESR (erythrocyte sedimentation rate) level.

LEARNING EXERCISES
1. What is the interpretation of Joey's blood tests?
2. What questions could have been asked of Joey and his parents to make a more informed nursing assessment of the state of health breakdown?

RICKETS

Rickets or childhood osteomalacia is a health breakdown involving softening and weakening of the bones, primarily caused by lack of vitamin D, calcium, and phosphate.

● Case study

Tui Tyuan's grandmother noticed the abnormally shaped wrists that he had had for the past year. Tui, 3, was interactive at the local play centre, wore a hat and played in the shade as instructed by adults. Tui's grandmother decided to take him to a local doctor. The doctor examined Tui, and ordered some blood tests and X-rays.

WHAT SHOULD YOU BE LOOKING AT IN THE LABORATORY AND OTHER TESTS?

Tui's blood results were as follows:

- Vitamin D = 4.2 mcg/L (normal = 14–76 mcg/L);
- Parathyroid hormone (PTH) = 46.2 pm/L (normal = 1–5 pm/L);
- Calcium = 2.5 (normal = 2.20–2.70 for Tui's age); and
- Alkaline phosphatase = 4310 U/L (normal = 30–350 μ/L for Tui's age).

There are advanced stages of rickets on Tui's X-ray involving the wrist and ankles. These joints display fraying, splaying (bone ends spread away from each other) and cupping of the epiphyses, which are markedly widened and poorly defined. The ankles are associated with angulation and some bowing of the tibia bilaterally. There is prominent periosteal new bone along the concavity of the shafts of the tibia and fibula.

WHAT IS THE PATHOPHYSIOLOGY?

Rickets is a condition caused by the deficiency of vitamin D, calcium and usually phosphorous. Vitamin D is required for normal calcium and phosphorous metabolism. It aids their absorption from the bowel and is required for normal bone formation[27]. Rickets develops in otherwise normal bone matrix when the critical ratio of calcium to phosphorous necessary for normal bone mineralisation is altered by inadequate amounts of calcium and/or phosphorous present in the extracellular fluid. Rickets is seen primarily in infancy and childhood. Bones affected are those that are growing fastest at the time of the deficiency[28] and occurs in the child's open growth plates[27]. Rickets is confirmed by X-ray, the changes being seen in wrists, ankles and tibia in Tui's case.

Tui's laboratory data typically shows a normal serum calcium level. There is insufficient calcium to be absorbed from the intestine because of the deficiency of available vitamin D, but the bones are serving as the reservoir to maintain a normal serum calcium level. The lack of calcium kept in bones contributes to the softening of bone.

Serum alkaline phosphatase is a bone isoenzyme produced by active osteoblasts; hence, this enzyme is present in serum during periods of increased growth, that is, childhood, puberty and any situation of bone healing[29]. As this isoenzyme is a marker of bone turnover, it becomes elevated as bone activity heightens during health breakdown, such as rickets. The raised PTH indicates increased hormonal activity to maintain normal serum calcium and phosphorous levels. The sustained higher level of PTH indicates a persistently low serum calcium, as Tui's results demonstrate.

WHAT IS THE TREATMENT?

Vitamin D deficiency rickets, once prevalent amongst children in industrialised cities, declined in incidence after the late 1920s when it became standard to fortify cow's milk and infant formula with vitamin D[30]. Today however, there are lifestyle behaviours such as: an avoidance of sun exposure to prevent skin cancer, adhering to strict vegetarian diets, and breastfeeding past six months without vitamin supplementation[30] that may contribute to a resurgence of rickets. Exposing the skin to daylight is the best way to produce vitamin D. Direct sunlight is not necessary, and the amount of sun exposure needed to produce enough vitamin D depends on light intensity, length of sun exposure and skin colour[31].

Exposure of the face and hands to sunlight for 2–3 hours produces sufficient vitamin D to prevent rickets. Most people receive more than this exposure during summer weather, and store enough vitamin D to see them through the darker months of the year[32]. The replacement of deficient calcium, phosphorus, or vitamin D will eradicate most symptoms of rickets. Important dietary sources of vitamin D include fish, liver, and milk.

NURSING IMPLICATIONS

The changing lifestyles of children over the last 10 years means less time is spent outside to avoid exposure to direct sunlight and there are progressively less calcium sources in our diets. For the clinician in primary health care or child health promotion, watching for vitamin D deficiency is a given. Understanding how the bone isoenzyme levels change with health breakdown is the most expedient way, coupled with X-rays of the affected limb, to watch how the rickets is reversed once treatment is commenced.

LEARNING EXERCISES

1. What is the role of UV light in generation of vitamin D?
2. How is the bone isoenzyme alkaline phosphatase useful in monitoring rickets?

OSTEOPOROSIS

Osteoporosis is typified by low bone density and increased fragility with thinning of bone[33]. This is due to the rate of bone resorption being greater than the rate of bone formation. Established osteoporosis includes the presence of fractures. Borderline low bone density is known as osteopenia.

 ## Case study

Lucy McDonald, 73, considers herself a healthy soul. However, she grew up in Europe during the Second World War when food, and particularly dairy foods, were not available. Food was still not freely available for about four years after the end of the war, so there were nearly ten years spanning Lucy's adolescence during which she endured malnutrition. Lucy has never been hospitalised. She leads a very active life and is busy with her grandchildren. It was during a boisterous episode with her granddaughter in the garden, while trying to kick a ball, that Lucy sustained a fracture in her foot. An X-ray confirmed the fracture but also revealed osteoporosis. In the emergency department, the staff put a support bandage on her foot and asked her to see her family doctor as soon as possible for proper diagnosis and to consider pharmacotherapeutic options.

WHAT SHOULD YOU BE LOOKING AT IN THE LABORATORY AND OTHER TESTS?

Demineralisation or decreased bone density can sometimes be detected by X-ray, but bones can appear normal despite loss of 30% of bone mineral. Bone density measurements using dual energy X-ray absorptiometry (DEXA) are much more accurate than X-rays. When a person is diagnosed as having osteoporosis, it is useful to have bone density checked, but more importantly, a thorough history should be taken to ascertain risk factors for fractures.

WHAT IS THE PATHOPHYSIOLOGY?

Osteoporosis is a form of health breakdown that involves calcium metabolism similar to rickets, but involves people at the other end of the life span. It is a chronic disorder of decreased bone mass causing an increased risk of fracture and a reduction in stature[34]. For those with osteoporosis, the rate of bone formation (osteoblast activity) is much lower than the rate of bone resorption (osteoclast activity). For any healthy adult, the bone remodeling cycle will take about 4–5 months[33,35], whereas remodelling for the adult with osteoporosis may take six times longer.

Bone mass is doubled between birth and about the age of two[35]. The mass doubles again up to the age of 10, but 10% will be lost by the time a person reaches late puberty.

For those with osteoporosis, the trabecular bone in particular is lost, more so than the hard outer portion of the cortical bone. With the loss of trabecular bone, the classical injuries seen are crushed vertebrae, fractured neck of femur and fractured distal radius.

The main factors affecting bone mass are: decreased oestrogen, nutrition, metabolic factors (calcium and phosphorous metabolism as detailed earlier in the section on rickets), and physical exercise[35]. Briefly, oestrogen stimulates osteoblast activity while suppressing osteoclasts. Satisfactory intake of calcium and vitamin D is essential to bone growth. Physical stress to bones stimulates bone remodelling.

Risk factors for osteoporosis[36] include

- Smoking, which can lead to rapid loss of calcium via the renal system;
- Diet lacking in calcium;
- Lack of exposure to the sun so vitamin D is not stimulated for calcium absorption;
- Increases in dietary sodium or protein can increase excretion of calcium;
- Caffeine and alcohol, which are diuretics which will increase calcium loss at the kidneys;
- Lack of exercise, which will reduce bone strength which is characterised by higher levels of calcium;
- Early menopause in women, and decreased oestrogen postmenopause;
- Steroid use;
- Poor health that alters calcium metabolism; and
- Small skeletal frame.

These risk factors are well discussed in the literature[33,35] in terms of their effect on bone remodelling.

Women can lose up to 10–15% of their bone mass in the five years following menopause[35]. By the time a woman reaches her 80s, she may only have half the bone mass she had when she was an adolescent. Primary osteoporosis is related to diminished oestrogen, so this tends to be a female health breakdown, after menopause. Premenopausal osteoporosis is caused by chronic glucocorticoid therapy, prolonged amenorrhoea and anorexia nervosa[37]. Secondary osteoporosis includes all other known etiologies pertaining to both men and woman as described in the risk factors list[36]. There are a number of treatments and medications that decrease bone mass, for example, anticonvulsants, corticosteroids and chemotherapy.

CORTICOSTEROIDS AND OSTEOPOROSIS

Corticosteroids have a specific effect on osteoblasts[38], blocking the vitamin D_3 induced osteoblastic activity, along with altering or stopping collagen production[39,40]. This effect of dampening effective bone remodelling can be reduced by discontinuing corticosteroid treatments.

WHAT IS THE TREATMENT?

Prevention starts with good nutrition and exercise. After menopause, oestrogen is the most important medication that can prevent osteoporosis. The literature[33,41] focuses on medications that are given to reduce the rate of bone loss, while consumer information tends to place high emphasis on lifestyle issues, such as diet and exercise. Both options are equally important.

APPLIED PHARMACOLOGY

Lucy was commenced on calcitriol (Rocaltrol), the vitamin D hormone in the pre-activated form. Calcitriol is well absorbed from the intestine, and the effects of a single dose last for several days. Metabolites of this drug are excreted through the faeces and urine; therefore, it is important to check the patient's renal function regularly. Lucy also would have been warned against taking other calcium supplements, as this may cause hypercalcaemia which would put her at risk of developing renal calculi. Eventually, Lucy was taken off calcitriol as she continued to have stress fractures. At present, she takes alendronate sodium 70 mg once a week. The bisphosphonates are a group of drugs that decrease bone turnover[39] suppressing osteoclast activity and are usually indicated for those with established osteoporosis[42]. Therapies with the best efficacy for fracture reduction in postmenopausal women with a fracture include bisphosphonates, raloxifene and PTH.

NURSING IMPLICATIONS

Good assessment for falls risk factors and management of appropriate drug therapies for those with osteoporosis are major nursing implications. This will potentially forestall any major fractures and avoid protracted hospitalisation.

LEARNING EXERCISES
1. Which drugs can potentially cause osteoporosis?
2. What are some of the risk factors for osteoporosis?

SKELETAL MUSCLE PATHOPHYSIOLOGY

This section describes the case of a person with fibromyalgia syndrome as an example of skeletal muscle health breakdown. There are many other muscle disorders that could be included in this section. However, fibromyalgia demonstrates how skeletal muscle pathogenesis can develop from the condition of 'chronic stress'.

FIBROMYALGIA SYNDROME

Fibromyalgia is a chronic form of health breakdown, with symptoms of fatigue and widespread pain in muscles, ligaments and tendons[43]. Previously, the condition was known by other names, such as fibrositis, chronic muscle pain syndrome and tension myalgia.

● Case study

Anne O'Sullivan, 37, complained of nondescript symptoms of muscle aches and 'tiredness' for the past 18 months. She works as a tailor, and there is great demand for her work. The nature of her work generates physical and mental tension. Anne saw her family physician who provisionally diagnosed fibromyalgia. Serum levels were checked for arthritis factor, but this returned negative.

The syndrome is delineated by generalised muscle aches, pain, stiffness, depression, fatigue and sleep disturbances[44,45] and diagnosis is often inaccurate[46,47]. This health breakdown appears to affect younger women, and is likely to be the result of a prolonged chronic stress response. The muscle aches and pains do occur at specific tender points: knee, greater trochanter prominences, gluteal muscle, muscle attachment to lateral epicondyle, some attachments to scapula, trapezius upper border, occiput, lower cervical spine at C5–C7 and at the second rib space[44].

WHAT SHOULD YOU BE LOOKING AT IN THE LABORATORY AND OTHER TESTS?

Fibromyalgia syndrome does not involve an inflammatory response, so none of the diagnostic markers used to measure an inflammatory response will be evident. There are general classification guidelines[48] for fibromyalgia to help in the assessment of the condition. This necessitates that a patient has extensive tenderness for at least three months in a minimum of 11 body locations[47].

WHAT IS THE PATHOPHYSIOLOGY?

The pathophysiology is likely to stem from a neurohormonal imbalance[43] relating to protracted stress. People with fibromyalgia have alterations in the regulation of neurotransmitters, such as serotonin, which is linked to depression, gastrointestinal symptoms and headaches. Fibromyalgia is also linked to substance P (a neurochemical linked to pain) associated with depression, stress and anxiety[49].

On biopsy, affected muscles have a deficiency in adenosine triphosphate (ATP), and red fibres appear tattered with mitochondrial changes, all suggesting growing hypoxia. The lack of sleep may cause the syndrome, or be a result of it. In any case, due to the lack of sleep, less serotonin is produced, perpetuating the depressive mood observed in those with fibromyalgia. Abnormally low hormone levels of somatomedin C (significant in stimulating body rejuvenation during the latter part of sleep) are also found in the blood of people with fibromyalgia.

WHAT IS THE TREATMENT?

Anne's treatment consisted of changes in lifestyle: changing her work patterns, reducing her work hours, and involvement in a program of gentle aerobic activity. She now works four days a week (not six), and goes swimming three times a week. It is felt that these activities improve serotonin levels and enhance oxygenation of musculature, so muscle strength is improved[45]. With the combination of mild daily aerobic exercise, a regular bedtime with adequate sleep, and one of several medications to improve deep sleep, the health breakdown of fibromyalgia improves.

APPLIED PHARMACOLOGY

Anne was asked to give up caffeine and other stimulants such as alcohol, as they tend to suppress deep sleep. Analgesics are often used to decrease pain for those with fibromyalgia. Tramadol, a non-opioid, non-steroidal anti-inflammatory drug is safe for long-term use[50]. Benzodiazepines are sometimes used to break the cycle of sleep disturbance and muscle spasm[44,50], but create problems of withdrawal.

Anne was commenced on low-dose amitriptyline, it being an effective medication to effect sleep. However, she had daytime side effects attributable to its long half-life, such as weight gain, dry mouth, and cognitive impairment. She was next prescribed low-dose doxepin, which has a shorter half-life and less side effects and successfully allowed her to sleep deeply.

NURSING IMPLICATIONS

Through continuing research[49], the assessment and diagnosis of fibromyalgia is now less complicated. Nursing goals are aimed at reducing pain, improving sleep and introducing gentle exercise to maintain muscle health. Pharmacotherapeutics are not always successful, although sedation can assist people in establishing a healthy deep sleep.

LEARNING EXERCISES
1. Why is fibromyalgia difficult to diagnose?
2. What other forms of health breakdown can fibromyalgia be confused with?

JOINT PATHOPHYSIOLOGY

The health breakdown of joints affects both young and old. This section introduces cases that consider joint pathophysiologies, such as gout, osteoarthritis and rheumatoid arthritis, as these are highly prevalent in most population groups.

GOUT

Gout is a metabolic disease caused by excess urate in the body, either over-produced, under-eliminated or due to an increase in purine intake[51]. It usually occurs in middle-aged men, but can peak in the mid-40s for some people. It is often associated with obesity, hypertension, high cholesterol and high alcohol use[51]. Only 3–6% of gout cases occur in women[28]; this is mostly related to menopause status, unless the woman has a strong family history.

● Case study

Paul Macfarlane, 66, has had a diagnosis of gout for about 20 years. He has a strong family history of gout (parents, brother and cousins). He also has hypertension and a chronic tophaceous ulcer on his right lateral lower leg. Paul decided to discontinue his medications because he was sick of taking them. They were

- allopurinol 300 mg mane and 100 mg nocte;
- colchicine 0.6 mg nocte; and
- prednisone 5 mg mane on a reducing scale.

WHAT SHOULD YOU BE LOOKING AT IN THE LABORATORY AND OTHER TESTS?

His latest urate levels have been

- 24/11/03   0.44 mmol/L (normal for an adult male = 0.20–0.42 mmol/L)[29]
- 18/2/04   0.39 mmol/L
- 18/3/04   0.45 mmol/L.

WHAT IS THE PATHOPHYSIOLOGY?

Gout is a disturbance in uric acid metabolism culminating in monosodium urate salt deposits in joints and eventually subcutaneous tissue. There is usually marked painful inflammation of the joints and urate deposits around the joints, and often excessive urate in the blood[52]. Urate is derived from purines ingested from food, and recycled from tissue breakdown or repair. The types of foods that are considered purine-rich are: sardines, beef, scallops, duck, and vegetables such as asparagus and peas. Purines are otherwise derived from nucleotide degradation and resynthesis.

Urates are excreted by the gut and kidneys. The renal system excretes two-thirds of urates that need to be eliminated. Urate is filtered by the glomeruli and then absorbed by the proximal convoluted tubules. The amount of secretion and reabsorption at this point determines the serum level. It is estimated that 10% of the filtered urate leaves the renal tubule to become part of urine[53]. The other third is excreted by the gut, metabolised by bacteria to form carbon dioxide and ammonia (uricolysis).

THE ROLE OF URATE

Serum becomes urate-saturated at 0.42 mmol/L. Beyond this point, when serum becomes supersaturated, the urate solidifies out into crystals. Sodium urate is less soluble at temperatures below 37°C. As peripheral tissues are usually cooler than core temperature, this explains why the deposits and related pain occurs in the periphery[28].

Gouty arthritis characteristically occurs in patients with hyperuricaemia, although clinical gout (symptomatic) cannot be equated with a raised serum urate[53]. Approximately 85% of people with hyperuricaemia can remain asymptomatic throughout their life, but this still remains a strong preclinical indicator to the development of gout. Hyperuricaemia can occur due to increased production of urate, limited excretion of urate or a combination of these processes. Under-excretion occurs in many cases of gout, whilst over-production of urate occurs only in about 10% of cases[53].

THE FOUR PHASES OF GOUT

Gout can be classified as idiopathic gout or secondary gout. The former occurs more frequently in men[28] at a ratio 20 : 1. It is not clear why this form of gout occurs. Secondary gout occurs when hyperuricaemia develops secondary to underlying conditions, such as renal, vascular or endocrine disease, or a hereditary cause. Drugs such as diuretics or antihypertensives can induce gout.

Gout is clinically divided into four stages of health breakdown. The first is asymptomatic hyperuricemia, second is acute gouty arthritis, third is intercritical gout, and finally chronic tophaceous gout. These four phases are summarised in Table 11.6.

First attacks of acute gouty arthritis seem to affect one joint (about 90%)[53]. Approximately 50% of those with acute gout involve the first metatarsophalangeal joint (podagra). One study reported that 50% of untreated patients with gout will develop tophi after a mean of 10 years[55].

During the intercritical gout phase, there can be a tendency for patients to be less cooperative in taking their medications. It is at this phase that the health professional has an opportunity to focus on secondary causes of hyperuricaemia. Medications need to be reassessed and checked for inducing acute episodes of gout (e.g., diuretics). The patient also should be reminded about alcohol and dietary habits that potentially contribute to acute gout episodes.

TABLE 11.6: FOUR PHASES OF GOUT		
Phase	**Description of Pathophysiology**	**Signs/Symptoms**
Asymptomatic hyperuricaemia	• Abnormally high serum urate • No arthritis, tophi or renal stones Treatment not needed except changes in diet[54]	Nil
Acute gouty arthritis	• Monoarticular arthritis with sudden or sustained hyperuricemia • Triggered by trauma, antihypertensive medication, diuretics and alcohol consumption[54]	Erythema, swelling of joint involved (e.g., metatarsophalangeal, instep, knee, ankle, wrist and fingers)
Intercritical gout	• Asymptomatic period between acute gouty arthritis attacks	Nil
Chronic tophaceous gout	• More frequent and prolonged acute gout episodes • Polyarticular • Result of inability to excrete urate as it is metabolically generated When hyperuricemia is high enough to precipitate out crystals of urate, tophi will also develop[54]	Tophi present as white blanched areas initially, where the urate amasses in the tissues Crystal deposition usually occurs in the peripheries such as ear pinna, or big toe

TOPHI FORMATION

The deposition of urate crystals in tissue induces a local inflammatory response with all the associated local immunological changes. Complications of tophi include pain, soft tissue damage, deformity of the joint, nerve compression (such as carpal tunnel syndrome) and finally, destruction of the joint[52]. Large tophi can also ulcerate and inevitably become infected chronic wounds.

WHAT IS THE TREATMENT?

Definitive diagnosis requires aspiration of the joint, and identification of crystals in the synovial fluid. Paul's gout could be effectively controlled by medical management, but frequently is not, as patients often become uncooperative with medication-taking. Paul needed to have his diet re-explained to him, why he needed to take a purine-free diet where possible. He also needed to reduce his alcohol intake, stressing how these habits exacerbate his hyperuricaemia. The rheumatologist reviewed his status and negotiated with him to return to his medications, as they take some time to become active and then will prevent some of the pain that he is likely to experience in future.

   A surgeon was consulted with regard to debridement and skin grafting of his tophi. Paul decided against this option as it was likely his grafts would not heal well. The prospect of a larger wound, and more time off work on bed-rest postoperatively, did not appeal to him. Paul's general practitioner was to further monitor his hypertension, renal status and general well-being. It is important for a wound expert to reassess the wound regularly.

PHARMACOLOGICAL CONSIDERATIONS

Treatment includes: non-steroidal anti-inflammatory medications, colchicine, cortico-steroids and analgesia[51,54]. Colchicine can have undesirable side effects (diarrhoea, nausea, vomiting), so may be stopped by the patient before any pain relief is experienced.

NURSING IMPLICATIONS

One of the major issues for those people with gout is the realisation that they can do much to prevent the sequelae of hyperuricaemia. Through education, patients can prevent the pain and the destruction of joints and soft tissue by managing their health breakdown with appropriate drug therapy and a diet low in purines. Interpreting the laboratory results and watching the trends is important, as is managing these results with ongoing support for appropriate medications.

LEARNING EXERCISES

1. How do purines affect the serum urate level?
2. Why is the monitoring of urate levels important in the care of those people with gout as health breakdown?

OSTEOARTHRITIS

Osteoarthritis is a degenerative joint disease of cartilage and is the most common form of arthritis. The process of health breakdown is as a progressive non-inflammatory disease, usually in the weight-bearing joints. The main pathophysiological changes include the loss of articular (hyaline) cartilage and establishment of dense subchondral bone[56,57].

● Case study

Mitsuyasu Jayasura, 53, complained about pain in his left hip. He explained that the pain subsided if he rested, and the pain was not really evident at the beginning of the day. He was a keen rower, but has not participated in sport since the pain in his hip started six months ago. On examination, the findings were:

- He had a limp (antalgic);
- No swelling, no deformity, no erythema of his left hip;
- No tenderness at the joint; and
- Movements were painful, and he had a restricted range of movements.

WHAT SHOULD YOU BE LOOKING AT IN THE LABORATORY AND OTHER TESTS?

X-rays were taken of Mitsuyasu's pelvis. To exclude rheumatoid arthritis, a full hematological profile was undertaken. The erythrocyte sedimentation rate, rheumatoid factor (RH) and C-reactive protein (CRP) should be measured, as these will be elevated for those with rheumatoid arthritis, but not for those with osteoarthritis.

RADIOLOGICAL FEATURES

The joint space is reduced between the acetabulum and head of femur. The X-ray also shows subchondral pseudocytes, bone which has been replaced by fibrous tissue due to chondrocyte proliferation[4,56,58]. Subchondral sclerosis is also noted on the X-ray, areas of segmental necrosis in the subchondral layer[56]. This stimulates osteoblast activity, giving rise to thickening at the subchondral plate and eventual sclerosis. Osteophytes appear at the joint margin due to bone remodelling. Remodelling of the femoral head causes head flattening, in turn restricting joint mobility.

WHAT IS THE PATHOPHYSIOLOGY?

The cause of osteoarthritis is unknown. There are conditions that predispose a person to the development of osteoarthritis, such as congenital dislocation of the hip, steroid use, infective arthritis, and avascular necrosis due to a fractured neck of femur (or other joint fractures).

Mechanical, immunological and inflammatory processes contribute to how osteoarthritis develops[57]. Synovial cells and chondrocytes are both stimulated to release enzymes (metalloproteinases) that break down protein and collagen from matrix[56]. The cartilage surfaces eventually become eroded, to the point that the articulating surfaces are rendered bald. At these surface changes, osteophytes (abnormal finger-like bone growth) develop, and subchondral sclerosis is common. As the disease advances, synovitis (inflamed synovial membranes) will occur. This inflammatory process encourages an over-production of synovial fluid and therefore, gives rise to joint swelling and effusion[57].

WHAT IS THE TREATMENT?

The major desirable outcome of treatment is to protect the joint from trauma and reduce inflammation. Non-steroidal anti-inflammatory drugs (NSAID) are the principal drug of choice to reduce swelling and pain. Today, people are encouraged to remain mobile and not rest their affected joints where possible. When all the options of drug therapy are exhausted, surgical replacement of the joint may become necessary. Hip and knee replacements are the most common joints to be replaced for those with osteoarthritis.

APPLIED PHARMACOLOGY

Mitsuyasu was encouraged to seek physiotherapy and to stay mobilised, even if painful. As the pain was managed with paracetamol, there may come a time that he will need to consider the use of NSAIDs (e.g., diclofenac), as they block prostaglandin synthesis[14,59]. The literature discusses the use of opioids for pain management, especially if surgery is delayed[57]. Surgical replacement of the entire hip joint (arthroplasty) is considered once the pain can no longer be managed with analgesics, or mobility and quality of life is severely impaired.

USE OF NON-STEROIDAL ANTI-INFLAMMATORY DRUGS

This group of medications has three major actions: analgesic, anti-inflammatory and antipyretic[14]. The compound is thought to decrease pain by inhibiting cyclo-oxygenase (COX)[5], the enzyme responsible for generating prostaglandin from tissue alterations such as trauma or inflammation.

The enzyme cyclo-oxygenase is found in two forms: COX-1 and COX-2[5,14]. COX-1 mediates prostaglandin formation and other functions such as platelet aggregation, gastric protection and renal vasodilation. COX-1 inhibition can result in gastric irritation[60], bleeding and renal prostaglandin inhibition. COX-2 relates to the prostaglandins that cause pain and fever so blocking COX-2 can have a desired consequence[14].

The older NSAIDs (e.g., indomethacin), the non–COX-2-selective compounds, inhibit both COX-1 and 2 so result in pain relief but also added potential side effects: gastric irritation which may proceed to ulceration. Renal insufficiency may also develop due to the loss of prostaglandin mediated renovasodilation. This problem is preventable and reversible[14]. Nursing implications are to observe patients at risk such as those with heart failure, renal failure and advancing age. These three groups of people are likely to develop side effects. Finally, it is useful to bear in mind that some people respond to only one of the numerous NSAIDs available. The drug may need to be taken for a few weeks before considered ineffective.

NURSING IMPLICATIONS

For all people with osteoarthritis, maintaining mobility is a major implication in nursing care. Mobility which is both free of pain and allows the person a quality of life is essential. This can be achieved by correct balance of activity and rest, sleep and appropriate analgesia. Pain relief such as the NSAID are excellent, especially when a COX-2-selective compound can be used in preference to the nonselective NSAIDS.

LEARNING EXERCISES
1. How is osteoarthritis best diagnosed?
2. Why are COX-2 selective medications best to alleviate pain for those with osteoarthritis?

RHEUMATOID ARTHRITIS

Rheumatoid arthritis (RA) is an immune-mediated systemic inflammatory[1] breakdown in health. It is not clear why people get rheumatoid arthritis, but trends show that women have a 3 : 1 greater chance[1] of developing RA, peaking between the fourth and sixth decade of life.

 Case study

Gloria Schwartz, in her late 50s, is a full-time teacher. Gloria noted, during a recent holiday with her husband, that she felt stiff in the mornings, and that she was getting painful swelling in her left wrist. She saw her family doctor after the holiday and he immediately suspected that she had developed RA because she has a family history of this breakdown in health.

WHAT SHOULD YOU BE LOOKING AT IN THE LABORATORY AND OTHER TESTS?

Gloria's blood tests revealed the following:

- Rheumatic factor = present
- CRP = present in diagnostic quantities during an acute episode of swelling in her wrist (CRP is defined previously in the case discussion of osteomyelitis in this chapter).

WHAT IS THE PATHOPHYSIOLOGY?

Currently, the principal aetiological theory regarding rheumatoid arthritis concerns the immunological activities that lead up to the development of the pathophysiology[28]. This may include an undiagnosed infection (antigen not identified as yet) in joints; or rheumatoid arthritis as a result of an autoimmune response. These two disease processes are likely to be interconnected, as an infectious agent may trigger the ongoing immunological events[61]. In the first theory, T cells react with the unknown antigen triggering the disease, resulting in the chronic inflammation[61]. The autoimmune theory places less emphasis on the role of the T cell, with chronic inflammation perpetuated by macrophage and fibroblast activity (T-cell independent). Gloria is positive for rheumatic factor, the antibody that reacts with a fragment of immunoglobulin G (IgG), an autologous or self-produced antibody[61]. She has had less presence of T cells, which suggests her disease is an autoimmune response (see Chapter 13) for which she has a genetic predisposition (relating to her familial history). For further information regarding genetic health breakdown, see Chapter 3.

Current literature links particular alleles of the major histocompatibility complex (MHC) to rheumatoid arthritis, especially human leucocyte antigens (HLA) of class II haplotyes DR4 and DR1[1,61-63]. In terms of immunological anomalies, there is also strong evidence that interleukin-1 and tumor necrosis factor alpha (TNFα) are key mediators of synovial inflammation[64] and degradation, as well as bone and cartilage destruction[65].

CHANGES TO SYNOVIUM

Initially, the pathological immune response is restricted to the synovium. As immunoglobulin IgG is formed, rheumatic factor (RF) antibodies are produced. When the IgG and RF react, complexes are formed that are not recognised by the body, setting up an autoimmune response. This is responsible for the commencement of an inflammatory response, first locally, then more systemically[61].

The complex progression of immunological events reaches an advanced local inflammatory process causing oedema, synovitis, and thickening of the synovial lining. Eventually, hypertrophy of the synovial lining invades surrounding tissues, encroaching upon the joint capsule, ligaments and tendons.

As noted earlier in this chapter, articular cartilage is avascular, and the synovium is responsible for the exchange of nutrients and waste. Consequently, antigens or cytokines that are present can maintain their effect on cartilage and synovium for longer[63].

A pannus refers to hypertrophied synovium which consists of macrophages, fibroblasts, mast cells and other less notable immunoresponsive cells. It can erode articular cartilage and sets the scene for osteophyte and bone spur development[1]. It is at this point that the similarities of osteoarthritis and rheumatoid arthritis are notable.

The main clinical manifestations of RA are related to symmetrical and multiple joint changes. These include: morning stiffness; soft tissue swelling; and swelling of fingers, wrists, hands, knees, feet, metacarpophalageal (MCP) or proximal interphalangeal (PIP) joints[61]. Other joints will become affected as the condition progresses. The 'swan neck'[66] deformity seen in those with RA occurs as joints become less stable and subluxation (dislocation) proceeds. The boutonniere deformity[1,61,66] can occur later in the disease progression; the PIP joints are flexed, but the distal interphalangeal joints are hyperextended. Other joints affected are: the knee, the ankle and sometimes the neck (dislocation of cervical vertebrae). People will experience other complaints apart from the changes to their joints, as RA has a systemic inflammatory effect including lethargy, weakness, and a low-grade fever while the immunological effects occur.

These clinical manifestations attributable to tissue changes cannot be satisfactorily captured by conventional radiography. As part of the treatment of rheumatoid arthritis, early diagnosis needs to be made of synovitis, which can only currently be achieved by magnetic resonance imaging[67].

WHAT IS THE TREATMENT?

Treatment goals for those with rheumatoid arthritis centre around early symptom control[56,68], such as minimisation of joint stiffness and swelling, mobility, reducing pain, and participating in their ongoing health care. Mrs Schwartz started wearing splints for both her wrists as they became more deformed. She also used hot wax applications to her wrists from the physiotherapist to relieve discomfort. She would start the day with warmed packs to her wrists (and eventually her ankles) especially during the winter, wearing the warmest socks and fingerless gloves.

APPLIED PHARMACOLY

An aggressive pharmacologic approach is favoured today[28,69]. Gloria was commenced on NSAID drugs, a cyclo-oxygenase-2 (COX-2) inhibitor which inhibits the production of prostaglandins responsible for damaging the joint structure. These particular drugs do not control disease progression, but give symptomatic relief. Other drugs used, such as the disease-modifying antirheumatic drugs (DMARDS), for example, sulphasalazine, gold and methotrexate, do affect disease advancement[14,66,69], but have considerable side effects for most patients. These drugs appear to have a more beneficial effect if combinations of DMARDs are used as opposed to monotherapy. Biologic agents to provide antibodies against cells known to have a destructive effect on cartilage and synovium are currently being developed[66]. Mrs Schwartz was still using just the COX-2 drugs a year after her diagnosis was made without side effects. She was never commenced on DMARDs, as her arthritis was too advanced and the benefit of these drugs would be minimal.

NURSING IMPLICATIONS

The major issues that affect the patient group with RA are: pain relief, dealing with loss of sleep, fatigue and limitations of mobility. Persistent pain has the corollary of sleep loss, fatigue and limited mobility[66]. Hence one of the main problems to overcome is relief of pain followed by appropriate drug treatment for the arthritis. While people are being commenced on DMARDS, NSAIDs are often used for analgesia particularly while DMARDS reach therapeutic levels. Heat and splinting of affected joints is useful to keep alignment and alleviate pain[66] of affected joints. This is balanced against a level of exercise that maintains mobility and relieves stiffness.

LEARNING EXERCISES

1. Apart from the musculoskeletal system, what other pathophysiological phenomena are linked to rheumatoid arthritis?
2. How does osteoarthritis differ from rheumatoid arthritis?

CONCLUSION

This chapter demonstrates the complexities of the musculoskeletal system as they exist within the composite of the body, remembering that the musculoskeletal system is only a small part of the 'whole'. Many of the health breakdowns introduced in this chapter affect the immune system, regulatory hormones, connective tissues and muscle; hence, we encourage you to read this chapter in conjunction with other relevant chapters in this book. All laboratory results were matched to normal laboratory ranges by Gill and colleagues[29], a very informative text in units that are relevant to New Zealand and Australia.

LEARNING EXERCISES

1. What are the two principal joints and describe them?
2. Compare the pathophysiology of osteoporosis and rickets.
3. What is the main cause of gout and how does this contribute to the breakdown of health?
4. Compare how bone heals for adults and older adults?

Recommended Readings

Gill, M, Ockelford, P, Morris, A, Bierre, T & Kyle, C. 2000; *The Interpretation of Laboratory Results*, Diagnostic Medlab, Auckland.

Hill, J (ed.). 1998; *Rheumatology Nursing,* Churchill Livingstone, Edinburgh.

Maher, AB, Salmond, SW & Pellino, TA. 2002; *Orthopaedic Nursing* (3rd ed.), Saunders, Philadelphia.

Schoen, DC. 2000; *Adult Orthopaedic Nursing*, Lippincott Williams & Wilkins, Philadelphia.

Staheli, LT. 2002; *Paediatric Orthopaedic Secrets* (2nd ed.), Hanley Belfus, USA.

References

1. Copstead, LC & Banasik, JL. 2000; *Pathophysiology: Biological and Behavioural Perspectives* (2nd ed.), W.B. Saunders, Philadelphia.

2. Rhoades, RA & Tanner, GA, (eds.). 2003; *Medical Physiology* (2nd ed.), Lippincott Williams & Wilkins, Philadelphia.

3. Gallo, A. 1996; 'Building Strong Bones in Childhood and Adolescence', *Paediatric Nursing*, 22 (5), 369–422.

4. Hansen, M. 1998; *Pathophysiology Foundations of Disease and Clinical Intervention*, W.B. Saunders, Philadelphia.

5. Smeltzer, SC & Bare, BG (eds.). 2004; *Brunner & Suddarth's Textbook of Medical-Surgical Nursing* (10th ed.), Lippincott Williams and Wilkins, Philadelphia.

6. Norman, AW. 1998; 'Sunlight, Season, Skin Pigmentation, Vitamin D, and 25-Hydroxy Vitamin D', *American Journal of Clinical Nutrition*, 67, 1108–1110.

7. Sills, I. 2001; 'Nutritional Rickets', *Topics in Clinical Nutrition*, 17 (1), 36–43.

8. Kumar, P & Clark, M. 1998; *Clinical Medicine* (4th ed.), W.B. Saunders, London.

9. Ganong, WF. 2001; *Review of Medical Physiology* (21st ed.), Lange Medical Books/McGraw Hill, New York.

10. Guyton, AC & Hall, JE. 1996; *Textbook of Medical Physiology* (9th ed.), W.B. Saunders, Philadelphia.

11. Altizer, L. 2002; 'Fractures', *Orthopaedic Nursing*, 21 (6), 51–59.

12. Goldacre, MJ, Roberts, SE & Yeates, D. 2002; 'Mortality after Admission to Hospital with Fractured Neck of Femur: Database Study', *British Medical Journal*, 325, 868–869.

13. Ministry of Health NZ. 2002; *Fracture of Neck of Femur Services in New Zealand Hospitals, 1999/2000*, Ministry of Health, Wellington.

14. Bennett, PN & Brown, MJ. 2003; *Clinical Pharmacology*, Churchhill Livingstone, Edinburgh.

15. Lew, DP & Waldvogel, FA. 1997; 'Osteomyelitis', *The New England Journal of Medicine*, 336 (14), 999–1007.

16. Peltola, H, *et al.* 1997; 'Simplified Treatment of Acute Staphylococcal Osteomyelitis of Childhood, *Pediatrics*', 99 (6), 846–850.

17. Rasool, MN. 2001; 'Primary Subacute Haematogenous Osteomyelitis in Children', *The Journal of Bone and Joint Surgery (British)*, 83–B (1), 93–98.

18. Ahmann, E. 1999; 'The Child with Musculoskeletal or Articular Dysfunction', in *Nursing Care of Infants and Children',* in DL Wong, *et al.* (eds.), Mosby, St Louis, 1947–1949.

19. Unkila-Kallio, L, *et al.* 1994; 'Serum C-Reactive Protein, Erythrocyte Sedimentation Rate, and White Blood Cell Count in Acute Hematogenous Osteomyelitis of Children', *Pediatrics*, 93 (1), 59–62.

20. Brook, IJ. 2002; 'Joint and Bone Infections Due to Anaerobic Bacteria in Children', *Pediatric Rehabilitation*, 5 (1), 11–19.

21. Lewis, AM. 1999; 'Orthopaedic and Vascular Emergencies', *Nursing*, 99, 29 (12), 54–56.

22. McCance, KL & Huether, SE. 2002; *Pathophysiology: The Biologic Basis for Disease in Adults and Children* (4th ed.), Mosby, St Louis.

23. Longjohn, DB, Zionts, LE & Stoll, NS. 1995; 'Acute Hematogenous Osteomyelitis of the Epiphysis', *Clinical Orthopaedics and Related Research*, 316, 227–234.

24. Ferguson, LP & Beattie, TF. 2002; 'Osteomyelitis in the Well-Looking Afebrile Child', *British Medical Journal*, 324, 1380–1381.

25. Markeas, N, *et al.* 2002; 'Clinical Microbiological Case: Acute Osteomyelitis in a Previously Healthy Child', *Clinical Microbiology and Infection*, 9 (2), 133–134.

26. Green, NE. 1999; 'Diagnostic Measures in Acute Osteomyelitis in Children', *The Journal of Musculoskeletal Medicine*, 16 (5), 272.

27. Berg, E. 2004; 'Rickets', *Orthopaedic Nursing*, 23 (1), 53–55.

28. Porth, CM. 2002; *Pathophysiology: Concepts of Altered Health States* (6th ed.), Lippincott Williams & Wilkins, Philadelphia.

29. Gill, M, *et al.* 2000; *The Interpretation of Laboratory Results*, Diagnostic Medlab, Auckland.

30. Hartmen, JJ. 2000; 'Vitamin D Deficiency Rickets in Children: Prevalence and Need for Community Education', *Orthopaedic Nursing*, 19 (1), 63–68.

31. Marks, R. 1999; 'Sunlight and Health', *British Medical Journal*, 319, 1066.

32. Wiseman, G. 2002; *Nutrition and Health*, Taylor & Francis, London.

33. Turkoski, B. 2002; 'Treating Osteoporosis without Hormones', *Orthopaedic Nursing*, 21 (5), 80–85.

34. Curry, LC & Hogstel, MO. 2002; 'Osteoporosis', *American Journal of Nursing*, 102 (1), 26–32.

35. Burke, S. 2001; 'Boning Up on Osteoporosis', *Nursing*, 31 (10), 36–43.

36. Geier, KA. 2001; 'Osteoporosis in Men', *Orthopaedic Nursing*, 20 (6), 49–56.

37. Gourlay, MLB, Brown, SA. 2004; 'Clinical Considerations in Premenopausal Osteoporosis', *Archives of Internal Medicine*, 164 (6), 603–614.

38. Crowther, CL. 2001; 'The Effects of Corticosteroids on the Musculoskeletal System', *Orthopaedic Nursing*, 20 (6), 33–38.

39. Bryant, B, Knights, K & Salerno, E. 2003; *Pharmamcology for Health Professionals*, Mosby, Sydney.

40. Rang, HP, Dale, MM & Ritter, JM. 1999; *Pharmacology*, Churchill Livingstone, Edinburgh.

41. Kessenich, CR. 2003; 'PTH Revisited for Osteoporosis Treatment', *The Nurse Practitioner*, 28 (6), 51–53.

42. Reid, IR. 2003; 'Biphosphonates: New Indication and Methods of Administration', *Current Opinion in Rheumatology*, 15 (4), 458–463.

43. Wilke, WS. 1996; 'Fibromyalgia: Recognising and Addressing the Multiple Interrelated Factors', *Postgraduate Medicine*, 96 (6), 73–81.

44. Groer, M & Jones, T. 2001; 'Common Disorders of the Musculoskeletal System', *Advanced Pathophysiology: Application to Clinical Practice*, in MW Groer (ed.), Lippincott, Philadelphia, 385–401.

45. Karper, WB, Hopewell, R & Hodge, M. 2001; 'Exercise Program Effects on Women with Fibromyalgia Syndrome', *Clinical Nurse Specialist*, 15 (2), 67.

46. Fitzcharles, MA & Poulos, B. 2003; 'Inaccuracy in the Diagnosis of Fibromyalgia Syndrome: Analysis of Referrals', *Rheumatology* (Oxford), 42, 263–267.

47. Wolfe, F. 1993; 'Fibromyalgia: on Diagnosis and Certainty', *Journal of Musculoskeletal Pain*, 1 (3), 17.

48. Douglas, J & Byrne, J. 1998; 'Skin and Nutrition', in *Rheumatology Nursing a Creative Approach*, Hill, J (ed.), Churchill Livingstone, Edinburgh, 173–193.

49. Aytekin Lash, A, Ehrlich-Jones, L & McCoy, D. 2003; 'Fibromyalgia: Evolving Concepts and Management in Primary Care Settings', *MEDSURG Nursing*, 12 (3), 145–160.

50. Bennett, R. 1997; 'The Fibromyalgia Syndrome', in *Textbook of Rheumatology*, Keley, W, et al. (eds.), W.B. Saunders, Philadelphia.

51. Kamienski, M. 2003; 'Gout: Not Just for the Rich and Famous! Everyman's Disease', *Orthopaedic Nursing*, 22 (1), 16–20.

52. Pittman, J & Bross, M. 1999; 'Diagnosis and Management of Gout', *American Family Physician*, 59 (7), 1799–1806.

53. Harris, M, Siegel, L & Alloway, J. 1999; 'Gout and Hyperuricaemia', *American Family Physician*, 59 (4), 925–934.

54. McDonald, E & Marino, C. 1998; 'Stopping Progression to Tophaceous Gout: When and How to Use Urate-Lowering Therapy', *Postgraduate Medicine*, 104 (6), 117–127.

55. Vazques-Mellado, J, et al. 1999; 'Intradermal Tophi in Gout: A Case Control Study', *Journal of Rheumatology*, 26 (1), 136–140.

56. Arthur, V. 1998; 'The Rheumatic Conditions: An Overview', in *Rheumatology Nursing: A Creative Approach*, Hill, J (ed.), Churchill Livingstone, Edinburgh, 21–58.

57. Baird, CL. 2001; 'First-Line Treatment for Osteoarthritis, Part 1: Pathology, Assessment, and Pharmacologic Interventions', *Orthopaedic Nursing*, 20 (5), 17–26.

58. Maher, AB, Salmond, SW & Pellino, TA. 2001; *Orthopaedic Nursing*, W.B. Saunders, Philadelphia.

59. Vallerand, AH. 2003; 'Treating Osteoarthritis Pain', *The Nurse Practitioner*, 28 (4), 7–17.

60. Moore, A, Edwards, J, Barden, J & McQuay, H. 2003; *Bandolier's Little Book of Pain*, Oxford University Press, Oxford.

61. Klippel, JH & Dieppe, PA. 1998; *Rheumatology* (2nd ed.), Mosby, St Louis.

62. Cope, AP. 2003; 'Exploring the Reciprocal Relationship between Immunity and Inflammation in Chronic Inflammatory Arthritis', *Rheumatology*, 42, 716–731.

63. Lasater, K & Groer, M. 2001; 'Arthritis', in M Groer (ed.), *Advanced Pathophysiology: Application to Clinical Practice*, Lippincott, Philadelphia, 245–265.

64. Dayer, JM. 2003; 'The Pivotal Role of Interleukin–1 in the Clincial Manifestations of Rheumatoid Arthritis', *Rheumatology*, 42 (supplement 2), ii3–ii10.

65. Goldring, SR. 2003; 'Pathogenesis of Bone and Cartilage Destruction in Rheumatoid Arthritis', *Rheumatology*, 42 (supplement 2), ii11–ii16.

66. Hill, J. 1998; *Rheumatology Nursing*, Edinburgh: Churchill Livingstone.

67. Ostergaard, M & Szkudlarek, M. 2003; 'Imaging in Rheumatoid Arthritis: Why MRI and Ultrasonography Can No Longer Be Ignored', *Scandinavian Journal of Rheumatology*, 32, 63–73.

68. Hazes, JMW. 2003; 'Determinants of Physical Function in Rheumatoid Arthritis: Association with the Disease Process', *Rheumatology*, 42 (supplement 2), ii17–ii21.

69. Breedveld, FC. 2003; 'Should Rheumatoid Arthritis Be Treated Conservatively or Aggressively?', *Rheumatology*, 42 (supplement 2), ii41–ii43.

12 | Haematological Health Breakdown

AUTHORS

YVONNE WHITE

FRAN OWEN

JOHN SIBBALD

PATRICK CROOKES

LEARNING OBJECTIVES

When you have completed this chapter you will be able to
- Outline the basic components of the blood and haematopoietic system;
- Describe common conditions which result in blood and haematopoietic dysfunction;
- Apply the goals of specific pharmacological management to common blood and haematopoietic dysfunctions; and
- Describe nursing actions relevant to the management of a person with a common blood or haematopoietic dysfunction.

INTRODUCTION

This chapter presents a review of the anatomy and physiology of blood and haematopoiesis, including components of plasma, blood cell types, haemostasis, and blood groups. Using a case-study approach, two general categories of common blood and haemopoeitic health breakdowns are then presented. These are red blood cell and coagulation disorders. Issues related to dysfunction of white blood cells or bone marrow, are discussed in Chapter 14 (see sections on leukaemia and myeloma).

HAEMOPOEITIC SYSTEM OVERVIEW

Blood is a viscous (sticky) fluid and its red colour is familiar to most people. The main reason blood is viscous is because it is not strictly true simply to call it a fluid. It is fact a liquid (plasma) with cells suspended in it (which is why blood is classified as a connective tissue). This can be demonstrated easily by taking a sample of blood, adding some heparin to it to prevent it from clotting and then spinning it in a centrifuge. After spinning a test tube of blood for a few minutes it can be seen that it separates into two parts. The top of the test tube will be seen to contain a yellowish fluid – the plasma, while at the bottom of the tube will be seen a solid red mass which can be demonstrated to be composed of cells. If one looks carefully at the test tube it will be seen that the plasma occupies approximately 55% of the total volume, and the cells approximately 45% of the total volume[1]. The measurement of of the percentage of cells to plasma is the haematocrit (Hct). The cell mass may also have a very thin top layer (less than 1% of the total volume) which consists of white blood cells (WBCs), whilst the rest of the cell mass will be red blood cells[1,2].

These red blood cells (erythrocytes; RBCs) account for 99% of cells in the blood. They are non–nucleated; biconcave discs approximately 7 μm in diameter. This shape gives the red cell a larger surface area to volume ratio, which enhances cell flexibility and ensures minimal membrane tension during volume changes, when the cells give up oxygen in the tissues and take it up in the lungs[1,2]. This flexibility enables the RBC to elongate when passing through capillaries, further increasing surface area for gas transport. Repeated deformation contributes to the limited life of erythrocytes.

Red cells contain haemoglobin, a large molecular weight protein – globin – each molecule of which contains four haem groups. Each haem group contain a ferrous iron (Fe^{2+}) atom that combines quickly and reversibly with one molecule of oxygen. Each molecule of haemoglobin can therefore carry up to four molecules of oxygen. The primary function of red cells is to transport oxygen, although globin also transports some carbon dioxide (CO_2). Red cells contain carbonic anhydrase, an enzyme important in CO_2 transport.

Red cell production (erythropoiesis) occurs in red bone marrow in adults; this is usually confined to the sternum (breastbone) and the iliac crest (hipbone). In children nearly all long bones contain red bone marrow. In the fetus red cell production also occurs in the liver and spleen. As children reach maturity red bone marrow is gradually replaced with yellow bone marrow until in the adult only the two sites of red cell production noted above remain. However, in times of need, for example following an accident with loss of blood, some yellow bone marrow may convert back to red marrow to assist in the replacement of lost red cells[1,2].

The rate of erythrocyte production is controlled by erythropoietin, a hormone produced by the kidneys. This hormone is secreted in response to a fall in the oxygen content of arterial blood. If you think about this for a moment you will appreciate that there are two main situations in which this occurs:

1. When there is a drop in the number of red cells – since they are the major means by which oxygen is carried in the blood; and
2. When the environmental oxygen pressure is low – for example, at high altitude. People living in the Himalayas have increased numbers of red cells – a condition called polycythaemia.

This condition is sometimes encountered in people who have chronic obstructive airways limitation (CAL), (see Chapter 6). Some essential dietary requirements for red cell production are iron, folic acid and vitamin B_{12}[1,2].

Because red cells have no nucleus they have a limited lifespan. Generally mature cells survive in the blood for up to 120 days. Aged red cells are extracted from the blood by macrophages of the reticuloendothelial system (i.e., macrophages in red bone marrow, liver, spleen, lymph nodes and loose connective tissue) and broken down. Globin is degraded into amino acids (which are recycled) while haem is converted to bilirubin (transported to the liver and excreted in bile) and iron is also recovered and recycled[1,2].

White blood cells (leucocytes; WBCs) are nucleated and much larger than red cells. There are comparatively few in the blood, around 1% of the total cell mass of the blood. Many of the white cells found in the blood are in transit to tissues. There are many types of white cells but all fall into one of two main classes – those that have granules in their cytoplasm (granulocytes) and those that don't (agranulocytes).

Granulocytes are further subdivided into three types depending on the sort of dye they stain with in a laboratory:

1. Neutrophils (stain with neutral dyes) account for 40–75% of WBCs, have a polymorphic (literally many shaped) nucleus and are phagocytes;
2. Eosinophils (stain with acid dyes) have a typical two-lobed nucleus, and inactivate histamine, phagocytose antigen-antibody complexes, and release fibrinolysin (an enzyme which breaks down fibrin); and
3. Basophils (stain with basic dyes) have a large nucleus generally obscured by granules, release histamine and heparin, and are sometimes referred to as mast cells[1,2].

Agranulocytes are divided into two groups – lymphocytes and monocytes. Lymphocytes may be small (7–9 μm) or large (8–16 μm) in diameter. Lymphocytes have a large dense nucleus and play a key role in humoral and cell-mediated immunity (see Chapter 13). Monocytes are the largest blood cells and are referred to as tissue macrophages (i.e., they have a largely phagocytic function[1,2]).

Thrombocytes (platelets) are also contained in the blood and are really small pieces of cytoplasm, 2–3 μm in diameter. They are derived from large cells in the red bone marrow called megakarocytes, and play an important role in the clotting of the blood[1,2].

Plasma forms approximately 55% of the blood. Its composition is 90% water, 8% protein, and 2% organic compounds and ions. As plasma is mainly water it carries many water-soluble substances around the body. The plasma also contains 'plasma proteins' – albumin, globulins and fibrinogen. Albumin is the most abundant of the plasma proteins (40 g/L), is produced in the liver and is a major contributor to the colloid osmotic pressure of blood. Albumin carries (in loose combination) hormones, bilirubin, fatty acids, bile salts, heavy metals and some drugs. It also buffers H^+ ions and transports a small amount of CO_2. Alpha-globulin (α-globulin) and beta-globulin (β-globulin) are also made in the liver and they transport various hormones, vitamins and minerals. Gamma-globulin (γ-globulin; also called immunoglobulins – some of the β-globulins are also immunoglobulins), are made in plasma cells. There are five types and each has a different function in immunity. Fibrinogen is also made in the liver. This is a large protein (the largest of all the plasma proteins) which is converted to insoluble fibrin during the clotting process[1,2].

HAEMOSTASIS

Haemostasis refers to the control and arrest of bleeding. It is a 'self defence' mechanism of the blood, and of the body, given the importance of the blood to the body. There are three components of haemostasis:

1. Blood vessel reactions;
2. Platelet reactions; and
3. Blood coagulation.

Tissue injury results in the release of products that cause local vasospasm and constriction of smooth muscle in the surrounding vessels resulting in an initial reduction in blood flow to the injured area. This compensatory mechanism lessens blood loss and assists in coagulation or clotting of the blood[1,2]. Injury also exposes collagen fibres in the sub-endothelial tissue, resulting in adherence of platelets and activation of several clotting factors. After adhering to the collagen, platelets release a number of substances: serotonin 5-HT (causes further vasoconstriction); ADP (which causes platelet aggregation and starts the process of formation of a plug at the site of the vessel damage); and thromboxane A2 (which also enhances platelet aggregation and vasoconstriction). Aspirin inhibits the synthesis of thromboxane[1,2].

Blood coagulation is a cascade or chain reaction of events where a stimulus changes circulating substances in the blood into an insoluble gel. There are 12 coagulation factors (proteins) synthesised by the liver. Vitamin K is an important co-factor for the synthesis of factors II, VII, IX and X. Calcium is also required in the coagulation, as it forms factor IV.

There are two paths by which coagulation occurs – the extrinsic and intrinsic pathways. Normally both pathways are required for haemostasis. The extrinsic pathway is activated principally by tissue factor (thromboplastin; factor III) and thromboxane A2, but may involve other factors that are released by damaged tissue. The intrinsic pathway is activated by substances 'intrinsic' to the vascular system when there is abnormal exposure of collagen fibres in the endothelial layer of the damaged vessel. Each pathway begins in a different way, but both lead to the final common path where the conversion of an active precursor prothrombin (factor II) to thrombin, and then thrombin to soluble fibrinogen (factor I) results in fibrin formation and coagulation[1,2].

Some important points to remember about coagulation are that:

- Calcium and vitamin K are necessary for synthesis of clotting factors and initiation of the coagulation cascade;[1,2]
- The chain reaction results in amplification and acceleration (a small stimulus results in an 'explosive' response);[1,2]

- Coagulation is normally controlled by antithrombins in plasma (which are potentiated by heparin)[1,2]; and
- Fibrin is eventually broken down by plasmin which is normally present as an inactive precursor plasminogen[1,2].

BLOOD GROUPS

Blood transfusion was attempted many times in the past. Sometimes it was successful but more often resulted in the death of the recipient. Why? Well, it is now common knowledge that there are different blood types and that donor and recipient blood have to be compatible for a successful transfusion. Incidentally, if you stop and think about it, a blood transfusion is a type of organ transplant and was indeed the first successful organ transplant[1,2].

Our modern system of blood typing (or grouping) dates back to the work of Landsteiner who in 1900 showed that all human blood could be divided into four groups on the basis of two antigens – A and B – present on the surface of the red cell. He further showed that there were also two antibodies corresponding to these antigens, present in the plasma – α and β. Thus based on this system four blood groups are possible (see Table 12.1)[1,2].

The incidence of these blood groups in the general population in Australia and New Zealand is A (38%), B (10%), O (49%), and AB (3%)[3,4]. There are however racial variations. For example, indigenous peoples have higher proportions of group A and lower proportions of group B[3,4], and group AB is more common in Asian people[1,2].

Donor cells must be compatible with the recipient's plasma. A little thought will show that it is possible to transfuse blood between groups safely as illustrated in Table 12.2[1,2]. Thus, group O are 'universal donors' and group AB are 'universal recipients'.

TABLE 12.1: BLOOD GROUPS		
Group	**Red Cells (Antigen)**	**Plasma (Antibodies)**
A	A	β
B	B	α
AB	A and B	–
O	–	α and β

TABLE 12.2: BLOOD TRANSFUSION COMPATIBILITY				
Group	**Recipient**			
Donor	**A**	**B**	**O**	**AB**
A	✓	×	×	✓
B	×	✓	×	✓
AB	×	×	×	✓
O	✓	✓	✓	✓

When incompatible blood is transfused the antibody(ies) present in the plasma react with the antigens on the red cell surface and cause them to agglutinate (stick together), lyse (break up) and thus liberate haemoglobin into the circulation. This causes kidney damage and death[1,2].

Since 1900 many other antigens and antibodies which affect compatibility have been discovered. There are now at least fifteen well established blood group systems. The most important of the other antigens is a red cell antigen D – otherwise known as the Rhesus factor (it was first discovered in the Rhesus monkey). Individuals who possess the D antigen are said to be Rh positive (85% of the general population); those who do are Rh negative (15% of the general population). There is no natural antibody to D but if an Rh^- person is given Rh^+ blood they will develop antibodies and any subsequent transfusion with Rh^+ blood will result in an incompatibility reaction[1,2].

If an Rh^- woman carries an Rh^+ fetus then at birth some of the baby's red cells may infiltrate the mother's circulation. If this happens she will develop D antibodies. If she carries a subsequent Rh^+ child, those antibodies will cross the placenta and will cause an incompatibility reaction in the fetus. The baby may die in utero, or may be born severely jaundiced (from excessive bilirubin due to the breakdown of haemoglobin from lysed red cells)[1,2]. Women who are Rh^- can be immunised to prevent Rh sensitisation.

In about 80% of people the A and B antigens are also present in secretions like tears, saliva, sweat, semen and breast milk. These people are called 'secretors'; the remaining 20% of the population are known as 'non-secretors'. Thus it is possible to classify secretors into ABO groups, a matter of great importance in forensic science[1,2].

KEY SUMMARY POINTS

1. Blood has two components, cellular components and a fluid component.
2. Red blood cells contain haemoglobin, which is vital for the transport of oxygen to the body tissues.
3. Both cellular components and plasma proteins play a vital role in haemostasis to reduce blood loss.
4. Haemostasis involves a complex chain reaction which is triggered by damage to endothelial tissue; an interaction of factors results in the formation of a platelet plug.

RED BLOOD CELL DISORDERS

ANAEMIA

Anaemia is a term that describes a decrease in or a dysfunction of red blood cells (RBC). Anaemia can be an acute or chronic condition. There are several causes of anaemia which can be classified as: a) RBC loss without RBC destruction; b) deficient RBC production; c) and increased RBC destruction over production[5,6]. Table 12.3 lists the common causes of anaemia)[5,6].

WHAT IS THE PATHOPHYSIOLOGY?

Homeostatic mechanisms normally ensure that the cardiac output delivers enough oxygen-carrying blood to the tissues to maintain normal functioning. The processes of ventilation, respiration and cardiac output are discussed more fully in Chapter 5 and Chapter 6. At

TABLE 12.3: CAUSES OF ANAEMIA[7]	
	Common Causes of Anaemia
RBC	• Haemorrhage (e.g., trauma, menstrual disorders, GIT bleeding, endometriosis, fibroids, parasitism)
Depressed RBC production	• Cancers (leukaemia, bone metastases, osteogenic sarcoma) • Lack of vitamin B_{12} (inadequate intake, malabsorption, lack of the intrinsic factor) • Iron deficiency (inadequate intake, chronic bleeding) • Decreased folic acid (inadequate intake, excessive alcohol intake) • Aplastic anaemia (may be associated with some medications, e.g., chloramphenicol administration) • Renal disease (lack of erythropoietin production)
Increased RBC destruction over production (haemolytic anaemias)	• Intrinsic abnormalities • Thalassemia • Sickle cell anemia • Hereditary spherocytosis • Extrinsic abnormalities • Infections • Malaria (*Plasmodiumm* species) • *Mycoplasma* • Disseminated intravascular coagulation (DIC) • Lead poisoning

rest, the body requires 250 mL of oxygen per minute to maintain normal functioning. Under normal conditions a cardiac output of 5 L/min maintains the required level of 250 mL of oxygen per minute more than adequately (in a young male adult, the standard for discussing human physiology)[7]. A less than adequate supply of oxygen leads to tissue hypoxia and hypoxaemia (reduced oxygen saturation). The kidneys play a vital role in the detection of hypoxaemia. The renal peritubular interstitial cells are sensitive to blood oxygen concentration and in response to hypoxaemia, produce erythropoietin (EPO). In combination with other factors, EPO increases RBC production by stimulating the bone marrow to produce pre-erythrocyte cells (reticulocytes)[2,7]. The number of RBCs per cubic millimetre of blood can be counted, and along with the haematocrit or packed cell volume, provides an indication of the numbers of RBCs in the circulation[2,7].

Iron deficiency anaemia is the most common anaemia globally[5]. As noted earlier, iron is a component of haemoglobin and is essential for an optimal oxygen–carrying capacity by RBCs. A full blood count (FBC) would show microcytic (small cell) and hypochromic (pale colour) RBCs with a decreased mean cell volume[5]. Deficiency in either vitamin B_{12} or folic acid leads to megaloblastic (large cell) anaemias. These chronic forms of anaemia would show large RBCs, a very low haemoglobin, but possibly with a normal haematocrit due to the large size of red cells[5].

Haemolytic anaemia (increased destruction over production of RBC) may occur as a result of internal (e.g., immune disorders) or external factors such as chemical (e.g., certain medications); physical (e.g., excess heat as in severe burns); or infectious agents (e.g., bacterial toxins, malaria)[5,6]. Sickle cell anaemia is an inherited haemoglobinopathy[6], which demonstrates sickle-shaped RBCs. This mishape impairs the RBC ability to adsorb oxygen and the RBC are seen as damaged which leads to clumping of the sickle cells and possibly a vascular occlusion can occur. This occlusion is related to the ability of the 'sickled' cells to clump together and block blood vessels[5,7].

WHAT ARE THE CLINICAL MANIFESTATIONS?

Tissue oxygenation is impaired because of the reduced oxygen carrying capacity of the RBCs. Symptoms occur in relation to the severity and onset of the anaemia and the degree of oxygen deficiency present. The most common clinical symptoms include fatigue and weakness – although anaemia may be asymptomatic especially if it develops over time, and the body is able to compensate for a period of time. All people with anaemia may have pallor, but this sign may be apparent earlier in the condition in people of Caucasian origin.[5,7] This may be especially noticeable in the conjunctiva of the eyes. As the anaemia becomes more severe, then shortness of breath, tachycardia and cardiac arrhythmias may occur as a result of tissue hypoxia. People with a pre-existing cardiac condition are more at risk of developing congestive cardiac failure if they have an associated anaemia. Anaemia is often a *symptom* of an underlying disease process (e.g., chronic renal failure, sickle cell disease)[5,7].

DIAGNOSTIC TESTS

As anaemia is a disorder of RBCs, the relevant diagnostic tests focus on assessment of the erythrocytes. These tests involve haemoglobin level, haematocrit, RBC volume, and the haemoglobin carrying capacity of the RBCs (MCH and MCHV) (see Table 12.4[5,7,8]). Other tests would involve assessment for underlying causes, for example iron studies and vitamin B_{12} levels.

WHAT IS THE TREATMENT?

Management strategies for anaemia differ depending on the underlying cause. Blood loss anaemia (RBC loss without RBC destruction) is most commonly related to haemorrhage, and is treated by the infusion of packed RBCs[5,7,9]. Anaemia resulting from acute blood loss may not be reflected in the haemoglobin (Hb) or haematocrit (Hct) levels in the early phases; it may be 48–72 hours[5,6,7] before an accurate and stable assessment of anaemia can be determined. This is because the blood cells and plasma are lost equally. As blood loss continues, body fluid will shift from the extracellular compartment to the intravascular compartment, which has a dilutional effect on Hb and Hct. A full blood count will show a normochromic (normal colour) and normocytic (normal size) anaemia and a normal mean cell volume. Chronic blood loss is common along the gastrointestinal tract, especially in aged people[5,7,9].

Deficient RBC production (e.g., related to nutritional deficiency) is treated according to the underlying cause. For iron deficiency anaemia, iron supplementation and EPO may be administered[5,7], although profound symptoms may also require packed cell infusions.

APPLIED PHARMACOLOGY

Iron is absorbed from the gut and is better absorbed if in the ferrous form. Iron can be given by oral, intramuscular and intravenous routes. If given orally, the administration of oral vitamin C increases iron absorption by reducing dietary ferric iron to ferrous iron[10,11].

TABLE 12.4: TESTS TO ASSESS HAEMATOLOGICAL FUNCTION[5,7,8]

Test	Normal Range*	Significance
Mean corpuscular volume (MCV)	80–100 fL	The average size of the erythrocytes. Result will be raised if cells are large (macrocytic), and decreased if cells are small (microcytic)
Total RBC count	$4.5–6.50 \times 10^{12}$/L	Normal RBC cell count varies with age, gender, altitude and exercise. Blood volume also affects results; hypervolaemia will show a dilutional effect with the RBC count being lower; in hypovolaemia a haemoconcentration effect will reflect a higher RBC count
Haemoglobin (Hb)	130–180 g/L	Normal values vary with age, gender, altitude and exercise. Blood volume will also affect the value; hypervolaemia will show a decreased level, and in hypovolaemia a high level
Mean Corpuscular Haemoglobin (MCH)	26–33 pg	The average amount of haemoglobin in each red blood cell
Mean Corpuscular Haemoglobin Concentration (MCHC)	310–360 g/L	The average weight (grams) of haemoglobin in each red blood cell
Serum Vitamin B_{12}	120–600 pmol/L	A vital factor in erythropoiesis; used to assess macrocytic anaemia
Serum Folate	7–25 nmol/L	A vital factor in erythropoiesis; used to assess macrocytic anaemia
Serum Ferritin	20–300 ug/L	Indicates total body store of iron
Red cell volume (Hct)	0.40–0.54	Volume of red blood cells expressed as a % of total blood volume
White blood cell count	$3.5–11 \times 10^9$/L	Measures the number and types of white blood cells
Bone Marrow Biopsies	n/a	Removal of a small amount of bone marrow by needle biopsy; allows evaluation of cellular components in the marrow and bone marrow iron stores; test is contraindicated in people with known coagulation defects[8]
Coagulation assays	Varies according to factor	Measures specific coagulation factors; used to assess the level of severity of the deficiency/ies[8]
Bleeding time	1–9 min	The time taken for bleeding to stop naturally
International Normalised Ratio (INR)	Variable according to therapeutic reason	Time for coagulation to occur after the addition of thromboplastin and calcium to the blood specimen

TABLE 12.4: (cont'd)		
Activated Partial Prothrombin Time (APPT)	30–40 sec; 60–70 sec (without activators) in an adult[8]	Evaluates the intrinsic clotting pathway; measures the time for a clot to form when activators are added to the specimen to shorten the clotting time
Erythrocyte Sedimentation Rate (ESR)	Varies	Alteration in blood proteins results in aggregation of RBCs; raised values indicative of an inflammatory process
Sickle-Cell Test	Negative	Demonstrates the presence of Haemoglobin S; RBCs that contain this are sickle shaped when deprived of oxygen
Direct Coombs' Test	Negative = no agglutination	Detects antibodies or complement bound to red blood cells and is indicative of haemolytic anaemias; RBCs are mixed with Coombs' reagent to test for agglutinins that lead to clumping and haemolysis
Indirect Coombs' Test	Negative = no agglutination	Used in routine cross matching of blood before transfusion and during pregnancy, as it detects antibody in the serum

Note: normal ranges may vary to a small degree due to different clinical laboratory reference values.

The majority of iron administered is bound to transferrin and transported to the bone marrow. The remaining iron will be stored as haemosiderin and ferritin[10].

EPO is a recombinant form of the natural occurring human EPO, and is administered either subcutaneously or intravenously. Currently there are two types of EPO for injection epoetin alpha and darbepoeitin alpha. The dosage is variable and titrated according to the individual response. Decreased responsiveness to EPO therapy is consistent with decreased vitamin B_{12}, decreased iron stores, aluminium toxicity and bone marrow fibrosis. During EPO therapy patients should have their Hb and iron stores monitored. This is usually done on a monthly basis in cases of anaemia associated with renal failure[10].

NURSING IMPLICATIONS

Any transfusion of blood products requires diligent checking to ensure the patient receives the correct unit of compatible blood[5,12]. Patient vital signs should be checked at the start of a transfusion, and every 15 minutes, and if there is any reaction experienced by the patient[12].

EPO administration is a safe therapy to promote erythropoiesis. Adverse reactions include flu-like symptoms, hypertension and seizure activity. Contraindications to the administration of EPO are hypertension, seizure activity and thrombotic events[9,10]. EPO can be administered either subcutaneously or intravenously. Subcutaneous injections are convenient for those who can self-administer. EPO is usually given intravenously in those persons with renal failure and who are on haemodialysis. The storage of EPO is very important in that it is prone to denature if it is frozen or becomes over heated. Therefore EPO should be kept at 2–8°C, and, if transport is required, this should be arranged to maintain the recommended storage guidelines[9,10].

Iron can be administered either by the oral, intramuscular or intravenous route. Oral iron should be administered with or immediately after food to reduce the risk of gastrointestinal irritation. There are several medications and foods that inhibit gastric absorption of iron (e.g., antacids, milk, and eggs). If administering intramuscularly, a deep intramuscular injection into the gluteus maximus should be undertaken using the Z-track technique to prevent skin staining and to promote absorption[10,11].

When administering iron intravenously (iron polymaltose), it should be diluted in normal saline and infused slowly to avoid the risk of anaphylaxis. Overdose of iron is treated by the use of chelating agents such as desferrioxamine, which binds with the iron and is excreted via the urine and the faeces[10,11].

LEARNING EXERCISES

1. What is the relationship between erythropoietin and eryhthropoiesis?
2. Why are the levels of vitamin B_{12} and iron important in the responsiveness to EPO therapy?
3. Why is Vitamin C administered with oral iron supplementation?

POLYCYTHAEMIA

Polycythaemia refers to a condition where there is an abnormal increase in RBC production. Polycythaemia can be either primary or secondary[5,7].

WHAT IS THE PATHOPHYSIOLOGY?

Primary polycythaemia is very rare and involves the over-production of RBC, leucocytes and platelets. Primary polycythaemia is a neoplastic disease with an unknown cause, which can lead to hypertension and venous stasis. Venous stasis can be noticed with a 'ruddiness' of the face, hands, feet and mucous membranes [7]. Secondary polycythaemia results from an increased production of EPO in response to hypoxia and is most commonly associated with an underlying cause (e.g., chronic hypoxia, high altitude, and chronic pulmonary and/or cardiac diseases)[5,7].

WHAT ARE THE CLINICAL MANIFESTATIONS?

Most symptoms are associated with the excess RBC, which results in hypervolaemia, and an increase in blood viscosity, which contribute to the development of hypertension and the development of thrombosis[5,7].

DIAGNOSTIC TESTS

A full blood count would demonstrate a high Hb level with a Hct greater than 55%[7].

WHAT IS THE TREATMENT?

The management of polycythaemia is related to control of the symptoms and the prevention of complications. Treatment includes episodic phlebotomy (venesection) to remove 200–500 mL of blood when required, as well as bone marrow suppression (e.g., interferon) to reduce RBC production[5,7].

APPLIED PHARMACOLOGY

Pharmacological management would include symptomatic control of complications related to polycythaemia (e.g., antihypertensives to aid the control of blood pressure). Pharmacological management would also be related to the control of underlying causes (e.g., pulmonary and cardiac disease – see Chapters 5 and 6)[5,7].

NURSING IMPLICATIONS

The risk of hypertension and thrombotic events are high in people with polycythaemia. Therefore, a thorough assessment of the individual for any signs of hypertension or thrombotic events should be undertaken. These would include regular monitoring of blood pressure and observation for any evidence of deep vein thrombosis, pulmonary emboli, cerebrovascular accidents, etc[5,7].

LEARNING EXERCISES
1. Explain why hypertension is a real risk in polycythaemia.
2. Why is phlebotomy used to treat polycythaemia?
3. Describe the compensatory mechanisms where patients with chronic airway limitation develop polycythaemia.

COAGULATION DISORDERS

THROMBOCYTOPENIA

Thrombocytopenia refers to a reduced number of platelets (normal range: 150–400 × 10^9/L)[13]. As platelets are a vital component of the clotting process, a reduced number of platelets may result in bleeding[5,7].

WHAT IS THE PATHOPHYSIOLOGY?

Thrombocytopenia or low platelet count can occur due to an under-production or increase in destruction of platelets. Destruction of platelets is commonly caused by the formation of gamma globulin (IgG) antibodies to platelets[13]. Idiopathic thrombocytopenia purpura (ITP) is characterised by a marked decrease in platelets as a result of an immune disorder. ITP can be either acute or chronic. Acute ITP presents as a sudden severe thrombocytopenia, and occurs commonly after a viral illness in children. In adults ITP is also associated with post-viral illness (mononucleosis), illicit drug use (cocaine, heroin), prescription drugs (quinine, sulpha-based drugs and salicylates), or with no identifiable underlying cause (idiopathic). Chronic ITP is a result of an autoimmune process of IgG-mediated phagocytosis, causing premature platelet destruction, particularly in the spleen, and is more common in young women[9].

ITP can be also classified as 'secondary' and is associated with several disorders such as systemic lupus erythomatosis, human immunodeficiency virus (HIV), sarcoidosis, and Hodgkin's lymphoma). The ITP may result in remission with the treatment of the underlying disease[9].

WHAT ARE THE CLINICAL MANIFESTATIONS?

Acute ITP may result in spontaneous bleeding when the platelet count falls below the normal range, and major haemorrhage is more likely to occur when the count is below $20 \times 10^9/L$. Patients with a low platelet count are more likely to have minor vascular bleeding from the nose and the mouth.

Chronic ITP often presents as a slow onset of bleeding symptoms. It can be an incidental finding in people who are having routine blood tests for other reasons[13].

● Case study

Sandy McPherson, 17, presented to her general practitioner with a sore throat two weeks ago, and was prescribed a penicillin-based antibiotic as well as aspirin 600 mg regularly for several days until her symptoms resolved.

Sandy then presented to the emergency department of her local hospital after noticing a fine pinpoint rash over her lower legs and buttocks. Sandy stated that she had also been bleeding from the gums over the past three days after brushing her teeth. She denied having any nosebleeds, or noticing any blood in her urine. On examination, it was noted that Sandy had several bruises on her thighs. Sandy denied any illicit drug use and the only medication she was now on was the contraceptive pill. She also stated that she had no allergies.

Further investigation showed Sandy's oral temperature was 36.5°C, her pulse rate was 80 beats/min and regular, blood pressure was 120/70 mmHg, and a routine urinalysis showed no abnormalities.

WHAT SHOULD YOU BE LOOKING AT IN THE LABORATORY AND OTHER TESTS?

During her presentation at the emergency department Sandy underwent several tests. These included a chest X-ray which demonstrated no abnormalities; a full blood count which revealed a Hb of 127, WBC 7.0, platelets $8 \times 10^9/L$. Serum urea, creatinine, electrolytes, coagulation studies and liver function tests were within normal range. A monotest was negative, IgG was positive, consistent with exposure to the Epstein Barr Virus, and IgM was negative. Sandy was also crossmatched in readiness for a blood product transfusion if required.

WHAT IS THE TREATMENT?

The treatment for ITP includes platelet transfusions (given only in the presence of significant bleeding), high-dose IgG, corticosteroids, and splenectomy (effective in 70% of patients). High-dose IgG is usually given in cases of acute ITP and will increase the platelet count by 70–80% of patients – however this may only be a transient rise. Corticosteroids (commonly prednisone) are administered at a high dose for several days to suppress immune function, and then weaned. This treatment will raise the platelet count in most patients[10,11]. As prednisone is a corticosteroid, all general issues related to steroid therapy apply[6,8].

Sandy was admitted to the haematology unit with the diagnosis of ITP. Management included medication (prednisone 50 mg/day, Mylanta 10 mL qid prn, and temazepam 1–2 tablets per night for sedation), and monitoring for complications and response to treatment. Monitoring included 4-hourly measurements of vital signs (T, PR, RR), twice daily blood sugar levels, ensuring a FBC was performed each day, and observing for any sign of overt or concealed haemorrhage. Sandy's doctor had also written an order to commence a platelet transfusion if any active bleeding was suspected.

Sandy was discharged two days later with a Hb of 124, WBC 7.5, platelets 24×10^9/L. There had been no obvious signs of bleeding. Sandy was discharged on prednisone 50 mg per day, with close follow up to be monitored by her general practitioner and specialist. Sandy was to continue to have a FBC performed second daily.

Over the next few weeks Sandy's platelet count continued to rise. One month after discharge Sandy was admitted to the day-stay ward for an infusion of disodium pamidronate, which inhibits osteoclastic bone resorption and prevents steroid-induced osteoporosis[10,11]. Sandy's dose of prednisone was gradually reduced and was ceased two months after presentation at the emergency department.

Within nine weeks Sandy's platelet count had returned to normal range, however she continued to be monitored on a monthly basis. Six months on, Sandy's platelet count was stable and her specialist felt that her ITP had completely resolved.

NURSING IMPLICATIONS

Anyone on steroid therapy should be monitored for the development of any of the multiple adverse effects of this therapy. People on steroid therapy need to be aware that they may be more prone to infections whilst undergoing therapy. Steroid therapy should not be suddenly stopped as this may induce adrenal insufficiency syndrome[10,11].

Disodium pamidronate must be diluted in 0.9% saline and administered over a period of two hours; it must never be given as a bolus dose due to the high risk of thrombophlebitis[10,11]. Patients should have serum calcium and phosphate levels monitored as hypocalcaemia is a potential adverse effect of disodium pamidronate administration[10,11].

LEARNING EXERCISES

1. What advice should be given to patients with ITP?
2. Why is hypocalcaemia a risk with disodium pamidronate therapy?

COAGULATION FACTOR DISORDERS

HAEMOPHILIA

Haemophilia is a genetically inherited bleeding disorder related to a lack of essential clotting factors. The types of haemophilia are: haemophilia A (decreased factor VIII), haemophilia B (Christmas disease; decreased factor IX), and as associated condition von Willebrand's Disease (vWD; a decreased factor that co-circulates with factor VIII)[5,7,9,14].

WHAT IS THE PATHOPHYSIOLOGY?

Haemophilia is a recessive inherited disorder transmitted via the X chromosome, and is therefore a disorder seen almost exclusively in males as they have only one X chromosome[14]. Von Willebrand's Disease is due to a lack of the von Willebrand's Factor (vWF), a protein that circulates with factor VIII and helps platelets bind to the endothelium at an injury site to result in haemostasis[5-7,9]. It is possible for the body to have decreased amounts of the vWF, or for the vWF that is present to be dysfunctional[5-7,9].

WHAT ARE THE CLINICAL MANIFESTATIONS?

Haemophilia is a disorder that is usually diagnosed in childhood as an incidental finding associated with a traumatic event. Suspicions are usually aroused in relation to the persistence of bleeding related to the extent of the trauma[5-7,9].

WHAT SHOULD YOU BE LOOKING AT IN THE LABORATORY AND OTHER TESTS?

In haemophilias it is vital to assess the coagulation ability of the blood, therefore coagulation studies, platelets levels and activated partial thromboplastin time (APTT, which is increased in haemophilias) should be assessed and monitored at regular intervals (see Table 12.4). Clotting factor assays should also be undertaken and expected results would be decreased level of factor VIII in haemophilia A and vWD, and decreased level of factor IX in haemophilia B[5-7,9].

WHAT IS THE TREATMENT?

Management of haemophilia relies on the early recognition of haemorrhage before overt symptoms occur, and the immediate administration of clotting factors (usually factor VIII or cryoprecipitate). Cryoprecipitate is prepared from fresh frozen plasma and contains fibrinogen and factor VIII. For vWD, bleeding is managed by the administration of desmopressin and cryoprecipitate. People with either haemophilia or vWD need to be aware of lifestyle limitations to reduce the risk of haemorrhage, and should be advised to wear an identity bracelet noting their disease[5-7,9].

APPLIED PHARMACOLOGY

The administration of desmopressin stimulates the release of body stores of the vWF[11]. Desmopressin should not be used in cases of vWD type IIB as it may lead to an increase in platelet aggregation[11].

NURSING IMPLICATIONS

The administration of cryoprecipitate has all the potential risks associated with the administration of blood products. Patients should also be advised to observe for any signs of haemorrhage such as swelling particularly around joints, and bruising[12]. If a joint is painful or there is overt swelling the joint should be immobilised and medical attention sought. Patient education to encourage effective self-management should be undertaken by the nurse. This education should include making the home safe, to use electric razors when shaving, soft bristle toothbrushes, how to administer clotting factors at home, and to avoid activities that may result in trauma[12]. Patients should also be advised that they should not take aspirin due to the increased risk of haemorrhage as a result of the pharmacological action of aspirin.[10]

ANTICOAGULANT TOXICITY

Anticoagulation therapy is used in a variety of medical conditions with the most common medications being warfarin and heparin. Warfarin inhibits the action of vitamin K on specific clotting factors (II, VII, IX and X) [8]. The action of warfarin is not immediate and occurs over 48–72 hours and the anticoagulation effect may persist for 4–5 days following the cessation of therapy[11]. The dosage of warfarin must be individualised and is adjusted depending on the international normalised ratio (INR) result. The INR range during warfarin administration is very narrow (see Table 12.5 for recommended reference ranges)[10].

The most common range for the INR is 2.0–2.5, however for those people who have undergone arterial or cardiac grafts and cardiac prosthetic valves require an INR range from 3.0–4.5[10]. This is due to the higher risk of thrombus formation in these groups. Response to warfarin is monitored by a daily INR until the patient becomes stable, and then at regular intervals following as set by the medical practitioner. Heparin has a direct anticoagulant action that potentiates the naturally occurring inhibitors of coagulation, antifactor Xa and antithrombin III, which then slows conversion of prothrombin to thrombin and fibrinogen to fibrin[10,11]. Heparin also impairs platelet function[11]. Low molecular weight heparin has a more specific effect with a reduced effect on thrombin and platelets[10]. Anticoagulant therapy carries a risk of anticoagulant toxicity.

WHAT IS THE PATHOPHYSIOLOGY?

Common conditions in which anticoagulation therapy is generally implemented include deep vein thrombosis and pulmonary emboli, persons with prosthetic cardiac valves, and people on haemodialysis. Haemorrhage resulting from anticoagulant toxicity may be as a result of an overdose of the drug or an interaction between the anticoagulant and another agent that potentiates the anticoagulation effect[5,7].

WHAT ARE THE CLINICAL MANIFESTATIONS?

Clinical manifestations of anticoagulant toxicity will be related to the anticoagulant agent itself, and the manifestations of either overt or hidden haemorrhage.

TABLE 12.5: INR REFERENCE RANGE FOR THE ADMINISTRATION OF WARFARIN

INR Range	Conditions
2.0–2.5	Deep vein thrombosis (DVT) prophylaxis
2.0–3.0	Pulmonary embolism, atrial fibrillation
3.0–4.5	Recurrent DVT, arterial grafts, cardiac prosthetic valves and grafts

Source: MIMS Online http://mims.hcn.net.au.ezyproxy.uow.edu.au:2048/ifmx-nsapi/mims-data/?MIval=2MIM (Viewed 4 May 2005).

WHAT SHOULD YOU BE LOOKING AT IN THE LABORATORY AND OTHER TESTS?

Once the patient is 'warfarinised', therapeutic levels should be monitored on a daily basis until a stable level is reached, and from then on at regular intervals, usually weekly using the INR[9].

WHAT IS THE TREATMENT?

Anticoagulant toxicity is managed by reducing or terminating the anticoagulant therapy, and using reversing agents if necessary. For heparin, if bleeding occurs then protamine sulphate may be administered to inactivate heparin. However as heparin has a short half life (approximately 4 hours), stopping an infusion may be sufficient to reduce the bleeding[10].

For warfarin toxicity, if bleeding occurs the administration of fresh frozen plasma (FFP) is beneficial to replace clotting factors. FFP is plasma frozen shortly after collection to preserve the clotting factors – particularly V and VIII. Vitamin K may be administered but may result in prolonged resistance to warfarin[11].

APPLIED PHARMACOLOGY

Heparin is a very commonly used anticoagulant with a half-life of four hours that will treble normal clotting time. Heparin can be administered intravenously or subcutaneously. When injecting via the subcutaneous route take care not to promote haematoma formation by injecting the dose slowly, and not applying pressure to the injection site. The therapeutic range for an effective anticoagulant effect should be to maintain the APPT at 1.5–2.5 times the control value[10,11].

NURSING IMPLICATIONS

Observing for haemorrhage is vital during anticoagulant therapy and bruising or painless swelling, particularly surrounding joints, should be noted. Daily testing of urine for haematuria is also a vital component of nursing care. If infusing heparin it should be administered alone because it is incompatible with many other drugs. If anticoagulant therapy is to be continued after the cessation of heparin, then warfarin (for example) should be commenced 3–5 days prior to the termination of the heparin. This allows time for an adequate anticoagulant effect to develop before the cessation of the heparin[10,11].

People who are on warfarin should be advised to avoid foods with high levels of vitamin K (e.g., green leafy vegetables, cereals, soybeans), as these will counteract the effect of the anticoagulation[10,11].

LEARNING EXERCISES

1. Explain how warfarin and heparin retard the clotting process, particularly in relation to the coagulation cascade.
2. Why should warfarin be commenced three days before the cessation of a heparin infusion to maintain the anticoagulant effect?
3. What is the range for an INR for someone on anticoagulation therapy (warfarin) for deep vein thrombosis?

DISSEMINATED INTRAVASCULAR COAGULATION

Disseminated intravascular coagulation (DIC) is a life-threatening condition, which is the result of several complex interactions. DIC is usually associated with a serious illness (e.g., sepsis, malignancy, shock, obstetric emergencies, and cardiac bypass surgery)[5–7,9].

WHAT IS THE PATHOPHYSIOLOGY?

In serious illness there is a pathological trigger (thought to be damaged endothelium) that results in excessive stimulation of the clotting cascade and the formation of multiple small emboli. This excessive coagulation results in clotting factors being depleted and therefore the patient will commence bleeding[5–7,9]. DIC is commonly associated with an overwhelming infection and a massive systemic reaction occurs with the release of inflammatory mediators, leading to the development of widespread capillary damage and organ dysfunction. Activated protein C plays a major role in the inhibition of coagulation factors and this is markedly decreased in DIC[6].

WHAT ARE THE CLINICAL MANIFESTATIONS?

Bleeding can occur from any site in the body and may be evident as multiple petechiae, and continual oozing from IV cannulae sites[5–7].

WHAT SHOULD YOU BE LOOKING AT IN THE LABORATORY AND OTHER TESTS?

A profound protein C deficiency (activity less than 40%), prolonged APPT and PT and a very low platelet count[6].

WHAT IS THE TREATMENT?

The major goal of treatment for DIC involves reducing the bleeding and the loss of clotting factors. Therefore, as well as treating symptoms and the underlying cause, heparin may be used to treat DIC by reducing the clotting cascade and the formation of microemboli. The treatment with heparin remains controversial. Transfusion with coagulation factors may also be instituted[6,9,14].

Recently the management of severe sepsis with the infusion of activated drotrecogin alfa (activated protein C) has had some success in acutely ill patients. The administration of Xigris according to strict criteria was found to decrease the mortality rate in some with severe DIC[13,15].

APPLIED PHARMACOLOGY

See the discussion on the use of heparin as an anticoagulant earlier in this chapter. The use of drotrecogin alfa has only recently commenced in Australia for very selective critically ill cases. It is administered via an intravenous infusion over 96 hours, and increases the level of Protein C and inhibits the coagulation cascade to reduce the use of coagulation factors[14,15].

NURSING IMPLICATIONS

Monitoring for the possibility of major haemorrhage is the primary aim of the care of a person with DIC. If DIC is being managed conservatively with the use of heparin the same nursing implications should be observed as mentioned previously in this chapter. If drotrecogin alfa is being administered then consideration should be given to any factor that promotes the risk of haemorrhage, prior to the commencement of drotrecogin alfa, as major bleeding has been reported with the use of this drug[6,14,15]. For example is the patient on any other anticoagulant? Have they undergone recent surgery? Is their platelet count low? Consultation with a pharmacist should be maintained when using this medication[15].

LEARNING EXERCISES

1. What signs in a patient would alert you that they might have a coagulation disorder?
2. Why is heparin used in DIC?

CONCLUSION

Haematological disorders commonly present as primary or secondary conditions in patients. Nurses require a sound knowledge of physiology, normal values and pathophysiology to provide a basis for assessment, monitoring, nursing care and treatment. Common disorders include anaemia, polycythaemia, thrombocytopenia, haemophilia, and anticoagulant toxicity. A less common but extremely severe condition is disseminated intravascular coagulation.

Major nursing activities associated with haematological health breakdown include monitoring laboratory values, blood and medication administration, and assessing the patient's response to treatments.

(The case study in this chapter was developed by nursing staff from Ward C7, Cancer Care Services, Wollongong Hospital, Wollongong, NSW. Used with permission.)

References

1. Marieb, EN. 2001; *Human Anatomy and Physiology* (5th ed.), The Benjamin/Cummings Publishing Company Inc., Redwood City, California
2. Silverthorn, DES. 2001; *Human Physiology: An Integrated Approach* (2nd ed.), Prentice Hall, Upper Saddle River, New Jersey.
3. Australian Red Cross Blood Service. 2001; *Blood Types*. Retrieved July, 2004 from http://www. giveblood.redcross.org.au.
4. New Zealand Blood Service. 2003; *What Are Blood Groups?* Retrieved July 2004 from http:// www.nzblood.co.nz.
5. Mantik Lewis, S, McClean Heitkemper, M & Ruff Dirksen, S. 2004; *Medical Surgical Nursing: Assessment and Management of Clinical Problems*, vol. 1 (6th ed.), Mosby, St Louis.
6. Stinson Kidd, P & Dorman Wagner, K. 2001; *High Acuity Nursing* (3rd ed.), Prentice Hall, Upper Saddle River, New Jersey.
7. Lemone, P & Burke, K. 2004; *Medical Surgical Nursing: Critical Thinking in Client Care* (3rd ed.), Prentice Hall, Upper Saddle River, New Jersey.
8. Jaffe, MS & McVan, BF. 1997; *Davis's Laboratory and Diagnostic Test Handbook*, F.A. Davis Co., Philadelphia.
9. Walsh, M (ed.). 2002; *Watson's Clinical Nursing and Related Sciences* (6th ed.), Bailliere Tindall, Sydney.
10. MIMS Online. Retrieved November 2003 from http://www.mims.hcn.net.au.
11. Tiziani, A. 2002; *Havard's Nursing Guide to Drugs* (6th ed.), Mosby, Sydney.

12. Australian Red Cross Blood Service. 2001; 'What Do You Want to Transfuse?'. Retrieved July 2004 from http://www.donateblood.com.au/clinical/WhatDoYouWant/.

13. Brain, M & Carbone, P. (eds.). 1995; *Current Therapy in Haematology–Oncology*, Mosby, St Louis.

14. McCance, KL & Huether, SE. 2002; *Pathophysiology: The Biological Basis of Disease in Adults and Children* (4th ed.), Mosby, St Louis.

15. Laterre, PF & Wittebole, X. 2003; 'Clinical Review: Drotrecogin Alfa (Activated) as an Adjunctive Therapy for Severe Sepsis – Practical Aspects at the Bedside and Patient Identification', *Critical Care*, 7: http://ccforum.com/inpress/cc2342.

13 | Immune Health Breakdown

AUTHORS

JULIE LEWIN

KATHY ROBINSON

MARIA CYNTHIA
    LEIGH

LEARNING OBJECTIVES

When you have completed this chapter you will be able to
- List all of the components of the immune system and describe their functions;
- Discuss different types of immunity and when they are employed;
- Discuss balance and control mechanisms of the immune system;
- Describe the pathophysiological changes associated with immune health breakdown;
- Identify and understand the use of diagnostic and therapeutic techniques associated with caring for the person with immune health breakdown;
- Describe the safe use of pharmacological agents in managing different aspects of immune health breakdown, and
- Discuss health care and lifestyle interventions required for people with immune health breakdown.

INTRODUCTION

Using a longitudinal case-study approach, different aspects of immune function and immune health breakdown across the lifespan will be presented. John, in the first case study, will be followed through burns trauma and healing, renal failure, kidney transplant and associated immunosuppression. Kim, in the second case study, will be followed though a typical inflammatory response, pregnancy, immunisation choices, the exaggerated immune response of autoimmune disease, ageing and cancer.

Specific learning exercises are listed at the end of each major subsection of this chapter.

THE NORMAL IMMUNE SYSTEM

Our bodies are constantly under threat of disease from external (e.g., bacterial and viral invasion) and internal (e.g., mutated cells such as cancerous cells) sources. If external invaders break through the *first line of defence* (e.g., anatomical barriers such as skin and mucosae), they encounter a *second line of defence* in the form of phagocytic cells and face death by toxic chemical assault. This is part of the inflammatory response that occurs whenever there is tissue damage, no matter the cause. Inflammation is a non-specific defence mechanism – if a cell or particle is detected as being damaged, infected, or otherwise 'not belonging', no matter how or why, it is considered hostile and is immobilised, destroyed and removed. The phagocytic cells of the non-specific defence mechanism also take chemical instructions from the much fussier specific defence mechanism, which is the *third line of defence*. All components of the non-specific immune system are modulated by products of the specific immune system, such as interleukins (IL), alpha and gamma interferon and antibodies (see Figure 13.1).

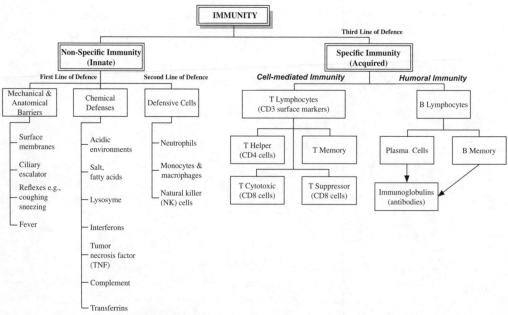

FIGURE 13.1 *Overview of immunity*

Lymphoid organs, tissues and cells form the main structural component of the immune system. Many of these lymphoid tissues are strategically located close to possible portals of entry for pathogens. The major organs contributing to the immune system are

- *Bone marrow*, which contains stem cells that eventually give rise to cells of the immune system;
- The *thymus*, which is involved in the education, selection and release of mature T lymphocytes;
- The *spleen*, which functions as an immunologic filter of the blood. It serves as an immunological sorting centre and produces large numbers of antibodies;
- *Lymph nodes*, which function as filters of lymph. Antigens are filtered out of the lymph in the lymph nodes and immune reactions take place here;
- *Tonsils, Peyer's patches* and the appendix, which are involved in the selective removal and destruction of antigens from the oropharynx and gastrointestinal tract; and
- *Lymphatic vessels*, which are thin-walled structures that drain lymph from most parts of the body.

Although the immune system is widely distributed and reliant on the many tissues that make up the lymphatic system, the immune system is better thought of in terms of its functions, rather than its anatomy.

Physically, the immune system consists of billions of individual lymphocytes (T and B cells), accessory cells of the non-specific immune system such as neutrophils and macrophages, and a vast array of chemical messengers or cytokines.

Lymphocytes, which normally account for 25–40% of the total leucocyte/white blood cell population, are capable of responding to specific antigens by either directly killing (on contact) the foreign cell (*cell-mediated immunity*, carried out by T cytotoxic cells), or by marking it 'for chemical destruction' when it encounters, and attaches to, a specific immunoglobulin (*humoral immunity*, involving activated B cells). Most lymphocytes (99%) reside in the lymphatic system. Activated B cells form clones of plasma cells, which secrete antibodies (immunoglobulins) into plasma and body fluids.

The specific immune response evokes the production of memory cells, allowing for an even speedier recognition and more effective response in case of further encounters. Specific immunity is the perennial student, constantly learning and adapting to personal immune experiences.

The immune system must be able to distinguish between antigens that 'belong' (self-antigens) and those that do not belong to the body (non-self). Self-tolerance develops during embryonic development. Those cells which would react against body components are not allowed to mature, and are destroyed. The selection process is so stringent that only about 1% of T cells are released.

Self-antigens are encoded by the *major histocompatibility complex (MHC)* genes, located on chromosome 6. When these antigens were first identified on the surface of human leucocytes, they were collectively called the *human leucocyte antigen (HLA)* complex. In transplant medicine, MHC compatibility testing is commonly referred to as *tissue typing*.

Balance and control of the immune system is critical for survival – hypersensitivities (allergies) and autoimmune disorders can result from an over-vigilant, over-responsive immune system, while immunodeficiency syndromes and increased susceptibilities to infections are typical of an under-active immune system. Immune activity is also influenced by activity of the neuroendocrine system, and thus subject to the influence of neural activity, neurotransmitters and hormones.

> ## LEARNING EXERCISES
> 1. Summarise the major homeostatic difficulties encountered by the immune system.
> 2. Outline the major divisions and homeostatic control of the specific immune system.

● **Case study**

John Groew, 25, weighs 70 kg and was involved in a motorbike accident late at night on a country road. He was not discovered until four hours later, by which time he was in moderate to severe shock. He had 40% deep partial and full thickness burns to his legs and back.

John was admitted to the burns unit and underwent intensive resuscitation effort, including the administration of 12 L of Hartmann's solutions (Parkland formula guidance) in the first 24 hours. His cardiovascular status stabilises, but his urinary output remains low. He has extensive lymphoedema.

At 36 hours, John's capillary seal is regained but he shows signs of acute pulmonary oedema. He has an external anteriovenous (AV) shunt[1] inserted and commences haemodialysis in order to maintain fluid and electrolyte balance while his kidneys convalesce from prerenal acute renal failure (ARF). (John's case will be reconsidered later in the chapter to address the immunological aspects of organ transplantation).

What are the basic prerequisites for a healthy inflammatory response?

* Adequate supply of water, nutrients and oxygen;
* Adequate drainage and elimination of cellular waste;
* Homeostatic balance and co-operation between the immune, nervous and endocrine systems; and
* A positive psychological outlook[1].

What raw materials are needed for John to mount an effective immune response? Adequate *hydration* and *nutrition* are essential if the inflammatory process/immune system is to be efficient and effective so the following are necessary:

* Water to constantly flush toxins and keep the cellular environment fresh;
* Kilojoules to provide energy for phagocytosis and cell proliferation;
* Essential amino acids for collagen and other protein synthesis;
* Fatty acids and cholesterol for synthesis of steroid hormones and cell membranes; and
* Vitamins and trace elements.

When tissue damage is extensive, the metabolic demands of the body for the inflammatory response and healing purposes can more than double. Unless protein supply matches demand, the body will rapidly catabolise (breakdown) muscles (including the diaphragm in severe cases), and recycle the amino acids to form more urgently-needed proteins such as albumin, fibrin, clotting factors, collagen and immunoglobulins. Matching supply with demand can be challenging, and critically ill patients often require Total Parenteral Nutrition (TPN) in addition to enteral feeds.

An adequate supply of *oxygenated blood* to body tissues is essential. Any condition that results in cell hypoxia will not only cause the accumulation of lactic acid (pro-inflammatory), but also dramatically reduce the cellular production of adenosine triphosphate (ATP). Without adequate ATP, the Na^+/K^+ pumps become less effective. Unable to maintain intracellular fluid and electrolyte balance, cells swell and finally burst, releasing enzymes that then cause further injury to nearby cells. The cycle of tissue destruction causing more tissue destruction will continue until oxygen supply meets cellular demand.

Disorders of the respiratory, cardiovascular and haematological systems have the greatest impact on the delivery of oxygenated blood.

Compared to non-smokers, the healing time for smokers is slow. Nicotine impedes the delivery of oxygenated blood by causing vasoconstriction, and chronic exposure to nicotine causes T cell unresponsiveness[2,3,4].

Venous and lymphatic drainage is crucial in keeping interstitial fluid clean from cell debris, inflammatory mediators and toxic metabolites. No cell can function properly if it is surrounded by its own (and neighbouring cells') waste products. Excess interstitial fluid normally drains into lymphatic capillaries, which join with others to form larger and larger lymphatic vessels, eventually emptying into the subclavian veins. En route, the lymph is filtered through a series of lymph nodes, each densely packed with B and T cells ready to react to anything suspicious. In this way, interstitial fluid is constantly cleansed – several times a day. The lymphatic system is fundamental to a properly functioning immune system.

If lymph nodes are diseased (e.g., cancer, parasites) or removed, (e.g., axillary dissection in radical mastectomy), lymphatic drainage is slowed. If the drainage basin (e.g., the affected arm) is suddenly flooded by interstitial fluid (e.g., inflammation-induced oedema from sunburn or bee sting), the lymphatic vessels cannot empty fast enough. The excess pressure causes them to irreversibly dilate, causing valvular incompetence. As a result, interstitial fluid cannot move into the (already full) lymphatic capillaries, so it lies stagnant between the cells. This is *lymphoedema*, and affected tissues will always be at risk of infection and have poorer healing ability.

The lungs have an extensive lymphatic drainage network which generally serves to keep the lungs 'dry', (i.e., free from *pulmonary oedema*). The lymphatics remove solutes, stray proteins and fluid from the interstitial space in the lungs.

An acute increase in volume or pressure may overwhelm the capacity of the lymphatic vessels to remove the excess fluid, and, as a result, pulmonary oedema occurs.

Why was John at risk of developing pulmonary oedema? John was susceptible to developing pulmonary oedema for several reasons. In burns and most other tissue damage situations, the greater the tissue damage the greater the inflammatory response. As a result of the increase in capillary permeability, fluids and even proteins escape into the interstitium, causing widespread oedema. When the capillary seal is regained, excess interstitial fluid is drained by the lymphatics and returned to the cardiovascular system. This adds to the workload of the heart and kidneys, and during this period pulmonary oedema may occur.

In this case study, John developed acute renal failure because of the prolonged time his kidneys went without adequate perfusion during shock. His decreased ability to make urine, combined with the return of excess interstitial fluid to the cardiovascular system, overloaded the capacity of the pulmonary lymphatics and caused the development of pulmonary oedema.

The immune system constantly treads a fine line between being over-vigilant and hyper-responsive (resulting in hypersensitivity and autoimmune disorders), and under-active and hypo-protective (resulting in immunodeficiency syndromes and a heightened susceptibility to infections and cancer). Appropriate *balance* and *coordination* between the various elements of the immune system, including appropriate levels of cellular activity, cytokine release and hypothalamic function are of the essence for normal function[5].

LEARNING EXERCISES

1. Discuss the basic requirements for normal immune function.
2. Explain why immune activity and the inflammatory process is so demanding of body resources, especially water, amino acids and oxygen.
3. Describe the role of the lymphatic system in reducing oedema.
4. Describe the function of lymph nodes and their role in the pathogenesis of lymphoedema.

NON-SPECIFIC IMMUNITY – FIRST AND SECOND LINES OF DEFENCE

The three major elements of non-specific immunity are

1. **Physical Defences**
   a. *Barriers* (anatomical and mechanical) are skin and mucosae (which line the respiratory, gastrointestinal and urogenital tracts) physically separate the external environment from the underlying tissues, and provide protection to internal structures. In addition, areas of the body subject to abrasion (e.g., skin or the mucosal layer of the rectum and vagina) are lined by stratified squamous epithelium and continually undergo desquamation, where the top layer of cells is shed to reveal the next layer of cells.

   Since burns cause the most severe loss of skin integrity, overwhelming infection remains the major cause of death and strict adherence to the principles of hygiene are important from the very onset of injury.

   Any condition that causes shock can result in the loss of integrity of the gastrointestinal mucosae. Compensatory mechanisms for shock include vasoconstriction of vessels supplying non-essential tissues – such as the gastrointestinal tract. If vasoconstriction is severe and prolonged, some cells in the blood-depleted areas become hypoxic, swollen and die. This causes defects in the anatomical barrier of the mucosae, and bacteria from within the gut wall can gain access to the capillaries and blood. This is called 'translocation of gut bacteria', and partly explains why critical illness and severe shock often result in septicaemia.

   b. *Oscillation* of bronco-pulmonary cilia moves mucus laden with inhaled micro-organisms, chemicals and dust, towards the mouth for expulsion or swallowing.

   Intubation temporarily hampers or renders useless ciliary function. Ciliary damage can be acquired, such as through inhaling cigarette smoke.

Primary Ciliary Dyskinesia is a genetic disorder (thought to be caused by mutation of a single gene, inherited in an autosomal recessive manner), where ciliary motion is erratic and uncoordinated[6]. Affected individuals have a lifetime history of chronic sinusitis, bronchiectasis, chronic cough, and recurrent pneumonia.

   c. *Reflexes* like coughing and sneezing help to expel foreign matter from the respiratory tract.

   d. *Fever* – in response to many viral and bacterial infections, macrophages release IL-1 and IL-2, which raise the hypothalamic temperature set-point. This may limit bacterial and some viral multiplication.

2. *Chemical defences*

In addition to flushing and diluting potential pathogens, bodily secretions (tears, saliva, gastrointestinal secretions, sweat) and plasma contain chemicals that help to defend the body against microorganisms:

   a. *Salt* and *fatty acids*, secreted by glands in skin, inhibit the growth of streptococci, fungi and most Gram-negative bacteria.

   b. *Gastric acid* – the acid concentration in the stomach is such that it effectively kills most bacteria. Antacids raise the stomach pH and make a person more susceptible to gastrointestinal infection.

   c. *Lysozyme*, an enzyme in secretions such as saliva and tears, breaks down the cell walls of some bacteria (especially Gram positive).

   d. *Tumour necrosis factor* (TNF), which is produced primarily by monocytes and macrophages, suppresses viral replication and activates phagocytes.

   e. *Complement* components and their products cause destruction of microorganisms directly, or with the help of phagocytic cells. Complement comprises a system of at least 20 proteins, which promote immune function and destroy foreign substances. Complement is self-regulating and also serves to limit immune function, as the molecules of the complement system help to remove immune complexes and prevent their accumulation[7].

   f. *Transferrin*, which is mainly produced in the liver, and *lactoferrin*, present in neutrophil granules and most secretions, deprive organisms of iron and also have a role as immune system modulators.

   • *Interferons* regulate growth and differentiation and exert immunological control. Alpha interferon is a small protein produced by virus infected cells which non-specifically inhibits all other virus replication by blocking protein synthesis. Interferons also activate macrophages and natural killer (NK) cells. Alpha interferon is currently being used to treat conditions as diverse as hepatitis C, melanoma and renal cancer[8].

   Why are interferons not more widely used in the management of viral infections? The answer is that interferons are expensive to produce, are administered by injection and unfortunately cause unpleasant side effects such as flu-like symptoms, nausea and headache.

3. **Defensive cells**

The following cells are involved in non-specific cellular defence mechanisms, and will thus attack a wide range of invading organisms. The most important defensive cells of the non-specific immune system are the neutrophils, macrophages and natural killer (NK) cells (not to be confused with T cytotoxic cells).

   • *Neutrophils* (polymorphonuclear leucocytes) are the most important phagocytes in bacterial destruction. Their granules and lysosomes contain *degradative* enzymes. In a non-specific immune response, neutrophils are the first cells to move out of dilating blood vessels as they are most easily deformed. Neutrophils respond to chemotactic factors or chemotaxins (chemicals released by bacteria and dead tissue cells) and move towards the area of highest concentration. They engulf the offending cell/particle, enclose it within a membrane, and release hydrolytic enzymes. Because this process (phagocytosis) consumes so much energy, the neutrophils' glycogen reserves become depleted and they soon die. When neutrophils die and their contents are released, remnants of their enzymes cause liquefaction of closely adjacent tissue. The accumulation of dead neutrophils, tissue fluid and other cell debris forms pus (often described as 'purulent discharge').

- *Macrophages*, derived from monocytes, are large mononuclear phagocytes. They are found in many body tissues and remove dead cell debris as well as attacking bacteria and some fungi. Since macrophages have greater glycogen reserves than neutrophils, they are able to replenish their lysosomal contents and therefore have a longer active life. Macrophages and other phagocytic cells such as the *dendritic cells* are known as *antigen presenting cells (APC)* because they display portions of what they have ingested on their surfaces and in doing so, communicate with and stimulate the specific immune system.
- *Natural killer (NK) cells* are non-specific aggressive lethal lymphocytes which have no immunological memory but attack and kill on contact anything which is recognised as foreign or abnormal. They target tumour cells and infectious microbes, particularly viruses. Granules inside NK cells contain cytolytic proteins such as *perforin*. These cells are involved in graft rejection and pose a major problem to transplant patients. NK cells that have been activated by lymphokines (such as interferon-gamma and IL-2) kill their targets more efficiently.

    Low NK cell activity seems to be associated with stress[9] of any type, poor nutrition, overwork, acute or chronic disease, emotional trauma and bereavement.

    Numbers of NK cells are reduced in cancer, severe viral infections, acquired immunodeficiencies and some autoimmune diseases. A drop in NK cells also occurs after significant blood loss.

LEARNING EXERCISES

1. Describe the three major elements of non-specific immunity.
2. Discuss the role of barriers in providing a first line of defence.
3. List examples of chemical defences and explain how they work.
4. List all of the cells engaged in non-specific cellular defence mechanisms and describe the role of each.

HEALING AND THE INFLAMMATORY RESPONSE

 Case study

Kim Casey, 5, had a splinter in her finger. Her father removed most of the wood, but the finger became sore, red, swollen and warm. The following day a small amount of pus was evident on the Band-Aid®, but two days later there was only a barely visible scar.

WHY THE INFLAMMATORY RESPONSE IS IMPORTANT TO SURVIVAL

Whenever there is tissue damage, be it from a period of hypoxia (e.g., myocardial infarction), physical trauma (e.g., traumatic brain injury) or invasion by a pathogen (infection), the innate and non-specific response of the body is to inflame the affected area. Inflammation is the process by which the body attempts to heal itself, and essentially consists of two stages:

- Removal of damaged tissue and offending substances; and
- Replacement with scar tissue.

Although the classical clinical manifestations of inflammation (redness, heat, oedema, pain and loss of function) may be uncomfortable, they nevertheless signal immune activity and responsiveness.

However, for someone who is severely immunodeficient, a simple splinter wound might lead to a life-threatening infection.

It is important to note that fever is not always a reliable indicator of infection. The elderly and those with immunodeficiencies cannot mount an adequate inflammatory response and thus may not display the classic systemic manifestations of infection such as fever. They are often misdiagnosed because they may only present with symptoms like confusion.

Small scale injuries (e.g., Kim's splinter) elicit a smaller immune response than large scale injuries (e.g., John's extensive burns), but the underlying process is similar, regardless of the cause or extent of tissue damage. The ability to generate an appropriate inflammatory response is crucial for healing and repair.

IMMUNE SYSTEM RESPONSE TO TISSUE DAMAGE

When cells are damaged, normally hidden parts of the cell membrane and intracellular components are suddenly exposed and released to the local environment. This initiates a chain of events, including the synthesis of many pro-inflammatory cytokines such as prostaglandins (PG) and leukotrienes (LT). Irritated mast cells (abundant in skin and respiratory mucosae), as well as neutrophils, basophils and platelets, release a mixture of other pro-inflammatory molecules including histamine, heparin and bradykinin.

PRO-INFLAMMATORY CHEMICALS DURING INFLAMMATION

- Histamine (H) is a powerful vasodilator released by mast cells and basophils. It increases vessel permeability and contributes to pain by sensitising nerve endings to other inflammatory mediators. Histamine also causes smooth muscle contraction of the bronchi.
- Prostaglandins (PG) are local hormones derived from membrane fatty acids. PG are highly potent substances that are not stored but rather produced as needed by cell membranes in virtually every body tissue. They have diverse actions dependent on cell type and may cause smooth muscle contraction, stimulate nociceptors, function as chemotaxins and promote the inflammatory response. Although highly potent, they are rapidly inactivated in the systemic circulation and the inactive metabolites are excreted primarily in urine.
- Leukotrienes (LT) are local, slow acting vasoactive substances released largely by white blood cells. LT are potent bronchoconstrictors and cause airway wall oedema. LT also attract eosinophils into the tissues and amplify the inflammatory process. Some asthma preventer drugs, such as montelukast (Singulair), act by blocking LT.
- Serotonin (5-hydroxytryptophan, or 5-HT) is capable of increasing vascular permeability, dilating capillaries and producing contraction of nonvascular smooth muscle.
- Bradykinin (BK) stimulates bare sensory nerve endings and is the most potent mediator of pain.
- Interleukins (IL) are chemical messengers released from lymphocytes and macrophages. They play a role in the inflammatory response (Il-5, IL-9, IL-11, IL-22), stimulate haemopoiesis (IL-3) and

allow communication between and stimulation of B lymphocytes (Il-1, IL-2, IL-4, IL-5, IL-6, IL-10, IL-13), T lymphocytes (IL-1, IL-2, IL-7, IL-16) and NK cells (IL-2, IL-12)[5].

WHAT IS THE PATHOPHYSIOLOGY?

The relationship between the physiological events involved in inflammation, the clinical manifestations and the beneficial effects of the inflammatory process are shown in Table 13.1.

HOW SCAR TISSUE IS FORMED

Following the neutrophils, monocytes leave the blood stream. Local macrophages are attracted to the area and ingest and destroy bacteria and cell debris. Monocytes and macrophages secrete cytokines (IL-1 and TNF), which stimulate the proliferation of

- Endothelial cells and the formation of new capillary networks; and
- Fibroblasts, which secrete collagen (protein) bridges to form a scar.

Excessive production of collagen leads to the formation of a raised keloid scar. Trauma to the skin, both physical (e.g., surgery) and pathological (e.g., lesions arising from acne vulgaris and varicella (i.e., chickenpox) is the primary cause identified for developing keloids. There are also familial tendencies and racial differences in the prevalence of keloid formation. The highest incidence of keloid scarring occurs in black Africans. The genetics of keloid formation are currently under investigation, and several genes seem to be involved[10,11].

However, due to the rising popularity in body piercing, there has been an increase in keloid formation of 'unusual' parts of the body such as the umbilicus and genitalia.

DAMPENING THE INFLAMMATORY RESPONSE

Problems arise if the inflammatory response is too strong, too weak, misdirected or otherwise damaging for the host, (e.g., allergic rhinitis, gastroenteritis, hepatitis or cellulitis). Basically, the inflammatory response may be dampened if it is excessive or when there is no significant protective benefit to the host.

Acute anaphylaxis[12] refers to a severe allergic reaction to a foreign protein or molecule such as penicillin, IV contrast media, bee or wasp venom, and certain foods (most notably, peanuts). Upon a second exposure to the allergen sensitised mast cells and basophils release large amounts of histamine. A cascade of biochemical and physiological events follows, which includes the involvement of many pro-inflammatory chemicals including PG and LT. Excessive vasodilation and increased capillary permeability lead to a dramatic drop in blood pressure, while bronchial smooth muscle contraction, airway oedema and mucus production cause acute respiratory distress.

In addition to providing support for the respiratory system (assisted ventilation, intubation) and cardiovascular system (IV fluids), the primary drug treatments for acute anaphylactic reactions are IV adrenaline and H1 antihistamines such as diphenhydramine (Benadryl, Unisom). (Corticosteroids are mainly effective in preventing biphasic i.e. delayed reactions, and are not considered as a first-line treatment).

TABLE 13.1: PHYSIOLOGICAL EVENTS UNDERLYING THE CLINICAL MANIFESTATIONS AND BENEFITS OF INFLAMMATION

Underlying Physiology	Clinical Manifestation	Benefit
1. Cytokines relax vascular smooth muscle and cause vasodilation 2. The increase in blood flow, together with an increase in capillary permeability, makes the area hyperaemic	Redness	1. Increases phagocytes such as neutrophils and macrophages and clotting factors in affected area 2. Increase the supply of O_2 and nutrients needed for repair
1. Increased metabolic activity by leucocytes and fibroblasts → an increase in the production of heat as a waste product of biochemical reactions → local warmth 2. Increased blood to area brings metabolic heat	Warmth	1. If microorganisms are present, the local increase in temperature may inhibit their growth or make them more vulnerable to attack 2. Haemoglobin alters its shape, releasing O_2 to the tissues more easily than normal 3. Many biochemical reactions become faster
Cytokines (especially histamine and PG) increase capillary permeability, making them more "leaky". The increased volume of interstitial fluid is oedema	Oedema	The influx of fluid dilutes: 1. Harmful chemicals and toxins in the area 2. Metabolic acids caused by anaerobic metabolism
1. Inflammatory cytokines (especially PG and BK) are released from damaged cells → irritate sensory nerves → perceived as pain 2. Oedema → presses on nerves → perceived as pain, numbness, tingling etc	Pain	1. Warning system that tissue is damaged 2. Inhibits movement and limits further damage
1. Cytokines can directly damage and inflame nearby muscle cells or motor nerves 2. Pain induces muscle guarding 3. Swelling and oedema impair function	Loss of function	1. Inhibits movement and limits further damage

ANTIHISTAMINES IN THE REDUCTION OF INFLAMMATION

Antihistamines antagonise histamine at H1 receptors and limit the effects of histamine. Unfortunately, many of the older drugs block histamine receptors in the CNS and cause drowsiness. Second-generation antihistamines such as loratadine (Claratyne, Claratin) and fexofenadine (Telfast, Allegra) have less ability to penetrate the CNS and are therefore non-sedating. These drugs are widely used as over-the-counter (OTC) medications for the control of allergic rhinitis.

OTHER INFLAMMATORY DRUGS IN THE REDUCTION OF INFLAMMATION

In Australia there are over 8 million prescriptions annually for non-steroidal anti-inflammatory drugs (NSAID)[13]; these drugs work by inhibiting the enzyme cyclooxygenase (COX), and in so doing, decrease the production of prostaglandins and leukotrienes. Some types of prostaglandins (those involved in the COX-1 pathway) are needed on a continuous basis and are stimulated by routine physiological events. The COX-1 prostaglandins stimulate physiological body functions, such as the production of protective gastric mucus and platelet maturation.

In contrast, the COX-2 pathway is induced by tissue damage/inflammation, and the resultant prostaglandins are pro-inflammatory. Inhibition of the COX-2 pathway dampens the inflammatory response, reduces oedema and alleviates pain.

Older NSAIDs such as aspirin (Asprin), indomethacin (Indocid), ibuprofen (Nurofen) and naproxen (Naprosyn, Naprogesic) inhibit both COX-1 and COX-2 pathways, thus lowering the production of the maintenance and pro-inflammatory prostaglandins. While the anti-inflammatory benefits come from the inhibition of the COX-2 pathway, many of the undesirable effects (such as susceptibility to gastric erosion) result from blockade of the COX-1 pathway. Second-generation NSAIDs such as celecoxib (Celebrex), selectively inhibit the COX-2 pathway (expressed in synovial cells and macrophages), and are thus becoming popular for the symptomatic control of arthritis, sports injuries and other forms of inflammation (see Figure 13.2).

Note that celecoxib (Celebrex) has a marked capacity for allergy owing to its sulphonamide structure[14].

The anti-inflammatory corticosteroids such as cortisol and prednisone inhibit the activation of phospholipase A2 by causing the synthesis of an inhibitory protein called lipocortin. It is lipocortin that inhibits the activity of phospholipases and therefore limits PG production[15] (see Figure 13.3). Steroids also impair lymphocyte function, which results in the production of less IL. This reduces communication between lymphocytes and lymphocyte proliferation. Hence, people on steroids long term have an increased susceptibility to infection.

Topical steroids are applied directly to a specific area of the skin. They are used to treat many inflammatory skin diseases, and are available in a variety of forms.

Absorption of topical steroids increases where the skin is inflamed at wound sites, and in other areas where the skin is not intact or is thin.

Paracetamol (Panadol, Pamol) may inhibit PG centrally rather than peripherally. It is analgesic and antipyretic but not an anti-inflammatory drug[16].

Maintenance (constitutive) Prostaglandins **Inducible Prostaglandins**

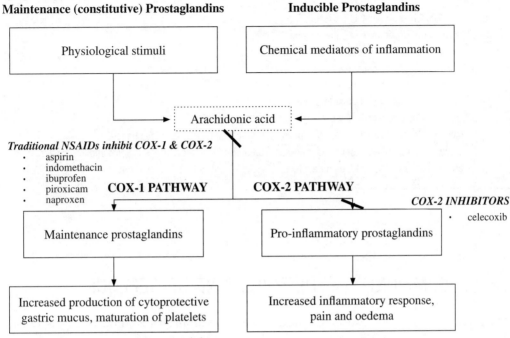

FIGURE 13.2 *Cyclooxygenase inhibitors*

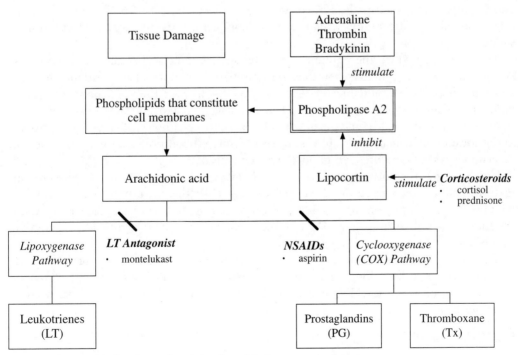

FIGURE 13.3 *Mechanism of action of anti-inflammatory drugs*

LEARNING EXERCISES
1. Discuss the importance of inflammation.
2. Identify the general conditions that cause inflammation.
3. Trace the physiological sequence of events that give rise to the classical clinical manifestations of inflammation.
4. Describe the benefits of inflammation.
5. Outline the process of fibrosis.
6. Identify circumstances in which the inflammatory response should be dampened.
7. Discuss the role of antihistamines, non-steroidal anti-inflammatory drugs (NSAID) and corticosteroid drugs in the reduction of inflammation.

SPECIFIC IMMUNITY – THE THIRD LINE OF DEFENCE

The immune response is a specific host defence mechanism that is stimulated by antigens. An *antigen* is a large, usually protein molecule, capable of generating an immune response. The specific immune response is antigen-specific, systemic and generates memory.

Each antigen may have one or more antigenic sites or epitopes. These epitopes are recognised by specific populations of lymphocytes. There are more than 10^{10} different B and T lymphocytes, each with different receptor molecules. Each B or T lymphocyte can only respond to antigens for which it has a complementary receptor molecule on its surface.

The process by which the immune system recognises and classifies antigens is complex. Antigens are best recognised when they are stationary. Therefore, phagocytic macrophages and dendritic cells (second line of defence) ingest whatever they recognise as foreign, perform a preliminary sort through of what they have ingested, and then display portions of the antigenic molecules on their surfaces. These *antigen presenting cells* are very important, as the location at which the 'trophy' antigen is displayed constitutes a signal or code and determines which type of T lymphocyte will be activated.

If the antigen is displayed next to a *major histocompatibility complex* (MHC) II protein, then it will be recognised by T helper cells (CD4); these, in turn, will activate B lymphocytes and a predominantly humoral immune response will take place. However, if the antigen is displayed next to a MHC I molecule, then it will be recognised by T cytotoxic cells (CD8) and a typical cell-mediated immune response will occur.

Thus, the MHC molecules, as well as serving as a unique fingerprint for the identification of cells belonging to self, also have a signalling function and allow the selective activation of those T lymphocytes best equipped to deal with bacterial, viral or other antigens.

HUMORAL IMMUNITY

The word 'humor' means fluid. Humoral immunity occurs when the immune system responds to an antigen by producing soluble antibodies that are transported around the body in the plasma. In general, this type of immunity is most effective when dealing with *extracellular antigens*.

B and T helper (CD4) lymphocytes recognise the antigen as it is presented in association with MHC II molecules. T helper cells respond by secreting a range of lymphokines – short range substances such as IL-2, which stimulates B and T lymphocytes to divide. B lymphocytes then proliferate to form clones of plasma cells which function as antibody factories and produce specific antibodies. While the functional plasma cells remain in the lymphoid tissues, the antibodies are transported around the body, bind to and inactivate the antigen. Memory cells retain information about the more effective antibodies.

CELL-MEDIATED IMMUNITY

Cell-mediated immunity is not systemic. The cell-mediated immune response involves activated T lymphocytes proliferating and then moving to the site of the antigen where they release short-range toxins. This is the typical response mounted by the organism to combat *intracellular antigens*, such as the hepatitis viruses that hide inside liver cells.

When antigens are presented in association with the MHC I complex, T cytotoxic (CD8) cells are activated. These T cytotoxic cells proliferate and produce a lethal lymphotoxin. T cytotoxic cells then move to the antigen bearing cells and release their short range lymphotoxin. As lymphotoxins are lethal substances, damage to other cells is minimised by the activated T cells travelling to their site of action. The lymphotoxin causes lysis of those cells bearing the relevant antigen, virus infected cells. The activated T cytotoxic cells also form memory cells. Another category of CD8 cells is the T suppressor cells. These cells play a regulatory role as they 'switch off' the immune response.

PRIMARY AND SECONDARY IMMUNE RESPONSE

The *primary immune response* follows the first exposure of a host to an antigen. It is a slow response that takes about two weeks, as a wide range of trial antibodies is produced by many different activated plasma cells. Initially, small quantities of large multivalent (many antigen attachment sites) polyclonal antibodies of the IgM type are typically produced. However, all five different classes of antibodies may be produced in response to one antigen. Over time, high affinity smaller antibodies of the IgG type replace the relatively inefficient antibodies of the IgM class. The cells that produce these efficient IgG antibodies are amplified or cloned, and memory cells for these higher-affinity and more effective antibody types are generated (see Table 13.2).

HOW ANTIBODIES WORK

The primary role of antibodies is to remove or inactivate antigens. When polyvalent antibodies bind to antigens, agglutination (clumping) occurs as each molecule of antibody binds to more than one molecule of antigen. The antigens become immobilised and neutralised as they lose function. Antibodies also activate the complement pathway and act as a signal for phagocytic or killer cells. This frequently culminates in death or destruction of cells/antigens.

TABLE 13.2: CLASSES OF ANTIBODIES		
Antibody Class	Valency (Number of Antigen Attachment Sites)	Location
IgM	Large, multivalent; cannot cross the placenta	Produced by activation of B lymphocytes during primary immune response
IgG	Small, bivalent; can cross the placenta	Produced largely by activation of memory cells during secondary immune response
IgA	Multivalent	Present in secretions, e.g., lining the gastrointestinal tract (GIT), breastmilk
IgE	Multivalent, reaginic; triggers mast cell degranulation	Released in situations of allergy
IgD	Small, similar to IgG	1% of antibodies

Infections in the gastrointestinal and respiratory system are prevalent in individuals with Down syndrome. This may be explained, in part, by low (20%) secretion rates of salivary IgA and IgG in these individuals[17].

The *secondary immune response* occurs on the second and all subsequent exposures to the same antigen. It is rapid and efficient, with specialised memory B and T cells becoming activated and generating large quantities of high-affinity identical monoclonal IgG within 2–3 days. During this process the immune response is reinforced as additional B and T memory cells are formed. This is essential for the maintenance of immunity as memory cells do not live forever.

Anaphylactic reactions are secondary immune responses involving IgE. On first exposure to the antigen (penicillin), mast cells and basophils become sensitised and display antigen-specific IgE on their cell surfaces. If exposed to the antigen a second time, the antigen and IgE bind together and cause the mast cells and basophils to almost immediately degranulate, releasing heparin, histamine and other chemical mediators. If left unchecked, the physiological cascade may continue to a state of collapse and irreversible shock.

Penicillin and cephalosporin antibiotics are the most commonly reported medical agents in anaphylaxis. Because of their molecular similarity, cross-sensitivity may exist. Since acute anaphylaxis is life threatening and parenteral administration of an allergen tends to result in a faster, more severe reaction, the first IV dose of an antibiotic must be attended by a medical officer. Although vaccine-associated anaphylaxis is a rare event, health care providers should be prepared to provide immediate medical treatment should it occur.

WHY MEMORY CELLS DO NOT LAST FOREVER

Lymphocytes deteriorate with age and need to be replaced. Some memory cells may live for over 20 years, but this is still not as long as a lifetime. When an individual is repeatedly exposed to an antigen, memory cells are repeatedly activated and renewed. If, however, the body is not repeatedly exposed to an antigen, (e.g., smallpox virus), all of the memory cells capable of responding may die and not be replaced.

IMMUNISATION

Vaccination is an attempt to use a non-pathogenic form of an antigen to elicit a primary immune response, with the generation of appropriate memory cells capable of producing effective antibodies. In this way, when a real infection occurs, the slow primary immune response is bypassed and the more rapid and efficient secondary immune response elicited.

Repeated or booster vaccinations are recommended to afford protection against diseases to which exposure is rare, as the number of memory cells is increased each time the organism responds to a specific antigen. If there is no exposure to an antigen, certain populations of memory cells may disappear due to lack of stimulation.

Unfortunately, vaccination itself does not guarantee the generation of appropriate memory cells and antibodies. The purpose of vaccination programs is to achieve *immunisation*, which is the generation of memory cells and the production of appropriate quantities of effective antibodies. The levels of specific antibodies in blood may be detected by simple laboratory tests. The results are reported as antibody titres.

DIFFERENCES BETWEEN VACCINATION AND IMMUNISATION

Vaccination is the administration of a vaccine, with no guarantee of outcome. There is individual variation in response and many individuals do not form appropriate antibodies (seroconvert) after a single vaccination. Immunisation refers to the formation/detection of measurable antibodies, that is, the success of a vaccination.

Active immunity is a long-lasting type of immunity in which antibodies and memory cells are produced. It may occur naturally, via infection, or artificially as a result of vaccination.

Passive immunity is immunity acquired by the transfer of antibodies from an immune person to a non-immune person. It is short-lived as no memory cells are transferred and antibodies are broken down over time.

The administration of anti-tetanus antitoxin is an example of passive immunity. Antibodies formed in other individuals are administered to non-immune persons who have potentially been exposed to tetanus.

TYPE OF VACCINES

The vaccines in widespread usage fall into three broad categories (see Table 13.3).

TABLE 13.3: TYPES OF VACCINES	
Type of Vaccine	Examples
Non-living extracts e.g., dead pathogens or inactivated toxins. These extracts are rapidly eliminated from the body	Pertussis, typhoid, tetanus, diphtheria
Living/attenuated pathogens e.g., pathogens weakened by continuous growth or mutation A stronger immune response is generated but such vaccines may not be suitable for use in the immunocompromised e.g., those with HIV	Measles, mumps, rubella, polio
Synthetic/recombinant vaccines e.g., vaccines prepared by genetic engineering Since only a small portion of the antigen is artificially created it is easily removed from the body and immunity may not be long lasting	Hepatitis A, hepatitis B, *Haemophilus influenzae* type B, chicken pox, meningococcus C

● Kim's case study (continued)

Kim, who at age 5 had the splinter removed from her finger, is now an adult. At 28, Kim decided that she wanted to start a family. She consulted her GP who advised her to have a blood test to determine her rubella titre.

PREGNANCY AND RUBELLA VACCINATION

As rubella is teratogenic (potentially harmful to the fetus), it is advisable that all women contemplating pregnancy ensure that they are adequately protected against this viral infection. A rubella titre is a measure of the amount of rubella antibody in a person's blood. Acceptable rubella titres depend on the type of test performed to determine antibody levels.

Due to the success of the widespread rubella vaccination campaign, very few people in most societies become infected with rubella. This minimises exposure for the whole population, and memory cells are not constantly restimulated and replaced.

Successful rubella vaccination leads to the active formation of antibodies and memory cells by the vaccinated individual. It is therefore a form of active immunity.

● Case study (continued)

Towards the end of an uneventful pregnancy Kim's placenta became a less effective barrier and her blood pressure increased rapidly.

PREGNANCY AND IMMUNOLOGY

Normally, the uterus is a site of 'privileged immunity' and the fetus is protected from immune attack by the mother[18]. However, as the placenta becomes a less effective barrier, Kim becomes exposed to fetal components. As is common during a first pregnancy, Kim then forms antibodies of the IgM class against certain fetal components. These antibodies seldom harm the baby as they are too large to cross the placenta, but the presence of large amounts of globular proteins does increase the viscosity of Kim's blood and hence her blood pressure.

PREGNANCY AND INFECTION

Pregnancy is not a disease, so Kim should not show an increased susceptibility to infection, even though aspects of her immune function may be dampened to prevent rejection of the fetus.

In some cases it is thought that repeated miscarriages may occur as a result of an over efficient maternal immune system rejecting components of the fetus. Studies have shown higher levels of tumour necrosis factor (TNF) in women experiencing repeated miscarriages[19,20].

Researchers have found that pregnant women with periodontitis were 7.5 times more likely to have a preterm low-birth-weight infant than were control subjects. Inflammation of the gums allows for the entry of bacterial cells and products into the circulation and causes an increase in cytokines[21-23]. Cleaning and scaling of teeth and resolution of periodontal disease can decrease the risk of preterm low-birth-weight in women with periodontal disease[24].

PREGNANCY AND INFLUENZA

There is no evidence that the influenza vaccine is teratogenic. The influenza vaccine has been recommended for all women who will be in their second and third trimesters of pregnancy during the influenza season[25]. However, the fact that Kim is pregnant does not place her in a high-risk category for influenza.

 Case study (continued)

One of Kim's pregnant friends tells her that she plans to save her baby's umbilical cord blood and have it kept in a cord bank.

CORD BLOOD CELLS

Cord blood contains undifferentiated cells (stem cells) that may be encouraged, by the judicious use of growth factors, to develop in a number of different directions. As stem cells have few surface antigens, they may be introduced into other persons without major rejection problems. In this way, stem cells may be used to replace damaged or diseased cells. Cord blood is therefore an alternative source of stem cells for bone marrow transplant. Processed cord blood is stored in liquid nitrogen (−196 degrees C) and can be kept for 20 years without loss of potency of the stem cells[26].

BREASTFEEDING

Breastfeeding allows the passive transfer of maternal antibodies to the baby and affords the baby protection against everything to which the mother is already immune. Unfortunately, the transferred antibodies only last a short time in the baby because they are removed and destroyed. Nonetheless, immunity transferred in this way affords very valuable protection to the newborn.

VACCINATION FOR INFANTS

Although Kim is affording her baby the best protection possible by breastfeeding, the baby has a juvenile immune system and is susceptible to many diseases against which Kim may not have developed antibodies. Infants are immunologically immature at birth. Therefore it is recommended to vaccinate the baby against many potentially fatal diseases.

● Case study (continued)

Kim's friend gave birth to a son and his cord blood was saved. During his first few months of life he suffered diarrhoea, had numerous skin and respiratory infections, and failed to thrive. He was diagnosed with severe combined immunodeficiency (SCID).

SCID

Severe combined immunodeficiency is a *primary immune deficiency*. The most common type is linked to the X chromosome, thus affecting only males. The defining characteristic is a severe defect in both B and T lymphocytes, which appears to be caused by a defect in IL-2. The lack of functional B and T cells usually results in the onset of one or more serious infections such as pneumonia, meningitis, skin infections and diarrhoea within the first few months of life. SCID is often called 'bubble boy disease'. It became widely-known during the 1970s and 80s, when the world learned of David Vetter, a boy with X-linked SCID, who lived for 12 years in a plastic, germ-free bubble. He died of a B cell lymphoma after receiving a bone marrow transplant from his sister. The first therapeutic replacement of defective genes has been performed in children with SCID[27,28].

DISORDERS OF IMMUNE FUNCTION

Disorders that affect the immune response can be divided into broad categories as shown in Table 13.4.

EXCESSIVE IMMUNE RESPONSE

Immune overactivity or hypersensitivity may be

- *Immediate* and occur within minutes or up to 24 hours. Clinically, three categories are recognised:
  1) Type 1 – classical allergy, (e.g., asthma, stings), mediated by mast cells and IgE;
  2) Type 2 – complement-mediated cytotoxicity, (e.g., incompatible blood transfusion); and
  3) Type 3 – immune complex reaction (autoimmunity, e.g., type 1 diabetes mellitus, rheumatoid arthritis).

TABLE 13.4: DISORDERS AFFECTING THE IMMUNE RESPONSE	
Inflammation & Infection	Lymphadenopathy Splenomegaly Lymphoedema Cellulitis Tonsillitis Infectious mononucleosis
Structural Disorders	Tumours such as Hodgkin's and non-Hodgkin's lymphomas
Excessive Response	*Allergies* e.g., hypersensitivity, anaphylaxis *Autoimmune diseases* e.g., Systemic lupus erythematosus Rheumatoid arthritis Type 1 diabetes mellitus Graves disease Pernicious anaemia Myasthenia gravis
Inadequate Response	*Congenital* e.g., Severe combined immunodeficiency disease (SCID) *Acquired* e.g., HIV *Induced* e.g., immunosuppressive drugs, lifestyle

• *Delayed* hypersensitivity occurs over several days. Sensitised T lymphocytes produce lymphokines and cause cell-mediated transplant rejection. There is initially no involvement of antibodies.

LEARNING EXERCISES
1. List the major categories of immune disorders.
2. Compare the problems associated with excessive and inadequate immune responses.
3. Explain the differences between immediate and delayed hypersensitivity reactions.

AUTOIMMUNE DISEASES

Autoimmune diseases involve excessive and inappropriate immune responses that damage the organism. Most autoimmune diseases involve recognition problems, as plasma cells mistakenly make antibodies against self-antigens (instead of foreign antigens).

In other autoimmune diseases, (e.g., systemic lupus erythematosus), immune complexes may block blood flow and damage and destroy organs, such as the kidney.

● Case study (continued)

In the busy lead up to her 30th birthday party, Kim felt tired and listless, had joint pain, and developed an annoying rash on her face after she tried to relax at the beach for a few hours. When she eventually consulted a doctor, he ordered several blood tests and joint X-rays. Kim's mother had developed rheumatoid arthritis in her 40s, so Kim was concerned that she may have similar problems.

X-rays demonstrated joint swelling without joint erosion. Blood tests showed that Kim had elevated immunoglobulins and antinuclear antibodies and reduced amounts of total complement and the complement proteins C3 and C4. Given her history and blood results, Kim was diagnosed with systemic lupus erythematosus (SLE)[29].

STRESS

Stress significantly affects the functioning of the immune system. Levels of pro-inflammatory chemicals such as IL-1 and IL-6 are increased while lymphocyte function is decreased.

ANTINUCLEAR ANTIBODIES

Antinuclear antibodies (ANA) are antibodies against normal cell nuclear components. These antibodies are present in 95% of people with SLE[30]. They are, however, not confined to people with SLE but may develop in a range of autoimmune diseases. The titre of ANA correlates with the severity of the disease[31].

PROTEINS C3 AND C4

Many people with SLE have reduced amounts of these proteins. This means that complement function is impaired, particularly the removal of immune complexes. Thus, immune complexes remain in the body for longer than they should and serve as an irritant.

PRESCRIBED STEROIDS

Glucocorticoids have an immunosuppressant effect (refer to Figure 13.3), and a reduction in immune activity will reduce some of the symptoms of SLE.

PLASMAPHERESIS

Plasmapheresis is similar to dialysis. It is a process whereby antibodies are removed from the blood, which is then returned to the body. This process may benefit Kim because it will reduce the number of immune complexes that may form in her body. Plasmapheresis is reserved for severe cases because it is expensive, time-consuming and there are associated risks.

RHEUMATOID ARTHRITIS AND SLE

Rheumatoid arthritis, which Kim's mother has, and SLE, which Kim has, are autoimmune diseases with a much higher incidence in females than males. There are also strong familial and tissue type tendencies, and it is quite common for a range of autoimmune diseases to manifest in the females from one family[7,32].

RHEUMATOID ARTHRITIS

Rheumatoid arthritis (RA) is a systemic autoimmune disorder, where antibodies formed against synovial cells lining the joints cause widespread inflammation, pain and impaired function. The disease may be inherited and many affected people display HLA-DR4[33]. Diagnosis is based on symptoms, X-rays and tests for rheumatoid factor. The rheumatoid factor test identifies abnormal, large IgM antibodies in about 80% of affected adults[31]. Other tests would include an erythrocyte sedimentation rate (ESR) – the higher the sedimentation rate, the greater the amount of inflammation – and a C-reactive protein test to monitor inflammation.

Treatment options include anti-inflammatory agents and analgesics, as well as disease modifying drugs such as the anticancer drug methotrexate and other immunosuppressive drugs.

SLE PROGNOSIS

SLE can be controlled through lifestyle changes and immunosuppressive medications, but it cannot be cured.

● Case study (continued)

Kim's symptoms improve. However, after several months of treatment Kim develops a cold, and then the 'flu', followed by conjunctivitis and vaginal candidiasis.

IMMUNOSUPPRESSION AND INFECTIONS

The pharmacological management of Kim's SLE has depressed her immune system. Consequently, she has reduced resistance to infection and is unable to effectively eliminate a range of pathogens from her body. Kim is also unable to ward off opportunistic infections such as candidiasis.

LEARNING EXERCISES

1. Define the term autoimmune.
2. Identify the components of the immune system that are involved in autoimmune disease.
3. List several different autoimmune diseases and explain how they occur.
4. Discuss gender differences in the incidence of autoimmune diseases.
5. Describe typical presenting symptoms of autoimmune diseases.
6. Identify laboratory investigations that aid in the diagnosis of autoimmune diseases.
7. Explain why systemic lupus erythematosus and rheumatoid arthritis are typical autoimmune diseases.
8. Discuss the pharmacological management of autoimmune diseases.

IMMUNODEPRESSION

Immunodepression refers to a reduction in number, or the impaired functioning, of cells involved in innate or acquired immunity. It is a compromised state in which the body's antigenic response is inappropriate. The immune system is finely tuned and may be adversely affected by

- Unhealthy lifestyle – too much stress, insufficient sleep or poor diet;
- Environment – factors include ionising radiation and toxins. Thyroid cancers and leukaemia often appear relatively soon after radiation exposure.
- Viruses – infections with viruses (e.g., HIV may harm the immune system). HIV ravages the immune system because it specifically binds to receptors on CD4 -T helper cells, multiplies inside these cells and destroys the T helper lymphocytes. As T helper cells play a central role in controlling both cell-mediated and humoral immunity, all aspects of specific immunity are impaired. The activity of the immune system is normally kept in balance by the joint actions of the CD4 and CD8 -T suppressor cells. Thus the CD4/CD8 ratio is an important determinant of the stage of HIV disease. HIV infection also impairs immune surveillance and increases the risk of cancers, in particular, Kaposi's sarcoma[34].
- Medical treatment – many medications, (e.g., most corticosteroid, antineoplastic and antiviral drugs) are immunosuppressive. Drugs such as cyclosporin (Neoral) are strongly immunosuppressive and decrease the functioning of the immune system, but have little effect the actual number of leucocytes. However, other drugs [all the cytotoxic drugs except vincristine (Oncovin) and bleomycin (Blenoxane)] also cause a reduction in the actual number of leucocytes and plasma cells by suppressing the activity of haemopoietic stem cells located in myeloid tissue (red bone marrow). Myelosuppression may reduce any or all blood cell populations.

Myelosuppression is often the limiting factor that determines how much cytotoxic therapy an oncology patient can tolerate. Anaemia may be corrected with infusions of red blood cells (RBC), while platelets are administered to address thrombocytopenia. Since neutropenia lowers defences against microorganisms, precautions such as reverse barrier nursing and stringent hygiene are essential to minimise exposure of the patient to pathogens.

• Genetic and chromosomal abnormalities – some individuals make incomplete or inappropriate antibodies or have defective B or T lymphocytes. Immunological abnormalities, including a high incidence of infection, autoimmune disease, and malignancy, are reported in those with Down syndrome[35,36].

• Psychological state – this plays a crucial role in how an individual combats disease and infection. Stress and anxiety impact on levels of cortisol, and elevated levels of cortisol reduce lymphocyte function. Catecholamines trigger the secretion of IL-10. Although multiple organ system failure is the leading cause of death in critically ill patients, 'immunoparalysis' is frequently overlooked. Following major surgery[37], shock and tissue injury, an initial excessive inflammatory response is followed by a paralysis of cell-mediated immunity[38].

● Case study (continued)

At 65, Kim is recently widowed. Although her SLE has remained under control, she is diagnosed with metastatic breast cancer. Kim read widely about the cancer and consulted the Internet where she found some exciting information about 'magic bullets'[39].

AGEING AND THE IMMUNE FUNCTION

Elderly people have deficient T cell function and antibody production in response to antigenic challenge. Impaired wound healing is associated with chronic illness. Many elderly people use medications that interfere with healing.

BEREAVEMENT AND MALIGNANCY

Bereavement and other emotional upsets dramatically affect the functioning of the immune system. All forms of stress increase the formation of cortisol and the sympathetic hormones. Chronic negative stress activates glucocorticoid pathways, and the resulting hormones reduce the function of the immune system by decreasing lymphokine production and retarding cell division. NK cells seem to be very susceptible to the effects of stress, and the body's natural surveillance mechanisms become less effective, thus allowing malignant cells to escape early detection and removal. Positive stress and positive mood, however, may increase immune function by elevating levels of endorphins and encephalins. There is a delicate balance, however, as top athletes seem to have a higher susceptibility to infections[40,41].

'MAGIC BULLETS'

'Magic bullets' was the descriptive term given to monoclonal antibodies in their early development in the 1980s[42]. It was hoped that antibodies with exquisite selectivity could be developed to selectively attach to cancer cells. If toxic agents could be attached to these magic bullets then selective cell death could be achieved[43]. A major problem has been that the early monoclonal antibodies were raised in animal cells and, when introduced into humans, the monoclonal antibodies themselves generated an immune response. Trastuzumab (Herceptin), a humanised monoclonal antibody for metastatic breast cancer, has recently been released with some reports of success[44].

LEARNING EXERCISES

1. List factors that may cause reduced function of the immune system.
2. Discuss problems that may be associated with reduced immune function.
3. Explain why untreated HIV devastates the immune system, and cite the cells involved.
4. Discuss the concept of psychoneuroimmunology.
5. Discuss the effects of ageing on immune function.
6. Explain why the risk of developing cancer increases with advancing age.
7. Discuss the significance of monoclonal antibodies and explain their potential clinical benefits.

TRANSPLANT

 John's case study (continued)

John, now 27, having developed end stage renal failure (ESRF), has been supported by haemodialysis three times a week for 3–5 h/session. John has had a series of pre-transplant tests (physical, psychological and practicality evaluations) to assess his suitability as an organ recipient.

KIDNEY TRANSPLANTS

Australia has the lowest organ donor rate of any country in the Western world[45]. It is estimated that up to 1% of people who die in a year might have the potential for organ donation, but only a small proportion of these actually become donors.

In 2003, 325 Australians and 67 New Zealanders received cadaveric kidney transplants but there are approximately 1500 Australians and 400 New Zealanders currently waiting for a kidney transplant. The average waiting period for a kidney transplant from a deceased donor is 4 years, although some people wait 15–20 years. Almost 40% of kidney transplants are now provided by living donors[46,47].

CANDIDATE SUITABILITY

In this case study, a psychological/psychiatric evaluation is necessary to determine John's understanding of the benefits and risks of transplant. The evaluation will consider how he might react to the transplanted kidney and assess his level of compliance with treatment.

Practical and social aspects are also considered. It is important that John has reliable transport at the time of transplantation, as well as clinical follow-up. Family or other support systems may be necessary to ensure the proper taking of medications, home testing, or other postoperative situations.

Note: the Northern Territory has one of the highest reported rates of kidney disease in the world and is 10 times higher than the national average. Over 80% of kidney patients are indigenous Australians and the majority come from distant communities[48,49]. Furthermore, recent research indicates that post-streptococcal glomerulonephritis (resulting from preventable streptococcal skin or throat infection) is implicated as a major risk factor for 40% of those indigenous Australians who have ESRF[50,51].

● Case study (continued)

John underwent a series of physical tests, including a CXR, ECG, echocardiogram and abdominal ultrasound (to exclude concurrent disease). Some minor nutritional deficiencies were detected and corrected, and his teeth were cleaned and scaled. Blood was drawn for a full blood count (FBC), blood grouping and tissue typing.

Test results showed that John's FBC was in the normal range, his blood group was O^+ve and his HLA types were identified.

John's sister and cousin volunteer to be tested to see if they were compatible donors.

ORAL HYGIENE IN TRANSPLANT RECIPIENTS

A suppressed immune system cannot mount a strong defence against invading micro-organisms. What might be asymptomatic mild gingivitis in a healthy individual can become a life-threatening septicaemia for the immunosuppressed. In addition, John has the best chance of accepting a compatible kidney if his immune system is relatively inactive. Furthermore, cyclosporin (Neoral), a commonly used anti-rejection drug, can induce gingival hyperplasia and inflammation.

Gingivitis is extremely common, affecting almost half of Australian adolescents and more than 90% of Australians in their 60s[52].

TISSUE TYPING (HLA/MHC MATCHING)

HLA marking is a process of identifying genetic markers (antigens) on leucocytes. Most successful transplants are those in which the donor and recipient have identical antigens (HLA)[53].

There are three general groups of HLA: A, B and DR. It is important to realise that each of the three HLA groups is inherited as part of a set, that is, one A, B, and DR from each parent. Each set is known as a 'haplotype'[54] (see Figure 13.4).

COMPATIBLE DONORS

John has a 1 in 4 chance of being an identical match with his sister (i.e., they share the same two haplotypes), and a 1 in 2 chance of being partly compatible (i.e., sharing one haplotype). He has a 1 in 8 chance of being compatible with his cousin.

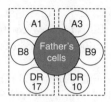
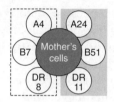
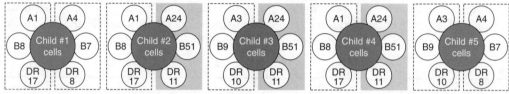

FIGURE 13.4 *Inheritance of HLA Haplotypes*

DIFFICULT OF FINDING UNRELATED COMPATIBLE DONORS

There are many different specific HLA proteins within each of these three groups. To date (March 2004) scientists have identified 325 different HLA-A, 592 different HLA-B and 451 different HLA-DR proteins[55].

Each of these HLA has a different numerical designation, for example, one person may have HLA-A1, while another might have HLA-A2. There are nearly 220 genes coding for MHC[56], so the chance of finding a match in the general population is much less than with immediate blood relatives. An individual's particular haplotype and its prevalence determines the degree of difficulty in locating a compatible donor.

GENDER

The gender of a donor is relevant. A recent study[57] looked at more than 124,000 kidney, 25,000 heart and 16,000 liver transplants on the Collaborative Transplant Study[58] database, and evaluated the graft survival according to donor and recipient gender. Overall, people who received an organ from a woman were less likely to have successful grafts, particularly if the organ donated was a kidney.

The study found that women receiving a kidney from a female donor were 15% more likely to reject the organ than if their donor had been a man. The situation was even more marked for men receiving kidneys from women, where the chance of rejecting the organ was 22% greater.

BLOOD GROUPS

For a successful transplant, blood types must be compatible but not necessarily identical (see Table 13.5). Blood types are commonly identified as A, B, AB, and O. People of blood group O (49% of the Australian population[59]) are described as universal donors, since their organs can be transplanted into a person with any blood type. A person with AB blood (the most rare in Australia) can receive a kidney from a person with any blood type (universal recipient). Various other combinations are possible for persons with A or B blood.

Whereas the antigens that determine blood group type are found on all cells, the antigens for the Rhesus factor (Rh) are only present on red blood cells. It is not necessary to match

TABLE 13.5: DONOR/RECIPIENT COMPATIBILITIES	
If the Blood Type of Recipient Is:	Donor Can be Type:
O	O
A	A or O
B	B or O
AB	A or B or AB or O

the Rh for solid tissue transplantations. However, since it is not possible to rid a transplanted organ of every single blood cell, a Rh⁻ recipient of a Rh⁺ donor organ may develop anti-Rh antibodies. This is unimportant except in the case of a Rh⁻ female, who wishes to bear children, receiving a solid organ transplant from a Rh⁺ donor. In this context the administration of anti-Rh antibodies prevents sensitisation of the Rh⁻ female. Anti-Rh antibodies promote the destruction of any Rh⁺ cells in the transplant recipient so that the woman is not stimulated to produce her own anti-Rh antibodies.

In terms of finding a compatible donor, is the fact that John's blood group is O⁺ve an advantage or a disadvantage? It is a disadvantage, because people with type O blood can only receive an organ from another person of type O. Since people of blood group O can donate to all groups, there is even greater demand for their organs. Most indigenous Australians have type O blood, whereas blood group A predominates in indigenous New Zealanders and Polynesians.

● **Case study (continued)**

While waiting for a suitable donor, John needs monthly blood tests to measure the general level of activity of his immune system. The tests performed include a full blood count (FBC), erythrocyte sedimentation rate (ESR), panel reactive antibody (PRA) and C-reactive protein (CRP).

PRA MONITORING

A transplanted organ is more likely to be accepted if the recipient's humoral immunity is relatively inactive. A high PRA indicates a high number of anti-HLA antibodies[60,61].

The types of antibodies a person develops depend on his medical history and exposure to antigens. For example, if John had previously received a blood transfusion from a donor with HLA-DR2, he could have developed antibodies to DR2. If he then received a transplant with DR2 antigens, his humoral response would be to immediately reject the organ (hyperacute rejection).

Those who have had several pregnancies, exposure to multiple blood transfusions, or previously received a transplant, will probably have high PRA readings. They are therefore more likely to react against otherwise compatible organs, and thus spend a longer time on transplant waiting lists.

ELEVATED CRP

CRP is a protein that is released by the liver under the influence of IL-1 and IL-6, in response to inflammatory stimuli. It plays a role inactivating the complement system. The level of CRP directly reflects the level of inflammation[31,62,63]. If John's CRP was high when a compatible kidney became available, he might not be considered a suitable recipient at that time.

LEARNING EXERCISES
1. Discuss immunological considerations relating to transplantation.
2. Explain the process and aims of tissue typing.
3. Discuss donor and recipient compatibilities.
4. Identify tests to monitor activity of the immune system.

● Case study (continued)

John's tissue type is not compatible with that of his sister or cousin. A potential donor is located in Perth and the kidney is kept on ice while being transported to Sydney. The transplant coordinator contacts John, who immediately presents to the Transplant Unit. Cross-matching between the donor and John is conducted. The cross-match is negative, meaning John does not have antibodies to the kidney.

John undergoes the kidney transplant. Unfortunately the transplanted kidney develops acute tubular necrosis. John requires temporary dialysis during the first post-surgical week.

POST-TRANSPLANT ACUTE TUBULAR NECROSIS

Post-transplant acute tubular necrosis (ATN) is the acute postoperative failure of a transplanted kidney. The condition is usually temporary and due to ischaemic damage of the nephrons. Dialysis may be necessary while the kidney recovers from the shock of transplant and reperfusion.

Ischaemic damage to any transplanted organ is correlated with the cold ischaemic time (CIT), that is, the time the organ is kept in cold storage. Different organs have different levels of CIT tolerance.

ORGAN REJECTION

The different types of organ rejection are

• Hyperacute – occurs when activated B cells generate plasma cells that produce antibodies against the transplanted tissue and cause the immediate destruction of the new kidney. This type of rejection may be avoided by cross-match testing immediately before transplant.

- Acute – this typically occurs during the first few months, usually around the 2nd or 3rd week. Sensitised T cytotoxic cells are responsible for attacking the organ and causing its destruction, and, for this reason, anti-rejection drugs are administered.
- Chronic – this may happen months or years after the transplant and is usually associated with an alteration in the total antibody load of the individual. This type of rejection is resistant to treatment with current medications.

MEDICATIONS TO REDUCE THE RISK OF REJECTION

- Glucocorticoids (e.g., prednisone) are the most commonly prescribed immunosuppressive drugs. They suppress both lymphocyte function and the inflammation associated with transplant rejection, and are frequently combined with other immunosuppressive medications.
- Cyclosporin (Neoral) and tacrolimus (Prograf) act by inhibiting T-cell activation, thus preventing T-cells from attacking the transplanted organ. Both drugs work in a similar way and limit the production of IL-1, IL-2, IL-3, IL-4 and gamma interferon.
- Sirolimus (also known as rapamycin) (Rapamune) is a new immunosuppressant that inhibits lymphocyte proliferation in response to cytokines. Since this action is distinct from that of cyclosporine and tacrolimus (that inhibit cytokine production), sirolimus can be combined with existing agents to produce a synergistic effect. Recent findings suggest that sirolimus could also possess anti-tumour potential[64].
- Azathioprine (Imuran) disrupts the synthesis of DNA and RNA and inhibits all immune cell populations.
- Mycophenolate mofetil (CellCept) inhibits the T and B lymphocyte proliferation that follows antigen presentation.
- Muromonab-CD3 (Orthoclone OKT3) is sometimes used to limit acute organ rejection. It is a specially engineered monoclonal antibody that targets the CD3 antigen on all T cells, and limits their proliferation and attack on antigens.
- Daclizumab (Zenapax) is an anti CD25 monoclonal antibody and IL-2 receptor antagonist. Used in combination with standard immunosuppressive agents, it is the first genetically engineered drug to reduce the risk of organ rejection in kidney transplant patients without increasing the incidence of opportunistic infections[65].

Immunosuppression may continue for months after drugs have been discontinued. Immunosuppression reduces immune surveillance by NK cells. The rate of certain malignancies in renal transplant recipients is 14 to 500 times higher than the rate in the general population[66]. In general, malignant tumours develop in 15–20% of graft recipients after 10 years, with skin tumours and lymphoproliferative disorders being the most frequent malignancies[64].

DRUGS TO PREVENT OR LIMIT INFECTION

In John's case study, these drugs are used to prevent or limit infection:

- Bactrim (trimethoprim, sulphamethoxazole) prevents and treats bacterial and protozoal infections. It is also used to prevent and treat *Pneumocystis carinii* pneumonia, a particularly troublesome opportunistic infection for those with a compromised immune system.
- Ganciclovir (Cytovene, Cymevene) is an antiviral drug used to prevent or treat cytomegalovirus (CMV) infection. The risk of CMV is highest in the first months after transplantation. Signs of infection include fatigue, high temperature, aching joints, headaches, visual disturbances and pneumonia.
- Acyclovir (Zovirax) is another antiviral, used to prevent or treat *Herpes simplex* and *Herpes zoster* (shingles). Acyclovir will not get rid of the herpes viruses, but it will inhibit multiplication, reduce pain and help heal the sores. It may be used to decrease the severity of CMV infections.

• Antifungal medications, (e.g., nystatin (Nilstat, Mycostatin) may be necessary to limit overgrowth of the opportunistic organism *Candida albicans* which causes thrush.

GAMMAGLOBULIN INJECTIONS

Gammaglobulin is a source of pooled human antibodies. When gammaglobulin is administered by injection to immunodepressed people it allows the passive transfer of antibodies. These antibodies afford protection against specific disease.

Since gammaglobulins are proteins, they would be digested in the stomach if administered orally and therefore most be injected. Most artificially administered gammaglobulins will be removed from the body in approximately three weeks, and therefore need to be readministered every 21 days.

 ## Case study (continued)

Because the risk of bacterial and fungal infection is greatest in the first few weeks after surgery, John was advised to take special precautions to prevent infections.

PATIENT PRECAUTIONS TO PREVENT INFECTION

Frequent hand-washing, stringent personal hygiene and good dental care will help John to limit infection. John should avoid large crowds in closed spaces, people with known infections or illnesses, and taking care of animals.

Case study (continued)

John celebrated the first anniversary of his kidney transplant. He had been compliant with his medications and had kept himself fit and active.

LONGEVITY OF TRANSPLANTED KIDNEY

The Australian survival rate for kidneys of people who have received a kidney transplant is more than 90% after one year and 77 per cent after five years[47]. Overall, 70% of transplanted kidneys that survive the one-year anniversary are still functional at the 10-year anniversary. Considering his age and general state of health, John's kidney may survive much longer.

CANCER

Malignancy following renal transplantation is an important medical problem during the long-term follow-up[67]. The overall incidence of malignancy is 3 to 5 times higher than in the general population, although the type of malignancy is different in various countries and dependent on genetic and environmental factors[68,69]. By 15 years post-transplant, more than one-third of cadaveric graft recipients in Australia will develop skin cancer, and one-fifth will develop a non-skin malignancy[70].

SKIN CANCER

As someone who is receiving immunosuppressants, John needs be extremely careful about protecting his skin and eyes from UV radiation, and should have regular skin screening.

LEARNING EXERCISES

1. Define and explain the process of graft rejection.
2. Identify immunosuppressive medications and explain their mode of action.
3. Discuss the problems associated with the administration of immunosuppressive medications.
4. List drugs that may be used to limit infection in those who are immunosuppressed.
5. Discuss the use of gamma globulins to promote immune function.

CONCLUSION

The immune system impacts on all aspects of health across the lifespan, from embryo to death. Lifestyle, genetics, physiological stress and mental state all contribute to the functioning of this system.

Overactivity of the immune system lends itself to hypersensitivities, including asthma, hayfever and other allergic responses, as well as autoimmune diseases such as SLE, type 1 diabetes mellitus and glomerulonephropathy. Reduced immune activity is characterised by heightened susceptibility to infection and poor wound healing. Over or underactivity of the immune system, whether it is induced by lifestyle or disease, results in significant health breakdown.

Recommended Readings

Ader, R, Felton, DL & Cohen, N. 2001; *Psychoneuroimmunology* (3rd ed.), Academic Press San Diego.

Benjamini, E, Coico, R & Sunshine, G. 2000; *Immunology: A Short Course* (4th ed), John Wiley, New York.

Martini. FH. 2004; *Fundamentals of Anatomy and Physiology* (5th ed,), Benjamin/Cummings, New Jersey.

Porth, CM. 2002; *Pathophysiology: Concepts of Altered Health States* (6th ed,), Lippincott, Philadelphia.

Roitt, IM, Brostoff, J & Male, DK. 2001; *Immunology* (6th ed.), Mosby, St Louis.

References

1. Dantzer R. 2004; 'Innate Immunity at the Forefront of Psychoneuroimmunology', *Brain Behaviour Immunology*, 18 (1), 1–6.

2. Manassa, EH, Hertl, CH & Olbrisch, RR. 2003; 'Wound Healing Problems in Smokers and Nonsmokers after 132 Abdominoplasties', *Plastic and Reconstructive Surgery*, 111 (6), 2082–2087.

3. Towler, J. 2000; 'Cigarette Smoking and Its Effects on Wound Healing', *Journal of Wound Care*, 9 (3), 100–104.

4. Sopori, ML & Kozak, W. 1998; 'Immunomodulatory Effects of Cigarette Smoke. *Journal of Neuroimmunology*, 83 (1–2), 148–156.

5. Hofmann, SR, Ettinger, R, Zhou, Y, Gadina, M, Lipsky, P, Siel, R, *et al.* 2002; 'Cytokines and Their Role in Lymphoid Development, Differentiation and Homeostasis', *Current Opinion in Allergy and Clinical Immunology*, 2 (6), 495–506.

6. Olbrich, H, Haffner, K, Kispert, A, Volkel, A, Volz, A, Sasmaz, G, *et al.* 2002; 'Mutations in DNAH5 Cause Primary Ciliary Dyskinesia and Randomization of Left-Right Asymmetry', *Nature Genetics*, 30 (2), 143–144.

7. National Institute of Autoimmune Disease. 1999; *Understanding Autoimmune Disease: How Does theImmune System Work?* http://www.niaid.nih.gov/publications/autoimmune/work.htm.

8. Jonasch E & Haluska FG. 2001; 'Interferon in Oncological Practice: Review of Interferon Biology, Clinical Applications, and Toxicities', *Oncologist*, 6 (1), 34–55.

9. Garland, M, Doherty, D, Golden-Mason, L, Fitzpatrick, P, Walsh, N & O'Farrelly, C. (2003); 'Stress-related Hormonal Suppression of Natural Killer Activity Does Not Show Menstrual Cycle Variations: Implications for Timing of Surgery for Breast Cancer', *Anticancer Research*, 23 (3B), 2531–2535.

10. Berman, B & Kapoor S. 2001; 'Keloid and Hypertrophic Scar', *eMedicine Journal*, 2 (11), 1–12. http://emedicine.com/derm/topic205.htm.

11. Bayat, A, Bock, O, Mrowietz. U, Ollier, WE & Ferguson, MW. 2003; 'Genetic Susceptibility to Keloid Disease and Hypertrophic Scarring: Transforming Growth Factor Beta₁ Common Polymorphisms and Plasma Levels', *Plastic Reconstruction Surgery*, 111 (2), 535–543, discussion 544–546.

12. Krause, RS. 2004; 'Anaphylaxis'. http://www.emedicine.com/emerg/topic25.htm.

13. Australian Government Pharmaceutical Benefits Scheme: Expenditure and Prescriptions. http://www.health.gov.au/pbs/general/pubs/pbbexp/pbmar04/index.htm.

14. Bengt, EW. 2001; 'Identification of Sulfonamide-like Adverse Drug Reactions to Celecoxib in the World Health Organization Database', *Current Medical Research Opinions*, 17 (3), 210–216. http://www.medscape.com/viewarticle/424620

15. Wallner, BP, Mattaliano, RJ, Hession, C, Cate, RL, Tizard, R, Sinclair, LK, *et al.* 1986; 'Cloning and Expression of Human Lipocortin: A Phospholipase A2 Inhibitor with Potential Anti-inflammatory Activity', *Nature*, 320 (6057), 77–81.

16. Galbraith, A, Bullock, S & Manias, E. 2003; *Fundamentals of Pharmacology*, Addison-Wesley Publishing Company, Sydney.

17. Chaushu, S, Yefenof, E, Becker, A, Shapira, J & Chaushu, G. 2002; 'Severe Impairment of Secretory Ig Production in Parotid Saliva of Down Syndrome Individuals', *Journal of Dental Research*, 81 (5), 308–312.

18. Jiang, S & Vacchio, MS. 1998; 'Cutting Edge: Multiple Mechanisms of Peripheral T Cell Tolerance to the Fetal "Allograft"', *Journal of Immunology*, 160, 3086–3090.

19. Clark, DA, Chaouat G & Gorczynski, RM. 2002; 'Thinking Outside the Box: Mechanisms of Environmental Selective Pressures on the Outcome of the Materno-Fetal Relationship', *American Journal of Reproductive Immunology*, 47 (5), 275.

20. Baxter, N, Sumiya, M, Cheng, S, Erlich, H, Ran, L, Simons, A & Summerfield, JA. 2001; 'Recurrent Miscarriage and Variant Alleles of Mannose Binding Lectin, Tumor Necrosis Factor and Lymphotoxin Alpha Genes', *Clinical Experimental Immunology*, 126 (3), 529–534.

21. Krejci, CB & Bissada, NF. 2002; 'Women's Health Issues and Their Relationship to Periodontitis', *Journal of the American Dental Association*, 133 (3), 323–329.

22. Lopez, NJ, Smith, PC & Gutierrez, J. 2002; 'Higher Risk of Preterm Birth and Low Birth Weight in Women with Periodontal Disease', *Journal of Dental Research*, 81 (1), 58–63.

23. Offenbacher, S, Lieff, S, Boggess, KA, Murtha, AP, Madianos, PN, Champagne, CM, *et al.* 2001; 'Maternal Periodontitis and Prematurity, Part I: Obstetric Outcome of Prematurity and Growth Restriction', *Annals of Periodontology*, 6 (1), 164–174.

24. Lopez, NJ, Smith, PC & Gutierrez, J. 2002; 'Periodontal Therapy May Reduce the Risk of Preterm Low Birth Weight in Women with Periodontal Disease: A Randomized Controlled Trial', *Journal of Periodontology*, 73 (8), 911–924.

25. Organisation of Teratology Information Services. 2003; 'Influenza and the Vaccine during Pregnancy'. http://www.otisprnancy.org/pdf/influenza.pdf.

26. Sydney Children's Hospital. 2003; *Australian Cord Blood Bank*. Acessed at: http://www.sch.edu.au/departments/acbb/donate.asp

27. Hacein-Bey-Abina, S, Le Deist, D, Carlier, F, Bouneaud, C, Hue, C, De Villartay, P, *et al.* 2002; 'Sustained Correction of X-linked Severe Combined Immunodeficiency by Ex Vivo Gene Therapy', *New England Journal of Medicine*, 346 (16), 1185–1193.

28. Onodera, M, Nelson, DM, Sakiyama, Y, Candotti, F & Blaese, RM. 1999; 'Gene Therapy for Severe Combined Immunodeficiency Caused by Adenosine Deaminase Deficiency', *Acta Haematologica*, 101, 89.

29. National Institutes of Health. 2003; *MEDLINEplus: Lupus*. www.nlm.nih.gov/medlineplus/lupus.html.

30. Lab Tests Online ANA: The Test. www.labtestsonline.org/understanding/analytes/ana/test.html.

31. Pagana, KD & Pagana, TJ. 1999; *Diagnostic Testing and Nursing Implications*, Mosby, St Louis.

32. National Institute of Arthritis and Musculoskeletal and Skin Diseases. 1999; *Handout on Health:*

Rheumatoid Arthritis. http://www.niams.nih.gov/hi/topics/arthritis/rahandout.htm.

33. Arthritis Foundation. 2003; *Rheumatoid Arthritis (RA)*. Accessed at: http://www.arthritis.org/conditions/DiseaseCenter/ra.asp.

34. Frisch, M, Biggar, RJ, Engels, EA & Goedert, JJ. 2001; 'Association of Cancer with AIDS-related Immunosuppression in Adults', *Journal of the American Medical Association*, 285,1736–1745.

35. Barroeta, O, Nungaray, L, Lopez-Osuna, M, Armendares, S, Salamanca, F & Kretschmer, RR. 1983; 'Defective Monocyte Chemotaxis in Children with Down Syndrome', *Pediatric Research*, 17, 292–295.

36. Levin, S. 1987; 'The Immune System and Susceptibility to Infections in Down Syndrome', *Progress in Clinical and Biological Research*, 246, 143–162.

37. Volk, HD. 2002; 'Immunodepression in the Surgical Patient and Increased Susceptibility to Infection', *Critical Care*, 6 (4), 279–281.

38. Angele, MK & Faist, E. 2002; 'Clinical Review: Immunodepression in the Surgical Patient and Increased Susceptibility to Infection', *Critical Care*, 6 (4), 298–305.

39. Eccles, SA. 2001; 'Monoclonal Antibodies Targeting Cancer: 'Magic Bullets' or Just the Trigger?', *Breast Cancer Research*, 3 (2), 86–90.

40. Mackinnon, LT. 2000; 'Chronic Exercise Training Effects on Immune Function', *Medicine and Science in Sports and Exercise*, 32 (supplement 7), S369-S376.

41. Mackinnon, LT. 1997; 'Immunity in Athletes: A Review', *International Journal of Sports Medicine*, 18, S62–S68

42. Halim, NS. 2001; 'Monoclonal Antibodies: A 25-Year Roller Coaster Ride', *The Scientist*, 14 (4), 16.

43. Panosian, C. 2001; 'Magic bullets fly again', *Scientific American*, October 2001. http://www.sciam.com/issue.cfm?issuedate=Oct-01.

44. Genentech. 2002; *Herceptin*. http://www.herceptin.com/herceptin/patient/e_about/about.htm.

45. Australian Bureau of Statistics: Australian Social Trends. 2002; 'Health: Health-related Actions – Organ Donation. www.abs.gov.au.

46. Australia and New Zealand Dialysis and Transplant Registry. 2004; *ANZDATA*. http://www.anzdata.org.au/ANZOD/ANZODReport/2004/2004ANZOD.pdf.

47. Central Sydney Area Health Service. 2003; http://www.cs.nsw.gov.au/mediacentre/mediareleases/2003/mr030606e.htm.

48. Gorham, G. 2003; *Prevention and Treatment Options for Renal Disease in the Northern Territory (with Particular Reference to the Barkly Region)*,

Cooperative Research Centre for Aboriginal & Tropical Health (CRCATH). http://www.crcah.org.au/crc/; or http://192.94.208.240//Crc/General/CRCPubs/reports/report files/Barkly.pdf. For more information, or copies of the report, contact: Cooperative Research Centre for Aboriginal and Torres Strait Islander Health, PO Box 41096, Casuarina, Northern Territory, 0811. Phone: (08) 8922 8106; Fax: (08) 8927 5187.

49. Cass, A, Cunningham, J, Wang, Z & Hoy, W. 2001; 'Regional Variation in the Incidence of End-Stage Renal Disease in Indigenous Australians', *Medical Journal of Australia*, 175 (1), 24–27.

50. White, AV, Hoy, WE & McCredie, DA. 2001; 'Childhood Post-Streptococcal Glomerulonephritis as a Risk Factor for Chronic Renal Disease in Later Life', *Medical Journal of Australia*, 174, 492–496.

51. Atkins, RC. 2001; 'How Bright is Their Future? Post-Streptococcal Glomerulonephritis in Indigenous Communities in Australia' (editorial), *Medical Journal of Australia*, 174, 489–490.

52. Health Division, Department of Public Services, Victorian Government. 1999; *Promoting Oral Health, 2000–2004: Strategic Directions and Framework for Action*. http://www.dhs.vic.gov.au/phd/9909034/index.htm.

53. Smith, S. 2002; 'Immunologic Aspects of Organ Transplantation', in *Organ Transplantation: Concepts, Issues, Practice, and Outcomes*, Medscape. http://www.medscape.com/viewarticle/436533.

54. Arbor, A; 'HLA Matching, Antibodies and You', University of Michigan Medical Centre, Department of Pathophysiology Histocompatibility Laboratory. http://www.med.umich.edu/trans/public/hla/hla_&_you.html.

55. HLA Database, European Bioinformatics Institute. 2004; http://www.ebi.ac.uk/imgt/hla/intro.html.

56. National Institutes of Health. 2000; News Release 6 September 2000. http://www2.niaid.nih.gov/newsroom/releases/ihwg.htm.

57. Zeier, M, Döhler, B, Opelz, G & Ritz, E. 2002; 'The Effect of Donor Gender on Graft Survival', *Journal of the American Society of Nephrology*, 13, 2570–2576.

58. Collaborative Transplant Study. 2003; *CTS: Collaborative Transplant Study*. http://www.ctstransplant.org/.

59. Australian Red Cross Blood Service. 2004; http://www.giveblood.redcross.org.au.

60. University of Maryland Medicine. 2003; 'High PRA Rescue'. http://www.umm.edu/transplant/kidney/highpra.html.

61. Montgomery, RA, Zachary, AA, Racusen, LC, Leffell, MS, King, KE, Burdick, J, *et al*. 2000; 'Plasmapheresis and Intravenous Immune Globulin

Provides Effective Rescue Therapy for Refractory Humoral Rejection and Allows Kidneys To Be Successfully Transplanted into Cross-Match-Positive Recipients', *Transplantation*, 70 (6), 887–895.

62. Listing, J, Rau, R, Muller, B, Alten, R, Gromnica-Ihle, E, Hagemann, D & Zink, A. 2000; 'HLA-DRB1 Genes, Rheumatoid Factor, and Elevated C-Reactive Protein: Independent Risk Factors of Radiographic Progression in Early Rheumatoid Arthritis', *Journal of Rheumatology*, 27 (9), 2100–2109.

63. Ridker, PM, Hennekens, CH, Buring, JE & Rifai, N. 2000; 'C-Reactive Protein and Other Markers of Inflammation in the Prediction of Cardiovascular Disease in Women', *New England Journal of Medicine*, 342 (12), 836–43.

64. Lutz, J & Heemann, U. 2003; 'Tumours after Kidney Transplantation', *Current Opinion in Urology*, 13 (2), 105–109.

65. Olyaei, AJ, Thi, K, deMattos, AM & Bennett, WM. 2001; 'Use of Basiliximab and Daclizumab in Kidney Transplantation', *Progress in Transplantation*, 11 (1), 33–39.

66. Haberal, M, Karakayali, H, Emiroglu, R, Basaran, O, Moray. G & Bilgin, N. 2002; 'Malignant Tumors after Renal Transplantation', *Artificial Organs*, 26 (9), 778–781.

67. Tremblay, F.; Fernandes, M, Habbab, F, de B Edwardes, MD, Loertscher, R & Meterissian, S. 2002; 'Malignancy after Renal Transplantation: Incidence and Role of Type of Immunosuppression', *Annals of Surgical Oncology*, 9 (8), 785–788.

68. Zeier, M, Hartschuh, W, Wiesel, M, Lehnert, T & Ritz, E. 2002; 'Malignancy after Renal Transplantation', *American Journal of Kidney Diseases*, 39 (1), E5.

69. Ramsay, HM, Fryer, AA, Hawley, CM, Smith, AG, Nicol, DL & Harden, PN. 2003; 'Factors Associated with Nonmelanoma Skin Cancer following Renal Transplantation in Queensland, Australia', *Journal of the American Academy of Dermatology*, 49 (3), 397–406.

70. Chapman, J & Webster, A. 2003; 'Cancer Report', in SP McDonald & G Russ (eds.), *The Twenty-Fifth Report: 2002*, Australia and New Zealand Dialysis and Transplant Registry, 83–90.

14 | Oncological Diseases

AUTHORS

KATE CAMERON

IAN OLVER

SALLY BORBASI

LEARNING OBJECTIVES

When you have completed this chapter you will be able to
- Describe the processes of cancer development (carcinogenesis);
- State the common causes of cancer and associated risk factors;
- Identify ways in which cancer is detected;
- Discuss differing treatment modalities for cancer including pharmacological agents and associated side effects;
- Describe the nursing implications of:
  a) a diagnosis of cancer; and
  b) treatment for cancer; and
- Understand key elements in the diagnosis and management of breast cancer, colorectal cancer, Hodgkin's disease, leukaemias, myeloma, lung cancer and prostate cancer.

INTRODUCTION

This chapter includes a detailed description of the anatomical and physiological changes that occur in cells to produce malignancy. The chapter continues by exploring common causal agents and risk factors associated with carcinogenesis. Diagnostic and treatment modalities are reviewed and the nurse's role in the care of the patient with cancer including chemotherapy, is discussed. The chapter concludes with a look at some specific cancers and uses a case study approach to illustrate aspects of care.

GLOSSARY OF TERMS

This chapter requires familiarity with the following terms:

- Biopsy – the surgical removal of tissue for examination to aid in diagnosis;
- Lymph nodes – small oval glands that form part of the defence against infection and cancer by filtering impurities picked up by lymphatic fluid;
- Adjuvant – therapy that is given in addition to primary local therapy, often when it is not certain whether any cancer cells are still present in the body;
- Metastasis – cancer that has spread from the original site to another part of the body;
- Malignant – a tumour that has the ability to metastasise or spread to other parts of the body;
- Palliative – care that is aimed at controlling symptoms rather than cure of disease;
- Cytotoxic – toxic to cells, commonly used to refer to chemotherapy treatment for cancer;
- Nadir – the lowest point, often used to refer to the lowest point of the cell count after chemotherapy treatment; and
- In situ – cells that have become cancer cells but haven't spread.

WHAT IS CANCER?

Cancer occurs because of changes, or mutations, in the genes in a cell that cause that cell to grow out of the control of signals from the remainder of the body. Cancer is really more than 100 different diseases because it can arise from any tissue in the body. Furthermore, cancer cells can spread to sites distant from their tissue of origin.

It is usually believed that at least four or five changes in the genes of DNA are needed over years for a cancer to develop from normal tissue in a process termed carcinogenesis. The first event that alters the DNA (deoxyribonucleic acid) may initiate the process, but further genetic 'insults' are required to promote the process so that a cancer is formed.

In order to be able to follow the processes of cancer development, we need to understand how the growth of normal cells is regulated and what can start and stop the process. From this we can see what changes are needed to escape from this normal pattern of growth and death of cells.

THE CELL CYCLE

At any one time, most cells in the body are not dividing (the G_o phase of the cell cycle), (see Figure 14.1).

Cells, however, can be stimulated to enter a cycle of division by growth factors or hormones. This ultimately results in the cell dividing into two daughter cells, each of which contains an identical copy of the DNA of the original cell. There are several phases to this cell cycle[1]. The first (G_1 or Gap 1 phase) is a time where proteins and ribonucleic acid are

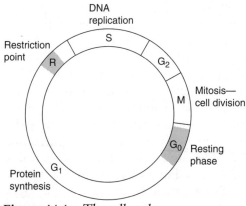

Figure 14.1 *The cell cycle*

synthesised in preparation for the replication (the process of duplicating or reproducing) of the DNA. At the end of this phase is a checkpoint or restriction point (R), which determines whether a cell will enter the next phase of the cycle, the S phase. This next phase is where the replication of the DNA occurs. There follows a second gap (G_2) in preparation for the mitotic phase (M). This second gap has a checkpoint to determine whether the cell will enter the mitotic phase. The mitotic phase is where a spindle of fibrin monomers (material resulting from the action of thrombin on fibrinogen) is formed which draws a copy of the duplicated sets of chromosomes to opposite sides of the cell in preparation for forming two daughter cells. Progression through the cell cycle depends on multiple factors, for example, proteins called cycline dependent kinases control the transitions through the cell cycle.

ONCOGENES

Oncogene translates as 'cancer causing gene'[2]. Why would the body have genes that cause cancer? There are normal genes in the body called proto-oncogenes. The products of these genes regulate the cell proliferation and growth and these genes are closely regulated. Oncogenes can be turned on because of a mutation in a proto-oncogene or a virus inserting an oncogene into the cell. Products of oncogenes behave abnormally, or are over-expressed and cause cells to divide independently of the normal body signals. Oncogene products can act in the cytoplasm of the cell to disrupt the signalling of growth factors or in the nucleus to alter the control of transcription of genes.

TUMOUR SUPPRESSOR GENES

Tumour suppressor genes are also part of the normal cell's DNA, but they have the opposite function to proto-oncogenes in that they suppress growth. In the normal body, old cells need to be able to die to be replaced. Such cells are programmed to die which is a process called apoptosis. The products made by tumour suppressor genes (e.g., p53the Rb gene) are involved in influencing the cell cycle. For example, Rb gene products are necessary for the transition from G_1 to the S phase of the cell cycle that was discussed earlier. p53 increases if there is DNA damage and can halt the cycle to either allow DNA repair to occur or to induce apoptosis. It is clear that either loss of a tumour suppressor gene or its mutation or inactivation could result in a cell that does not die when it should, that is, it transforms the cell into a cancer cell. Furthermore, anti-cancer therapies will try to induce apoptosis. If p53 is intact, higher rates of therapy induced apoptosis would be expected.

GROWTH FACTORS

Growth factors are signals that reside outside the cell and many are products of oncogenes. To impact on cell function, growth factors have to attach to a receptor (like a key fitting into a lock) that straddles the membrane of a cell and activates transmembrane proteins called tyrosine kinases. Activation of these proteins initiates a cascade, enabling the signal to travel from the outside of the cell, through the cytoplasm of the cell to the DNA in the nucleus of the cell, where the reading of genes and the duplication of DNA are controlled. This flow of information is called signal transduction. Having a receptor activated by a growth factor can cause proliferation of a cell or differentiation, or migration of the cell, or confer protection from programmed cell death and sometimes even growth arrest. These signalling pathways are not just single events but multiple paths interacting with each other, and the outcomes can differ, depending on the duration and intensity of the signals and the cooperation between pathways[3]. This creates some overlap in signalling pathways, which explains why a minimum of 4 or 5 hits on oncogenes or tumour suppressor genes (which code for the growth factors, their receptors and the signal transducers) are needed to disrupt the normal regulation of cell function which then leads to cancer.

TUMOUR GROWTH

Theoretically, a cancer cell population that keeps dividing into two daughter cells will exhibit exponential growth, with doubling of the cell population after every cycle. If this were the case, after 30 cycles from each cell, there would be 2^{30} (10^9) cells or 1 gram (or $1\,cm^3$) of tissue. This is the minimal size for detection of a tumour on current scanning machines. Only ten more doublings would produce 10^{12} cells or $1\,kg$ tissue, which could be lethal. However, since some cells will die if a tumour outgrows its blood supply and some will differentiate into non-dividing cells so the rate of growth will not be as rapid. In fact, the peak growth rate of a tumour occurs just before it is clinically detectable and then slows down. This pattern produces what is known as a Gompertzian growth curve, where the growth fraction (the number of dividing cells) of the tumour declines over time[4].

However, when a tumour is treated, a constant percentage of cells is killed (log kill), and as the tumour shrinks, its growth fraction can increase and the rate of growth increase. The observed time in which solid tumours actually double their volumes is variable. Lymphomas usually have volume doubling times of 22 days, while a bowel cancer might be 90 days and some adenocarcinomas may double only each year. The clinical importance of this is that tumours will have started to grow months to years before they are detected, so that any event that a patient may cite as occurring immediately before the detection of a tumour (e.g., trauma), cannot be the causal factor.

Various methods are used to measure the growth of tumours. One method is radioactive labelling of a DNA base (thymidine) and measuring how much of the label is incorporated into the DNA of the tumour. The non-invasive methods involve using proteins made at various stages of the cell cycle as markers of proliferation. One example would be the cyclins mentioned earlier which appear at checkpoints in the cell cycle.

ANGIOGENESIS

A tumour could not grow beyond $2–3\,mm^2$ without new blood vessels growing to provide it with nutrients. Angiogenesis is the growth of new blood vessels from existing vessels and occurs during processes such as the healing of wounds. Cancer cells can produce angiogenic factors (such as vascular endothelial growth factor and basic fibroblast growth factor) that stimulate the formation of new blood vessels. These are balanced with anti-angiogenic factors (such as angiostatin and endostatin)[5].

Several things happen in response to an angiogenic stimulus. The cells around the outside of blood vessels shrink back and the endothelial cells that line blood vessels release proteases (such as the matrix metalloproteinases), which break down the supporting matrix around the vessels. New endothelial cells can migrate into the degraded matrix and form tubes that bud off from the blood vessels to form new blood vessels. Some of the regulation of this occurs when oncogenes in cancer cells are activated, particularly the ras oncogene. Macrophages in the extracellular matrix release angiogenic factors and the cell adhesion molecules (integrins and cadherins) are involved in the adhesion, migration and control of the endothelial cells. If the cancer grows too quickly for the new blood vessel formation, only the outer rim of the cancer will be viable and the inner and middle areas, lacking blood supply, will become necrotic.

These new blood vessels not only provide a means for nutrients to reach the cancer cells but also provide a mechanism for the cancer cells to escape from their original site of growth out into the blood stream so they can spread throughout the body. This process of new blood vessel formation also happens with these secondary deposits of cancer cells.

METASTASES

One of the features of cancer is its ability to spread from one part of the body to another[6]. One way that tumours can cause problems is to directly invade from the primary site into surrounding tissues. Cancer cells can also travel via the blood vessels or via lymphatic vessels which are drainage channels between lymph nodes but also connect with the blood vessels. Another route of tumour invasion is transcoelomic spread, where cancer cells can invade the peritoneal cavity or pleural space.

Not all cells in a cancer are capable of spreading, but every time a cancer divides, it is more likely that it will produce a colony or clone of daughter cells with the ability to metastasise. Even if these cells reach the bloodstream, there is no guarantee that a secondary deposit will result since it appears that not only is there a need for the correct type of cells (seeds), but also to find the right organ (soil) in which to grow. The primary cancer can metastasise to different organs, but there are established patterns of spread for many cancers which means the metastases must only be able to survive in certain environments. The cells also need to be able to survive the journey, migrate to an area and be accepted by surrounding cells.

For tumours to spread, the cancer cells must be able to detach themselves from each other. This is regulated through adhesion proteins (cadherins) on the cells' surfaces which then attach to the membrane separating them from the adjacent extracellular matrix where they want to go. This basement membrane is a scaffold with collagen fibres containing proteins such as laminins and a coating of fibronectin. The cancer cells bind to these fibres in preparation for breaking through. There are many adhesion molecules, such as immunoglobulin adhesion molecules, intergrins and selectins, which all take part in regulating the binding of cells to each other and to the extracellular matrix through which they must move. Cancer cells move through the matrix in response to chemicals in the tissues which attract them or which they produce themselves in order to move independently. The cells move by a series of adhesion and release of the surrounding tissues. They can move into blood and lymph vessels or directly into adjacent organs.

In order to invade surrounding tissues, enzymes called proteases must dissolve the tissue to create a passage. Such enzymes are the serine proteases, the matrix metallaoprotienases and the aspartyl proteinases such as cathepsin D, and there must be a balance between activating and inhibiting factors to regulate this process. Interestingly, cathepsin D concentrations are a prognostic factor in breast cancer and all of these processes are potential targets for the development of new anti-cancer agents.

When the cancer cell reaches another organ it must move from, for example, a blood vessel into the organ in a reverse process to which it escaped. There are many stages of the journey all regulated by adhesion molecules and proteases. Having looked at factors that affect the development and growth of cancer, let us look at the causes of cancer.

WHAT CAUSES CANCER?

In the chain of events that results in cancer, the initiating event may be a change in a single gene in a cell. A person can inherit a defective gene. An example is the discovery that inherited mutations in the BRCA 1 or 2 genes (breast cancer 1 and 2 genes) make women susceptible to developing breast cancer[7]. Carcinogens can also come from the environment, such as the cancer causing agents found when tobacco is burned. In the early stages a cell may not be cancerous, but other agents may promote the process by causing the altered cells to form lumps (such as occurs with polyps in the bowel) which progressively become larger and more abnormal. The agents that promote this change may be viruses or chemicals or even hormones in the case of breast and prostate cancer. Eventually, the pre-cancerous cells will become malignant, either by loss of genes when dividing or further exposure to tumour-promoting agents. Not all damage to the DNA results in the eventual development of cancer, as sometimes, cells can repair the DNA before becoming cancerous. We see then that cancer is caused if a cell is genetically susceptible, perhaps because of inheriting a mutated gene and then, either further mistakes occur when it divides, or agents in the environment trigger the cell to become malignant over time.

AGENTS THAT CAUSE CANCER

In our environment, there are many agents that can cause cancer. These have been discovered by studying large populations of people or in instances where rare cancers cluster together and have in common exposure to a particular agent. Here we will look at the more common cancer causing agents[8].

SMOKING

Smoking tobacco has been associated with 1 in every 3 cancer deaths, and up to 8 in 10 lung cancer deaths. It is also strongly associated with other cancers, such as those of the head and neck or bladder. Burning tobacco creates carcinogens and susceptibility to this agent (and others) varies between individuals because of inherited characteristics. If smokers stop smoking, their risk of lung cancer progressively drops over a period of up to 25 years, proportional to their tobacco usage.

ALCOHOL

In combination with smoking, heavy alcohol intake has been implicated in the development of head and neck cancer. It can also cause liver damage that will lead to liver cancer and may have a smaller role among other factors for common cancers, such as breast cancer.

WORKPLACE EXPOSURE

Perhaps the best known association between exposure to agents in the workplace and cancer is the exposure to asbestos and the development decades later of mesothelioma or lung cancers. There are many other examples, including aniline dye workers being susceptible to bladder cancer, exposure to arsenic in smelting promoting lung and skin cancers and exposure to wood dust resulting in cancers of the sinuses.

DIET

The associations between diet and cancer have been more difficult to establish. High fat consumption, particularly of animal fats, has been linked to colon, breast and prostate cancer. It has been suggested that dietary fibre protects against bowel cancer. Fresh fruit and vegetables contain antioxidants and vitamins that help prevent cancer by aiding DNA repair and slowing cancer promotion. Contaminants of food such as aflatoxins contaminating peanuts are associated with liver cancer, while salting fish or frying food produces carcinogens.

RADIATION

The exposure to ionising radiation from nuclear accidents or war has been well documented to cause cancer. More subtle exposure can result from radon gas arising from the ground where there is underground uranium and the exposure from diagnostic or therapeutic radiation. The risk from non-ionising radiation from power lines or mobile phones has been more difficult to establish.

SUN

Exposure to ultraviolet rays from the sun can cause DNA damage and immunosuppression, particularly in non-pigmented skin. Long-term exposure is associated with non-melanoma skin cancers, while the development of melanoma is more associated with brief bursts of intense sunburn.

INFECTIONS

Most infections do not cause cancer and cancer is not infectious, which is a very important message for patients with cancer who should be able to maintain close personal contact with others as part of coping with the disease. There are specific associations between some infections and particular types of cancer. The human immunodeficiency virus (HIV) is associated with lymphomas and Kaposi's sarcomas. The papilloma virus is linked with cancer of the cervix, hepatitis B with liver cancer and the Ebstein-Barr virus which causes glandular fever with lymphomas. *Helicobacter pylori* in the stomach is associated with stomach cancer and lymphoma while a parasite *Schistosoma haematobium*, in developing countries, causes a rare type of bladder cancer.

HORMONES

Over-stimulation of hormone-sensitive organs such as the breast or endometrium may promote cancer in those where a gene mutation is already present. Sometimes, these may be greater production of hormones or from taking hormone medications.

MEDICATION

Hormone replacement therapy and oral contraceptives have been linked to endometrial cancer. Cytotoxic drugs, particularly alkylating agents, have been associated with the development of secondary cancers several years after their use.

RISK FACTORS

Some groups of people may be at higher risk of developing cancer, such as older people. Additionally, there are some groups at risk of developing specific types of cancer, due to genetic or cultural factors. For example, Japanese people are more likely to develop stomach cancer due to their high intake of pickled foods. In developed countries, the incidence of cancer is increasing as the incidence of other diseases such as infections decreases, and the population tends to live longer. The lifestyle of developed countries may contribute to a higher incidence of certain cancers, for example colorectal and breast cancer related to a high-fat, low-fibre diet.

HOW ARE CANCERS DETECTED?

Cancers generally present as a new lump or a sore that does not heal. Screening programs are used to assist in the early detection of common cancers (mammography to detect breast cancer) or to detect abnormal cells before they become cancerous (Pap smears to detect abnormal cervical cells).

The test used to confirm a diagnosis of cancer is a biopsy of the lesion or lump. If it is suspected that the cancer may have spread from this area, other tests may be used to check cancer spread, such as biopsy of surrounding lymph nodes, chest X-ray, bone scans, computerised axial tomography (CAT) scans and positron emission tomography (PET) scans.

NURSING IMPLICATIONS

A diagnosis of cancer is likely to be a traumatic event for the person concerned, as well as for their family and friends. While the word 'cancer' can be simply defined as an abnormal proliferation of cells, as previously explained cancer can actually be more than a hundred different diseases, depending on the cells and organs affected. More importantly however, the meaning of the word cancer can be interpreted in many different ways by those affected, and their response will be influenced by various factors, such as their experiences leading up to the diagnosis, their perception of the meaning of cancer, their cultural background, their knowledge of treatment and treatment effects, how they have coped with traumatic events in the past and their individual coping styles[9]. Thus, it is important not to make assumptions about 'cancer patients', but rather to approach people diagnosed with cancer on an individual basis. It is also important to dispel any myths associated with cancer, for example, that cancer can be caught by kissing or touching.

Patients diagnosed with cancer face the daunting task of learning about the disease and possible treatments, as well as making a decision about treatment, usually within a relatively short time. Nurses caring for patients with cancer may play a role both in helping the person adjust to their diagnosis and in supporting them through the decision-making process. Nurses can teach patients to self-advocate for quality cancer care through teaching communication skills, how to find and manage information, as well as decision-making and negotiation skills[10]. Nurses can assist the person adjust to the diagnosis of cancer through: checking what information has been given by medical staff (to aid consistency); asking if they need more information, what support they need and how they are feeling; and above all, listening to their responses. Additionally, it is important to provide information at the pace and in the level of detail as preferred by the person concerned. Repetition of information may be needed, as it has been shown that patients may retain only a portion of the information provided, due to factors such as their emotional and psychological response to the diagnosis of cancer, any cognitive impairment, or a lack of motivation to learn (for whatever reason)[11].

Providing practical information about support is also an important nursing role. There are many support agencies, such as the Cancer Council of Australia (TCCA) and the Leukaemia Foundation, which offer support and assistance to people affected by cancer as well as health care professionals. Additionally, there are national and state consumer support and advocacy groups, as well as services that may be offered by local councils and districts. It is important to remember that newly diagnosed patients are often reliant on health care professionals to refer them to these services, particularly if they do not know they exist!

LEARNING EXERCISES

1. Describe the changes occurring at cellular level that give rise to cancer.
2. Outline some of the common causes of cancer.
3. Discuss some of the cancer screening mechanisms currently in use.
4. Explain the role of nurses in the prevention and detection of cancer.

THE TREATMENT OF CANCER

Cancers that are in a localised area may be treated using locally targeted therapies. Surgery can cure a cancer if it has not spread beyond the tissue of origin. Radiotherapy can cover a local area and can be curative as a single modality of treatment, or given in addition to surgery to improve the chances of local control. If there is spread of a tumour beyond its site of origin, or there is a strong chance of microscopic spread beyond, then a systemic treatment is required. This can be chemotherapy, hormone therapy or newer biological or targeted therapies. This section focuses on chemotherapy, radiotherapy, hormone therapy and biological and targeted therapies.

CHEMOTHERAPY

The first scientific development of anti-cancer drugs was during the Second World War. when the alkylating agent nitrogen mustard was used to treat lymphomas. This followed the observations of the effects on individuals' lymphoid tissue of nitrogen mustard gas when an Allied ship was bombed in Bari Harbour in Italy, exposing the servicemen and townspeople to this gas[12].

Most of the cytotoxic drugs that we use today work by disrupting the DNA in cells[13]. If cells cannot replicate their DNA and divide, they die. These drugs do not specifically target cancer cells, but affect any cell that is dividing at the time, which explains why they are toxic to the bone marrow, hair follicles and mucosal cells, as these are populations of cells that are constantly dividing. Usually, the proportion of a cancer that is growing is higher than normal tissues and has less ability to repair itself, and that is why the drugs have a differential effect on cancers. Chemotherapy drugs are classified by how they act (see Table 14.1).

Alkylating agents work by bonding to the bases on DNA and cross-linking the chains of DNA that are wound around each other. This causes breaks in the DNA chains and stops them unwinding to be replicated. This cross-linking can occur wherever the cell is in the cell cycle.

TABLE 14.1: ANTI-CANCER DRUGS

Alkylating Agents	Antimetabolites	Anthracyclines
Amasacrine	Methotrexate	Daunorubicin
Busulphan	Raltitrexid	Doxorubicin
Carmustine	Cladribine	Epirubicin
Chlorambucil	Fludarabine Phosphate	Idarubicin
Cyclophosphamide	Mercaptopurine	Mitozantrone
Fotemustine	Thioguanine	
Ifosfamide	Capecitabine	**Platinum Compounds**
Lomustine	Cytarabine	Carboplatin
Melphalan	Fluorouracil	Cisplatin
Temozolomide	Gemcitabine	Oxaliplatin
Thiotepa	Colaspase	
	Hydroxyurea	**Antineoplastic Antibodies**
Topoisomerase Inhibitors		Gemtuzumab
Irinotecan	**Miscellaneous**	Rituximab
Topotecan	Altretamine	Trastuzumab
	Anagrelide	
Taxanes	Arsenic Trioxide	**Hormones**
Docetaxel	BCG	Tamoxifen
Paclitaxel	Bleomycin	Toremifene
	Dacarbazine	Aminoglutethimide
Vinca Alkaloids	Dactinomycin	Anastrozole
Vinblastine	Interferon	Letrozole
Vincristine	Mitomycin	
Vindesine	Procarbazine	
Vinorelbine	Thalidomide	
Podophyllotoxins	**Tyrosine Kinase Inhibitors**	
Etoposide	Imatinib	
Teniposide	Gefitinib	

Antimetabolites are another class of cytotoxic drugs. These bear a close relationship to the building blocks of DNA and RNA. Drugs like methotrexate can substitute for folic acid in DNA production and 5 fluorouracil can substitute for one of the bases that make RNA. Once substituted, they disrupt the synthetic process because they do not have the same function as the native components.

Antitumour antibiotics, such as bleomycin and doxorubicin, are isolated from bacteria. They slide between the chains of DNA and prevent them dividing.

Other drugs are derived from plants. Vincristine comes from the periwinkle plant and works by stopping the microtubules joining together to form the spindle to which the identical copies of DNA attach to be drawn to opposite sides of the cell during mitosis. Only cells that are in this phase of the cycle will be able to be killed by this drug. Another class of drugs from plants, the taxanes, are made from the bark of yew trees and actually work in the opposite way by stopping the spindle disaggregating and therefore stopping the process of cell division. Drugs originally derived from chemicals in the mandrake plant, the podophyllotoxins, etoposide and teniposide, stop the cell cycle before the spindle forms. They affect the way the DNA is folded and cause breaks in the DNA, which stops it dividing.

RESISTANCE TO CHEMOTHERAPY

Cancer can be or become resistant to chemotherapy. Every time a cancer cell divides, there is the possibility that a mutation may occur that confers resistance to particular drugs. If the drugs are not present, there will be no advantage to this, but in the presence of the chemotherapy these resistant cells will survive. In another mechanism of resistance, there is a multi-drug resistant gene that can be turned on in response to exposure to certain types of drugs including doxorubicin, vincristine and paclitaxel It codes for a protein called p-glycoprotein which acts as a pump in the cell's membrane and pumps the drug out of the cell before it can kill the cell. Resistance to one of these drugs by this mechanism implies resistance to all the others. An even simpler way in which cancer can avoid being killed by chemotherapy is through being sheltered. There are some sites in the body, particularly the brain and testes, which appear to provide sanctuary from chemotherapy. There are many other such mechanisms of resistance, or a cancer cell can simply repair the damage done by chemotherapy drugs before it dies. There is still much to learn about the pathways to cell death and predicting which cells are likely to respond or be resistant to chemotherapy.

TOXICITIES OF CHEMOTHERAPY

The side effects of chemotherapy are best considered in the sequence in which they occur, although it is beyond the scope of this text to consider them in detail. The most immediate effects are hypersensitivity reactions, which if common, as with paclitaxel, can be reduced by premedication with steroids and antihistamines. Extravasation injuries, where chemotherapy leaks from the vein into the surrounding tissue (sometimes referred to as tissuing), can be generically treated with ice, but drugs such as doxorubicin, which can cause severe continuing tissue damage, should have specific antidotes used. Some cytotoxic agents are irritating to the veins and should be administered in diluted form. With tumours such as leukaemias, which may have rapid breakdown after chemotherapy, a tumour lysis syndrome can occur which is characterised by hyperkalaemia, hyperphosphataemia and hypocalcaemia, hyperuricaemia, renal impairment and acidosis. Where this is a possibility, patients should be pretreated with hydration and uric acid lowering drugs such as allopurinol and bicarbonate as necessary if acidosis develops. Acute post-chemotherapy nausea and emesis occur within the first 24 hours, but the advent of the $5HT_3$ receptor antagonist class of antiemetics, such as ondansetron and the new neurokinin receptor antagonist, have improved the control of delayed emesis over the following days.

The next group of toxicities occurs between 10 and 14 days after the administration of chemotherapy. The dividing cells which are due to replace mature white blood cells or mucosal cells when they die at approximately 10 days have been killed by the chemotherapy, and the blood counts fall and mouth ulcers can occur. There are several different types of white blood cells, which have different roles in preventing and fighting infection. One of the most important types is the neutrophils, which chiefly work against bacterial infection. The white cell counts recover within a few days as stem cells are turned on and new mature cells result. The danger of low white blood cell count is that any bacterial infection that occurs at this time can be life threatening. Any fever at this time or suspicion of infection is treated immediately with broad spectrum antibiotics. To minimise this risk, a granulocyte colony stimulating factor (G-CSF) can be given after chemotherapy to stimulate quicker recovery and avoid the period of low counts. There are no such growth-stimulating factors for the mucosal cells, so mouth ulcers are simply treated with local anaesthetics and antiseptics until they heal within about 10 days. Taste changes may be caused by chemotherapy drugs, but are managed with dietary adaptation as preferred. Likewise, diarrhoea is treated symptomatically. Hair loss also occurs in this period. Anaemia is common and is one cause of fatigue, which can be corrected by transfusion. Delayed emesis, which occurs with drugs such as cisplatin, may be controlled by a new class of drugs, the neurokinin$_1$ receptor antagonists.

Several months later, cumulative organ toxicities can occur. Doxorubicin, for example, damages the heart slightly with each dose, but it is not until eight or nine doses that a decrease in the pumping function of the heart can be detected. Cisplatin causes progressive kidney damage and sometimes tinnitus, high-frequency hearing loss and neuropathy. Vincristine damages the long nerves to the limbs, causing numbness of the feet and hands.

Finally, there are the late toxicities that occur in a small number of patients years after their therapy. Patients may become infertile after chemotherapy. Some women may become prematurely menopausal. Secondary cancers caused by the chemotherapy (particularly alkalyting agents) may start to appear 2 to 5 years later.

NURSING IMPLICATIONS

Nurses use their skills in assessment, problem solving and clinical judgement to make decisions about the optimal care of patients. It is important that the patient undergoing cytotoxic chemotherapy treatment understands the potential and anticipated effects; however, as you can see from the previous section, these effects are many and learning about them could be overwhelming. Initially, as cytotoxic therapy is by its very nature toxic, the patient should be fully assessed in terms of physical condition, nutritional status, renal, pulmonary, liver and cardiac function, bone marrow function and performance status before chemotherapy is administered[14].

Safe and effective administration of the drugs themselves is also critically important, and nurses administering these should have a full understanding of how to protect themselves and the patient from unwanted exposure to the drugs. Tied in with this is the need to manage the intravenous access devices used to administer the drug, whether a peripheral intravenous line, peripherally inserted central catheter (PICC), or a centrally inserted line (e.g., implanted, tunnelled or centrally exiting). At times, patients are discharged home with an intravenous line in situ for ongoing use. Nurses are responsible for educating the patient and family in the care and maintenance of the line, and must have a good understanding themselves in order to both use the line and to educate the patient in care and maintenance as needed[15].

The nurses' role in chemotherapy administration lies in providing information about the treatment and ensuring this is understood, anticipating and managing side effects and toxicities, administering the chemotherapy, and educating the patient and family to be safely discharged to the home or other environment. Indeed, discharge planning is incorporated into the nursing care plan/care pathway from day 1. Additionally, nurses are frequently responsible for referring to other disciplines, due to complications or problems arising which require care outside the boundaries of nursing practice[14]. Advanced practice nurses are specialists in an area who are increasingly taking on extended roles. Patients may well be managed by an oncology nurse practitioner or clinical nurse specialist who will have extensive knowledge and skill in the field.

The importance of full and ongoing assessment cannot be overstated. Through this, toxicities can be prevented, or detected early in their development and effectively treated.

• *Management of immediate patient problems*: Hypersensitivity reaction kits should be available when cytotoxic drugs are administered, and ongoing assessment should include information about whether premedication is required for further cycles.

Nausea and vomiting may be the most distressing side effects experienced by patients undergoing cytotoxic therapy. Poor management of nausea and vomiting in initial chemotherapy cycles can lead to ongoing problems for the remainder of treatment, due to anticipatory association[16]. Factors predicting a greater degree of nausea and vomiting include younger age, female gender, and previous motion and/or pregnancy associated sickness, while a history of heavy alcohol intake is associated with less emesis. It is important to assess whether nausea alone is present, as frequently health professionals may believe that the absence of vomiting means that these symptoms are well controlled, whereas for the patient, nausea may be the more distressing side effect. Nausea and vomiting can be well managed through nurses communicating with the patient to assess the frequency and severity of nausea and vomiting and its effect on quality of life and daily activities, then using this information to more effectively manage these side effects[17]. Patients receiving high dose metoclopramide or prochlorperazine should be observed for related dystonic reactions. Patients who understand the use and mechanism of anti-emetic agents are likely to manage this effect more effectively, so education is a major part of the nursing role. Additionally, advising patients on strategies such as avoidance of stimuli, adjusting eating habits (e.g., smaller portions) and increasing intake of nourishing fluids to ensure adequate nutritional intake can be useful. Engaging the family in patient education is an important strategy to strengthen understanding and support.

• *Management of delayed patient problems*: Bone marrow suppression frequently occurs and may be life threatening. The nadir (i.e., lowest point) of the white cell count usually occurs between 7 and 14 days after chemotherapy administration. Patients should be advised to take precautions throughout the neutropenic period, including being aware of the signs of infection and reporting to health care professionals should these become evident, avoiding those with infections, avoiding crowded places including cinemas and public transport, avoiding damaging the body's defence mechanisms against infection such as skin and mucous membranes (e.g., by using a soft toothbrush), avoiding cuts and bruises and maintaining a good nutritional intake. Good personal hygiene should also be maintained.

The nursing role in relation to prevention and management of mouth ulcers is also important. There are few effective preventive measures and these are mostly drug specific (e.g., oral administration of ice chips for those receiving intravenous 5-fluorouracil). The most important strategy is to ensure regular oral hygiene, which does not damage the mucous membrane[18]. Should mouth ulcers develop, pain relief should be used as needed, including anaesthetic mouthwashes before meals, as well as antiseptic mouthwashes to reduce the risk of systemic infection. Taste changes can also be experienced by those undergoing chemotherapy treatment, which can occur over an extended period and may impact on the patient's nutritional intake and enjoyment of eating as a social event[19]. When present, taste changes can be managed through altering foods eaten to preference.

Lethargy and fatigue are frequently experienced by patients, to a degree that cannot be explained by anaemia alone. There is currently a great deal of interest in this area, as one that impacts significantly on patients' quality of life. Research shows that a regular exercise regimen may counteract feelings of fatigue[20].

One chemotherapy effect that is experienced by many, but not necessarily discussed by health professionals, is the effect that cancer chemotherapy may have on sexuality and fertility. A loss of libido is frequently experienced, due both to the psychological and physical impact of the treatment, yet this is frequently not raised with or by health care professionals[21]. Male patients have the option of sperm storage to support long-term fertility. Research is ongoing into oocytestorage techniques for female patients undergoing cancer treatment, however this is not yet widely available. Both men and women should be advised to avoid pregnancy due to the risk of deformities in the fetus.

Finally, hair loss can be one of the most devastating side effects from the patients' perspective, partly because it is a visible sign of illness, as well as causing a significant change in body image. Nurses can offer practical assistance by informing patients where they can purchase wigs and/or scarves, providing information on reimbursement schemes if available, and by offering emotional support. Referral can be made to programs such as 'Look Good . . . Feel Better', a free service offered by volunteers from the cosmetic industry which provides an opportunity for patients to experiment with make-up, to receive advice on skin care and to be pampered[22]. For those with young children, the experience of hair loss can be particularly traumatic and again, there are support agencies which nurses can refer patients to.

RADIOTHERAPY

Radiotherapy is a localised form of treatment that may be defined as 'the use of ionising radiation for therapeutic purposes'[23], where radiation is used to damage and/or kill cells in a specified treatment area. Radiotherapy treatment is commonly administered over a period of one to six weeks; however, this is influenced by the treatment dose and intent. A variety of methods are used for delivery of radiotherapy treatment, the most commonly used being external beam radiotherapy (or teletherapy), which is delivered using a machine such as a linear accelerator. The type of treatment used depends on the location, size and type of tumour, and the treatment intent may be definitive (the sole mode of treatment used), adjuvant (used in conjunction with other treatment), prophylactic (used in areas which may harbour cancer cells), control (to limit the growth of disease) or palliative (when cure is not predicted)[24].

Specialised treatment delivery methods have been developed to administer high doses of radiotherapy to specific areas, such as the use of brachytherapy (internally delivered radiotherapy treatment) in prostate cancer. There are resulting potential side effects, including urinary and rectal morbidity and erectile dysfunction[25].

Despite its administration to a localised area, radiotherapy causes both localised and systemic effects, including skin reactions, fatigue, and loss of appetite. The systemic effects are likely to overlap with those caused by the cancer itself; however, for example, fatigue is likely to be experienced by the patient with cancer as a 'universal symptom of illness'[26], and may be exacerbated by radiotherapy. The incidence of radiotherapy-related fatigue is high (up to 80% experience fatigue during or shortly following treatment and up to 30% experience chronic fatigue following treatment). Patients receiving radiotherapy on an outpatient basis may experience greater levels of fatigue due to the need to travel and wait for treatment.

Site-specific radiotherapy side effects include bone marrow suppression, hair loss, diarrhoea, mucosal inflammation and ulceration, and nausea and vomiting[27], which are treated as needed. These complications can be severe, for example, as when curative doses of radiotherapy are delivered to the head and neck region. This can cause xerostomia (loss of saliva), dental deterioration and most commonly, oral mucositis, which may be severe and is treated similarly to those receiving chemotherapy, i.e., assessment pre-treatment, frequent mouth washes and ongoing assessment[28]. From a patient perspective, interviews conducted with patients undergoing radiotherapy treatment have shown that patients feel it is important that they are well informed by health care professionals about radiotherapy treatment and its effects[29].

HORMONE TREATMENT

Hormones are chemical messengers and some organs are under the control of hormones released from distant sites. For example, the pituitary gland at the base of the brain releases hormones, which in women stimulates the ovary to produce the hormone oestrogen, and in men the testis to produce the hormones androgens. These in turn stimulate the breast tissue, the endometrium and the prostate gland. Cancers in these organs can also be stimulated by these hormones, and blocking that stimulus can cause death of the tumour. For example, tamoxifen is an antioestrogen medication, which will stop the body's oestrogen from stimulating breast cancer cells that have oestrogen receptors on their surfaces. Similarly, in prostate cancer, either removing the source of androgens by removing the testes or blocking the androgens with drugs, such as flutamide, will shrink this tumour.

PROTEIN THERAPIES

Some proteins produced by the body are known to have effects on the immune system and can be produced in large quantities and given as anti-cancer therapy. Such a drug is interferon, which has multiple sites of action and is a treatment option for melanoma. Attempts have also been made to use proteins on the surface of cancer cells to make vaccines, but these are still experimental, as are therapies based on inserting genes into cancer cells to cause them to die.

TARGETED THERAPIES

A new approach to systemic therapy targets products of gene expression that are specific to cancers, rather than targeting DNA non-specifically. The initial examples of these treatments were rituximab (Mabthera)[30], trastuzumab (Herceptin)[31], imatinib mesylate[32] (Glivec) and gefitinib[33] (Iressa). The first two are monoclonal antibodies used for lymphomas and breast cancer respectively, which were produced by fusing mouse and human antibodies. The general side effects are fevers, chills, 'flu-like' symptoms, nausea and asthenia, and allergic reactions. Rituximab can be associated with heart arrhythmias and trastuzumab exacerbates cardiac failure in some patients. The targets CD 20 and HER 2-Neu over-expression are measured respectively to determine whether the therapy is useful. Imantanib (Glivec) and gefitinib (Iressa) are small molecules which target the tyrosine kinases associated with over-expression of specific gene products. Imatanib is used for chronic myeloid leukaemia, and is the only therapy that is effective in treating the rare gastrointestinal tumour (GIST). Gefitinib has been associated with symptomatic responses in non-small cell lung cancer, even when given after two lines of chemotherapy. Again the side effects are mild, including rash, diarrhoea and myalgias.

NURSING IMPLICATIONS

Patients come from a variety of backgrounds with different understanding and expectations of cancer treatment. It is important for nurses not to assume that once the initial education is complete the patient will go through the rest of chemotherapy treatment uneventfully, but instead to keep checking with the patient as to how he/she is, as well as checking with family and friends. Those from rural and remote areas may experience particular difficulty in travelling to treatment centres and managing side effects during travel. Cancer treatment can also be expensive due to time off work, travel required, and particularly for those from rural areas, time for the spouse or partner away from work as well. Issues that arise during treatment may not be volunteered by patients and can cause unnecessary distress, so it is important to advise that many support groups are available for those undergoing cancer treatment.

AFTER TREATMENT: ISSUES OF CANCER SURVIVORSHIP

The experience of cancer does not end with the completion of treatment. Survivors of cancer treatment may be expected to feel thankful and happy at having been faced with potential death and surviving. While this is true of some, there is a range of reactions seen in cancer survivors. Australian researchers describe the experience of survivors as living through an illness experience, but then not returning to a 'normal' world[34]. This is understood to be due to three main elements. First, the label of 'cancer patient' persists, both in the minds of the patient and those around the patient, and is reinforced by the need for ongoing assessment and vigilance. Second, the patient is aware of the body's mortality and its capacity for serious illness. Third, there is the sense that the patient has lived through an extraordinary experience (cancer) and is in a way alone in that experience. Added to this is the difficulty that patients may feel when finishing treatment. Usually, they have come to know the staff and may have seen treatment as a life-saving intervention, which can add to difficulties experienced at the end of treatment. Good communication with the patient and his/her family from diagnosis onwards can assist the transition through identifying these perceptions and issues and reassuring the patient that a range of responses and feelings is normal.

SPECIFIC CANCERS

BREAST CANCER

Breast cancer is the most common cause of cancer deaths in women. Most are sporadic, but some are inherited due to mutations in genes such as BRCA 1 and BRCA 2. Breast cancer may be confined to the ducts in the breast before becoming invasive, and sometimes this will show as calcifications in screening mammograms. The initial treatment is surgery, either to remove the breast or just the lump and then to sterilise the rest of the breast with radiotherapy. Breast cancer often spreads to the lymph glands under the arm, which are often sampled or removed, both as part of therapy and to predict the likelihood of later widespread disease (this correlates with the number of nodes involved). Follow-up with radiotherapy improves local control, and chemotherapy or hormone therapy after surgery reduces the chance of distant relapse. Breast cancer most commonly spreads to the liver, lungs, bone or brain. Once widespread it is incurable, with a median survival of two years. Chemotherapy is used to control the disease and bone symptoms may be alleviated with bisphosphonates or radiotherapy. Trastuzumab may be used for breast cancers that over-express HER 2.

COLORECTAL CANCER

Unless detected early by screening with a test to measure blood in the stools, bowel cancer on the right side of the bowel tends to be quite advanced before symptoms such as anaemia, from slow blood loss or occasional pain arise. Left-sided tumours usually present with frank per rectal bleeding or obstruction. Colon cancer is cured by surgery if detected early when it is confined to the bowel wall. If it has spread through the wall or into the surrounding lymph nodes, additional (known as adjuvant) chemotherapy following surgery improves the likelihood of survival. With rectal cancer, adjuvant radiotherapy is also used. Follow-up after treatment involves checking using colonoscopy and a blood test for the carcinoembryonic antigen (CEA). The first site of distant metastases is often the liver, then lungs, and once metastatic, bowel cancer is incurable but progression of the disease can be controlled by drugs such as 5 fluorouracil with irinotecan or oxaliplatin.

HODGKIN'S DISEASE

This cancer involving the lymph nodes tends to spread along nodes in the midline of the body and was named after Thomas Hodgkin who first described the disease. It has two peaks of incidence, in young adults and in those over 60 years of age, and is associated with infections such as with the Epstein-Barr virus. It can be associated with general symptoms of weight loss, drenching night sweats and fevers. It was one of the first cancers to be cured by multi-agent chemotherapy (nitrogen mustard, vincristine, procarbazine, prednisone [MOPP] or adriamycin, bleomycin, vinblastine and dacarbazine i.e., [ABVD]). If localised to a small group of nodes on one side of the diaphragm, Hodgkin's disease can be cured with radiotherapy. The development of a second cancer years after therapy is more common if both radiotherapy and chemotherapy have been used.

LEUKAEMIAS

These are malignancies of the white blood cells in the bone marrow and are categorised as acute or chronic depending on their time course, and are further classified by their cell of origin, either myeloid or lymphatic. Acute leukaemias can occur years after exposure to radiation, cytotoxic drugs or benzene derivatives. Acute lymphocytic leukaemia is the most common leukaemia in childhood and has a high cure rate with chemotherapy. The spinal fluid also requires treatment as leukaemic cells may be harboured there. Acute myeloid leukaemia in adults requires intense induction chemotherapy to eradiate the leukaemic cells in the bone marrow, and 15–30% of people are cured. Maintenance chemotherapy is often given. If the leukaemia relapses, high dose chemotherapy with bone marrow transplants from normal donors can be used.

Chronic myeloid leukaemia has a classic abnormality, the Philadelphia chromosome, which is formed when one part of chromosome 9 relocates to chromosome 22. It has a chronic phase, then an accelerated phase, followed by what is known as a blast crisis when it transforms into acute leukaemia. The chronic phase, which usually lasts for four or five years, can be treated with oral chemotherapy or interferon. More recently, Imatinib has been found to be active. High-dose therapy may also be used to attempt cure. Chronic lymphatic leukaemia on the other hand is a more indolent disease, which is associated with an increasing rate of infection and may eventually need palliation treatment using oral chemotherapy agents.

MYELOMA

Myeloma is an incurable malignancy of the plasma cells in the bone marrow. Plasma cells usually produce immunoglobulins to help fight infection. In myeloma, abnormal proteins are produced which can be measured in the blood and part of which can be excreted in the urine as Bence-Jones protein. Myeloma often presents as multiple lytic (or eroded) areas in the bones that can cause pain, fractures or high blood calcium levels and ultimately kidney failure. Increasingly, intense chemotherapy regimens, including stem cell transplantation, have improved the control of this disease.

LUNG CANCER

Small–cell lung cancer is the most chemosensitive form of lung cancer and is likely to spread by the blood stream very early in its history; hence, it is often initially treated with chemotherapy with a cure rate of 5–10% of patients. For the remainder, including for those with non-small-cell carcinoma, lung cancers remain localised to the lung for longer and therefore the initial treatment is surgery, which in early stage disease can be associated with five-year survival rates of 45%. In more extensive disease, surgery, radiotherapy and chemotherapy may be used. Metastatic disease is incurable but more active drugs are being discovered and there are multiple agents based on cisplatin, the taxanes, and gemcitabine or vinorelbine. There is also potential for the epidermal growth factor receptor (EGFR) tyrosine kinase inhibitor Gefitinib to improve the outcome.

PROSTATE CANCER

The natural history of prostate cancer is variable, with more men dying with the disease than of the disease. This makes the issue of screening using the presence of PSA (prostate specific antigen) in the blood problematic, because although screening will be life saving for some men, it may lead to over-treatment of others. The treatment choices for localised disease are surgery or radical radiotherapy, particularly in older patients. For advanced disease, hormone therapy is the treatment of choice. The main site of metastasis is the bone. Radiotherapy can be used to relieve pain in localised areas or injected isotopes can alleviate widespread pain. Bisphosphonates can reduce bone complications. When the disease becomes hormone insensitive, chemotherapy has only had very limited impact.

● Case study

Elizabeth Thompson, 34, was recently diagnosed with invasive ductal carcinoma (breast cancer) in her left breast. She is married with two children, a girl aged six and a boy aged two. The lump was detected when she attended her general practitioner for a routine biennial check up, including a Pap smear. A biopsy of the lump showed it was cancerous and had probably been there for some time. Elizabeth had an appointment with the surgeon to discuss her results.

Elizabeth is likely to be feeling shock at her diagnosis and may find it helpful to take a family member or friend with her to the appointment as support and to help with asking questions and listening to the answers. She may ask about: the extent of the disease; what further information is needed and how this will be obtained; treatment options and their risks and benefits; the prognosis; the time and cost involved in treatment; any significant long-term effects; and any entitlements to services and supports (such as reimbursement for travelling or prostheses). The surgeon will order tests of the breast cancer pathology and the axillary lymph nodes, and may order other tests such as X-rays, depending on Elizabeth's clinical symptoms. The results of the pathology of the tumour or its spread to the lymph glands will dictate the need for additional treatment with hormone therapy or chemotherapy. The results in Elizabeth's case indicate that she should receive chemotherapy, as the pathology indicates it is an aggressive tumour and there is a possibility it may have spread. Elizabeth is referred to an oncologist and prescribed cytotoxic chemotherapy for six months. One of the key concerns she focuses on is her hair falling out.

Elizabeth should be given information about options of wigs and scarves to help her manage her hair loss, should she have chemotherapy. She should be referred to sources for these, as well as programs such as 'Look Good . . . Feel Better'. She may need referral to a social worker or psychologist for counselling on handling discussion with her children on her hair loss and being sick. Practical advice is also available through pamphlets and children's literature.

 Case study

Mr Antonio Corelli, 72, emigrated from Italy 50 years ago and has a strong and supportive family. He is diagnosed with colon cancer, which at operation was found to have spread to the local lymph glands. The surgeon told Mr Corelli that the entire tumour was removed, but has recommended chemotherapy treatment after surgery. Furthermore, the surgeon discussed the treatment options with him during a ward round when no family members were present. Mr Corelli now appears apprehensive and confused about the treatment plan and why chemotherapy is needed.

It is critical that Mr Corelli understands the treatment offered and the potential side effects. The specialist should be advised that Mr Corelli needs more information, and an interpreter should be offered. He should be informed about the risks and side effects of chemotherapy, including the need to minimise his risk of infection, the risk of experiencing nausea and vomiting and mucositis and what to do should these occur, fatigue, and the impact on personal relationships. One strategy, which may be useful in checking his level of understanding, is to ask him to recount his understanding of the treatment.

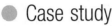

Case study

Ms Anne Shaw, 67, is a pensioner who lives on her own in a home unit. She is currently 10 days following her third cycle of ABVD chemotherapy, which is being used to treat her Hodgkin's disease. After the first cycle of ABVD, her neutrophil count dropped to $500/mm^3$ (normal range 1500–4000 mm^3). She has not had a blood test taken after the second or third cycles. She has been taking her temperature daily as advised, and her temperature reading is currently 38.2°C. She rings the ward for advice.

LEARNING EXERCISES

1. Why is Ms Shaw's temperature likely to be raised?
2. What advice should the nurse on the ward give her?

Ms Shaw's neutrophil count was significantly lower than normal, which put her at risk of infection. She should be advised to seek medical treatment as soon as possible, and should be prescribed broad-spectrum antibiotics immediately to treat the infection and avoid life-threatening sepsis.

CONCLUSION

This chapter has shown that the development of cancer is a complex process of genetic aberration, influenced by risk factors such as lifestyle choices. An understanding of this process including cellular changes allows a better understanding of the treatments used and their effects.

Cancer treatments are toxic and it is important that patients undergoing these understand the principles of their side effects to better enable them to care for themselves safely. The nurses' role is often to ensure that patients have the information they require at a level and pace they can access effectively. Cancer and its treatment also do not take place in isolation, but has an impact on the patient, family and friends. This chapter has used case studies to demonstrate the variety of circumstances and needs of patients that nurses can encounter.

Nurses working in any area are likely to care for those affected by cancer, particularly in the context of an ageing population such as currently seen in Australia. For this reason, it is advantageous for nurses to have knowledge and insight into the effects of cancer and its treatments.

Recommended Reading

Corner, J & Bailey, C. (eds.). 2001; *Cancer Nursing: Care in Context*, Blackwell Science, London.

DeVita, VT, Hellman, S & Rosenberg, SA. 2001; *Cancer: Principles and Practice of Oncology*, Lippincott Williams and Wilkins, Philadelphia, 335–460.

Olver, I. 1998; *Conquering Cancer: Your Guide to Treatment and Research*, Allen & Unwin, Sydney.

Poulton, G. (ed.). 1998; *Nursing the Person with Cancer*, Ausmed, Melbourne.

Souhami, RL, Tannock, I, Hohenberger, P & Horiot, J-C. 2002; *Oxford Textbook of Oncology* (2nd ed.), Oxford University Press, Oxford.

Yarbro, CH, Goodman, M, & Hansen Frogge, M, (eds.). 2000; *Cancer Nursing: Principles and Practice* (5th ed.), Jones and Bartlett, Boston.

References

1. Elledge, SJ. 1996; 'Cell Cycle Checkpoints: Preventing an Identity Crisis', *Science*, 274, 1664–1672.
2. Bishop, JM. 1995; 'Cancer: The Rise of the Genetic Paradigm', *Genes and Development*, 9, 1309–1315.
3. Cross, M & Dexter, TM. 1991; 'Growth Factors in Development, Transformation and Tumourigenesis', *Cell*, 64, 271–280.
4. Laird, AK. 1965; 'Dynamics of Tumour Growth: Comparison of Growth Rates and Extrapolation of Growth Curves to One Cell', *British Journal of Cancer*, 19, 278–291.
5. Folkman, J. 1990; 'What Is the Evidence that Tumours are Angiogenesis Dependent?', *Journal of the National Cancer Institute*, 82, 4–6.
6. Hart, IR. 2002; 'Metastases', in RL Souhami, I Tannock, P Hohenberger & J-C Horiot (eds.), *Oxford Textbook of Oncology* (2nd ed.), Oxford University Press, Osford, 103–113.
7. Easton, DF, Ford, D & Bishop, DT. 1995; 'Breast Cancer Linkage Consortium: Breast and Ovarian Cancer Incidence in BRCA 1-Mutation Carriers', *American Journal of Human Genetics*, 56, 265–271.
8. Olver, IN. 1998; *Conquering Cancer: Your Guide to Treatment and Research*, Allen & Unwin, Sydney.
9. Wells, M. 2001; 'The Impact of Cancer', in J Corner & C Bailey (eds.), *Cancer Nursing: Care and Context*, Blackwell Science, London 63–85.
10. Gomez, EG & McHale, M. 2002; 'The Advocacy Needs of Patients with Cancer and Cancer Survivors', in EG Gomez & M Gullatte (eds.), *Advocacy in Health Care: Teaching Patients, Caregivers and Professionals*, Oncology Nursing Society, Pittsburgh, 9–13.
11. Dodd, MJ. 1999; 'Self-Care and Family Teaching', in C Henke Yarbro, M Hansen Frogge & M Goodman (eds.), *Cancer Symptom Management* (2nd ed.), Jones & Bartlett, Sudbury, Massachusetts, 20–32.
12. Alexander, SF. 1944; *Final Report of Bari Mustard Casualties*, Allied Force Headquarters, Office of the Surgeon, Washington DC, APO 512, 20 June 1944.
13. DeVita, VT, Hellman, S & Rosenberg, SA. 2001; *Cancer: Principles and Practice of Oncology*, Lippincott Williams and Wilkins, Philadelphia.
14. Dougherty, L & Bailey, C. 2001; 'Chemotherapy', in J Corner & C Bailey (eds.), *Cancer Nursing: Care and Context*, Blackwell Science, Oxford, 179–221.
15. Gorski, LA & Grothman, L. 1996; 'Home Infusion Therapy', *Seminars in Oncology Nursing*, 12 (3), 193–201.
16. Marek, C. 2003; 'Antiemetic Therapy in Patients Receiving Cancer Chemotherapy', *Oncology Nursing Forum*, 30 (2), 259–269.
17. Wickham, R. 1999; 'Nausea and Vomiting', in C Henke Yarbro, M Hansen Frogge & M Goodman (eds.), *Cancer Symptom Management* (2nd ed.), Jones and Bartlett, Sudbury, Massachusetts, 228–263.
18. The Joanna Briggs Institute. 1998; *Best Practice: Prevention and Treatment of Oral Mucositis in Cancer Patients*, Joanna Briggs Institute for Evidence Based Nursing and Midwifery, Adelaide.
19. Cameron, K, Borbasi, S, Quested, B & Evans, D. 2003; 'A Matter of Taste: The Experience of Chemotherapy-related Taste Changes', *The Australian Journal of Cancer Nursing*, 4 (1), 3–9.
20. Mock, V, Pickett, M, Ropka, ME, Muscari Lin, E, Stewart, KJ, Rhodes, VA, *et al.* 2001; 'Fatigue and Quality of Life Outcomes of Exercise during Cancer Treatment', *Cancer Practice*, 9 (3), 119–127.
21. Hughes, MK. 2000; 'Sexuality and the Cancer Survivor: A Silent Coexistence', *Cancer Nursing*, 23 (6), 477–482.
22. 'Look Good . . . Feel Better'. Accessed 20 July 2003 at: http://www.lgfb.org.au/home.html.
23. *Churchill's Illustrated Medical Dictionary*. 1989; Churchill Livingston, New York.
24. Haas, ML & Kuehn, EF. 2001; 'Teletherapy: External Radiation Therapy', in D Watkins-Bruner, G Moore-Higgs & M Haas (eds.), *Outcomes in Radiation Therapy*, Jones and Bartlett, Sudbury, Massachusetts, 55–66.
25. Abel, L, Dafoe-Lambie, J, Butler, WM & Merrick, GS. 2003; 'Treatment Outcomes and Quality-of-Life Issues for Patients Treated with Prostate Brachytherapy', *Clinical Journal of Oncology Nursing*, 7 (1), 48–54.
26. Moore, GJ & Hayes, C. 2001; 'Maintenance of Comfort (Fatigue and Pain)', in D Watkins-Bruner, G Moore-Higgs & M Haas (eds.), *Outcomes in Radiation Therapy*, Jones and Bartlett Publishers, Sudbury, Massachusetts, 459–492.
27. Maher, KE. 2000; 'Radiation Therapy: Toxicities and Management', in C Henke Yarbro, M Hansen Frogge, M Goodman & SL Groenwald (eds.), *Cancer Nursing: Principles and Practice*, Jones and Bartlett, Sudbury, Massachusetts, 323–351.
28. Shih, A., Miaskowski, C., Dodd, MJ., Stotts, NA & MacPhail, L. 2002; 'A Research Review of the Current Treatments for Radiation-induced Oral Mucositis in Patients with Head and Neck Cancer', *Oncology Nursing Forum*, 29 (7), 1063–1080.
29. Long, LE. 1998; 'Getting through Radiation Therapy: A Hermeneutic Inquiry of the Experience of Undergoing Radiation Therapy', in *Faculty of Health Sciences, School of Nursing. . . .* Flinders University of South Australia, Adelaide.
30. Plosker, GL & Figgitt, DP. 2003; 'Rituximab: A Review of Its Use in Non-Hodgkin's Lymphoma

and Chronic Lymphocytic Leukaemia', *Drugs*, 63, 803–843.

31. Mokbel, K & Elkak, A. 2001; 'Recent Advances in Breast Cancer', *Current Medical Research Opinion*, 17, 116–122.

32. Capdeville, R, Silberman, S & Imatinib, A. 2003; 'A Targeted Clinical Drug Development', *Seminars in Hematology*, 40, 21–25.

33. Sridhar, SS., Seymour, L., Shepherd, FA. 2003; 'Inhibitors of Epidermal-Growth-Factor Receptors: A Review of Clinical Research with a Focus on Non-Small Cell Lung Cancer', *Lancet Oncology*, 4, 397–406.

34. Little, M, Sayers, EJ, Paul, K & Jordens, CFC. 2000; 'On Surviving Cancer', *Journal of the Royal Society of Medicine*, 93 (10), 501–503.

15 | Ageing and Health Breakdown

AUTHORS

MELISSA SINFIELD

DEBORAH HATCHER

DEBRA JACKSON

LEARNING OBJECTIVES

When you have completed this chapter you will be able to
- Describe the major physiological systemic changes that accompany ageing and how these play a part in health breakdown;
- Discuss polypharmacy and why older people are vulnerable to it;
- Explain the importance of thorough health assessment in the care of older people; and
- Develop nursing interventions to promote safety and reduce hazards associated with ageing and the use of medications.

INTRODUCTION

THE AGEING POPULATION

Australia and New Zealand, along with the rest of the world, have ageing populations. People are living longer than ever before due to various factors, including improved health services, and scientific and medical developments that have led to improvements in pharmacology as well as other technologies that promote longevity. In addition, increasing consumerism has resulted in an enhanced awareness of the role of diet, exercise and general health maintenance among people in general, including older people. These factors, coupled with a declining birth rate, mean that Australia's population will continue to age at least until the middle of the century[1]. From a health perspective, people are considered old once they are 65 years and *old,* old when over 85 years.

TERMINOLOGY

The branch of medicine concerned with the elderly is called geriatric medicine, or gerontology. *Geriatrics* is a word derived from the Greek word *geras*, meaning old age[2]. *Gerontology* is also derived from Greek (*geron* = old man) and is the umbrella term used to describe the study of ageing and its problems, and encompasses biophysiologic as well as social and psychological aspects[2]. More recently, the term *gerontic nursing* has become part of the health care lexicon and is a broad term to describe the range of caring acts associated with nursing older people[2].

Nursing care of the aged, or *gerontic nursing* is a specialist area of health care and there are many courses available to nurses at postgraduate level. While many older people remain in good health well into old age, health care providers encounter older people in almost all clinical settings. With the exception of paediatrics and midwifery, all clinical areas are seeing increasing numbers of older people. Therefore, despite the status of gerontic nursing as a specialty, the demands of the ageing population require all nurses to have proficiency in gerontic nursing – that is, be cognisant of biophysical, experiential and psychosocial aspects of ageing, and how ageing affects and is affected by disease and its management, including surgical and pharmacological interventions.

This chapter introduces you to some of the major health-related changes that accompany ageing, with a particular focus on applied pharmacology, polypharmacy and health assessment.

SYSTEMIC CHANGES ASSOCIATED WITH AGEING
CARDIOVASCULAR SYSTEM

The cardiovascular system is the system most likely to deteriorate as people age[3]. Structural changes may include dilation and increased rigidity of the aorta[3,4], fibrosis of the endocardium[5], left ventricle hypertrophy[4], and thickening and rigidity of the atrioventicular valves[5]. There may be loss of pacemaker cells and an increase in fibrosis and adipose tissue both in and around the heart[4,5]. Rigidity of the aorta and ventricle walls leads to a decrease in myocardial contractility[3]. There is a decrease in the amount of blood filling the heart and therefore in the amount that is pumped out with each beat (reduced stroke volume)[4]. In older people, the contraction and relaxation phase of the left ventricle are prolonged, resulting in reduction of the heart's pumping ability[3,4,6] and reduced cardiac output[3]. There may be calcification of the coronary arteries that impedes blood flow and causes hypertrophy of the left ventricle[4].

As people age, changes in the lining of blood vessels frequently occur. The middle layer of the vessel, tunica media, becomes rigid due to the thinning and calcification of the elastin fibres. Fibrosis and an accumulation of fats and lipids lead to atherosclerosis in the inner layer, tunica intima[6]. Some common examples of health breakdown in the elderly due to age-related changes in the cardiovascular system include atherosclerosis, and hypertension or hypotension.

ENDOCRINE SYSTEM

In the endocrine system, there are many diverse changes that can be attributed to ageing[6]. Structural changes include fibrosis and atrophy of glands and an increase in nodularity[4,6]. These changes may lead to a decrease in activity, basal metabolic rate, and less thyrotropin secretion and release. There may be a decrease in iodine clearance rates[4,6], excretion of 17-ketosteroids and thyroid function due to a loss of adrenal function[6].

Secretion of glucocorticoids, progesterone, androgen, oestrogen and aldosterone are all reduced[6]. The volume of the pituitary gland decreases[6], there is atrophy and fibrosis, and a decrease in vascularity, mass and weight. There is increased interstitial fatty tissue in the parathyroid gland[4]. Age-related changes to the pancreas lead to a decrease in glucose tolerance[4] and insufficient release of insulin by the beta cells leads to a decrease in the older person's ability to metabolise carbohydrates[6].

Some examples of health breakdown due to changes in the endocrine system include diabetes mellitus, hyperthyroidism and hypothyroidism.

GASTROINTESTINAL SYSTEM

Problems associated with the gastrointestinal system are common in older people[7]. Changes in function include decreased gastric emptying and increased gastric pH[8], decreased peristaltic action of the oesophagus, reduction in the production of ptyalin, hydrochloric acid and pepsin and a tendency for faulty absorption of vitamins B_1, B_{12}, K, calcium and iron[9]. Many older people experience poor appetite[10]; which may be due to a reduction in taste bud acuity and a decline in their ability to detect sweet and salty food[10]. Older people can also experience problems with their dentition[6] which decreases their ability to enjoy eating. Impaired swallowing increases with age[11] and has been attributed to decreased salivation to moisten food[5,6]. This may also be due to medications such as antihistamines and antidepressants that have anticholinergic effects[11]. Their gag reflex may be diminished resulting in dysphagia[6] and nearly half the people aged over 80 years have diverticulitis due to weakening of the intestinal wall[12]. Other physiological changes include a tendency to constipation or faecal incontinence. The latter is caused by loss of muscle tone of the internal sphincter of the large intestine and diminished awareness of a forthcoming bowel evacuation[9].

GENITOURINARY SYSTEM

A number of structural changes of the genitourinary system occur as people age. Within the kidneys, renal mass[4,6], renal tissue growth, renal blood flow and glomerular filtration rate decrease and creatinine clearance falls with age[6]. Tubular reabsorption and renal concentrating ability decline, resulting in less efficient tubular exchange of substances, conservation of water and sodium and antidiuretic hormone secretion. Adaptive mechanisms to maintain blood volume and extracellular fluid composition are impaired as people get older and plasma renin and plasma aldosterone levels decrease[4]. In the bladder, smooth muscle is replaced by fibrous connective tissue, the muscles weaken and bladder capacity decreases[4,6]. There may also be loss of striated muscle in the external urethral sphincter and decrease in closing pressure[4]. Older people may experience decrease in the force of the flow of urine[4,6], difficulty in bladder emptying and delay in micturition reflex[3,4,6].

In older men, fibrosis of seminiferous tubules can occur, as well as reduced fluid retaining capacity in the seminal vesicles[6], and erections may be slower and more difficult to maintain[4]. The prostate enlarges with age[3,5] and testosterone production may be reduced[6]. In ageing women, a decrease in eostrogen levels weakens the skeletal pelvic floor muscles and urethra smooth muscle[3,5]. There may be atrophy of the vulva, cervix, uterus, fallopian tubes and labia, and the vagina may atrophy and shorten with thinning of the mucous lining and loss of elasticity[6].

Age-related health breakdown related to the genitourinary system includes urinary incontinence, benign prostatic hypertrophy and urinary tract infection[3,4,5,6].

INTEGUMENTARY SYSTEM
The older person's skin differs significantly from the skin of a younger person[13]. Reduction in skeletal muscle mass and subcutaneous fat leads to loose, wrinkled and fragile skin[8]. Skin elasticity is reduced[12] and the time taken for an older person's wounds to heal is usually longer due to reduction in epidermal turnover and repair[14]. Sweat and oil secreting glands atrophy and the older persons' skin loses its ability to retain moisture and is likely to become dry and scaly[15]. Cellular changes can range from uneven pigmentation[16] through to the development of malignant melanoma[14]. Nearly half the people aged 65–75 years of age have at least one significant skin problem, and the majority of people over 75 have between one and four disorders[12]. These include pruritis (severe itching), lentigos (liver spots), eczema, purpura, seborrheic keratoses[12], fungal infections and other skin disorders such as scabies and herpes zoster[17].

MUSCULOSKELETAL SYSTEM
As a consequence of the ageing process, there is decreased bone and muscle mass, and muscle weakness[6]. Older people's bones become brittle due to reduction in calcium absorption[6] and because the rate of bone reabsorption is greater than the rate of new bone formation[4,5]. The number of skeletal muscle fibres decreases with age[3,4,5,6] and there can often be atrophy and decrease in muscle fibre size[3,4,6]. Older people may experience a decrease in height due to a loss of bone mass in the vertebrae and thinning of the intervertebral discs[4,5,6]. Joints may become enlarged[6] and tendons and ligaments can shrink and harden, resulting in reduction of joint mobility[3]. In addition, synovial fluid in the joints can become more viscous and membranes more fibrotic[6]. Reflexes become slower, largely due to shrinkage of muscles and tendons[4].

Age-related alterations to the musculoskeletal system can lead to changed appearance and slower movements in the older person[4]. As a consequence of these changes, their movement is often more cautious, they may experience difficulty maintaining their balance[3], and can be prone to falls[6]. Three examples of health breakdown due to changes in the musculoskeletal system are osteoporosis, osteoarthritis and fractures.

NERVOUS SYSTEM

Nervous system changes attributed to ageing are diminished brain weight[18], and a reduction in the size and density of neurones[19]. The number of synapses is reduced, as well as the concentration of neurotransmitters[7,19]. As the body ages, there may be an accumulation of neurofibrillary tangles and neuritic plaques associated with dementia[20], and cognitive function can diminish, although this varies widely between individuals[21]. It is important to remember that one way in which older people's cognitive function can be maintained is by presenting them with interesting and challenging learning activities[15]. Alterations in normal sleep patterns can occur with age, and the older person may experience increased wakefulness and arousal from sleep[8]. Some examples of health breakdown associated with the ageing nervous system are dementia, delirium, depression, insomnia, epilepsy and Parkinson's disease[17].

RESPIRATORY SYSTEM

Respiratory function is affected by advancing age[14]. Hardening of the airways and supportive tissue can occur, and degeneration of the bronchi, reduction in the elasticity and mobility of intercostal cartilage, and reduction in the strength and elasticity of the respiratory muscles are common[9]. Pulmonary function tests are likely to reveal a decrease in vital capacity and reduction in forced expiratory volume[8]. Older people may be unable to take deep breaths, have decreased cough reflex and dry mucous membranes[4]. Respiratory disorders common in the elderly are asthma, chronic obstructive pulmonary disease, pneumonia and influenza[17].

SENSORY SYSTEM

As people age, the acuity of the five senses, hearing, sight, smell, taste and touch, tends to diminish[7].

- Hearing: By age 65, one person in three has some hearing loss; by age 75, the incidence is one person in two[15]. Age-related hearing deficits include increased sensitivity to loud sounds, tinnitus, increased effort required to recognise speech[22]; impaired sound localisation[23] and presbycusis can lead to hearing loss for high-frequency sounds[6,24]. Conduction deafness is common in older people; they hear outside sounds as muffled and their own voice may seem louder. Hearing loss may lead to the older person experiencing social isolation[15].
- Sight: Older people's eyesight is often diminished, their pupils are smaller[25] compared to younger people and their eye lens tends to lose elasticity resulting in a reduction in the accommodation capacity of the lens[25]. There is a decreased ability to adjust to darkness and glare, a reduction in peripheral vision[7], and an inability to focus on near objects[26]. There is a decrease in retinal image quality, a decline in contrast sensitivity, and difficulties in distinguishing between the colours, blue and green[27,28]. They may also experience a reduction in tear production[7,8,15].

  Disorders associated with the ageing eye are macular degeneration[27], which can lead to loss of central vision and difficulty seeing detail, and diabetic retinopathy, which may result in loss of parts of the visual field, blurring and patchiness of vision. Glaucoma often produces a loss of peripheral vision[24], and cataracts result in blurred vision, sensitivity to bright light and changes in colour vision[15]. Vision impairment can impact negatively on the older person's ability to interact with others, and may lead to functional difficulties, loss of independence, social isolation, loneliness and decreased quality of life[27].

- Smell: The sense of smell diminishes with advancing age due to reduction in the cells of the olfactory bulb in the brain and in the number of sensory cells in the nasal lining[9,15].
- Taste: Atrophy of the tastebuds and decline in their number results in a reduction in the efficacy of the tastebuds[9]. Older people frequently have decreased ability to detect sweet and salty foods[10].
- Touch: Peripheral neuropathy is common in the elderly[29] and leads to overall reduction in touch sensation.

PHARMACOLOGY

Pharmacokinetics may be affected in older people and this is due to systemic changes affecting drug absorption, distribution, metabolism and excretion (see Table 15.1). Altered pharmacokinetics are attributable to age-related changes, such as decreased cellular activity, reduced blood flow to major organs, decreased renal and hepatic function, reduced gastric motility, decreased muscle activity, and altered homeostatic responses[30].

Older people are vulnerable to *polypharmacy*[31,32], a phenomenon that has been linked to health problems as diverse as constipation[33] and delirium[34]. There are various definitions of polypharmacy. Galbraith, Bullock and Manius[35] state that it is 'the excessive or unnecessary use of medications'. Patel[36] takes a different view and defines it as the use of multiple medications by an individual that can cause drug-to-drug interactions, and links it to the presence of multiple disease processes. Older people tend to have more health problems both in number and complexity than younger people[37], and so have legitimate reasons for increased drug use.

Hayes[37] asserts that polypharmacy accounts for 30% of hospital admissions of older people. It is of vital importance therefore that clinicians have an awareness of existing medication intake before prescribing or administering a new agent. In some situations, an individual's health status is such that a risk/benefit analysis will support the introduction of a new agent, despite any known hazards associated with concurrent use of certain agents. The responsibility then is on clinical staff to be aware of the nature of the possible reactions, and to monitor older people closely and regularly for any evidence of the presence of adverse reactions.

Many pharmaceutical agents have adverse affects that may compromise the general health of older people and it is important that nurses maintain a sound knowledge of the adverse reactions of commonly prescribed drugs. Consider oral health as an example; many prescribed drugs have the potential to cause xerostomia (dry mouth), reduced salivary secretion, ulceration and/or discolouration of the oral mucosa, oral pain and swelling, oral infections and altered taste sensations[31]. Any or all of these adverse affects have the capacity to contribute to difficulties with appetite and food intake, and, therefore, compromise nutritional status. Sometimes, additional medications are prescribed to treat adverse reactions or iatrogenic disease.

Certain social factors are identified as influencing older persons' adherence to drug regimens. Older people are more likely than other age groups to be on a fixed income, and this can mean that affording prescribed medication might be difficult at times. Older people also have high usage of over-the-counter medications such as laxatives and analgesics, and this may increase the likelihood of adverse reactions and drug interactions[30].

TABLE 15.1: PHYSIOLOGICAL CHANGES OF AGEING AND PHARMACOLOGICAL IMPLICATIONS

System	Physiological Changes	Some Specific Tests Relating to This System	Some Pharmacological Implications
Cardiovascular System	• Dilatation and rigidity of aorta • Fibrosis of endocardium • Hypertrophy of left ventricle • Reduction of pacemaker cells • Atrioventricular valves become thick and rigid • Decrease in myocardial contractility • Prolonged contraction and relaxation phase of left ventricle • Reduced cardiac output • Calcification of coronary arteries • Increase or decrease in blood pressure • Increase in peripheral resistance • Decrease in baroreceptor function	• Arterial blood gases (ABGs) • Red blood cell count (RBC) • Haemoglobin (Hb) • Bronchoscopy • Chest X-ray • Sputum analysis • Pulse and ear oximetry • Pulmonary angiography • Magnetic resonance imaging (MRI)	• Slower distribution of medications • Exaggerated effects of some medications • Reduced rate and extent of absorption
Endocrine System	• Atrophy and fibrosis of thyroid • Reduced thyroid activity and function • Decrease in basal metabolic rate • Decrease in radioactive iodine uptake • Diminished thyrotropin secretion and release • Decrease in iodine clearance rates • Reduction of glucocorticoids, 17-ketosteroids, progesterone, androgen and oestrogen in adrenal glands • Diminished aldosterone levels • Atrophy and fibrosis of pituitary gland	• Serum cortisol, catecholamines, parathyroid hormone, calcium and phosphorous. • Oral glucose tolerance • Blood sugar level (BSL)	

System	Age-related changes	Diagnostic tests	Implications
	• Increased interstitial fatty tissue in parathyroid • Decreased glucose tolerance in pancreas • Insufficient release of insulin • Reduced testosterone production • Decrease in oestrogen level post menopause		• Slower absorption of oral medications • Slower transit time of medications • Alteration in the half-life of some medications • Increased potential for drug interactions • Slower metabolism contributing to accumulation
Gastrointestinal System	• Loss or absence of teeth • Decline in saliva production • Decreased peristaltic action and relaxation of the lower oesophageal sphincter • Decrease in the production of ptyalin, hydrochloric acid and pepsin • Tendency for faulty absorption of vitamin B_1, B_{12}, calcium, iron, and vitamin K • Decrease in taste acuity • Decline in ability to detect sweet and salty food	• Serum alkaline phosphatase, bilirubin, amylase and lipase • Plasma ammonia • Urinary bilirubin • Upper gastrointestinal endoscopy • Lower gastrointestinal endoscopy • Barium swallow test • Barium enema • Cholangiography • Ultrasonography	
Genitourinary System	• Decrease in renal mass and renal tissue growth • Reduction in renal blood flow • Reduced glomerular filtrate rate • Decreased nephron and tubular function • Reduced ability to concentrate and dilute urine • Impairment of adaptive mechanisms to maintain blood volume and extracellular fluid composition • Decline in renin and plasma aldosterone levels • Diminished bladder capacity • Loss of striated urethral muscle	• Urinalysis • Blood urea nitrogen • Creatinine clearance • Electrolytes • Serum creatinine • Serum proteins • Urea clearance • Cystourethroscopy • Nephrotomography • Renal computed tomography • Retrograde cystography • Ultrasonography • Intravenous pyelography • Renal angiography • Cystometry	• Decreased filtration and excretion rates • Increased serum levels • Increased toxicity of some medications at normal levels

TABLE 15.1: (cont'd)

System	Physiological Changes	Some Specific Tests Relating to This System	Some Pharmacological Implications
	• Penile erections slower and more difficult to maintain • Atrophy of vulva, vagina, cervix, uterus, fallopian tubes and labia	• Voiding cystourethrography • Pap test • Semen analysis • Colposcopy • Laparoscopy • Hysterosalpingography • Pelvic ultrasonography	
Integumentary System	• Decrease in elasticity of the skin • Thinning of the skin • Xerosis • Loose and wrinkled skin • Uneven pigmentation • Easily torn skin • Traumatic purpura • Dermal atrophy	• Patch test • Skin biopsy • Gram stain and cultures • Tzanck test • Phototesting	• Altered rate of drug absorption with some topical preparations
Musculoskeletal System	• Loss of bone mass in vertebrae • Thinning of intervertebral discs • Bone absorption rate higher than bone formation rate • Reduced muscle mass, strength and movements • Reduction in number of skeletal muscle fibres • Decrease in capillary supply to muscles • Increase in adipose cells • Enlarged joints • Tendons and ligaments shrink and harden • Slower reflexes • Reduced bone mineral mass • Decrease in calcium absorption	• Arthrocentesis • Skeletal X-rays • Bone scan • Computed tomography • Magnetic resonance imaging • Arthroscopy • Serum calcium • Serum phosphorous • Rheumatoid factor	• Altered adipose tissue levels can affect the responses to some fat-soluble drugs

System		Diagnostic tests	
Nervous System	• Neuronal density diminishes • Brain weight diminishes • Neurones get smaller • Reduction in the number of synapses with a reduction in the concentration of neurotransmitters • Reduction in cognitive function, although this varies widely between individuals • Accumulation of neurofibrillary tangles and neuritic plaques	• Skull X-rays • Spinal X-rays • Cerebral angiograph • Myelography • Computed tomography • Brain scan • Magnetic resonance imaging • Electroencephalography • Lumbar puncture	• Increased concentrations of medications in the brain • Increased/absorption of some medications may cause dizziness and confusion
Respiratory System	• Hardening of the airways and supportive tissue • Degeneration of the bronchi • Reduction in elasticity and mobility of the intercostals cartilage • Reduction of strength and elasticity of respiratory muscles • Breathlessness during physical exertion • Reduction of vertical dimension of the thorax • Stiffening of the lung tissue	• Arterial blood gases • Red blood cell count • Pulmonary function tests • Bronchoscopy • Pulmonary angiography • Chest X-ray • Thoracic computed tomography • Magnetic resonance imaging • Sputum analysis • Thoracentesis • Pulse and ear oximetry	
Sensory System	**Hearing** • Increased sensitivity to loud sounds • Tinnitus • Increased effort required to recognise speech • Impairment of sound localisation • Presbycusis can lead to hearing loss for high-frequency sounds **Sight** • Decrease in retinal image quality • Decline in contrast sensitivity • Decrease in pupil diameter	• Fluorescein angiography • Orbital computed tomography • Orbital radiography • Ocular ultrasonography • Refraction • Slit-lamp examination • Tonometry • Accoustic immittance test • Pure tone audiometry • Rinne test • Weber's test • Word recognition test	• Impaired vision can impact on the older person's ability to read medication labels. • Reduction in nerve sensations of finger tips and palms may impede the older person when they are removing lids from medication bottles

TABLE 15.1: (cont'd)

System	Physiological Changes	Some Specific Tests Relating to This System	Some Pharmacological Implications
	• Reduction in the accommodation capacity of the lens • Increase in sensitivity to glare • Impaired dark adaptation • Decreased depth perception and visual field • Reduced colour discrimination • Age-related macular degeneration can lead to loss of central vision and difficulty seeing detail • Diabetic retinopathy may result in loss of parts of the visual field, blurring and patchiness of vision • Glaucoma often produces a loss of peripheral vision • Cataracts result in a loss of contrast vision **Smell** • Loss of cells in the olfactory bulb in the brain • Decrease in the number of sensory cells in the nasal lining **Taste** • Atrophy of taste buds, lose efficiency and decline in number **Touch** • Loss of nerve endings particularly in finger tips, palms of hands and lower extremities		

Adapted from.4,5,7,9,10,16,19–24,35

● Case study

Mrs Joy Anderson, 75, lives at home with her husband of 50 years. She is 155 cm tall and weighs 49 kg. Over the past five years, her husband, Reg, has had three right cerebral vascular accidents (CVAs), which have resulted in him experiencing significant left-sided weakness, difficulty with walking, eating and grasping objects. Sometimes, Mr Anderson has urinary incontinence at night. The Andersons have three adult children, two sons and a daughter. Their daughter, who lives close by, is in daily contact with her parents by telephone and visits every second day. Both sons are in contact with their parents approximately weekly.

Mrs Anderson finds the responsibilities of caring for her chronically ill husband very stressful and has had trouble sleeping. She says that she has no trouble falling asleep, but then wakes up a few hours later and is unable to settle back to sleep. Twelve months ago, a sedative was prescribed by her doctor. She finds that it is sometimes effective. Mrs Anderson has been taking the same antihypertensive medication for the past five years. Her general practitioner checks her blood pressure at every visit and though Mrs Anderson did not know the latest reading, she said the doctor was happy with it. Lately, Mrs Anderson has lost interest in eating and often cannot be bothered to cook a meal for herself and her husband.

At her daughter's insistence, Mrs Anderson has agreed to a fortnightly community home-care visitor who cleans the house and does the heavy laundry. The home-care visitor also takes Mr and Mrs Anderson to medical appointments and to do their shopping.

Over the past three weeks, Mrs Anderson has been experiencing frequency of urine and dysuria. Early one morning, as she rushed to the toilet, she tripped on a floor mat and fell heavily on her right hip. Unable to get up, she was forced to lie on the floor until her daughter arrived later that morning, by which time she had been lying on the floor for nearly three hours.

Mrs Anderson was transported to the emergency department of the local hospital where a physical examination revealed that she had pain on passive motion of her right hip and shortening and external rotation of her right leg. During the initial examination, Mrs Anderson described how her urinary frequency had, she believed, caused her to fall the previous night. A urine sample obtained from Mrs Anderson was noted to have a strong odour and was dark in colour. A ward urinalysis revealed leucocytes, protein and blood. A mid-stream specimen of urine (MSU) was collected and sent to the laboratory for analysis.

An anteroposterior (AP) X-ray of the pelvis confirms a diagnosis of a fracture to the right intracapsular femoral neck. An intravenous line was inserted, intravenous fluids commenced, an indwelling urinary catheter inserted, and Mrs Anderson was nil-by-mouth in preparation for surgery later that morning. The results of the MSU indicated a diagnosis of cystitis and Mrs Anderson was prescribed a course of intravenous antibiotics.

Mrs Anderson's daughter contacted her brothers to discuss their father's care while their mother was hospitalised. The siblings agreed that their father should spend one week at each of their homes, during which time they would investigate the possibility of nursing home respite care for their father. Mr Anderson was furious when his children informed him of the arrangements they had made and refused to leave his home. He shouted at them that he could manage very well, with the assistance of his daughter and the fortnightly home-care visitor, while his wife was in hospital.

LEARNING EXERCISES

1. What are Mr and Mrs Anderson's main health concerns at the present time?
2. Identify the sources of social support Mr and Mrs Anderson have at the present time.
3. What are the main factors that make Mr and Mrs Anderson vulnerable to injury and illness?
4. What resources could the nurse draw on to assist Mr and Mrs Anderson in their current situation?
5. What resources are available to assist Mr and Mrs Anderson maintain optimal health in the community?

HEALTH ASSESSMENT

Thorough and rigorous health assessment provides the baseline information upon which nursing care and nursing interventions are planned. Thus, it is an essential step in effective care planning and delivery. There are many approaches to health assessment, with the functional health assessment[38] and head-to-toe approach[39] being two of the most common. Regardless of the framework used, a systematic approach is necessary. When assessing older people, the same techniques are applied as for all adults. Sound communication skills are essential, and care should be taken to minimise distractions. In multicultural societies, care must be taken to ensure that resources such as health care interpreters or Indigenous health workers are available if needed to facilitate effective and culturally appropriate communication.

When working with older people, it is necessary to have an awareness of normal age-related changes, and it is important to avoid ageist stereotypes and misconceptions about ageing that may create bias and impair accurate assessment and conclusions[37]. For example, incontinence is not a normal aspect of ageing, and should be subject to further investigation in persons of all ages. Similarly, confusion should not be considered to be a normal part of ageing – it can be symptomatic of polypharmacy as well as a variety of acute conditions, and should be comprehensively investigated.

Health assessment has several interrelated components including client history, physical assessment, social assessment, and mental health assessment; these are discussed below.

CLIENT HISTORY

The client history is a crucial aspect of assessment. Theoretically, taking the history of an older person is the same as for any other adult. In the client history, information is derived from a range of sources, such as referral letters from health and welfare workers, and laboratory results. However, the primary source of information is the client interview. The interview is crucial because it is an opportunity to engage the client and to gain insights into their own perspectives and health concerns. This approach positions client concerns as central to the assessment process. The interview also provides an opportunity to assess the client's affect, and how they are able to interact and articulate their issues and concerns.

A private and quiet setting should be selected and the client's comfort needs should be attended[39]. Older people may not report symptoms because they may themselves attribute these to the ageing process, and so careful and thorough questioning is necessary. Closed-ended questions may be useful to help direct the interview in a focussed way[37]. Appropriate techniques such as questioning, probing and clarifying should be used to elucidate accurate and detailed information[40]. When assessing older people, special care must be taken to provide for the possibility of sensory impairment, such as deafness or difficulty hearing, or cognitive impairment, such as short-term memory loss. Individuals with cognitive impairment present special challenges during assessment, but even in the presence of such impairments, it is still important to include the individual and to gain the perspectives of older people themselves. Additional information can be gained from relatives and carers to give a more detailed picture if necessary.

Individuals should be asked about their history of medication use, and to describe any side effects they have experienced. A thorough medication history includes information about prescription medications, over-the-counter medications, herbal preparations and vitamin or mineral supplements[36] because of older persons' susceptibility to polypharmacy.

Nurses should be aware that a client might not consider over-the-counter products as medication. Therefore it is important to ask clarifying questions, such as:

• Do you take anything that you buy from the chemist or the supermarket, such as pain killers, laxatives or vitamins?
• How often would you take any non-prescribed medication such as painkillers, antacids or cough mixture?

In some situations, such as when a person is uncertain of the name or dosage of medications, it can be useful to ask older people themselves, or their relatives or carers, to bring medications into the health care setting so they can be viewed and accurately identified.

PHYSICAL ASSESSMENT

Older people can have multiple, complex needs which vary amongst individuals and are different from those in other age groups. When assessing the older person in any setting, it is important to understand the changes associated with ageing so that this information can be used to suit the functionality of the person[3,41]. This will assist the nurse to recognise the changes that occur with ageing and those relating to health breakdown. In addition, an older person may have atypical presentation of health breakdown[41,42]; the symptoms may not be specific on presentation and the problems associated with health breakdown are often interrelated[41].

When conducting a physical assessment with an older person, it is important to gain the person's consent, maintain privacy and level of comfort. Consideration of their energy levels and attitude, their level of communication and environment is important. The framework for assessment suggested here is to use a general top-to-toe assessment and a major systems approach. Inspection, palpation, percussion and auscultation are the means used to collect information during the assessment[3,42].

To begin, the general assessment involves an examination from head to toe for appearance, level of consciousness and mood, signs of distress and mobility[3,42]. It includes taking vital signs such as temperature, pulse, respirations, blood pressure, height and weight.

An older person's *cardiovascular* system should be assessed in the same way as any other adult[41]. Palpate the point of maximal impulse, which may be displaced in older people with left ventricular hypertrophy. Palpate for neck vein jugular venous distension, carotid artery bruit, and trophic changes in arms and legs, for example oedema, loss of hair[4,41]. Palpate pulses for rate, rhythm, volume and symmetry. Check fingers for clubbing and capillary refill for information about circulation[41].

In assessing older people, it is important to be aware that large variations in cardiac rhythm occur. Pulses may be difficult to palpate due to atherosclerotic changes in vessels and the resultant narrowing of the lumen; however, pulses should be symmetrical in strength. Arteries may be stiff or appear kinked. There should be no deterioration in colour in the extremeties[3].

When assessing the *endocrine* system, it is important to remember that endocrine health breakdown often resembles changes associated with ageing[3]. Assess the older person for signs of hypothyroidism, including fatigue, depression, muscle weakness, constipation, weight gain, dry hair and skin. Conversely, assess for signs of hyperthyroidism, such as anxiety, tiredness, sleeplessness, feeling hot and sweaty, shortness of breath, weight loss, difficulty focusing eyes and bulging of one or both eyes. Diabetes should be considered and older people need to be assessed for polyuria, polydipsia, weight loss, blurred vision, alterations in weight and tiredness[3,4,5,6].

Assessment of the *gastrointestinal* system is the same as an assessment for younger people. However, the oral examination is more important for older people[41] with the oral cavity, mouth, larynx, pharynx, lips, teeth, and lymph nodes assessed for normality[4]. The shape and symmetry of the abdomen should be observed. Other observations include checking for a pulsating abdominal aorta, visible peristalsis[41,42], abdominal distension and hernia protrusion[41]. Auscultation for vascular bruits and bowel sounds should be performed in all four quadrants. Percuss for tympany or dullness to determine if air or fluid is present. Palpate for tenderness, masses and organ enlargement[4,41,42]. In assessing older people, abdominal palpation is easier due to a thinner abdominal wall and relaxed muscle tone. However, abdominal distension[3] and aortic aneurysms[41] are usually more common.

When assessing the *genitourinary* system of the older person, palpate kidneys for tenderness and percuss and palpate the abdomen for a full bladder[4]. Perform a urinalysis. Examination may also include checking the scrotum and prostate in men, and breasts and vagina (pelvic) in women. These assessments may be viewed as extended skills with specific consent and a second health professional required to act as a witness. Assess external genitalia for dryness and atrophic changes, vaginal discharge and for stress incontinence during coughing[41]. Assess hydration status[4]. Older people are susceptible to infection due to ageing changes and immobility and a urinary tract infection is frequently asymptomatic.

When assessing the *integumentary* system, the entire body surface including nails, hair and mucous membranes needs to be examined[41]. Older people are more susceptible to skin health breakdown and this can be detected in a change of skin colour[3]. It is important to check skin folds and look for tears, lacerations, redness over areas of pressure and pressure ulcers. Check for oedema. Skin turgor and dryness of lips is particularly important for assessing hydration[42].

It is important to note any asymmetry when examining the *musculoskeletal* system. The stature and posture of the older person should be assessed, as well as voluntary and involuntary movement[2]. Inspect bones for deformities, range of motion, tenderness, enlargement, soft tissue swelling or crepitation in joints. Inspect muscles for tone, signs of atrophy, and evaluate the strength of each muscle group[41]. Assess reflexes and general coordination, gait, posture and static balance[42]. Observe for evidence of past or recent injuries.

An older person tends to take smaller, slower steps, have a reduced arm swing and flexed elbows and knees[3]. Consider if the person uses a stick, walker, frame or prosthesis[4] as problems with balance or gait increases the risk falls.

The same technique as for assessing a younger person should be used when assessing the *nervous* system. Assess the level of consciousness, mental status, affect and mood and speech and language of the older person[3,4]. Check the reaction of pupils and sensation to light, touch and pain. Assess cranial nerves and all reflexes[4,41]. Assess balance, tremor, coordination and gait in combination with the musculoskeletal assessment. Cognitive function should be assessed using mental status instruments, for example, Folstein Mini Mental State Examination. Assess for depression using the Geriatric Depression Scale. Test cerebellar function by using the Romberg test and use the 'get up and go' test for assessing gait[41]. In assessing the older person, remember medications may cause neurologic changes. Generally, due to the ageing process, the speed of response may be slower[3] and it is not unusual to detect a change in one or more senses.

When assessing the *respiratory* system, inspection of the anterior and posterior shape and symmetry of the chest is required. Observe for barrel chest and use of accessory muscles[41]. Assess the rate and rhythm of respirations, cough, and colour and consistency of sputum[4]. Palpate for tenderness for musculoskeletal injury[41] or lumps[42]. Percuss the lung fields for dull or flat sounds. Auscultate for breath sounds, crackles, fluid, wheezes, constricted airway, or rub-inflamed pleura[4,41].

When assessing the older person, it is important to remember that they have a greater risk of health breakdown of the respiratory system and that signs and symptoms may present differently from those experienced by younger people. Consider that palpation may be more difficult due to loose skin over the chest; the loss of elastic recoil produces a hyper-resonance on percussion; and reduced mobility may cause crackles at bases of lungs – a cough will clear this[3].

SOCIAL ASSESSMENT

Social assessment is an essential aspect of an holistic approach when caring for older people, and consists of assessment of their past and current social status and their physical environment. Sensitive and systematic social status assessment enables nurses to understand the context in which the older person ages and should be undertaken in conjunction with physical and mental health assessments. The advantages of social status assessment from the older person's perspective include the opportunity to identify their own needs for professional and informal support and make explicit their personal views on the maintenance of their current lifestyle, recreation and leisure activities[43].

Hamilton Smith[44] argues that social assessments that focus on the lifestyle and relationship issues important to older people help nurses understand the unique needs of the older person and serve as a reminder that older people are not an homogenous group and that their past experiences and current physical, financial and living circumstances can potentially impact on their experience of ageing. Information gathered during social assessment should be detailed and comprehensive and take account of the older person's life-long experiences and habits[45]. Issues such as key events that have shaped their life, usual daily routines, normal lifestyle including community activities, friendships, work, beliefs, values and interests need to be considered. Information gathered from social assessments can provide insights that directly impact on decisions about the type and appropriateness of interventions the older person receives[46]. A number of geriatric social assessment tools have proved useful, including the Philadelphia Centre Geriatric Morale scale (PCGMS)[47], Sickness Impact Profile (SIP) and Geriatric Quality of Life Questionnaire (GQLQ)[48].

An assessment of the physical environment in which the older person lives encompasses assessment of the internal and external home environment. Data gathered for the assessment of their residential environment can include the following aspects: security and lighting; safety of external walkways and stairs; the condition and appropriateness of furniture; accessibility of bathrooms, laundries and kitchens; placement of telephones and power points; the use of floor rugs; and installation of home modifications such as grab-rails, raised toilet seats, thermostatic heating systems and modified bench heights[49,50].

MENTAL HEALTH ASSESSMENT

Deterioration in mental status is not a normal part of ageing[37], and any changes should be investigated. Among the common problems seen in older people are memory deficits[32], confusion, depression, delirium, or dementia[51]. Acute confusion or delirium can signify a medical emergency, and are considered to be reversible conditions, as they often present as a result of polypharmacy and drug interactions. McGarry Logue[32] identifies memory deficit as being one of the major contributors to medication errors in the self-medicating older person. Dementia generally presents with a slower onset and is accepted as a chronic condition[37].

Depression is a relatively common condition in old age[51]. Older people are faced with a number of issues that can give rise to depression including loss of their partner or friends, chronic pain, disease processes, poverty, social isolation and biochemical changes. Issues around spirituality such as hope, feelings of connectedness, values and belief systems are also important considerations when undertaking a mental health assessment.

There are a number of portable and user-friendly tools available to assess the mental status of older persons, including particular problems. The Mini Mental Status Examination (MMSE) is a short and simple 10-item tool with well established validity and reliability[51,52]. The Geriatric Depression Scale (GDS) is a 30-item scale used to identify and rate depression in older people[51]. The Spiritual Well-Being Scale (SWBS) is a 21-item tool that covers a range of issues, including purpose and meaning in life[52].

DEVELOPING TREATMENT PLANS

Treatment plans are based on thorough and rigorous assessment, and individualised to meet the specific needs of those for whom they are developed. This is so for people of all ages. Principles to consider in developing effective treatment plans in older people include environmental safety, pharmacological interventions and management.

As noted earlier in this chapter, older people are vulnerable to polypharmacy and to the potential hazards that are associated with the use of multiple medications. An effective plan will incorporate measures to avoid negative outcomes of medication use through monitoring for early detection of any problems. These measures are likely to include

• Regular and on-going review of medications. Particularly in the presence of chronic health conditions, there is the potential for people to continue to take medications for long periods of time, even though their condition or need for the drug may have changed since its initial prescription. In addition, use of over-the-counter medications may change over time, and it is important therefore to regularly review all medications;

- Simplification of therapeutic regimens. Older people are being placed on progressively more complex therapeutic regimens, and this means that healthcare providers are challenged to find new and effective ways of ensuring that regimens are kept as simple and as compatible with an individual's lifestyle as is possible. Nurses and other health professionals should make use of available technology to assist older people to safely manage their treatment plans[32];
- Monitoring for signs of toxicity. Some common drugs such as digoxin and phenytoin have a narrow therapeutic range, and levels in excess of the therapeutic range will result in toxicity. Therefore, regular blood monitoring is needed to ensure that values are in the therapeutic range. This monitoring will also detect if values are sub-therapeutic. Values that are sub-therapeutic or toxic indicate a need for urgent medical review. It is also important to provide relevant and accessible information to older people and their families about the signs and symptoms of toxicity, and advise them to seek immediate attention from a health care professional should they experience or observe any of the signs or symptoms; and
- Alertness to drug interactions and adverse effects. Polypharmacy makes older people susceptible to drug interactions and adverse reactions. Client teaching and the provision of information about interactions and adversity specific to medications they are taking should form a part of any on-going treatment plan. These can take many forms, depending on the substances involved and therefore, it is wise to monitor general health, and be prepared to review medications in light of observed or self-reported changes in health including sleeping patterns, bowel patterns, energy levels, appetite and weight.

LEARNING EXERCISES

1. What are the physiological changes of ageing that relate to Mr Anderson?
2. What are the physiological changes of ageing that relate to Mrs Anderson?
3. Why is Mrs Anderson more likely to experience falls, fractures and cystitis?
4. What are the predisposing factors that led to Mr Anderson suffering a cerebrovascular accident stroke?
5. What are the pharmacological implications of the medications Mrs Anderson has been taking?
6. What are some of the environmental factors that predispose Mr and Mrs Anderson to injury?
7. What physical disorders does Mrs Anderson experience?
8. What physical disorders does Mr Anderson experience?
9. How do these physical disorders impact on Mr and Mrs Anderson's quality of life?
10. What are some important considerations to consider when conducting an assessment on Mr and Mrs Anderson?
11. What might be an example of some ageist stereotypes in this case study?
12. What are the main issues in the case study?
13. What are some of the attitudes that underpin this case study?
14. How would you feel if you were the people in the case study?
15. How do you think you might respond in this situation?
16. Considering safety issues, how would you encourage the autonomy of Mr and Mrs Anderson?
17. What, if any, specific issues does medication use present to Mr and Mrs Anderson?

18. Does a member of the family have the right to make Mr Anderson live with them, or go to respite care?
19. Do you include clients in the decision-making processes concerning their care?
20. As a nurse, in what ways could you be an advocate for Mr and Mrs Anderson?
21. Are there any issues related to equity and access to services that might be of particular relevance to Mr and Mrs Anderson?
22. What particular assistance might they be able to access due to their status as older people, and/or as pensioners?
23. What specific cultural issues are raised in relation to the case study?

CONCLUSION

With an ageing population, nurses are increasingly likely to care for older people in a range of clinical settings. Knowledge of the changes associated with ageing and of gerontic health assessment is therefore essential for nurses delivering care to this vulnerable population. As ageing is an individualised process, the ability to conduct rigorous and systematic health assessment will enable nurses to plan, deliver and evaluate appropriate care for older people with careful attention to gerontic pharmacokinetics, polypharmacy and adverse drug events.

The reader is encouraged to apply the knowledge gained in this chapter to the case study and to carefully consider each question included as part of the student activities. Application of this knowledge to their clinical practice will help ensure that nurses provide optimal care to older people and their families, care which honours the individual needs and preferences of the older person within the context of the pathophysiological and pharmacological alterations associated with ageing. These issues can have a profound effect on improving the quality of life of the aged.

Recommended Reading

Annells, M & Koch, T. 2002; 'Older People Seeking Solutions to Constipation: The Laxative Mire', *Journal of Clinical Nursing*, 115, 603–612.

Australian Medical Handbook Drug Choice Companion: Aged Care. 2003; Commonwealth Department of Veterans' Affairs, Canberra.

Coleman, Y. 2001; 'Nutrition Assessment and Screening', in S Koch & S Garratt (eds.), *Assessing Older People: A Practical Guide for Health Professionals*, MacLennan & Petty, Sydney, 171–192.

Koch, S. 2001; 'Holistic Assessment', in S Koch & S Garratt (eds.), *Assessing Older People: A Practical Guide for Health Professionals*, MacLennan & Petty, Sydney, 21–35.

Patel, R. 2003; 'Polypharmacy and the Elderly', *Journal of Infusion Nursing*, 263, 166–169.

Yeung, K. 1998; 'Overview of the Quality of Life Instruments in the Elderly', *Journal of the American Geriatrics Society*, 469, 28–38.

References

1. Australian Bureau of Statistics (ABS). 1999; *Australian Social Trends 1999, Population Projections: Our Ageing Population*. http://www.abs.gov.au/ausstats/abs@.nsf/.
2. Lueckenotte, A. 2000; *Gerontologic Nursing*, (2nd ed.), Mosby, St Louis.
3. Springhouse. 2002; *Better Elder Care: A Nurse's Guide to Caring for Older Adults*. Springhouse, Pennsylvania.
4. Matteson, M, McConnell, E & Linton, A. 1997; *Gerontological Nursing: Concepts and Practice* (2nd ed.), W. B. Saunders, Philadelphia.
5. Chop, W & Robnett, R. 1999; *Gerontology for the Health Care Professional*, F.A. Davis, Philadelphia.
6. Eliopoulos, C. 2001; *Gerontological Nursing* (5th ed.), Lippincott, Williams and Wilkins, Philadelphia.
7. Andresen, G. 1989; 'A Fresh Look at Assessing the Elderly', *Registered Nurse*, 526, 47–56.

8. Nowazek, V & Neeley, M. 1996; 'Health Assessment of the Older Patient', *Critical Care Nursing*, 19, 1–6.

9. Ebersole, P & Hess, P. 1998; *Toward Healthy Ageing: Human Needs and Nursing Response* (5th ed.), Mosby, St Louis.

10. Coleman, Y. 2001; 'Nutrition Assessment and Screening', in S Koch & S Garratt (eds.), *Assessing Older People: A Practical Guide for Health Professionals*, MacLennan & Petty, Sydney, 171–192.

11. Kayser-Jones, J & Pengilly, K. 1999; 'Dysphagia among Nursing Home Residents', *Geriatric Nursing*, 202, 77–82.

12. MD Consult. Accessed at: http://home.mdconsult. com/das/patient/view/32347979-2.

13. Weinstock, M. 1991; 'Ageing and the Skin', *Intern Med World*, 619, 32–34.

14. Khanna, P & Geller, J. 1992; 'Clinical Implications in the Elderly' *Topics in Emergency Medicine*, 143, 1–9.

15. Koch, S. 2001; 'Holistic Assessment', in S Koch & S Garratt (eds.), *Assessing Older People: A Practical Guide for Health Professionals*, MacLennan & Petty, Sydney, 21–35.

16. Palmissano, C & Norman, R. 2000; 'Geriatric Dermatology in Chronic Care and Rehabilitation', *Dermatology Nursing*, 122, 116–123.

17. *Australian Medical Handbook Drug Choice Companion: Aged Care*. 2003; Commonwealth Department of Veterans' Affairs, Canberra.

18. Keefover, R. 1998; 'Ageing and Cognition', *Neurological Clinics*, 16, 635–648.

19. Brody, H. 1992; 'The Ageing Brain', *Acta Neurological Scandinavian Supplement*, 137, 40–44.

20. Minichello, V, Alexander, L & Jones, D. (eds.). 1992; *Gerontology: A Multi-Disciplinary Approach*, Prentice Hall, Sydney.

21. Morris, J & McManus, D. 1991; 'The Neurology of Ageing: Normal versus Pathologic Change', *Geriatrics*, 46, 47–54.

22. Allen, N, Burns, A, Newton, V, Hickson, F, Ramsden, R, Rogers, J, et al. 2003; 'The Effects of Improving Hearing in Dementia', *Age and Ageing*, 322, 189–193.

23. Katz, J. 2001; 'Issues of Concern for the Ageing Anesthesiologist', *Anesthesia and Analgesia*, 926, 1487–1492.

24. Osborn, R & Rapson, W. 2001; 'Assessment of the Vision and Hearing Function of Residents in Aged Care Facilities', in S Koch & S Garratt (eds.), *Assessing Older People: A Practical Guide for Health Professionals*, MacLennan & Petty, Sydney, 223–237.

25. Artal, P, Guirao, A, Berrio, E, Piers, P & Norrby, S. 2003; 'Optical Aberrations and the Ageing Eye', *International Ophthalmology Clinics*, 432, 63–77.

26. Roberts, A. 1989; 'The Normal Eyeball: Systems of Life – no. 177, senior systems 42', *Nursing Times*, 85, 55–58.

27. Houde, S & Huff, M. 2003; 'Age-related Vision Loss in Older Adults: A Challenge for Gerontological Nurses', *Journal of Gerontological Nursing*, 294, 25–33.

28. Marshall, M. 1997; 'Therapeutic Design for People with Dementia', in S Hunter (ed.), *Dementia Challenges and New Directions*, Athenaeum, Gateshead, 181–193.

29. Thomas, D & Edelberg, H. 2003; *Falls STAT!Ref Online Medical Data base*. http://online.statref.com/search.aspx.

30. Paterson, R, Rees, N, Czarniak, P, Reiss, B & Evans, M. 1993; *Pharmacological Aspect of Nursing Care in Australia*, Thomas Nelson Publishers, Melbourne.

31. Fitzpatrick, J. 2000; 'Oral Health Care Needs of Dependent Older People: Responsibilities of Nurses and Care Staff', *Journal of Advanced Nursing*, 326, 1325–1332.

32. McGarry Logue, R. 2002; 'Self-Medication and the Elderly: How Technology Can Help', *American Journal of Nursing*, 1027, 51–55.

33. Annells, M & Koch, T. 2002; 'Older People Seeking Solutions to Constipation: The Laxative Mire', *Journal of Clinical Nursing*, 115, 603–612.

34. Insel, K & Badger, T. 2002; 'Deciphering the 4 Ds: Cognitive Decline, Delirium, Depression and Dementia – a review' *Journal of Advanced Nursing*, 38 (4), 360–368.

35. Galbraith, A, Bullock, S & Manias, E. 1997; *Fundamentals of Pharmacology* (2nd ed.), Addison-Wesley, Melbourne.

36. Patel, R. 2003; 'Polypharmacy and the Elderly', *Journal of Infusion Nursing*, 263, 166–169.

37. Hayes, K. 2000; 'Geriatric Assessment in the Emergency Department', *Journal of Emergency Nursing*, 265, 430–435.

38. Gordon, M. 1987; *Nursing Diagnosis: Process and Application* (2nd ed.), McGraw-Hill, New York.

39. Bickley, LS. 2000; *Bates' Pocket Guide to Physical Examination and History Taking* (3rd ed.), Lippincott, Philadelphia.

40. Stein-Parbury, J. 2005; *Patient and Person* (3rd ed.), Churchill Livingstone, Sydney.

41. Stone, JT, Wyman, JF & Salisbury, SA. 1999; *Clinical Gerontological Nursing: A Guide to Advanced Practice* (2nd ed.), W.B. Saunders, Sydney.

42. *Handbook of Geriatric Nursing Care*, (2nd ed.). 2003; Lippincott, Williams & Wilkins, Sydney.

43. Jones, D, Sloane, J & Alexander, L. 1992; 'Quality of Life: A Practical Approach', in V Minichiello, L Alexander & D Jones (eds.), *Gerontology: A*

Multidisciplinary Approach, Prentice Hall, New York, 224–265.

44. Hamilton Smith, E. 1991; 'Social and Lifestyle Assessment', in S Koch & S Garratt (eds.), *Assessing Older People: A Practical Guide for Health Professionals*, MacLennan & Petty, Sydney, 21–35.

45. Clipp, E & Steinhauser, K. 2003; 'Psychosocial Influences on Health in Later Life', STAT!Ref Online Medical Database. http://online.statref.com/search.aspx.

46. Lilly, M, Richards, B & Buckwalter, K. 2003; 'Friends and Social Support in Dementia Caregiving', *Journal of Gerontological Nursing*, 29 (1), 29–36.

47. Lawton, M. 1975; 'The Philadelphia Centre Geriatric Morale Scale: A Revision' *Journal of Gerontology*, 30, 85–89.

48. Yeung, K. 1998; 'Overview of the Quality of Life Instruments in the Elderly', *Journal of the American Geriatrics Society*, 469, 28–38.

49. Sutherland, B. 2001; 'Assessing Environment', in S Koch & S Garratt (eds.), *Assessing Older People: A Practical Guide for Health Professionals*, MacLennan & Petty, Sydney, 21–35.

50. Lachs, M, Feinstern, A & Cooney, L. 1990; 'A Simple Procedure for General Screening for Functional Disability in Elderly Patients', *Annals of Internal Medicine*, 112, 699.

51. Pritchard, E. 1999; 'Screening for Dementia and Depression in Older People', *Nursing Standard*, 14 (5), 46–52.

52. Krach, P, DeVaney, S, DeTurk, C & Zink, M. 1996; 'Functional Status of the Oldest-Old in a Home Setting', *Journal of Advanced Nursing*, 24 (3), 456–464.

16 | Mental Health Breakdown

AUTHORS

LOUISE O'BRIEN

SCOTT FANKER

LEARNING OBJECTIVES

When you have completed this chapter you will be able to
- Identify the epidemiology and clinical features of schizophrenia and depression;
- Review key pathophysiologic findings in relation to schizophrenia and depression;
- Identify pharmacological and other treatments for schizophrenia and depression; and
- Identify the implications for nursing patients with breakdown in mental health.

INTRODUCTION

Biological processes have been suspected to play a role in the aetiology of mental illness since antiquity. Hippocrates, for example, proposed that depression or 'melancholy' resulted from a systemic excess of 'black bile'[1]. Interest in pursuing possible biological foundations of mental illness increased in the 1950s and 1960s, with a number of independent observations and discoveries related to the development of pharmacological agents targeting disorders such as tuberculosis and hypertension. Fortuitously, these drugs had an effect on either psychotic or depressive symptoms. The resulting use of drugs such as chlorpromazine, imipramine and iproniazid provided further impetus to interest in identifying the neurochemical mechanism of action of these agents, and the development of theories of the biological foundations of psychiatric illness. The modern era of psychopharmacology was thus born, and from the 1960s onwards, significant research effort has been applied to increasing our understanding of the biological substrates and, importantly, treatment of mental disorders.

Mental disorders are often conceptualised, diagnosed and treated at the broad 'syndrome' rather than specific 'disease' level. Unlike in, say, pneumonia where diagnosis can be confirmed radiologically via a chest X-ray and a specific infectious agent can be identified through bacterial culture, there are no diagnostic tests to confirm a particular discrete mental disorder. Diagnosis is based, in the main, upon assessment of the presence or absence of certain symptoms. It is likely that mental illnesses such as schizophrenia and depression are broad syndromes that encompass a number of related disorders. Therefore, in most of the mental disorders, biological research findings need to be considered and interpreted with some caution. Biological processes in mental illness may be influenced by clinically heterogenous samples. Interpreting grouped data, possibly affected by the presence of several types of a disorder (such as subtypes of depression), needs to proceed with some caution. The presence of a particular biological abnormality does not necessarily confirm that it is pathophysiologically relevant to the disorder in question. It is possible that a biological finding may relate to another physiological disturbance, such as sleep abnormalities or weight loss, or represent the confounding effect of a biological factor known to influence body systems, for example, age, sex, menstrual cycle, and nutritional status. Having acknowledged these caveats, significant advances have been made in the biological understandings of mental illness related to biochemical, genetic, and neurological abnormalities.

This chapter will provide an overview of some of the key pathophysiological findings related to depression and schizophrenia. While biological factors are discussed primarily, it should be noted, and emphasised, that the environment within which a person develops a mental illness is also important. Although the vulnerability to a particular mental illness may be able to be demonstrated biologically, the expression of the illness is very likely multifactorial.

SCHIZOPHRENIA

PATHOPHYSIOLOGIC PROBLEMS RELATED TO SCHIZOPHRENIA

Schizophrenia is a psychotic illness that can affect a person's functional and cognitive ability, perception and expression of emotion. A psychotic illness is one where the individual's mental state is disturbed to the extent that they have difficulty distinguishing external reality from their internal perceptions[2]. Schizophrenia is perhaps best described as a syndrome that is identifiable by a cluster of signs and symptoms, which have diverse pathogenic bases[3]. The symptoms of schizophrenia can be debilitating in that they affect the person's ability to think, to concentrate, to relate, and to function in usual day-to-day activities. The symptoms can be divided into two groups: positive and negative. Positive symptoms include disorders of thinking and perception including delusions, hallucinations and bizarre behaviour. Negative symptoms include reduced levels of energy and motivation, attention deficit, blunted affect, passive social withdrawal and impairment in social functioning, loss of motivation, poverty of speech and poor rapport[2,4,5].

The criteria for diagnosing schizophrenia include the presence of characteristic symptoms:

- Delusions;
- Hallucinations;
- Disorganised speech;
- Disorganised behaviour and negative symptoms;
- Social/occupational dysfunction with diminishment of work, interpersonal and self-care functions; and
- The symptoms need to be present for at least 6 months and not be due to mood disorders or substance abuse[6].

The presentation of an acute episode of schizophrenia is often a critical event that requires an immediate and comprehensive response. People with schizophrenia also frequently suffer emotional symptoms, such as depression and anxiety. Suicidal ideation may be present, with 10% of people with schizophrenia completing suicide[7].

A number of subtypes of schizophrenia have been identified. The *Diagnostic and Statistical Manual of Mental Disorders*[6] identified five subtypes: paranoid, disorganised, catatonic, undifferentiated and residual. A number of biological researchers use subtypes of type I or positive schizophrenia, which has a preponderance of positive symptoms; and type II or negative schizophrenia, which has a preponderance of negative symptoms[2].

COURSE OF THE ILLNESS

The course of schizophrenia is often marked by a prodromal phase in which there may be changes in the person's social behaviour. Some of these changes, particularly those of withdrawal, irritability and anger, moodiness, and loss of interest in appearance and social relationships, may seem to be related to age-specific behaviours in adolescence. Other symptoms during the prodromal phase may include depression, suspiciousness, anxiety, and sleep disturbance. The first episode of schizophrenia usually occurs between the late teens and early thirties. The trajectory of the illness is highly variable. It may be brief (up to 2 years) with remission, or may last much longer with residual symptoms. Around 25% of people with the illness have a full remission following one or more episodes[5]. Around one third of people with schizophrenia will have a recovery from the acute phase that is marked by fewer relapses and fewer hospitalisations for acute episodes than those who retain residual symptoms. While this group may still require ongoing treatment and support, they will be able to function in the community[8]. Positive symptoms of delusions and hallucinations and disorders of thinking predominate in the early episodes of the illness, but tend to decrease in intensity over time. Loss of social and work skills, self-care and relationships may feature in the residual phase.

Better outcome is associated with

- Good pre-morbid adjustment;
- Acute onset;
- The presence of triggering events (stress) prior to the acute episode;
- The presence of affective symptoms;
- Brief duration of active symptoms;
- Few residual symptoms;
- A family history of affective disorder; and
- Being a woman[6].

Relapse following treatment is associated with

- Use of non-prescribed drugs and alcohol;
- Stressful environments; and
- Lack of social role and failure of social reintegration[9].

AGE OF ONSET AND INCIDENCE OF SCHIZOPHRENIA

The age of onset of schizophrenia peaks for men at 18–24 years, and peaks for women at 24–32 years. The overall lifetime prevalence for schizophrenia of 1% is the same for men and women; however, better outcome is related to older age at onset[2,4]. The prevalence of schizophrenia has been shown to be similar across gender, race, religion, population density, and level of industrialisation[7].

● Case study

Frank Martinez, 20, was brought to the emergency department by his parents. He presents as a slightly built, casually dressed and anxious young man. For 3 months, Frank has been neglecting his personal care, withdrawn and not attending university where he is a second-year science student. He currently spends most of his time lying on his bed. In the past week, he has become distressed, claiming that someone is pumping toxic fumes into his room. His parents report that he has been talking to himself, and occasionally shouting. He has stopped eating with the family, eating tinned food after everyone is in bed. Today he threatened his mother when she tried to talk to him. Prior to the onset of these symptoms, Frank had become less communicative, moody and isolative; changes attributed to his age. He had been a conscientious student, with above-average academic success, who socialised with a small group of friends. He has not been involved in any social activities for the past six months.

PATHOPHYSIOLOGY OF SCHIZOPHRENIA

The early descriptions of schizophrenia by Kraepelin and Bleuler in the early 1900s described it as a biological disorder[10]. Later theories ventured into psychological and familial explanations, focusing attention on the psychology of the person, or family communication. These explanations have not been supported by scientific studies and recent research has focussed on genetics, brain pathology and brain chemistry.

GENETIC FACTORS

There is evidence that genetic factors play a role in the development of schizophrenia. Twin studies have indicated a clear genetic link. Studies of monozygotic (identical) twins demonstrate a concordance (both twins having the same illness) rate of 40–55%, compared with a concordance rate for dizygotic (non-identical) twins of around 10%[11,12]. If one parent has schizophrenia, there is a 10% risk that offspring will develop the disorder. This risk rises to around 45% if both parents have the disorder[11]. If schizophrenia were a purely genetically inherited disorder, the concordance rate for monozygotic twins would be around 100% since they share 100% of their genes with each other. It must be concluded that other factors are implicated in the development of the disorder. The possibility of one gene being responsible for schizophrenia has been ruled out[13]. Genetic studies of people with schizophrenia and their biological parents indicate that altered calcineurin signalling could contribute to a susceptibility to schizophrenia[13]. The genetic effect is complex and probably involves multiple genes as well as non-genetic factors. Other illnesses with this pattern of genetic effect include insulin-dependent diabetes mellitus, multiple sclerosis and coronary artery disease[14].

BRAIN PATHOLOGY

Schizophrenia has been described as a neurodevelopmental disorder and a number of influences on brain development have been implicated[11]. No specific brain development problem has been identified, and it is possible that schizophrenia may be the result of the interaction or combined effect of several neurodevelopmental events in utero. Environmental factors that may have contributed to brain pathology include maternal exposure to viral illness, malnutrition, birth difficulty and injury[11]. Gestational and birth problems have been identified as more frequent in people who develop schizophrenia. People with schizophrenia are more likely to have been born in winter, and influenza epidemics are linked to higher rates of schizophrenia[11]. Maternal influenza in the third trimester of pregnancy, or very poor maternal nutrition in the first trimester, has been identified as risk factors. It is suspected that these perinatal insults may result in a lack of oxygen to some brain regions, and with that, the hippocampal and parahippocampal areas being implicated[5]. These areas play a major role in the reception and distribution of sensory stimuli and subsequently the organisation of thinking processes.

Neuroimaging studies of young people newly diagnosed with schizophrenia show a pattern of brain abnormality similar to people who have had schizophrenia for a much longer time, implying that brain changes may relate to the pathophysiology of the diagnosis rather than the effect of having the diagnosis for a long period of time. These abnormalities include enlargement of the ventricles, enlargement of the sulci on the cortex of the brain, reduction in brain size, and reduction in size of specific areas, such as hippocampal and prefrontal areas[11,15]. The loss of cells over time in early-onset schizophrenia has also been demonstrated. A group of young people with schizophrenia showed progressive loss of brain cells in the parietal lobes, spreading to other areas of the brain over time. The study correlated the greatest loss of cells with the worst symptoms of the disorder[11]. Velakoulis and colleagues (2000) suggest a model for neurodevelopmental understanding of schizophrenia involving a lesion in the hippocampal area that creates a vulnerability to further injury during the early stages of psychosis that may be linked to stress or marijuana use[15].

BIOCHEMICAL CHANGES

The neurotransmitter dopamine was first implicated in the development of schizophrenia in the 1960s and was accepted as a key biochemical abnormality. Evidence that dopamine is implicated in schizophrenia includes the observation that drugs such as amphetamines and cocaine, which increase dopamine levels in the brain, cause psychotic symptoms such as hallucinations and bizarre behaviour. The dopamine receptors D2 and D4 are thought to be implicated in positive symptoms; D3 receptors are thought to be implicated in negative symptoms. Drugs used to treat schizophrenia, the antipsychotics, block dopamine receptors and thus decrease the activity of the dopamine system. Other neurotransmitters implicated in schizophrenia include glutamate, serotonin, glycine, gamma-aminobutyric acid (GABA), acetylcholine (ACh) and noradrenaline. It is probable that there is a chemical imbalance associated with schizophrenia that is related to multiple neurotransmitters that affects the ability to receive, organise and transmit sensory messages[2,4,11].

VULNERABILITY-STRESS MODELS

The biological defects related to genetic factors, brain pathology and biochemical changes, while showing consistent and strong association with schizophrenia, are not a sufficient condition for the occurrence of the disorder[16]. The occurrence of a particular mental disorder in a particular individual needs to be understood by the presence of interacting biological, psychological, and social factors. The vulnerability-stress model is based on the understanding that a certain percentage of the population will, because of particular genetic and brain development factors, be vulnerable to schizophrenia. In certain psychological and environmental conditions, this vulnerability will be expressed as an episode of schizophrenia. Having a vulnerability to schizophrenia does not necessarily imply that the person will develop an episode of the disorder. Whether or not the person will experience the disorder, and whether or not the person will suffer relapses of the disorder, is dependent upon

- The level of vulnerability: high vulnerability will predispose the person to the disorder with very little stress; low vulnerability will require very high levels of stress in order for symptoms to be expressed;
- The resilience of personality: people who are competent and adaptive to varying social and environmental factors are better able to withstand stress; and
- The level of stress: a certain level of stress needs to be present for the symptoms to be expressed.

These three factors interact, thus providing a model for aetiology of schizophrenia that recognises biological, psychological and sociological influences[5,16].

TESTS TO CONFIRM SCHIZOPHRENIA

While changes in brain structure and chemistry have been identified as vulnerability factors related to schizophrenia, there is no specific biological marker, and thus no biochemical test or brain scan that can identify schizophrenia at this point in time[17].

NURSING IMPLICATIONS

The diagnosis of schizophrenia is made by careful and comprehensive psychological and biological assessment including assessment of presenting problems, history of the illness, premorbid personality and functioning, corroborating information, family history, and observation. The presence of delusions, hallucinations, disorganised speech and behaviour are characteristic symptoms of acute psychosis that may indicate a schizophrenic process. Positive symptoms tend to fluctuate over time and the client may be unwilling to discuss delusional material until there is a level of trust. The negative symptoms of loss of interest, withdrawal, anergia, poverty of speech, poor self-care and a blunted emotional response may be observed. The person presenting with a range of symptoms indicative of schizophrenia may also present with high levels of anxiety, depression, or aggressive responses related to delusional material. There is a high level of substance misuse and dependency in people presenting with schizophrenia[8].

● Frank's case study (continued)

Frank presents with a range of symptoms that may indicate a psychotic process. On assessment Frank complained that he has had trouble thinking clearly for over 12 months. He has not been attending university as he was convinced that other students, even those he knew well, were conspiring to have him excluded. He cited evidence of this as seeing students in small groups laughing, and he thought that they were making disparaging remarks about him. He also had experienced hearing voices in his bedroom and thought that these were coming through the airvents. He described two voices talking about him saying he was 'stupid, a loser', and commenting on what he was doing. He thought his parents might be part of this conspiracy.

LEARNING EXERCISES

1. What evidence is there that Frank is suffering a psychotic illness?
2. How is his illness affecting his current social and familial relationships as well as his ability to develop psychosocially?
3. Frank and his parents want to know about his illness. What explanations would you provide?

TREATMENT

Treatment for schizophrenia involves a combination of pharmacological and psychotherapeutic interventions[5,18]. Early treatment of schizophrenia is important. The duration of untreated psychosis has been associated with cognitive deterioration. Early treatment may increase the likelihood of symptomatic relief, reduce cognitive deficits[19], and decrease the adverse effects on family and social networks[20]. The place of treatment needs to be assessed in light of the person's safety, the ability of the family to provide containment and support, and the availability of community mental health services.

Hospitalisation should be considered if there is any concern for the safety of the person, family and community.

PHARMACOLOGY

Drugs, which aim to reduce the symptoms of schizophrenia, are called antipsychotics. Traditional antipsychotic drugs, such as chlorpromazine, haloperidol and trifluoperazine, block D2 receptors and have an effect on positive symptoms, but little effect on the negative symptoms that can have a significant impact on the person's quality of life and functional status. These drugs may also produce sedation, emotional settling, and psychomotor slowing. In addition, these drugs have a range of peripheral and central nervous system side effects that range from minor effects, such as constipation and dry mouth, to chronic movement disorders and life-threatening neuroleptic malignant syndrome[2].

Atypical antipsychotic drugs such as olanzapine, risperidone, and quetiapine are much better tolerated, although patients taking these drugs still need monitoring for neuroleptic malignant syndrome, extrapyramidal and a range of other side effects, including significant weight gain. In addition, atypical antipsychotics have been significantly associated with the onset of diabetes mellitus[21]. This group of drugs is called atypical because of their difference from the earlier antipsychotic agents. The atypical antipsychotic agents differ in terms of their neurotransmitter and neuroreceptor activity and their effect on negative symptoms. These drugs have less effect on D2 receptors, but antagonise other dopamine and serotonin receptor sites. They are being increasingly favoured in clinical practice. First-episode psychosis is usually treated with one of the atypical antipsychotic drugs. Monitoring of effectiveness includes observation of both positive and negative symptoms. An anxiolytic, such as diazepam, can be added in the short term to reduce distress levels of anxiety, agitation and insomnia. Monitoring for side effects includes observation for signs of dystonia (impaired muscle tone, often in the head, neck and tongue) shaking, stiffness and restlessness. Physical observations should include temperature, blood pressure and pulse as medication may alter cardiovascular function or have toxic effects. In the longer term, maintenance doses of atypical antipsychotics can be used, with continued monitoring. Clozapine may be effective when other treatments have failed. The use of clozapine is limited to registered centres, and in addition to the previously mentioned adverse effects, there is need to monitor for the severe adverse effects of neutropenia, agranulocytosis, and myocarditis[2,20].

PSYCHOTHERAPY

Psychotherapeutic treatment is as important to recovery from a psychotic illness as medication. An episode of schizophrenia can render the person's view of themselves and their world as confusing, unreliable and chaotic. At the very least, the person needs someone who is empathetic and knowledgeable about the illness and the human response to the illness, about the pharmacological treatments and about recovery.

COGNITIVE BEHAVIOURAL TECHNIQUES

Cognitive behavioural techniques have proved effective in teaching coping skills for the management of symptoms of schizophrenia and the development of problem-solving responses. A more detailed discussion of cognitive behavioural therapy is included later in this chapter. Trygstad *et al.* demonstrated that behavioural management of persistent auditory hallucinations was clinically effective[22]. Rector and Beck reviewed studies of cognitive behavioural therapy and schizophrenia and concluded that cognitive behavioural therapy, in conjunction with pharmacology and other psychosocial treatments, improves outcomes of treatment of positive and negative symptoms[23].

Further interventions are considered in the section on *Nursing Implications* at the end of this chapter.

DEPRESSION

Depression represents a significant public health issue. The World Health Organization's (WHO) recent *Global Burden of Disease* study has estimated that by 2020, depression will contribute the largest share of disability in the developing world, and the second largest share of disability worldwide[24,25]. The incidence of depressive disorders is relatively similar worldwide in terms of distribution and impact at individual and community levels[26].

Depression causes significant distress and suffering, and can lead to impairment in educational, social, family, interpersonal and employment functioning. There is a well established link between depression and suicide, and it is a grim fact that each year upwards of 2,300 Australians[27] and 500 New Zealanders[28] die by suicide. Rates of suicide in Australia and New Zealand are similar and rank high in comparison to international rates[28]. The direct cost of treating depression in the Australian context is estimated to be in the region of $500 million annually, of which approximately $60 million is spent on pharmaceuticals. The true cost of depression to individuals and the community defies quantification[27].

In Australia, depression has been identified as a National Health Priority Area, and the *National Action Plan for Depression* has been developed to provide a strategic direction for the prevention, early intervention, assessment and treatment of depression[29]. These initiatives aim to elevate depression to the ranks of heart disease and cancer in terms of community awareness and government commitment to prevention and treatment.

PREVALENCE, NATURAL HISTORY AND COURSE OF DEPRESSION

Depression is disconcertingly prevalent in the community, an observation that has been confirmed by the findings of a number of large-scale epidemiological studies conducted internationally. In Australia, the National Survey of Mental Health and Wellbeing estimated that some 5.8% of the adult population (or approximately 778,000 adults) had an identifiable depressive disorder in the 12 months prior to the survey[30]. The National Co-morbidity Survey, a second large survey of the epidemiology of mental disorders in the USA, found the overall lifetime rate of major depressive episode to be 17.1% (12.7% among males, and 21.3% among females)[31].

Differences in the prevalence rates reported between epidemiological studies are likely to be accounted for by differing methodologies employed in each study, for example the use of different survey questionnaires. However, it can be stated with some confidence that between 5 and 10% of the adult population will experience a major depressive episode in a 12-month period[26].

Depression frequently co-occurs with other mental disorders, for example anxiety symptoms or disorders occur in approximately 30% of patients with depression, and approximately 30% of people with depression experience panic attacks[32]. There are a number of medical illnesses where depression is a frequent concomitant condition, or where there seems to be evidence of the primary medical illness precipitating depression – either through a biologically mediated process and/or due to the stress associated with chronic, disabling or life-threatening illness. The incidence of depression among medically ill populations has been found to be as high as 15%[33]. Medical illnesses or syndromes where there is evidence of an association with depression include, but are not limited to, the list in Table 16.1.

TABLE 16.1: SOME MEDICAL ILLNESSES OR SYNDROMES ASSOCIATED WITH DEPRESSION	
Cancer	Migraine
Myocardial infarction	Multiple sclerosis
Cerebrovascular accident	Parkinson's disease
Diabetes	Rheumatoid arthritis
HIV/AIDS	Systemic lupus erythematosus
Epilepsy	Chronic fatigue syndrome
Dementia	Pain

The average age of onset of major depressive disorder is in the late 20s; however, depression can occur at any age[34], with depression in the elderly and childhood depression being common and sometimes under-recognised by health professionals[35,36]. The onset of symptoms of major depression can be insidious, with symptoms increasing in frequency and severity over several weeks or months, or onset can be sudden. The duration of an episode of major depression is variable, lasting from weeks to years. Left untreated an episode of major depression can last for six to nine months[34,37].

While many people experience only a single episode of major depression and recover fully, approximately 50–85% of people will experience subsequent episodes of major depression[38]. Approximately 20% of people who experience a major depressive episode will experience a relapse within 12 months[39], an important consideration for planning preventative treatment, such as maintenance antidepressant medication or 'booster sessions' where psychological treatment has been used.

ASSESSMENT AND CLINICAL FEATURES OF DEPRESSION

Depressed, sad or dysphoric mood is a normal response to hearing bad news or experiencing a loss of some kind. This normal response does not constitute evidence of 'clinical depression'. One of the key challenges for clinicians assessing people who report depressed mood is to evaluate whether such experiences are 'normal' responses to circumstances or events, or possibly represent evidence of a clinical or 'major' depressive episode, where definitive treatment is required[40].

Major depression is distinguished from 'normal' depression on the basis of the presence of certain characteristic symptoms, and by the severity, duration and persistence of these symptoms. There is no single symptom upon which a diagnosis of major depression can be made but, as a general principle, pervasively lowered mood is frequently a key feature, and people who report depressed mood for two weeks, and anyone who reports suicidal ideation, should be evaluated for the presence of a depressive disorder.

The American Psychiatric Association (2000) identifies the following diagnostic criteria for a major depressive episode[6]. Five (or more) of the following symptoms must be present during the same two-week period and represent a change from the person's previous level of functioning. At least one the symptoms must be either depressed mood or loss of interest or pleasure:

1. Depressed mood, present for most of the day, nearly every day, as indicated by either subjective report (e.g., feels sad or empty) or observation made by others (e.g., appears tearful). In children and adolescents, the mood state can be irritable;
2. Markedly diminished interest or pleasure in all, or almost all, activities most of the day, nearly every day (as indicated by either subjective account of observation made by others)';
3. Significant weight loss when not dieting (e.g., a change of more than 5% of body weight in a month), or decrease or increase in appetite nearly every day. Note: In children, consider failure to make expected weight gains;
4. Insomnia or hypersomnia nearly every day;
5. Psychomotor agitation or retardation nearly every day (observable by others, not merely subjective feelings of restlessness or being slowed down);
6. Fatigue of loss of energy nearly every day;
7. Feelings of worthlessness or excessive or inappropriate guilt (which may be delusional) nearly every day (not merely self-reproach or guilt about being sick);
8. Diminished ability to think or concentrate, or indecisiveness, nearly every day (either by subjective account or as observed by others); and
9. Recurrent thoughts of death (not just fear of dying), recurrent suicidal ideation without a specific plan, or a suicide attempt or a specific plan for committing suicide.

SUB-TYPES OF DEPRESSION AND THEIR SIGNIFICANCE

The classification of depressive disorders has been the subject of considerable debate for close to a century[41,42.] However, there is agreement that depression is likely to represent either a range of disorders, or that there are meaningful sub-types of depression. Two of the types or subtypes of depression that are clinically significant are melancholia (or the melancholic subtype) and psychotic depression (or major depression with 'psychotic features').

'Melancholic' depression is characterised by the presence of significant mood disturbance, psychomotor agitation or slowness (psychomotor retardation), and a profound inability to experience pleasure. Identifying melancholia is significant as there is some evidence that melancholia is specifically responsive to biological treatments (antidepressant medication, electroconvulsive therapy [ECT]). In 'psychotic depression', delusions or hallucinations and profound feelings of guilt are often present. There is often severe psychomotor slowing or agitation, and the mood disturbance is severe. Psychotic depression usually requires hospitalisation and treatment with a combination of antidepressant and antipsychotic medication, or ECT[34,41,43].

● Case study

John Smith, 49, married with two adult children, and employed as an accountant in a large city firm, has presented to the Community Health Centre for assessment, after having been referred by his general practitioner. Mr Smith gave a history of 'not feeling himself' for the past 4 weeks. He described periods of tearfulness, (which he stated was out of character), and irritability, both at home and work. Mr Smith stated that there has been a decline in his work performance, with his manager recently commenting that Mr Smith did not seem to be able to focus on his work. Mr Smith expressed frustration that he felt 'tired all the time,' spending many hours awake each night worrying whether he would have sufficient funds for his retirement. Mr Smith stated that he had previously been a keen golfer, regularly organising and competing in amateur competitions. In recent weeks, he had been unable to 'get the energy or motivation' to play. At the assessment, Mr Smith seemed restless, constantly wringing his hands and tapping his feet. He avoided eye contact and spoke with a soft and hesitant voice. At one point, Mr Smith apologised for becoming tearful when discussing his family, with whom he stated he had a very close relationship. Mr Smith admitted to occasional thoughts of wishing he were dead, but he denied thoughts of suicide, stating that he would 'never do that to his family'. When asked about the severity of his depressed mood, Mr Smith stated, 'I am at my lowest ebb, I have never felt so bad in all my life'.

PATHOPHYSIOLOGIC ORIGINS OF DEPRESSION

Depression is a complex and multifaceted disorder, or set of disorders, that, as yet, is not fully understood. No single pathophysiologic basis for depression has been identified. It is likely that it is an interaction between biological and psychological or psychosocial factors that contributes to the development of depression.

BIOLOGICAL FOUNDATIONS

GENETIC FACTORS

The possible role of genetic transmission in the mood disorders has been, and remains, a target of research effort. Evidence for genetic associations in the mood disorders is strongest for bipolar disorder, although there is some evidence for a hereditary component to depression. Family studies have indicated that first-degree relatives of those with major depressive disorder are two to three times more likely to have depression. This finding is supported by adoption studies that have shown that the increased risk of developing depression remains even in circumstances where offspring of those with major depressive disorder have been raised in adoptive families. In twin studies the rate at which monozygotic twins are concordant for depression is approximately 50%, while the rate of concordance for dizygotic twins is between 10–25%. Molecular biology techniques are being used in an attempt to identify specific genes or gene markers that are relevant to the genetic transmission of mood disorders (genetic linkage studies). At this stage, no consistent findings have emerged, but associations between mood disorders (principally bipolar disorder), and genetic makers have been reported for chromosomes 5, 11, 18 and X.

BRAIN PATHOLOGY
IMAGING RESEARCH

To date, consistent and replicable findings from imaging research have not been reported for major depressive disorder. Some studies using functional imaging techniques (SPECT and PET) have reported reduced cerebral blood flow in the cerebral cortex, especially in the frontal cortical region.

BIOCHEMICAL CHANGES
NEUROTRANSMISSION AND DEPRESSION

Serotonin is the neurotransmitter that has been most frequently been implicated in the pathophysiology of depression. Serotonin has both inhibitory and facilitatory functions, playing a role in the regulation of biological functions such as sleep, appetite and libido. Data from a number of studies have provided support for the hypothesis that depleted serotonin levels may underlie some depressive disorders. Of note, a number of antidepressant medications, for example the selective serotonin reuptake inhibitors or SSRIs (fluoxetine, paroxetine, sertraline, fluvoxamine, citalopram), increase levels of serotonin in the CNS. Other evidence for the role of serotonin down-regulation in depressive disorders has come from studies that have demonstrated that depletion of serotonin can precipitate depression. Low concentrations of serotonin in cerebrospinal fluid, and low concentrations of serotonin binding sites on platelets in patients with suicidal impulses, have been reported in a number of studies. Such data provides additional support for the serotonin hypothesis in depression and raises the possibility that serotonergic dysfunction may play a role in mediating suicidal impulses.

Interest in the potential role of noradrenaline in the pathophysiology of depression has taken a number of lines. Noradrenaline has an important role in the control and regulation of a number of autonomic nervous system responses, including regulating arousal and the 'flight or fright' response. Research has been directed to identifying whether noradrenaline levels are lowered in depressed versus non-depressed groups. Findings from these studies have been equivocal. The role of synaptic beta-receptor activity and sensitivity has also been studied. Activation of beta-receptors (located on the noradrenaline and serotonin neurons) reduces neurotransmitter release. Some antidepressant agents (e.g. the selective serotonin-noradrenaline reuptake inhibitor [SNRI], venlafaxine) increase noradrenaline levels, providing further support that noradrenaline may be involved in the pathophysiology of at least some forms of depression.

Dopamine levels in the CNS are correlated with levels of serotonin. Dopamine has a role in the regulation of a number of biological processes, including motor activity, emotional, learning and memory, goal-directed activity, attention, and social behaviour. Not surprisingly, then, some studies have demonstrated lowered CNS levels of the dopamine metabolite (homovanillic acid [HVA]) in some depressed patients. Elevated dopamine levels have been reported in patients with psychotic depression, an interesting finding given that dopamine hyperactivity is a robust research finding in schizophrenia and other psychotic disorders[44].

NEUROENDOCRINE REGULATION

There is interest in the possible role of altered neuroendocrine function as a potential cause of depressive disorders, with melatonin, prolactin, thyroid function, growth hormone, testosterone being a focus for research attention[45].

PSYCHOLOGICAL AND PSYCHOSOCIAL FOUNDATIONS

Many psychological theories have been advanced to account for the cause and pathophysiology of depression. Freud considered that depression was a function of introjected hate towards the self, while more recently cognitive models of depression have been developed. The cognitive theory of depression suggests that certain people are predisposed to the development of depression due to the presence of certain cognitive distortions, or patterns of thinking called schemata, which influence the way people think, feel and behave. According to the cognitive model of depression some people use 'depressogenic' schemata, in other words patterns of thinking, feeling and behaviour that inherently provoke or maintain depression. Aaron Beck (1979), a pioneer of cognitive theory and therapy, proposed that people prone to depression use a triad of cognitive distortions: a negative view about the self, a negative view about their environment, and a negative view about the future[46]. Cognitive therapy and cognitive-behavioural therapy are effective psychotherapeutic techniques that aim to modify these and other cognitive distortions.

LIFE EVENTS AND STRESS

There appears to be a relationship between life events (e.g., divorce, death of a loved one, loss of employment) and the development of depression. Various theories have been proposed to explain the relationship between life events and the development of depression, including suggestions that the stress associated with the life event may cause functional changes in the brain that precipitate a depressive episode.

PERSONALITY FACTORS

Personality style has been considered as a factor that may increase an individual's vulnerability for the development of depression. It is possible that people with certain personality types may using internalising defence mechanisms like self-blame, and these patterns of coping may increase risk of psychological disturbance, including depression.

● John Smith's case study (continued)

Mr Smith stated that there had been a number of stressors in his life in recent months. He had been promoted at work into a role that meant that he had to supervise the work of a team of colleagues. Mr Smith's daughter had recently left home to live with friends in a suburb across the city, and Mr Smith's wife had discovered a lump in her breast that was currently being investigated. Mr Smith denied having had any psychiatric symptoms or treatment in the past, but he stated that his mother suffered from 'nerves' for many years, and his sister had suffered from postnatal depression after the birth of each of her children. Mr Smith described himself as having a strong work ethic (he worked up to 60 hours each week), and he stated that he was a perfectionist. He also stated that he had tended to be a 'gloomy person' by nature, always worrying about the possible negative consequences of events or decisions. Mr Smith stated that he was in good health, although for several months he had noted that he was excessively tired, and had experienced tremors, palpitations and excessive perspiration. He had also experienced some weight loss. Mr Smith stated that he had not discussed these symptoms with his general practitioner, believing that they were nothing serious and would pass of their own accord.

LEARNING EXERCISES

1. Does Mr Smith currently have symptoms suggestive of a major depressive episode?
2. Are there any clinical indications that Mr Smith may have a major depressive sub-type?
3. What factors could be relevant to Mr Smith's current depression?
4. What additional information would need to be sought in relation to Mr Smith's symptom report?
5. Mr Smith asks, 'What has caused my depression?' What would be the approach to answering this question?

PHARMACOLOGICAL TREATMENT OF DEPRESSION

One of the most significant advances in the treatment of depressive disorders has been the development of antidepressant medications, beginning in the late 1950s with imipramine and continuing to the present day with the introduction of an array of 'new generation' antidepressant agents. The tricyclic antidepressants (TCAs) have been used widely in clinical practice since the 1960s, and have been evaluated in hundreds of clinical trials. The TCAs have a wide side effect profile and are not routinely used as first-line treatments for depression; however, there is some evidence to suggest that the TCA's may be more effective in the treatment of severe subtypes of depressive disorder (e.g., melancholic or psychotic depression). Examples of TCA agents include, imipramine, amitriptyline, nortriptyline and desipramine. The selective serotonin reuptake inhibitors (SSRIs) are a class of antidepressants used extensively in the treatment of depression, obsessive-compulsive disorder, and panic disorder. The SSRIs (fluoxetine, fluvoxamine, sertraline, paroxetine, citalopram) are often used as first-line treatments for major depression. Other agents that are used in the treatment of depression include mirtazapine and venlafaxine (inhibitors of serotonin and noradrenaline reuptake), nefazodone (a serotonin antagonist), and moclobemide (a reversible monoamine oxidase inhibitor).

An antidepressant is usually indicated in circumstances where the mood disturbance is severe, persistent or recurrent, where suicidal ideation is present, in situations where the person has had a favourable response to medication in the past, where there is a strong family history of depression or another mood disorder, and where there has been no response to a psychological (psychotherapy) intervention[40]. Additionally, the presence of melancholic or psychotic features would always require antidepressant medication to be commenced[26,34,43]. Selection of an antidepressant agent would usually be determined on the basis of consideration of the following factors[47]:

- Efficacy (the likelihood that the agent will work);
- Tolerability (the likelihood that the patient will be able to tolerate the adverse effects of a particular agent);
- Symptom profile (e.g., choice of a more sedating agent if insomnia is clinically significant); and
- Medical history (e.g., avoiding an agent that is associated with effects on blood pressure if patient has a history of or risk factors for hypertension or hypotension).

NON-PHARMACOLOGICAL APPROACHES TO MANAGING DEPRESSION

While antidepressant medication plays a significant role in the management of depressive disorders, there are a number of other non-drug treatments that are also used in the treatment of disorders.

ELECTROCONVULSIVE THERAPY

Electroconvulsive therapy (ECT) continues to play a role in the treatment of depression, although less frequently due to the range and effectiveness of available antidepressant medications. ECT involves the application of electrical stimulation to an anaesthetised patient in order to induce a brief generalised (tonic-clonic) convulsion. The therapeutic efficacy of ECT is not well understood, but is believed to relate to convulsion itself, rather than the electrical stimulation. ECT remains an effective and safe treatment option in clinical situations where rapid resolution of symptoms is required (e.g., presence of a very severe mood state, high suicide risk, dehydration or nutritional compromise), or where other treatments have been unsuccessful or cannot be tolerated due to adverse effects[48].

REPETITIVE TRANSCRANIAL MAGNETIC STIMULATION

Repetitive transcranial magnetic stimulation (rTMS) is a treatment that is currently receiving significant research interest. rTMS involves small, highly focused currents being introduced into outer brain structures. Unlike ECT, rTMS does not require an anaesthetic. Evidence for the efficacy of rTMS in the treatment of depression is equivocal, and further studies are required before definitive conclusions and treatment recommendations can be made. It is likely, though, that rTMS will play some role in the treatment of depression in the future[49].

COGNITIVE-BEHAVIOURAL THERAPY

Cognitive-behavioural therapy, (CBT) is a robust psychotherapeutic modality targeting thinking, feelings and behaviour that has been extensively evaluated in the treatment of depression and anxiety disorders. Evidence suggests that CBT is as effective as medication in the treatment of depression of mild to moderate severity[50].

ST JOHN'S WORT

The herb St John's wort (SJW)(*Hypericum perforatum*) has recently received considerable attention in both the popular media and scientific literature for its purported antidepressant properties. While there is certainly some evidence that SJW offers potential as an antidepressant, many questions concerning the safety and efficacy of the compound remain unanswered. There is, as yet, insufficient evidence from well designed randomised controlled studies to recommend SJW as a treatment for depression. There is also evidence that SJW possesses enzyme-inducing properties and can interfere with the metabolism of a number of commonly prescribed medications[34,51,52].

NURSING IMPLICATIONS

There are important roles for nurses providing care to people who are suffering from breakdown in mental health. Nurses working in both hospital and community-based settings are well placed to provide interventions designed to improve mood, manage distressing thoughts and emotions and maintain safety, and to minimise the negative consequences of mental illness.

THERAPEUTIC ALLIANCE AND SUPPORTIVE PSYCHOTHERAPY

How a person understands their mental illness, and how other people respond to it makes a difference to their recovery. Mental illness has been stigmatised across time and many cultures. The findings that some mental illnesses are caused, at least in part, by biological vulnerability can provide relief but may also render people helpless. The idea that they have a genetic 'abnormality' may seem like an inheritance that they cannot change. The person can become 'self-stigmatising' turning nihilistic beliefs about mental illness upon themselves[12]. Self-stigmatisation is reinforced by social stigmatisation as the person with a mental illness is frequently 'blamed' for their plight and families are caught in the web of responsibility[53].

The formation of a therapeutic alliance with the person with a mental illness and their family is crucial to positive outcomes of treatment. A therapeutic alliance can affect their sense of self, engagement with treatment, compliance with medication, success of psychosocial interventions and the ability to negotiate with services.

The establishment of a relationship with a person who has recently suffered a psychotic or depressive episode is a skilled process requiring an understanding of the nature of the disorder and the nature of human response to such experience. The person may be highly suspicious and fearful and require a consistent and persistent, gentle and empathic approach in order to develop a climate of trust. Developing a therapeutic alliance allows assessment of the way the person views their illness and thus what approach may be most beneficial. Thompson, McGorry & Harrigan (2003) found that people who had suffered a psychotic episode tended to 'seal over' the experience, however interventions that encouraged integrating the experience into their understanding of themselves was helpful to recovery[54]. People who have suffered an acute episode of mental illness need to have a person in the clinical setting who has an ongoing understanding of their illness history and treatment, of their social and family situation, of their current stresses, their goals, hopes, and ambitions. Such a person can provide coordination of services, ongoing support, and hope for the future.

MEDICATION MANAGEMENT

Nurses need knowledge of the medications that are prescribed for a specific client, the target symptoms and how to assess them, the dosage range, and the side effect and drug-interaction profile. Most psychotropic drugs work on neurotransmitters and neuroreceptor sites. Nurses need an understanding of the specific neurotransmitters and receptors involved and the way drugs act upon them.

A rapid and sympathetic response to clients suffering side effects of medication is important. Nurses should be able to assess and intervene in the management of side effects. Issues of weight gain in response to psychotropic medication should be treated seriously as this may affect self-esteem, activity, and may be a precursor to the development of diabetes mellitus.

Knowledge of the factors that affect individual response to medication and dosage range is important. The cytochrome P-450 enzyme system is linked to the metabolisation of psychotropic drugs and is characterised by variations in individuals and ethnic groups. African Americans, and Asians have been identified as more likely to poorly metabolise psychotropic drugs[2]. Inhibition of metabolism of drugs, leading to increased plasma levels and delays in clearance, may be also be affected by body constitution, other drugs, and by medical illness.

EDUCATION

Education should target the person with the illness, their family and significant others. Education has been demonstrated to improve knowledge of mental illness, to reduce stress levels and to influence recovery[55].

Education should be titrated to the ability of the client and family to absorb new knowledge, and provide information on

- A multifactorial understanding of the illness including vulnerability factors, the role of environment and stress, and the role of self;
- The illness process;
- The use of medication;
- The need for time and support to recover from the illness; and
- Strategies that may assist recovery.

Medication information should include the targeted symptoms of the illness, and side effects and their treatment. In addition nurses need to develop a collaborative approach, to work with the client to develop an acceptable regime, and to explore feelings and beliefs about medication[56]. Relapse prevention plans can be developed in conjunction with the client and the family. Plans should identify early warning signs of illness/relapse (for instance: insomnia, withdrawal, depressed mood, increased delusional thinking, bizarre speech patterns, suicidal thoughts) and identify a first-line response.

ONGOING ASSESSMENT

Assessment is an ongoing part of the management of a person experiencing an episode of depression or psychosis. Nursing assessment should be directed to evaluating the severity, type and persistence of the cognitive, emotional, social and biological features of the illness, the extent to which symptoms are responding to treatment and the efficacy and acceptability of the medication regime. Risk assessment is a key component of assessment, and nurses should evaluate suicide risk on an ongoing basis. Suicide assessment involves making sensitive but honest enquiries as to whether a person has had thoughts about harming themselves or taking their own life, whether they have made or are considering active means of taking their life, consideration of the lethality of identified methods, and determining the intent with which the person is committed to ending their life.

PROMOTING ACTIVITY AND EXERCISE

Inactivity is a common feature of depression. Activity and exercise have what can be regarded as natural antidepressants because activity distracts people from their problems and negative thinking, reduces feelings of tiredness, promotes sleep, and is inherently motivating. Strategies for increasing activity and exercise can include assisting people to identify a list of pleasant activities (e.g., walking around the block, swimming for 30 minutes) graded in terms of their complexity and completion time required, and then encouraging the client to commence with the easiest task on the list. It can then be useful to review completion of the tasks, how it made the person feel, and to use positive feedback that encourages attempts at the next activity on the list.

It has been hypothesised that exercise may reduce depression through stimulation of neurotransmitters in the brain. It is important to consider issues around a person's exercise tolerance and level of fitness when encouraging exercise.

PROMOTING SLEEP

Sleep disturbance is a very common feature of mental illness. Providing advice in relation to good sleeping habits can be helpful, for example:

- Avoiding alcohol, caffeine and nicotine;
- Use of regular exercise in the late afternoon or early evening;
- Avoid reading or watching television in bed;
- Only go to bed when feeling sleepy;
- Do not lie in bed tossing in turning, get up and do an activity in another room, returning to bed when feeling sleepy again;
- Reduce stimuli in the bedroom;
- Avoid daytime napping; and
- Learn and use relaxation techniques, such as progressive muscular relaxation[40].

DEALING WITH DEPRESSIVE THINKING

Nurses working with clients with depression can apply communication strategies designed to help correct some of the distorted cognitions depressed people commonly use. For example, depressed people often experience difficulty in making decisions. Assisting with the use of a step-by-step problem-solving approach can be helpful:

1. Break the problem down into a specific issue or goal;
2. Identify the range of strategies or solutions that could be applied;
3. Evaluate each option in terms of its likely benefits and risks;
4. Implement the strategy/solution; and
5. Review outcome.

Strategies for dealing with the negative thinking patterns that some depressed people have can involve assisting the person to consider a more balanced or alternative viewpoint. For example, in response to a depressed person stating, 'I am never going to get better' it could be helpful to say something like 'You have been able to participate in some of the group discussion today, which you haven't been able to do previously. This is a sign that you are starting to get better'. In response to a negative statement like 'Nothing is changing, I still feel terrible' it might be helpful to reply in a way that acknowledges the person's feelings but conveys a positive outlook, such as 'I understand that you feel that it is taking some time for you to get better, let's look at what we could do together to make the afternoon enjoyable'[40].

THOUGHT DISTURBANCE RELATED TO PSYCHOSIS

Hallucinations and delusions can be extremely distressing for clients. It is useful to discuss these phenomena in a straightforward way. Be vigilant in observing for behaviour that may indicate the client is concerned with hallucinations. This may be pre-occupation, muttering, talking aloud, or hyper-vigilance. Ask directly about hallucinations 'Are you hearing voices?' and 'Tell me what the voices are saying to you.' This gives the client permission to talk about the experience. Utilise problem-solving skills in the management. Encouragement to focus on your voice and what you are saying, or listening to a radio with a headset at other times may be useful. Similarly, asking clients to describe delusions or discussing their suspicions can be helpful although this should be time-limited. Acknowledging the frightening aspects of both hallucinations and delusions and encouraging problem-solving to manage these phenomena is useful. Identifying the triggers for delusional thinking and hallucinations can help pinpoint triggers in the environment.

CONCLUSION

Mental health breakdown is multifactorial. This chapter has demonstrated that breakdown in mental health is likely to be related to both a biological vulnerability to a mental illness and developmental and stress factors in the environment. The role of nursing in such disorders focuses on understanding the illness, monitoring pharmacological and other physical treatments, education of the client, family and the community, and specific interpersonal and psychodynamic interventions.

SUMMARY OF KEY POINTS

- Pathophysiology of mental illness is related to biological vulnerabilities that may be genetic, brain abnormality or neurochemical in origin;
- Biological vulnerability is insufficient alone to predict the onset of mental illness;
- Schizophrenia has a multifactorial aetiology: vulnerability factors, including genetic predisposition, biochemical changes or brain pathology interact with resilience and stress;
- Treatment of schizophrenia involves both pharmacological and psychotherapeutic interventions;
- Depression is a major public health issue;
- Depression co-occurs with many medical disorders;
- Depression has a multifactorial aetiology: biological factors, genetics, brain pathology and biochemistry interact with life events and personality;
- Treatment of depression involves pharmacology, and possibly other physical treatments, and psychotherapeutic interventions; and
- Nursing implications for breakdown in mental health includes: specific knowledge about mental health, mental illness and its treatment and human response to stress, therapeutic alliance and supportive psychotherapy, ongoing assessment, education, collaboration and specific interventions aimed at ameliorating symptoms.

Recommended Readings

Blows, WT. 2003; *The Biological Basis of Nursing: Mental Health*, Routledge, London.

Gamble, C & Brennan, G. 2000; *Working with Serious Mental Illness: A Manual for Clinical Practice*, Bailliere Tindall & RCN, Edinburgh.

Keltner, NL & Folks, DG. 2001; *Psychotropic Drugs* (3rd ed.), Mosby, St. Louis.

Keltner, NL, Folks, DG, Palmer, CA & Powers, RE. 1998; *Psychobiological Fundations of Psychiatric Care*, Mosby, St Louis.

Meadows, G & Singh, B. 2002; *Mental Health in Australia: Collaborative Community Practice*, Oxford University Press, Oxford.

References

1. Jackson, S. 1986; *Melancholia and Depression from Hippocratic Times to Modern Times*, Yale University Press, Newhaven.

2. Keltner, NL & Folks, DG. 2001; *Psychotropic Drugs* (3rd ed.), Mosby, St Louis.

3. Trimble, MR. 1996; *Biological Psychiatry* (2nd ed.), Wiley, Chichester.

4. Blows, WT. 'Schizophrenia', in WT Blows, 2003; *The Biological Basis of Nursing: Mental Health*, Routledge, London, 158–179.

5. Provencher, HL, Fournier, JP & Dupais, N. 1997; 'Schizophrenia Revisited', *Journal of Psychiatric and Mental Health Nursing, 4,* 275–285.

6. American Psychiatric Association. 2000; *Diagnostic and Statistic Manual of Mental Disorders* (4th ed., text revision), American Psychiatric Association, Washington, DC.

7. Turner, SM & Hensen, M. 1997; *Adult Psychopathology and Diagnosis* (3rd ed.), Wiley, New York.

8. Mueser, KT, Drake, RE & Bond, CR. 1997; 'Recent Advances in Psychiatric Rehabilitation for Patients with Severe Mental Illness', *Harvard Review of Psychiatry*, 5 (3), 123–137.

9. Brennan, G. 2000; 'Stress Vulnerability Model of Serious Mental Illness', in C Gamble & G Brennan (eds.), *Working with Serious Mental Illness: A Manual for Clinical Practice*, Baillière Tindall & RCN, Edinburgh.

10. Craig, TKJ. 2000; 'Severe Mental Illness: Symptoms, Signs and Diagnosis', in C Gamble & G Brennan (eds.), *Working with Serious Mental Illness: A Manual for Clinical Practice*, Baillière Tindall & RCN, Edinburgh.

11. Andreasen, NC. 2001; *Brave New Brain: Conquering Mental Illness in the Era of the Genome*, Oxford University Press, Oxford.

12. Faraone, SV, Tsuang, MT & Tsuang, DW. 1999; *Genetics of Mental Disorders: A Guide for Students, Clinicians and Researchers*, The Guilford Press, New York.

13. Gerber, DJ, Hall, D, Miyakawa, T, Demars, JA, Karayiorgou, M & Tonegawa, S. 2003; 'Evidence for Association of Schizophrenia with Genetic Variation in the 8p21.3 Gene, PPP3CC, Encoding the Calcineurin Gamma Subunit', *Proceedings of the National Academy of Sciences of the United States of America*, 100 (15), 8993–8998.

14. Moldin, SO. 1997; Genes and Schizophrenia. *Journal of the California Alliance for the Mentally Ill*, 8 (3), 84–86.

15. Velakoulis, D, Wood, SJ, McGorry, P & Pantelis, C. 2000; 'Evidence of Progression of Brain Structural Abnormalities in Schizophrenia: Beyond the Neurodevelopmental Model', *Australian and New Zealand Journal of Psychiatry*, 34 (Suppl.), S113–S126.

16. Kiesler, DJ. 1999; *Beyond the Disease Model of Mental Disorders*, Praeger, Westport, Connecticut.

17. Copolov, D & Crook, J. 2000; 'Biological Markers and Schizophrenia', *Australian and New Zealand Journal of Psychiatry*, 34 (Supplement), S108–S112.

18. Gould, RA, Mueser, KT, Bolton, E, Mays, V & Goff, D. 2001; 'Cognitive Therapy for Psychosis in Schizophrenia: An Effect Size Analysis', *Schizophrenia Research*, 48, 335–342.

19. Amminger, GP, Edwards, J, Brewer, WJ, Harrigan, S & McGorry, PD. 2002; 'Duration of Untreated Psychosis and Cognitive Deterioration in First-Episode Schizophrenia', *Schizophrenia Research*, 54, 223–230.

20. Therapeutic Guidelines. 2000; *Therapeutic Guidelines: Psychotropic, Version 4*. Therapeutic Guidelines Limited, Victoria, Australia, 116.

21. Sernyak, MJ, Leslie, DL, Alarcon, RD, Losonczy, MF & Rosenheck, R. 2002; 'Association of Diabetes Mellitus with Use of Atypical Neuroleptics in the Treatment of Schizophrenia', *American Journal of Psychiatry*, 159 (4), 561–566.

22. Trygstad, L, Buccheri, R, Dowling, G, Zind, R, White, K, Griffin, JJ, et al. 2002; 'Behavioural Management of Persistent Auditory Hallucinations in Schizophrenia: Outcomes from a 10 Week Course', *Journal of the American Psychiatric Nurses Association*, 8 (3), 84–91.

23. Rector, NA & Beck, AT. 2001; 'Cognitive Behavioural Therapy for Schizophrenia: An Empirical Review', *The Journal of Nervous and Mental Disease*, 189 (5), 278–287.

24. Murray, C & Lopez, A. 1997a; 'Global Mortality, Disability, and the Contribution of Risk Factors: Global Burden of Disease Study, *Lancet*, 349, 1436–1442.

25. Murray, C & Lopez, A. 1997b; 'Alternative Projections of Mortality and Disability by Cause 1990–2020: Global Burden of Disease Study', *Lancet*, 349, 1498–1504.

26. Bauer, M, Whybrow, P, Angst, J, Versiani, M, Moller, H-J, World Federation of Societies of

Biological Psychiatry (WFSBP) Taskforce on Treatment. 2002a; 'Guidelines for Biological Treatment of Unipolar Depressive Disorders, Part 1: Acute and Continuation Treatment of Major Depressive Disorder', *World Journal of Biological Psychiatry*, 3 (1), 5–43.

27. Commonwealth Department of Health & Aged Care and Australian Institute of Health and Welfare. 1999; *National Health Priority Areas: Mental Health – A Report Focusing on Depression*, Canberra.

28. Ministry of Health (Manatu Hauora). 2004; *Suicide Facts: Provisional 2001 Statistics* (all ages). Ministry of Health, New Zealand. www.moh.govt.nz, accessed 30 July 2004.

29. Commonwealth Department of Health & Aged Care. 2000; *National Action Plan for Depression*, Mental Health and Special Programs Branch, Publications Production Unit, Canberra.

30. Australian Bureau of Statistics. 1998; *Mental Health and Wellbeing: Profile of Adults,* Australian Government Publishing Service, Canberra.

31. Kessler, R, McConagle, K, Zhao, S, Nelson, C, Hughes, M, Eshleman, S, *et al*. 1994; 'Lifetime and 12-Month Prevalence of DSM-III-R Psychiatric Disorders in the United States', *Archives of General Psychiatry*, 51, 911–918.

32. Ballenger, J. 1996; 'Comorbidity of Panic and Depression: Implications for Clinical Management', *Psychopharmacology*, 13 (Supplement 4), 13–17.

33. Stevens, D, Ries Merinkangas, K & Merinkangas, J. 1995; 'Comorbidity of Depression and Other Medical Conditions', in E Beckham & W Leber (eds.), *Handbook of Depression* (2nd ed.), Guildford Press, New York.

34. American Psychiatric Association. 2002; *Practice Guideline for the Treatment of Patients with Major Depression*. www.psych.org, accessed 10 June 2003.

35. Burns, J, Andrews, G & Szabo, M. 2002; 'Depression in Young People: What Causes It? Can It Be Prevented?' *Medical Journal of Australia*, 177, S93–96.

36. Sawyer, M, Arney, F, Baghurst, P, Clark, J, Graetz, B, Kosky, R, *et al*. 2002; 'The Mental Health of Young People in Australia: Key Findings from the Child and Adolescent Component of the National Survey of Mental Health and Well-Being', *Australian and New Zealand Journal of Psychiatry*, 35, 806–814.

37. Solomon, D, Keller, M, Leon, A, Mueller, T, Shea, M, Warshaw, M, *et al*. 1997; 'Recovery from Major Depression: A 10-Year Prospective Follow-up Across Multiple Episodes', *Archives of General Psychiatry*, 54, 1001–1006.

38. Mueller, T, Leon, A, Keller, M, Solomon, D, Endicott, J, Coryell, W, *et al*. 1999; 'Recurrence after Recovery after Major Depression Disorder during 15 Years of Observational Follow-up', *American Journal of Psychiatry*, 156, 1000–1006.

39. Lee, A & Murray, R. 1998; 'The Long-Term Outcome of Maudsley Depressives', *British Journal of Psychiatry*, 153, 741–751.

40. Treatment Protocol Project. 1997; *Management of Mental Disorders* (2nd ed.), Sydney: World Health Organization Collaborating Centre for Mental Health and Substance Abuse.

41. Parker, G. 2000; 'Classifying Depression: Should Paradigms Lost Be Regained? *American Journal of Psychiatry*, 157 (8), 1195–1203.

42. Roth, M. 2001; 'Unitary or Binary Nature of Classification of Depressive Illnesses and Its Implications for the Scope of Manic Depressive Disorder', *Journal of Affective Disorders*, 64, 1–18.

43. Bauer, M, Whybrow, P, Angst, J, Versiani, M, Moller, H-J, WFSBP Taskforce on Treatment. 2002b; 'Guidelines for Unipolar Depressive Disorders, Part 2: Maintenance Treatment of Major Depressive Disorder and Treatment of Chronic Depressive Disorders and Subthreshold Disorders', *World Journal of Biological Psychiatry*, 3 (2), 69–86.

44. Thase, M & Howland, R. 1997; 'Biological Processes in Depression: An Updated Review and Integration', in E Beckham & W Leber (eds.), *Handbook of Depression* (2nd ed.), Guildford Press, New York.

45. Sadock, B & Sadock, V. 2003; *Kaplan and Sadock's Synopsis of Psychiatry, Behavioural Sciences / Clinical Psychiatry* (9th ed.), Lipincott, Williams and Wilkins, Philadelphia.

46. Beck, AT. 1979; *Cognitive Theory of Depression*, Guildford Press, New York.

47. Mendelwicz, J. 2001; 'Optimising Antidepressant Use in Clinical Practice: Towards Criteria for Antidepressant Selection', *British Journal of Psychiatry*, 179, (Suppl. 42), S1–S3.

48. Fink, M. 2001; 'Convulsive Therapy: A Review of the First 55 Years', *Journal of Affective Disorders*, 63, 1–15.

49. George, M, Nahas, Z, Kozel, A, Kozel, F, Li, X, Denslow, S, *et al*. 2002; 'Mechanism and State of the Art of Transcranial Magnetic Stimulation', *The Journal of ECT*, 18 (4), 170–181.

50. DeRubeis, RJ, Gelfand, LA, Tang, TZ & Simons, AD. 1999; 'Medications Versus Cognitive-Behaviour Therapy for Severely Depressed Outpatients: Mega-Analysis of Four Randomised Controlled Trials', *American Journal of Psychiatry*, 156 (7), 1007–1013.

51. Maidment, I. 2000; 'The Use of St John's Wort in the Treatment of Depression', *Psychiatric Bulletin*, 24, 232–234.

52. Therapeutic Goods Administration. 2000; 'Information Sheet for Health Care Professionals:

Interactions of St John's Wort Preparations'. www.health.gov.au/tga, accessed 30 May 2003.

53. Epstein, M & Olsen, A. 2002; 'Mental Illness: Responses from the Community', in G Meadows & B Singh (eds.), *Mental Health in Australia: Collaborative Community Practice*, Oxford University Press, Oxford, 11–17.

54. Thompson, KN, McGorry, P & Harrigan, SM. 2003; 'Recovery Style and Outcome in First-Episode Psychosis', *Schizophrenia Research*, 62, 31–6.

55. Mueser, KT, Corrigan, PW, Hilton, DW, Tanzman, B, Schaub, A, Gingerich, S, *et al.* 2002; 'Illness Management and Recovery: A Review of the Research', *Psychiatric Services*, 53 (10), 1272–1284.

56. Gray, R, Wykes, T & Gourney, K. 2002; 'From Compliance to Concordance: A Review of the Literature on Interventions to Enhance Compliance with Antipsychotic Medication', *Journal of Psychiatric and Mental Health Nursing*, 9, 277–284.

17 | Palliative Care and Health Breakdown

AUTHORS

AMANDA JOHNSON

KATHLEEN HARRISON

DAVID CURROW

MEGAN LUHR-TAYLOR

ROBERT JOHNSON

LEARNING OBJECTIVES

When you have completed this chapter you will be able to
• Understand the core components of a palliative care approach and their application to an individual and family;
• Identify the cluster of symptoms commonly experienced by an individual requiring palliation;
• Understand the pathophysiology underpinning the cluster of common symptoms;
• Assess an individual for the presence of the common symptoms;
• Select the appropriate interventions inclusive of pharmacology to be implemented following identification of the common symptoms; and
• Develop foundation knowledge and generic skills in palliative care to assist in the support of an individual and their family receiving palliation.

INTRODUCTION

This chapter is designed to provide undergraduate nursing students and nursing professionals with an understanding of the cluster of symptoms and the existence of a terminal pathway most commonly shared by individuals who are dying, irrespective of the underlying pathophysiology. Case studies are used to illustrate that the manifestation of symptoms and the presence of the terminal pathway are not exclusive to any one particular disease entity but can be derived from cancer, neurological, cardiac, respiratory, renal and/or age-related chronic illnesses, such as dementia.

The case studies aim to enhance the capacity of a beginning nurse to provide effective nursing care embracing a palliative care approach. This approach is based on the premise of early assessment, intervention and management to improve the individual and their family's quality of life. The two primary needs expressed by individuals dying and their families are

1. The desire to be comfortable and free from symptoms, allowing them to have ongoing interaction with family and friends; and
2. Maintaining a quality of life in which they can achieve meaningful goals.[1,2]

REFLECTIVE EXERCISE

1. What aspects does a nurse find most challenging when providing nursing care to an individual, who is dying, and their family?
2. Why are these aspects challenging to a nurse?

DEMOGRAPHICS OF DEATH IN AUSTRALIA

Australia's life expectancy in the 21st century has significantly improved for both genders, with the exception of Indigenous Australians[3,4]. With advancements in medicine and public health (food, water and sanitation), the opportunity to live longer is created, resulting in an increasingly aged population[5]. The main causes of death in our adult population are related to malignancy and circulatory disorders (acute myocardial infarction, cerebrovascular accidents).[6] This leads to an increased incidence of chronic illness in our aged population that will see more people dying from diseases that are chronic, and with multiple pathologies present[3,4,6,7], than ever before.

An increased life expectancy brings innate gains for individuals, but nationally, this situation provides a significant challenge for government to provide a comprehensive health care system responsive to the needs of our ageing population.

WHY IS THERE A NEED FOR A PALLIATIVE CARE APPROACH?

Worldwide, the incidence and mortality from cancer and chronic disease is expected to increase significantly over the next 20 years[8-10], creating more demand for palliative care than ever before[5]. Cognisant of this changing health pattern, the World Health Organization (WHO) now defines palliative care as

an approach that improves the quality of life of patients and their families facing the problem associated with life-threatening illness, through the prevention and relief of suffering by means of early identification and impeccable assessment and treatment of pain and other problems, physical, psychosocial and spiritual[9] (p. 84).

The WHO definition reflects the shifting of palliative care and explicitly identifies that the approach can now begin at the time of diagnosis or at any other point along the illness trajectory, and may be implemented in a range of health care settings[10].

THE CHALLENGE FOR NURSES

The nature of the death experience now faced by nurses is significantly shaped by the changing demographics of disease morbidity and mortality, and the increasing age of the Australian population. Nurses will be caring for individuals who will commonly have more than one disease state and/or disability present at the time of death[3,4]. This co-morbidity of disease results in increased acuity and complexity in the management of symptoms, thus placing additional demands on the nurse's knowledge and skill mix. The need for nurses to develop a palliative approach inclusive of core knowledge and generic skills, and to transfer this knowledge and skill across acute, community and residential aged care facilities, is paramount[6]. Ensuring nurses have this capacity will enable individuals and their families to be better managed during their chronic illness and palliation.

A sound knowledge base of the underlying disease pathophysiology, an understanding of the cluster of common symptoms experienced by the individual, and the capacity to undertake a nursing assessment to formulate the effective management of these symptoms, are required. The opportunity to normalise this significant life event, and to facilitate meaning and understanding of the experience for the family during and after the individual's death, is an important contribution for nurses. Having the opportunity to participate in such an experience affords the family a greater chance to engage with their grief in an uncomplicated manner during the individual's illness and subsequently in their bereavement.

The nurse is central in the provision of symptom assessment and management for individuals and their families requiring palliation[11-16]. Throughout this chapter, we explore specifically those symptoms most commonly identified as having the potential to compound suffering in individuals who are dying.

THE COMMON CLUSTER OF SYMPTOMS

Individuals who experience a chronic, life-threatening illness where curative and restorative outcomes are no longer viable often share a common cluster of symptoms at the end of their life. Evidence is now emerging acknowledging that individuals dying from chronic illnesses may also experience a similar set of symptoms to those experienced by an individual who is dying from cancer[6,8,17]. The symptoms most commonly identified[12,18] are:

- Fatigue;
- Pain;
- Nausea with or without vomiting;
- Constipation; and
- Dyspnoea.

This list of symptoms is not exhaustive, and you will encounter many other symptoms experienced by individuals in your nursing practice. However, the symptoms listed are representative of those *shared* by many people who are facing a life-limiting illness, regardless of the underlying disease, and which may be present in varying degrees. These symptoms have the greatest potential to adversely affect an individual and their family's quality of life if not treated effectively. An understanding of the symptoms, their cause and the ongoing management will provide you with the skills to intervene appropriately to promote comfort and a quality of life for the individual and their family.

The use of pharmacology in conjunction with non-pharmacological interventions can prove to be invaluable to the individual requiring palliation. Combined, these interventions may promote an improved quality of life for not only the individual experiencing the symptom but also for the family. The important issue to remember here when implementing non-pharmacological interventions is to review their efficacy and interactions with the prescribed medications through discussion with the individual's medical specialist and/or pharmacist[5,19,20].

Three case studies are introduced below which examine a variety of symptoms and their related initial management. The case studies are then re-introduced after further discussion of the above symptoms.

● Case study one

Kathy Anderson, 45, presented to the community health services via a referral for assistance with symptom management. Her symptoms were dull constant pain in her lower back and right rib area, decreased mobility, spasmodic slight nausea, decreased bowel elimination and decreased appetite.

Kathy had recently been diagnosed with breast cancer and bony metastases (right 5th rib/right hip). Kathy had been seen at the local cancer centre and had completed four cycles of chemotherapy, with no further plans for treatment. She agreed with the stated symptom management issues, but it was noted that she appeared breathless on minimal exertion.

● Case study two

Jane Cartwright, 52, had frequent admissions to the local teaching hospital over the past four years. She then presented with an exacerbation of her chronic obstructive pulmonary disease.

When the nurse attended her, Jane was propped up in a recliner presenting with severe dyspnoea and oxygen therapy in situ via nasal prongs. Jane stated that she had had a constant dull pain in her chest, which worsened when she got periods of increased breathlessness. She also stated that she could not eat much, and that going to the toilet was a real problem. You noted that she also had blue discolouring in her upper and lower extremities, as well as swelling in her lower extremities.

● Case study three

Antonio Renaldi, 78, migrated to Australia from Italy in 1955. Antonio worked as a market gardener since his arrival on a one-hectare site near a busy city road. His property had recently been subdivided, and Antonio had been experiencing moderate to severe short-term memory loss. Most recently, Antonio had experienced depression, early waking, and social withdrawal from his family. Following psychogeriatric assessment, including a Mini Mental Assessment (score 22/30) and a CT brain scan, he was diagnosed with Alzheimer's disease.

Antonio and his wife were visited by a community nurse, after he was referred following a fall. He had a long history of rheumatoid arthritis affecting his ankles and knees. The fall had left him with severe bruising to the left side of his body and face. He sustained a fractured right wrist and was unable to shower himself. The nurse assisted with showering and assessed his pain requirements.

LEARNING EXERCISES
1. Examine the three case studies and identify the symptoms shared by all these individuals.
2. How are these shared symptoms manifested within each of the individuals presented in the case studies?

On review of the case studies, the initial issue that should be apparent to you is that the people, their context and the underlying disease processes are all different. What should also be evident is the sharing of common symptoms between the case studies that are expressed differently as a result of their unique situations.

In case study one, Kathy is relatively young, has cancer and is receiving treatment; her cancer is aggressive and she has metastases. She wants help with her pain, due to the debilitating effect of the pain and her metastases – the reduction in her mobility, her nausea, her decreased bowel activity and her poor appetite. The nurse's role is to assess each of these areas, and to create a plan of care that is acceptable to, and can be managed by, Kathy and her carers.

In case study two, Jane's disease process is chronic obstructive pulmonary disease. Her key symptoms are dyspnoea, pain and constipation. The chronic nature of this disease means that Jane has suffered for a period of time and is likely to continue to suffer. The nurse's role is to ease or minimise that suffering, and give Jane a plan of care so that she can obtain assistance when she requires it. As in Kathy's case, education about her symptoms, their cause and their management will be an essential element of the care being provided by the nurse.

In case study three, Antonio's disease process is different again; however, he too will be treated using a palliative approach because his condition is incurable and has complex needs. Antonio is experiencing pain but no longer understands why. The nurse's aim is to provide interventions that will maintain his level of function and provide his wife and carers with the means to manage his behaviour and symptoms.

CLUSTER OF SYMPTOMS

FATIGUE

Fatigue is the first symptom that is the most frequently encountered symptom individual's and their families who experience a chronic illness and or who are dying experience, regardless of the underlying cause[21–22]. No one agreed definition exists for fatigue, but it is generally accepted that it is a subjective feeling of easy tiring, reduced capacity to perform activities, generalised weakness; impaired cognitive function; and emotional lability[22–25]. Fatigue may also be referred to as asthenia.

In the majority of individuals experiencing a chronic or end-stage illness, fatigue will be experienced, particularly towards the terminal stages. The underlying mechanisms of why fatigue develops in these individuals are not widely understood[22], but it is known that the impact of fatigue is significant on the individual's well-being, relationships with others, and their ability to perform cognitive and physical tasks[21,23]. Several contributing causes have been identified:

- The underlying disease;
- Treatment modalities;
- Stress and the effect on the central nervous system;
- Personal characteristics;
- Environmental factors;
- Drugs;
- Anaemia;
- Infection;
- Sleep disturbance;
- Cachexia; and
- Psychological, for example, depression, anxiety, boredom[5,21,23,25].

Fatigue is both multifactorial and multidimensional, and the individual's experience of the symptom is shaped by the degree to which biological, psychological, social and personal factors impact and affect the individual[18]. Several theories have been proposed to explain the underlying pathophysiology of this symptom[21]:

1. Accumulation theory suggests that fatigue is related to the accumulation of muscle metabolites that interfere with normal cellular function;
2. Depletion theory, where the individual experiences a significant loss of red blood cells leading to a reduction in their oxygen-carrying capacity and hypoxaemia;
3. Central nervous system model demonstrates the interface of more than one mechanism where a reduction in intracellular calcium in the peripheral nervous system has an impact on the central nervous system and subsequent muscular performance;
4. De-conditioning effect, where patients reduce their activity levels when they become ill which has a biochemical, physiological and behavioural effect on their perception of fatigue; and
5. Tumour effect, where lipolytic and proteolytic factors are produced by the tumour's cell membrane and cause disruption to the host's metabolic functions[5,21,22,24,25].

The complex and multidimensional nature of this symptom requires a comprehensive physical and mental health assessment to identify potential strategies to support the individual. Nurses have a responsibility, as with all other symptoms requiring palliation, to consider a variety of approaches for implementation and to undertake a holistic evaluation of their effectiveness[23]. Adoption of this approach into the nurse's practice has the potential to improve the symptom for the individual.

The use of medications to manage this symptom is often viewed as being limited, although the following have some beneficial effects: corticosteroids, megestrol acetate, and methylphenidate[21,22,23].

More commonly, it is the non-pharmacological interventions that are more frequently used as first line management, for example, balancing activity and rest, counselling, adaptation of physical activities, changing medications, education, promotion of sleep, controlling other symptoms[21,22,24].

As the end of life nears, increasing fatigue and drowsiness signal a natural decline towards death. It is at this time that no active fatigue management strategies are instituted but rather, the individual and their family are supported holistically by the nurse[21].

PAIN

Pain is consistently ranked highly in studies by individuals and their families as the symptom they most fear and find distressing[5,26,27]. Pain reportedly occurs in 75% of individuals with cancer and 65% of individuals dying from other causes[28], and yet, relief of pain and suffering can be achieved for most individuals who are dying[26]. The palliation of pain is achieved through accurate and continuous assessment undertaken by health professionals initially on presentation, regularly throughout the course of treatment, when changes in the individual's pain state occurs and by acting as the individual's advocate[27,29].

Collectively, the following two definitions convey the multidimensional nature of pain and therefore, the complexity in managing this symptom. Pain is 'an unpleasant sensory and emotional experience associated with actual and potential tissue damage, or described in terms of such damage'[30](p. 249). Importantly, 'pain is whatever the person says it is, and existing whenever the person says it does'[31](p. 95). The two definitions show how an individual has the capacity to express the impact of their pain in a number of ways: psychologically, behaviourally, psychosocially and/or spiritually[27]. In particular, the second definition highlights that the symptom of pain is a highly personal and subjective experience for the individual.

Pain arises for individuals who are dying from three sources:

1. As a direct consequence of the disease process, for example, infiltration of the malignancy to surrounding tissues, or following a myocardial infarction;
2. By the treatment which is undertaken, for example, chemotherapy, radiotherapy, surgery that subsequently causes injury to the surrounding nervous, muscle and visceral tissues[32]; and
3. As a consequence of concurrent problems worsening as the body changes, for example, chronic lower back pain worsened by deconditioning, ischaemic heart disease[5].

For some individuals, their pain may occur as a combination of all three sources, making their pain management a more complex entity.

Pain can be classified in several different ways. A brief review of the main categories of pain (acute, chronic) are described below, along with the three main physiological types (somatic, visceral and neuropathic)[5,28,32]. Some examples accompany the description and are related to individuals receiving palliation. A more detailed examination of pain theory and pathophysiology can be obtained from the recommended reading, listed at the conclusion of the chapter.

Acute pain is the result of recurrent or progressive tissue damage or inflammation, which serves to warn the individual of the injury and is usually a time-limited experience[32,33].

Pain of this nature has a rapid onset and is usually self-limiting once treatment is initiated, with a predictable outcome[5]. Acute pain produces the following signs reflecting a sympathetic nervous system response: tachycardia, tachypnoea, hypertension, sweating, pupillary dilatation and pallor[5,28].

By contrast, chronic pain results from a chronic pathological process and from repetitive stimulation of the central nervous system[28]. Chronic pain has an ill-defined onset, with the individual appearing withdrawn and depressed[5]. This type of pain continues to occur and may increase in its intensity, becoming more severe over time[5].

Somatic pain occurs as a result of the activation of nociceptors in cutaneous and deep musculoskeletal tissues that are stimulated by physical factors such as heat, pressure, distension, or chemical reactions such as injury and inflammatory processes[32]. This pain is often described as a constant, gnawing or aching sensation felt superficially and is mostly localised in its origin[5,27,28]. Examples may include bone metastases, soft tissue inflammation.

Visceral pain results from the infiltration, compression, distension, or stretching of the thoracic and abdominal viscera, and is often accompanied by other symptoms, such as nausea, vomiting and sweating[32]. This pain is often described as cramping, wavelike, deep, squeezing or pressure, and is often referred to cutaneous sites remote from the existing lesion[5,27,28,32]. An example may include liver metastases causing liver capsule distension resulting in referred shoulder tip pain.

Neuropathic pain is a consequence of an injury sustained to the peripheral and/or central nervous systems, where nerve impulses fail to be transmitted and alternate pathways established are painful[32]. The pain is often described as a numb, radiating, burning sensation, shock-like or electric[5,27,28]. Examples may include radiation-induced brachial plexopathy, spinal cord compression, cisplatin neuropathy. These descriptions support the nurse's assessment of how the pain is being felt by the individual, and allow for an accurate determination by the nurse of the type of pain the individual is experiencing (somatic, visceral, neuropathic) and therefore assist in the selection of the most appropriate treatment strategies for the individual.

New pain in an individual dying must be investigated thoroughly, as it may be the sign of infection, fracture, or a neurological problem that may be reversible[33].

The primary issue for individuals who are dying is that they are fearful of their pain and the potential impact the pain relief may have on their capacity to engage in normal activities of daily living. Unrelieved pain significantly impacts on all aspects of their quality of life and well-being – their physical, psychological, social and spiritual dimensions[27,34]. Unresolved pain becomes in itself a disease entity with physical changes occurring on the nervous system and leading to the exacerbation of the individual's suffering. Furthermore, if pain is not controlled, disruption to the individual's capacity to engage holistically within their social context potentiates the development of dysfunctional relationships[35,36].

For this reason, the nurse has a responsibility to undertake a systematic and comprehensive pain assessment to evaluate the pain needs of the individual, the effect of their responses on their family and to provide advocacy in this process[33]. This is achieved through: collection of the person's history; undertaking a physical assessment; utilising a pain scale; determining the level of interference to 'normal' function; a description of the pain and its location; an assessment of how their pain feels over a period of time; identification of any behavioural factors affecting their pain and social interaction capacity;

determining the effect of pain on their mood, sleep, capacity to cope, goals and finances; and assessing the ongoing impact the suffering has had on their spirituality[27,33].

Underpinning the pain management of individuals who are dying is the need for a comprehensive pain assessment that embraces The World Health Organization principles of: *by the ladder; by the clock* and *by mouth*[37]. The principle of *by the ladder* refers to a graduated step approach to the use of pharmacology, commencing with milder agents in the beginning and leading to the use of opioids when stronger pain is evident. In addition, adjuvant analgesics and non-opioids are used collectively along each step. Adjuvant analgesics are widely used in palliation and have the capacity to

1. Have an independent analgesic effect; or
2. Work synergistically with other agents to enhance comfort; or
3. Relieve other symptoms associated with pain, for example, anxiety[27].

See examples of adjuvant analgesics in Table 17.1. The *by the clock* principle operates on the premise that pharmacology is administered across a 24-hour time span and not according to an 'as needed basis'. This is particularly significant for palliative care clients; given the incurable nature of their disease, the impetus causing the pain is not able to be removed or reversed. Utilising the *by the clock* principle results in a constant flow of analgesia for the individual and prevents peaks and troughs. Where possible, it is preferred that pharmacology be administered *by mouth* as this is the simplest and least invasive route for the individual and in many instances, the most cost effective[27].

There are many pharmacology agents available for use by individuals experiencing pain when they are dying. Detailed below are some examples of pharmacology you may see in practice.

TABLE 17.1: SUMMARY OF PHARMACOLOGY USED TO MANAGE PAIN[5,28,29,38]	
Type of Pain Pathway	**Drug Groups and Examples**
Somatic	Non-opioids: paracetamol, ibuprofen, piroxicam, indomethacin, naproxen
	Opioids: morphine, oxycodone, codeine, fentanyl, methadone, hydromorphone, tramadol
Visceral	Non-Opioids: paracetamol, hyoscine butylbromide
	Opioids: morphine, oxycodone, codeine, methadone, hydromorphone, tramadol
Neuropathic	Opioids: morphine, oxycodone, codeine, hydromorphone, tramadol
	Anti-inflammatories: dexamethasone, ibuprofen, piroxicam, indomethacin, naproxen
	Anti-depressants: nortriptyline, amitriptyline, imipramine, doxepin, dothiepin
	Membrane stabilisers: sodium valproate, carbamazepine
	Spinal and regional analgesia: Epidural and Intrathecal: opioids, bupivacaine, clonidine

Constipation is the most commonly reported side effect in the use of opioids, and one that is preventable with the commencement of appropriate aperient regimes following accurate and regular assessment of bowel function undertaken by the nurse. It is also useful to note that any drug with an 'anti' prefix can exert anticholinergic effects, the result being a demonstrable effect on the gastrointestinal tract motility. When used as adjuvant analgesics, drugs such as antiemetics, antidepressants and anticonvulsants can further exacerbate the predilection to obstinate constipation in this client group caused by opioids. The goal in symptom management is to promote comfort and relieve suffering. Our responsibility lies in the prevention of this additional problem for the individual[27,29]. Further discussion on constipation as a symptom is discussed below.

As well as the individual use of pharmacology agents, there are other pharmacology preparations used to assist individuals with their pain management. These agents are known as adjuvant analgesics or co-analgesics[28,29]. They are often drugs used for other indications but which may produce an analgesic effect in certain situations[28,29]. In individuals requiring palliation, they are especially useful as they often possess an independent analgesic property in addition to their primary action; they have the capacity to work in combination with other agents to promote comfort or to relieve the associated symptoms of pain, for example, anxiety[27]. They are often used with drugs from all steps of the analgesic ladder. Examples of adjuvant analgesics include anti depressants, anti convulsants, membrane stabilizing drugs; corticosteroids, skeletal muscle relaxants, antispasmodics, bisphosphonates and local anaesthetics[27–29].

In addition to the extensive use of available pharmacology, non-pharmacological interventions are also used to assist in modifying the individual's perception of pain and may support the promotion of comfort and relief of suffering[27,29]. Some examples are presented below in Table 17.2. It is important for the nurse to remember that pain is

TABLE 17.2: SUMMARY OF NON-PHARMACOLOGICAL PAIN INTERVENTIONS[27,29]

Education

Counselling

Relaxation/meditation

Massage

Transcutaneous electrical nerve stimulation (TENS)

Heat/cold therapy

Acupuncture

Acupressure

Aromatherapy

Reflexology

Music therapy

Pet therapy

Hypnosis

multidimensional, and includes both physiological and emotional components. While pharmacological intervention primarily addresses the physiological component, many of the non pharmacological interventions may support the emotional component of pain. Often these interventions are used in conjunction with the pharmacological agents to enhance the efficacy of the pain management strategies collectively for the individual[27,28,34].

The most significant role a nurse can play when working with an individual experiencing pain is to be able to assess their pain effectively, and ensure that the appropriate treatments are implemented as a priority. The individual's description of the pain, and the intensity of the pain being described, becomes the most significant prompt for action, and will assist the nurse to review the appropriateness of the treatments that may already have been implemented. The description gives an indication of the type of pain being expressed. Once the nurse knows that the type of the pain may be somatic, or visceral or neuropathic or combinations of type in differing locations, the nurse has an indication of the physiological cause and the nature of the pathways being activated. It is then possible to review the current treatment(s) for efficacy, and assist in ensuring that appropriate pharmacological and non-pharmacological interventions are commenced specific to the type of pain and the amount or intensity being expressed[27,29].

NAUSEA WITH OR WITHOUT ASSOCIATED VOMITING

For most individuals, nausea and/or vomiting will be experienced at some point in their disease trajectory, either emanating from the underlying disease pathology or as a consequence of their treatment. Nausea and/or vomiting is significantly distressing to the individual and their family, and has the potential to severely impact on their quality of life[39–41].

By definition, nausea is when the individual experiences an unpleasant sensation that is often described as a feeling experienced in the back of the throat or epigastrium[40–42]. Nausea is often accompanied by vomiting or retching. Vomiting is a forceful expulsion of gastric contents through the mouth, while retching is the rhythmic, spasmodic contraction of the diaphragm and abdominal muscles[40–42].

The physiology of nausea and vomiting is a complex process and is controlled by the vomiting centre located in the brainstem[5,40]. The vomiting centre is stimulated by the central and peripheral neural pathways. The central pathways include the midbrain afferents, for example, anxiety, increased intracranial pressure; and the chemoreceptor trigger zone (CTZ), for example, medications, chemicals, biochemical abnormalities[5,40,41]. The peripheral pathways consist of: vagal afferents, for example, upper gastrointestinal tract, mechanical; the pharyngeal afferents, for example, irritation in the pharynx such as cough; and the vestibular system, for example, medications, brain tumours[5,40,41].

The vomiting centre, in response to the stimulation of one or all of the above pathways, reacts by stimulating the autonomic efferents to the gastrointestinal tract[5,39]. This interaction produces the typical autonomic symptoms of sweating, pallor, salivation and tachycardia[5,39], commonly associated with an episode of nausea and or vomiting.

Essential in planning the care for the individual experiencing nausea and or vomiting is to listen to the individual's story about their symptoms and through this, to ascertain potential causes. Additionally, a history of associated symptoms, dietary changes, current disease state, current medications and physical examination is undertaken, to provide a holistic assessment to determine the relevant nursing interventions[5,40,41].

The first-line management of nausea with or without vomiting is to identify and treat the underlying cause. In the individual receiving palliation, it is quite likely that their nausea and vomiting will be the result of the interplay of a number of pathways together, depending on the underlying disease pathology and/or treatment modality[18,39,40,41].

Even with the treatment of reversible causes, nausea often persists. As is the case in previously discussed symptoms, the management of nausea and vomiting must also be addressed holistically as the underlying cause is often multifactorial, therefore requiring the use of more than one pharmacological and/or non-pharmacological intervention being implemented concurrently[5].

The range of non-pharmacological interventions may include, but is not limited to: acupressure; relaxation therapy; therapeutic touch and massage; herbal remedies (e.g., ginger, slippery elm); meditation; reflexology; distraction; acupuncture[5,40-43].

As the specific cause of nausea and/or vomiting is so varied, no one pharmacological agent will provide resolution of the symptoms and frequently, combinations are used. Table 17.3 summarises some of the common pharmacology used in practice.

TABLE 17.3: SUMMARY OF PHARMACOLOGY USED TO MANAGE NAUSEA WITH OR WITHOUT VOMITING[5,40-43]

Type of Nausea/Vomiting Pathway	Drug Examples
Cerebral cortex (central)	Promethazine, haloperidol, lorazepam
Chemoreceptor trigger zone (central)	Haloperidol, promethazine, metoclopramide, $5HT_3$ antagonists e.g., ondansetron
Vestibular apparatus (central)	Cyclizine, hydroxyzine, promethazine, hyoscine, prochlorperazine
Gastrointestinal tract (peripheral)	Antacids, sucralfate, domperidone, metoclopramide, cisapride, promethazine, hyoscine, ondanestron

CONSTIPATION

By definition, constipation is when the individual experiences infrequent or difficult defaecation in comparison to their normal bowel movements[44-46]. For individuals who are dying, constipation is reported as one of the most common and distressing symptoms experienced (78%), regardless of the underlying cause.[46] However, this symptom has the capacity to be prevented when effectively assessed and management interventions implemented by the nurse.

When individuals are receiving palliation, it is a popular belief that, because individuals eat very little or do not eat at all, the outcome should be little or no faeces production. This in itself is untrue. The amount of production may slow down, but just as a baby consumes only fluid in its early life, it still produces faeces on a daily basis, so too does the individual who is dying[5,45].

In individuals who are dying, the most likely cause of their constipation is multifactorial[5,44]. These factors may be related to the individual's lifestyle, for example, diet, age, mobility, directly from the disease and/or from drug therapy, in particular opioid analgesia[44]. Listed below are some examples of factors that may lead to constipation in the individual requiring palliation:

1. Medications, such as opioids, antiparkinsonian drugs, $5HT_3$ antagonists, some types of chemotherapy, iron, antidepressants, diuretics, phenothiazines and antacids;
2. Metabolic issues, such as dehydration, fever, poor oral intake, vomiting, hypercalcaemia, hypokalemia and hyperthyroidism;
3. Psychological issues, such as depression, lack of privacy, changes in life routines, fear of incontinence/diarrhoea and a history of sexual abuse;
4. Nutritional issues, such as a low-residue diet, high in fats and sugars, low in fibre, poor fluid intake, nausea and vomiting;
5. Immobility, decreasing peristaltic action of the bowel;
6. Colorectal obstruction, and anal conditions, such as fissures, perianal abscess and haemorrhoids; and
7. Neurological issues, such as sacral nerve root infiltration, spinal cord compression and cerebral tumour[5,44–46].

Individuals who experience constipation may exhibit one or more of the following clinical signs: malaise, anorexia, abdominal bloating and distension, nausea, abdominal and/or rectal pain, urinary retention, incomplete rectal emptying, difficulty in evacuating stools, restlessness and confusion, and rectal diarrhoea (overflow)[5,44,45]. Nurses therefore have a responsibility to promote the individual's comfort, and to alleviate any distress associated with this symptom[45,46]. In addition, the potential complications of unresolved constipation consist of psychological, cognitve and physical consequences[45,46] and further exacerbate the individual's suffering.

Assessment of constipation is primarily directed at preventing complications and promoting the individual's comfort[45,46]. The assessment includes identification of risk factors, history of previous bowel function, presence of bowel sounds, history of aperient usage, physical assessment and function of the individual, review of lifestyle factors, the impact of the disease state, and a rectal examination to determine the presence or absence of faeces in the lower rectum[45,46].

Similar to previously discussed symptoms, the symptom of constipation is also multifactorial, and therefore requires the implementation of a variety of pharmacology and non-pharmacological interventions, to be used either singularly or concurrently. Table 17.4 summarises some of the common pharmacology used in practice.

Liquid-based medications can be contraindicated in palliative care clients who are in the end stage of their disease and who are exhibiting symptoms associated with the

TABLE 17.4: SUMMARY OF PHARMACOLOGY USED TO MANAGE CONSTIPATION[5,44–46]	
Type of Laxative	**Drug Examples**
Stimulant laxatives	Bisacodyl, senna, danthron
Osmotic laxatives	Sulfate, hydroxide, lactulose, sorbitol
Lubricants	Liquid paraffin, olive oil
Bulk-forming laxatives	Psyllium, methylcellulose
Saline laxatives	Magnesium hydroxide, magnesium citrate
Suppositories	Glycerine, bisacodyl, saline enemas

common terminal pathway, particularly weakness and fatigue. This is due to the potential for aspiration to be increased in this client group where their levels of consciousness vary and their weakened state precludes them from being able to protect their airway adequately.

DYSPNOEA

Dyspnoea is one of the common symptoms experienced by individuals with end-stage disease, regardless of the underlying cause. By definition, dyspnoea is when the individual experiences difficulty in breathing, manifesting as shortness of breath and/or laboured breathing[47–49]. While the breathing is due to altered physiology, it is also determined by the subjective experience of the individual. Depending on the underlying disease pathology, the nature of the respiratory problems experienced consist of one or more of the following with varying degrees of intensity: dyspnoea, cough or haemoptysis. The respiratory problems displayed by the individual may be acute or chronic, and are often a source of distress for the individual, the family and health professionals observing and providing care.

The cause of dyspnoea is related to one or more altered respiratory physiological processes as a result of the disease state increasing ventilatory demand, and may include

1. Increased respiratory effort to compensate for increased load, such as pleural effusion or obstruction of large airways;
2. Increased proportion of respiratory muscle required to maintain respiration, such as in muscle weakness, ascites;
3. Increased ventilatory requirements, such as hypoxaemia, hypercapnia, anaemia, congestive cardiac failure, haemorrhage; or
4. Reduced functional lung tissue leading to impaired ventilatory movement, such as pleural effusion, embolism and emphysema[47,50].

Commonly, the characteristic 'death rattle' sound is noted in the final phase of their disease. This symptom manifests when air passes over or through pooled secretions located in the oropharynx or bronchi. The audible gurgling, which may also be present, occurs because of the individual's lack of ability to expectorate pooled salivary secretions in the oropharyngeal region. The accompanying sound that emerges is very distressing to both the individual and the family. For many nurses, the symptom creates a sense of anxiety, as it has become synonymous with death in the clinical setting[47–52].

In planning for care in the palliative phase, the nurse undertakes an assessment of the individual to identify the interventions to implement, and subsequently evaluates their responsiveness. This consists of: determining the history of the symptom; the nature of onset (acute or chronic); whether it is affected by position or physical activity; responsiveness to current pharmacological agents; and identifying any precipitating factors, such as anxiety, fear[48–50].

The first-line management of dyspnoea is treatment of the underlying cause and symptoms, for example, primary obstruction due to lung cancer requiring surgery, or a blood transfusion to resolve an anaemic state secondary to disease pathology. From a palliative care perspective, care focuses on enabling individuals to have a degree of control over their dyspnoea so as to increase their capacity to re-engage in activities of living. The degree to which this is achievable is determined by the progressive nature of the disease and subsequent deterioration being experienced by the individual.

Management of dyspnoea consists of non-pharmacological and pharmacological interventions. The range of non-pharmacological interventions implemented is extensive and includes: optimising physical positioning; limiting and prioritising physical activity; use of relaxation techniques to manage anxiety; use of a room with cool, humidified air; a physical environment allowing a breeze, for example, open window, use of a fan; use of loose clothing; and oxygen therapy[5,47–50]. Other supportive measures, such as nebulised saline, steam, and physiotherapy, may also contribute to having a positive impact on the comfort of the individual and their family[5,47–50]. See Chapter 6 for further discussion of dyspnoea and its management.

As the disease progresses, the effectiveness of the supportive measures may be reduced and additional interventions or pharmacology may be required (see Table 17.5).

TABLE 17.5: SUMMARY OF PHARMACOLOGY USED TO MANAGE DYSPNOEA[5,47,49]	
Drug Group	**Drug Examples**
Opioids	Morphine via nebulizer, systemic morphine
Anxiolytics	Diazepam, lorazepam
Bronchodilators	Salbutamol via aerosol, aminophylline, theophylline
Corticosteroids	Prednisolone, dexamethasone
Mucolytics	Acetylcysteine via nebulizer, humidified air (steam, saline)
Anticholinergics	Hyoscine hydrobromide, haloperidol

COUGH

In some instances, dyspnoea may be accompanied by a cough. A cough occurs naturally to remove foreign pathogens from the respiratory system. The nature of the cough can be either dry or productive; this is principally determined by the underlying disease state. In a person experiencing end-stage disease, the cough results from stimulation of receptors located in the larynx, pharynx, or tracheobronchial tree[47,49].

A productive cough is often the result of hyperactivity of the receptor sites causing excess secretions to be produced. The individual may also be more susceptible to infective pathogens, resulting in an increased sputum production due to an inflammatory response[49]. Therefore, an infective process needs to be excluded or treated with an appropriate antibiotic[5]. The presence of cough for the individual contributes to their debilitated state by disturbing their sleep, causing fatigue and pain. Persistent coughing can also cause increased blood pressure, headache, ruptured vessels and pathological fractures[5,49,50].

The management of a cough is directly related to treating the underlying cause, and consists of non-pharmacological interventions and pharmacology (see Table 17.6).

Some examples of non-pharmacological interventions that may also support the individual, either independently or concurrently with pharmacological agents, include: avoidance of the stimuli that triggers the coughing; chest physiotherapy; avoidance of dehydration; humidification of room or inspired air; suctioning; positioning the individual into the most comfortable position[5,49,50].

TABLE 17.6: SUMMARY OF PHARMACOLOGY USED TO MANAGE COUGH[5,47-49]	
Drug Group	**Drug Examples**
Opioid (exert an antitussive effect)	Codeine, hydrocodone, morphine
Non-opioid antitussive	Dextromethorphan, pholcodine
Local anaesthetics	Lidocaine via nebulizer, bupivacaine via nebuliser
Mucolytics	Nebulized saline, inhalations e.g., menthol
Antitussive	Benzonatate

HAEMOPTYSIS

At times, blood streaks may be present in the individual's respiratory secretions as a result of blood vessels rupturing, usually due to a coughing episode and/or underlying disease pathology. In this context, a cough suppressant to reduce the incidence of coughing supports the individual adequately. In the case of severe haemoptysis, a very rare occurrence, the individual needs to be managed with opioids and anxiolytic pharmacology. The presence of severe haemoptysis signifies the terminal phase for the individual[47,50].

● Case studies (continued)

Twelve months have passed since the first contact with the individuals in the case studies.

In case study one, Kathy has regularly sought assistance from the local cancer centre. Centre staff over time have come to know her two teenage children well, with occasional contact with her husband who works full time. Kathy visits the local cancer centre for monthly pamidronate infusions, to treat her multiple bony secondaries. She is also having chemotherapy for a large liver metastasis, diagnosed only two weeks ago. Today, Kathy is complaining of severe, constant abdominal pain localised to her right upper quadrant. On observation, she is extremely pale, sweaty, tachycardic and tachypnoeic. She also complains of increased episodes of nausea and her bowels have not been open for the last five days.

In case study two, Jane has had seven admissions to hospital in the past year. On initial examination today, the nurse finds Jane still requires oxygen via nasal prongs but at a higher concentration. She is now unable to walk due to breathlessness, and still has the constant dull chest pain, which at times becomes quite sharp and radiates down her left arm. She appears to have lost a lot of weight and her extremities are a dark blue/purple colour. Many areas on her extremities have skin breaks noticeable, and there is a large area of ulceration on her left medial malleus. Eating has now become a major problem for her because she is unable to chew due to dyspnoea. Jane states she has suffered with constipation for the past three months and takes occasional laxatives.

In case study three, it is revealed that five months after initial contact, Antonio was referred to the community health services because his wife had become increasingly concerned about his behaviour, including becoming lost in his local area. He now requires continued prompting in his personal hygiene, and he is no longer able to dress himself. There are days when his arthritis leaves him unable to move freely. His wandering has increased, and his wife can no longer leave him alone to go shopping. He becomes agitated especially in the early evening, and spends his time looking for his brother Giovanni.

LEARNING EXERCISES

1. After reviewing each of the case studies, compare and contrast your initial contact to their current presentation.
2. How do you perceive their progression?
3. Identify the common issues and symptoms common to all three case studies.

In case study one, Kathy now presents the nurse with a different set of pain descriptors. She has severe, constant pain located within her abdominal region. The nurse must ascertain by physical and verbal assessment what is occurring. Could these descriptors be due to increasing size of secondary tumour growth causing increased abdominal pressure and pain? Could Kathy be experiencing haemorrhage of some description? Or does she have a severe constipation/bowel obstruction? The severity of Kathy's pain makes the nurse believe that Kathy is suffering a subcapsular bleed around her liver. This situation constitutes a palliative medical emergency due to the acute on chronic nature of the pain being experienced. Immediate medical and current analgesic review is required.

Discussion and education must occur with Kathy and her carer to maintain their awareness of causal issues and from this, Kathy and her carer have an increased ability to make informed decisions surrounding their own care outcomes.

In case study two, Jane has experienced changes to her whole health presentation. She describes a constant dull ache in her central chest region, but also describes spasmodic sharp radiating pain at times throughout the day. A medical and nursing physical and verbal assessment must be attended, due to the potential cardiac (angina) origin of this pain. The nurse may also look at other causal factors contributing to this pain, for example, extensive utilisation of inspiratory and expiratory muscle groups. But in this instance, the pain is due to cardiac insufficiency. Treatment is usually a combination of cardiac agents and opioid-based medications. See Chapter 5 for further discussion of ischaemic chest pain.

In case study three, Antonio has deteriorated since your last contact with him. He is becoming more dependent and less physically able. The pain he experiences in his knees and hands has diminished his ability to perform tasks; this pain overlaid on dementia is causing greater concerns for his wife and family. In assessing his pain and its impact, the nurse must review the type, location, intensity, causative and any exacerbating or relieving factors. The nurse must also consider nonverbal cues that Antonio may present which indicate his level of pain, such as aggression when he is walked or has his hand held. For Antonio, rest, heat and analgesia are likely to lead to the best outcomes for the relief of his pain and increased functionality. Assessment of his behaviour may also lead the nurse to recommend a review of his medications, and perhaps to begin discussions with his wife and family of residential placement for Antonio, either for respite or permanent care.

THE COMMON TERMINAL PATHWAY

At the beginning of the chapter, the concept of the *common terminal pathway* was introduced. The common terminal pathway is a trajectory almost totally independent of the underlying disease and evident in the final stage of the palliation continuum. The concept consists of the presence of the following symptoms, for which a reversible, treatable causative factor is not identifiable:

* Catabolic state (not simply not eating);
* Cachexia (anorexia and weight loss);
* Fatigue, lethargy and profound weakness; and
* Significant alteration in functional mobility[35,53–55].

From this, the terminal pathway is defined, is irreversible and allows accurate prediction of the individual's prognosis. The common terminal pathway, once evident within the individual, is used to re-orientate care approaches and options for the individual and their family. It is often at this time that the symptom needs for the individual may alter, either increasing, resolving or new ones being created, which require that the nurse continues to be diligent in undertaking holistic assessments of the individual and their family, so that their needs may be met[53,54].

As death approaches, individuals tolerate symptoms very poorly as a result of their significant weakness and general debility. In conjunction with the physical and psychological assessments being undertaken at this time, it is very necessary that all pharmacology and other treatment interventions be re-evaluated and their efficacy determined[53–55].

PATHOPHYSIOLOGY OF END-STAGE DISEASE

A common perception exists that people ultimately die because of a single body system stopping – 'his heart gave out', 'her kidneys failed', 'they got pneumonia from lying in bed'. These processes can indeed cause death and clearly do in some people. However, for the individual experiencing predictable death as the result of a progressive, chronic end-stage disease, death is rarely due to single organ failure. Within these individuals, there are in effect a number of systemic changes that occur, linked to the underlying irreversible disease pathology that by its very nature continues to assault or injure its host as the disease progresses[50,53].

Factors, such as loss of weight, loss of appetite, cachexia and loss of energy, are present regardless of the disease pathology. The presence of these factors co-existing in the individual's body signals a physical deterioration known as catabolism. A catabolic state exists when energy metabolism pathways are no longer functioning normally and energy is expended in large amounts. This systemic change is mediated, in part, by the response of the body to the insult, that is, the existence of disease that can no longer be effectively controlled (neoplasm, organ failure, viral load from AIDS)[50,53,56].

The process of catabolism is mediated by chemicals secreted by the body in response to a number of both normal and pathological processes. These chemicals, known as cytokines, include tumour necrosis factor, interleukin 1 and interleukin 6. It is important to understand that cytokines are secreted normally as a homeostatic response to maintain normal function, and are released in larger amounts in response to infection or inflammation. In processes of overwhelming insult resulting from chronic illness or irreversible disease, the body continues to secrete increasing amounts of these cytokines, as the normal triggers to stop production are inhibited. In individuals with chronic progressive disease, the continued production of cytokines actually initiates a cascade of decline denoting the common terminal pathway (loss of weight, loss of appetite and markedly reduced energy). Once the common terminal pathway is evident, attempts to curb the weight loss and subsequent anorexia are futile, as the process cannot be reversed without effective treatment of the underlying cause. Care approaches that attempt to increase dietary and fluid intake are inappropriate and ultimately enhance the burden of the end-stage phase for the individual and their family[53, 56].

In individuals where the common terminal pathway is evident, the disease prognosis can be reasonably well delineated by looking at the systemic changes being displayed in the individual, for example, the speed of the weight loss and complete absence of interest in any food. Once this is determined, assessment of the changes and the level of function able to be sustained by the individual can be used to guide the development of appropriate supportive care[54,56].

When the individual moves into the terminal phase of their illness, the nurse has a responsibility to reassess the symptoms being experienced by the individual and their associated management. Due to the changing physical and psychological state of the individual, all current pharmacology and other interventions require ongoing review, to ensure that the most appropriate and effective interventions are implemented at this time, to ensure optimal outcomes for the individual and their family[5,12–16].

REFLECTIVE EXERCISE

In trying to conceptualise the cellular changes occurring at the time that the common terminal pathway becomes evident, recall how you felt when you last had the 'flu'. Exhausted? No energy? No appetite? How you feel at the height of the flu is how many of these individuals feel every day during the terminal phase of their life.

When you have the flu, the tumour necrosis factor is being released in moderated amounts as a normal response to the infection; when the infective process begins to reverse you feel better as the infection resolves. In individuals exhibiting the common terminal pathway, there is no resolution because of the presence of progressive disease; therefore, the process is not self-limiting[54,56].

● Case studies (continued)

More time has passed and it is relevant to examine the progress of each of the individuals in the three case studies.

In case study one, six weeks have passed since the last visit. This time, the nurse finds Kathy in bed, where she states she now spends most of her time. She says it takes a lot of energy to get up and do things in the house, but on a positive note, her pain seems well controlled at the moment. She also states she is not eating much and has no interest in food. The nurse notes Kathy has lost a lot of weight over the past six weeks. The nurse also notes that the children are at home with their mother, her husband has reduced his work to part-time, and Kathy's mother is living in the house when he is away. Her friends have organised a roster to help with cooking and to be there when her mother or husband are not. Kathy is dying, and expresses that she is now resigned to her death and is actively making plans for her funeral. Her dearest wish is to die at home, with her family and friends around her. The nurse feels that Kathy will get her wish and that it will not be very long before she dies.

In this case, Kathy's wishes are well known and should be respected. There is no advantage in her being admitted to hospital or palliative care unit with the support structure that has been created at home. She is being kept comfortable and is having her physical, psychosocial and spiritual needs well met. The nurse should focus on and address any of Kathy's symptoms, and provide support to the network of carers that have amassed. For Kathy, a comfortable death in the company of her family should be a shared goal for the nurse.

In case study two, Jane is examined in hospital again. She is now completely bedbound and states she cannot talk for too long, as it is too exhausting. Her breathlessness is extreme on minor movement, and her anxiety levels rise very quickly with minimal interaction. She cannot eat any solid food, only consuming fluids and ice to suck. Her urine output is low and dark in colour; she appears cachectic and is sleeping for long periods. Jane says she feels she 'can't go on much longer, she is so tired and each breath is an effort'. Jane too is dying, and the nurse believes she will not see out the end of the week.

Jane will die comfortably in the hospital; the nursing staff will aim to ease her suffering and may find positioning her out of bed with oxygen via nasal prongs more useful than bed rest. Jane should be moved gently and without effort on her part. Discussion with her about her spiritual needs should take place and the availability of a pastoral care worker may be helpful. In any case, Jane should feel comfortable about dying and be given permission to let go.

In case study three, Antonio is admitted to your nursing home. He has had repeated respite care in the facility over the past year, and has had a steady decline in self-care, to the point where he is now requiring full-time care. He has recently wandered in the night onto the busy road outside his home and is in danger of injury.

Three weeks ago, Antonio had a fall and fractured his right femur. He was treated at the local hospital with open reduction and internal fixation (pin and plate) of the shaft of femur, and has been unsuccessful in regaining full mobility despite physiotherapy.

Today, Antonio is in a chair for his safety, refusing breakfast or fluids. He is confused and babbling in Italian. You note that Antonio is thin, weak and pale, with obvious muscle wasting to his legs and arms. On further inspection, his temples are hollowed, eyes sunken, shoulders bony, collarbones prominent, and he has a dry tongue. He is becoming more cachectic and looks like he may not survive the rest of the week. His family spend time with him keeping vigil at his bedside.

Antonio's immobility has reduced his need for food, and he has reached the end-stage of his dementia. He is disinterested in eating and will only tolerate small sips of water before dropping off to sleep again. He winces when turned every second hour and when his knees are moved. He has generalised weakness and no energy. Cachexia has reduced his muscle mass, and his skin is now thin and easily broken, and shows evidence of skin tears on his lower legs. The nurse must continue to treat Antonio gently, to ensure that his skin does not break, and try to encourage him to drink.

His wife and family are constant visitors, and the nurse should encourage them to become involved in his care and to talk about their concerns. It is also important to encourage them to look after themselves and ensure they get adequate rest. Suggesting that they visit in shifts is a good idea, especially when there is a large number in the family.

LEARNING EXERCISES

1. Identify the presence of the common terminal pathway in each of the case studies.
2. How does it present?
3. What are the similarities for each of the case studies?

When caring for an individual in end stage-disease, consider any change in functional status. If they have been mobile and able to function relatively independently one week, and then become chair or bed fast the next week due to deterioration in energy levels and strength, this is significant in terms of prognosis. This pattern denotes that ultimate death can be potentially predicted in relation to the speed of the deterioration. By applying this principle, the nurse is more able to guide appropriate care and goal setting for the individual and their family[55].

As the presence of the terminal pathway continues, a more systemic effect is apparent and you will notice a significant deterioration in the individual just prior to their death. Generally, the key indicators of impending death are

- Weakened pulse;
- Gradual fall in blood pressure;
- Shallow and slower respirations;
- Consciousness is slowly lost;
- Peripheral skin becomes colder and clammy; and
- Skin around the mouth and extremities becomes cyanotic[35,50,54,55].

It is during this time that pharmacology previously prescribed for symptom management is reviewed in the light of changing symptoms and deteriorating function[53,54].

Continuation of medication regimes designed to alleviate or minimise suffering in the individual, utilising the principles of by the clock and by the ladder described earlier, remain paramount during this phase. During this period of the disease trajectory, as death becomes more imminent, you will also need to review the appropriateness of the prescribed route of pharmacological interventions. It is at this time that individuals may require their drug therapy delivered in a different form or via a different route, for example, subcutaneous delivery of opioids, liquid versus tablet form of medications where appropriate[35,54,55].

Individuals are frequently unconscious in the last days to hours of life, and no longer possess the ability to express their levels of pain and discomfort. This has the potential for their pain management not to be maintained according to the best practice principles outlined in this chapter. Remember that the irreversible disease process in these individuals continues until death; therefore, vigilant continuation of all appropriate strategies aimed at the amelioration of their cluster of symptoms must continue until death occurs[54,55].

CONCLUSION

Caring for an individual dying and their family can be a challenging and confronting experience for both the beginning and experienced nurse irrespective of the underlying disease. The principles outlined in this chapter are related to the assessment and management of the more common cluster of symptoms shared by individuals dying from a chronic, life threatening illness where curative and restorative outcomes are no longer viable. They include: developing an understanding of the pathophysiology involved in the disease trajectory; actively listening and being responsive to the needs expressed by the individual dying and their family, ensuring a palliative care approach is implemented at an appropriate point along the illness continuum for that individual and their family; and understanding the cultural, psychosocial and spiritual context in which your individual and their family live. Adopting these principles into your nursing practice will enable you to deliver individually tailored, culturally sensitive palliative care to all individuals dying, regardless of the disease state or health care setting. The following words will help:

> Conversation, openness and willingness to discuss death might be part of the new courage. The courage of talk and tears. It is through this that we lift the taboo . . . a gentle death, a strong death, near those you love and who care for you, knowing you have lived and, in dying, been allowed to live creatively'[57] (p. 346).

Recommended Readings

Atkinson, J & Videe, A. 2001; 'Promoting Comfort for Patients with Symptoms Other Than Pain', in S Kinghorn & R Gamlin (eds.), *Palliative Nursing Bringing Comfort and Hope*), Ballière Tindall, Edinburgh, 43–62.

Barham, D. 2002; 'The Last 48 Hours', *Contemporary Nurse*, 13 (2), 179–191.

Faull, C & Hirsch, C. 2000; 'Symptom Management in Palliative Care', *Professional Nurse*, 16 (1), 840–843.

Payne, R, Gonzales, GR. 2003; 'Pathophysiology of Pain in Cancer and Other Terminal Diseases', in D Doyle, G Hanks, N Cherny & K Calman (eds.), *Oxford Textbook of Palliative Medicine* (3rd ed.), Oxford University Press, Oxford, 288–298.

Porock, D. 2003; 'Fatigue', in M O'Connor & S Aranda (eds.), *Palliative Care Nursing: A Guide to*

Practice (2nd ed.), Ausmed, Melbourne, 137–152.

Wildiers, H & Menten, J. 2002; 'Death Rattle Prevalence, Prevention and Treatment', *Journal of Pain and Symptom Management*, 23 (4), 310–317.

Woof, R, Carter, Y, Harrison, B, Faull, C & Nyatanga B. 1998; 'Terminal Care and Dying', in *Handbook of Palliative Care*, Blackwell Science, London, 307–332.

References

1. Klinkenberg, M, Willems, DL, van der Wal, G & Deeg, JH. 2004; 'Symptom Burden in the Last Week of Life', *Journal of Pain and Symptom Management*, 1, 5–13.

2. Steinhauser, KE, Christakis, NA, Clipp, EC, McNeilly, M & Mcintyre, L. 2000; 'Factors Considered Important at the End of Life by

Patients, Family, Physicians and Other Care Providers', *Journal of American Medical Association*, 284, 2476–2482.

3. Najman, J. 2000; 'The Demography of Death: Patterns of Australian Mortality', in A Kellehear (ed.), *Death & Dying in Australia*, Oxford University Press, Melbourne.

4. Australian Institute of Health and Welfare. 2002; *Australia's Health 2002*, Australian Institute of Health and Welfare, Canberra.

5. Woodruff, R. *Palliative Medicine* (4th ed.), Oxford University Press, Melbourne.

6. Skillbeck, J & Payne, S. 2003; 'Palliative Care in Chronic Illness', in M O'Connor & S Aranda (eds.), *Palliative Care Nursing: A Guide to Practice* (2nd ed.), Ausmed, Melbourne.

7. Taylor, GJ, Kurent, JE, Heffner, JE & Brescia, FJ. 2003; 'Palliation for Chronic Illness', in GJ Taylor & JE Kurent (eds.), *A Clinician's Guide to Palliative Care*, Blackwell Science, Malden, MA.

8. Fallon, M. 2004; 'Palliative Medicine in Non Malignant Disease', in D Doyle, G Hanks, N Cherny & K Calman (eds.), *Oxford Textbook of Palliative Medicine* (3rd ed.), Oxford University Press, Oxford.

9. World Health Organization. 2002; *National Cancer Control Programs Policies and Managerial Guidelines* (2nd ed.), World Health Organization, Geneva.

10. Currow, D. 2002; 'State of Palliative Service Provision', *Journal of Pain and Symptom Management*, 2 (24), 170–172.

11. Brodsky, J, Habib, J, Hirschfeld, MJ (eds.). 2003; *Key Policy Issues in Long Term Care*. http://www.who.int/ncd/long_term_care/index.htm

12. Aranda, S. 2003; 'A Framework for Symptom Assessment', in M O'Connor & S Aranda (eds.), *Palliative Care Nursing: A Guide to Practice* (2nd ed.), Ausmed, Melbourne.

13. Roberts, A & Bird, A. 2001; 'Assessment of Symptoms', in S Kinghorn & R Gamlin (eds.), *Palliative Nursing Bringing Comfort and Hope*, Baillière Tindall, Edinburgh.

14. Glass, E, Cluxton, D & Rancour, P. 2001; 'Principles of Patient and Family Assessment', in BR Ferrell & N Coyle (eds.), *Textbook of Palliative Nursing*, Oxford University Press, New York.

15. Faull, C. 2000; 'Symptom Management in Palliative Care', *Professional Nurse*, 16, 840–843.

16. Abrahm, J. 1998; 'Promoting Symptom Control in Palliative Care', *Seminars in Oncology Nursing*, 14 (2), 95–109.

17. Connolly, M. 2001; 'The Disadvantaged Dying – Care of People with Non Malignant Conditions', in S Kinghorn & R Gamlin (eds.), *Palliative Nursing Bringing Comfort and Hope*, Baillière Tindall, Edinburgh.

18. Atkinson, J & Virdee, A. 2001; 'Promoting Comfort for Patients with Symptoms Other Than Pain', in S Kinghorn & R Gamlin (eds.), *Palliative Nursing Bringing Comfort and Hope*, Baillière Tindall, Edinburgh.

19. Zollman, C & Thompson, E. 1998; 'Complementary Approaches to Palliative Care', in C Faull, Y Carter & R Woof (eds.), *Handbook of Palliative Care*, Blackwell Science, Oxford.

20. McCabe, P & Kenny, A. 2003; 'Complementary Therapies', in M O'Connor & S Aranda (eds.), *Palliative Care Nursing: A Guide to Practice* (2nd ed.), Ausmed, Melbourne.

21. Porock, D. 2003; 'Fatigue', in M O'Connor & S Aranda (eds.), *Palliative Care Nursing: A Guide to Practice* (2nd ed.), Ausmed, Melbourne.

22. Sweeney, C, Neuenschwander, H & Bruera, E. 2004; 'Fatigue and Asthenia', in D Doyle, G Hanks, N Cherny & K Calman (eds.), *Oxford Textbook of Palliative Medicine* (3rd ed.), Oxford University Press, Oxford.

23. Woof, R. 1998; 'Asthenia, Cachexia and Anorexia', in C Faull, Y Carter & R Woof (eds.), *Handbook of Palliative Care*, Blackwell Science, Oxford.

24. Dean, GE & Anderson, P. 2001; 'Fatigue', in BR Ferrell & N Coyle (eds.), *Textbook of Palliative Nursing*, Oxford University Press, New York.

25. McKinnon, S. 2002; 'Fatigue', in KK Kuebler, PH Berry & DE Heidrich (eds.), *End of Life Care Clinical Practice Guidelines*, W.B. Saunders, Philadelphia.

26. Yurk, R, Morgan, D, Franey, MA, Stebner, JB & Lansky, D. 2002; 'Understanding the Continuum of Palliative Care for Patients and Their Care Givers', *Journal of Pain and Symptom Management*, 24, 459–470.

27. Brant, J. 2003; 'Pain Management', in M O'Connor & S Aranda (eds.), *Palliative Care Nursing: A Guide to Practice* (2nd ed.), Ausmed, Melbourne.

28. Forbes, K & Faull, C. 1998; 'The Principles of Pain Management', in C Faull, Y Carter & R Woof (eds.), *Handbook of Palliative Care*, Blackwell Science, Oxford.

29. Paice, JA & Fine, PG. 2001; 'Pain at the End of Life', in BR Ferrell & N Coyle (eds.), *Textbook of Palliative Nursing*, Oxford University Press, New York.

30. International Association for the Study of Pain, Subcommittee on Taxonomy. 1979; 'Pain Terms: A List with Definitions and Notes on Usage', *Pain*, 6, 249–252.

31. McCaffery, M. 1968; *Nursing Practice Theories Related to Cognition, Bodily Pain and Man-Environment Interactions*, UCLA Press, Los Angeles.

32. Payne, R & Gonzales, GR. 2004; 'Pathophysiology of Pain in Cancer and Other Terminal Diseases', in D Doyle, G Hanks, N Cherny & K Calman (eds.), *Oxford Textbook of Palliative Medicine* (3rd ed.), Oxford University Press, Oxford.

33. Fink, R & Gates, R. 2001; 'Pain Assessment', in BR Ferrell & N Coyle (eds.), *Textbook of Palliative Nursing*, Oxford University Press, New York.

34. Farrer, K. 2001; 'Pain Control', in S Kinghorn & R Gamlin (eds.), *Palliative Nursing Bringing Comfort and Hope*, Baillière Tindall, Edinburgh.

35. Woof, R, Carter, Y, Harrison, B, Faull, C & Nyatanga, B. 1998; 'Terminal Care and Dying', in C Faull, Y Carter & R Woof (eds.), *Handbook of Palliative Care*, Blackwell Science, Oxford.

36. Kissane, D & Yates, P. 2003; 'Psychological and Existential Distress', in M O'Connor & M Aranda (eds.), *Palliative Care Nursing: A Guide to Practice* (2nd ed.), Ausmed, Melbourne.

37. World Health Organization (WHO). 1990; *Cancer Pain Relief and Palliative Care. Report of a WHO Expert Committee.*

38. Hanks, G, Cherny, N & Fallon, M. 2004; 'Opioid Analgesic Therapy', in D Doyle, G Hanks, N Cherny & K Calman (eds.), *Oxford Textbook of Palliative Medicine* (3rd ed.), Oxford University Press, Oxford.

39. Mannix, K. 2004; 'Palliation of Nausea and Vomiting', in D Doyle, G Hanks, N Cherny & K Calman (eds.), *Oxford Textbook of Palliative Medicine* (3rd ed.), Oxford University Press, Oxford.

40. Millership, R. 2003; 'Nausea and Vomiting', in M O'Connor & S Aranda (eds.), *Palliative Care Nursing: A Guide to Practice* (2nd ed.), Ausmed, Melbourne.

41. King, CR. 2001; 'Nausea and Vomiting', in BR Ferrell & N Coyle (eds.), *Textbook of Palliative Nursing*, Oxford University Press, New York.

42. Griffie, J & McKinnon, S. 2002; 'Nausea and Vomiting', in KK Kuebler, PH Berry & DE Heidrich (eds.), *End of Life Care Clinical Practice Guidelines*, W.B. Saunders, Philadelphia.

43. Fallon, M & Welsh, J. 1998; 'The Management of Gastrointestinal Symptoms', in C Faull, Y Carter & R Woof (eds.), *Handbook of Palliative Care*, Blackwell Science, Oxford.

44. Sykes, N. 2004; 'Constipation and Diarrhoea', in D Doyle, G Hanks, N Cherny & K Calman (eds.), *Oxford Textbook of Palliative Medicine* (3rd ed.), Oxford University Press, Oxford.

45. Bailey, B. 2003; 'Constipation', in M O'Connor & S Aranda (eds.), *Palliative Care Nursing: A Guide to Practice* (2nd ed.), Ausmed, Melbourne.

46. Economou, DC. 2001; 'Bowel Management: Constipation, Diarrhoea, Obstruction and Ascitities', in BR Ferrell & N Coyle (eds.), *Textbook of Palliative Nursing*, Oxford University Press, New York.

47. Chan, KS, Sham, MK, Tse, D & Thorsen, AB. 2004; 'Palliative Medicine in Malignant Respiratory Diseases', in D Doyle, G Hanks, N Cherny & K Calman (eds.), *Oxford Textbook of Palliative Medicine* (3rd ed.), Oxford University Press, Oxford.

48. Bredin, M. (2003); 'Breathlessness', in M O'Connor & S Aranda (eds.), *Palliative Care Nursing: A Guide to Practice* (2nd ed.), Ausmed, Melbourne.

49. Dudgeon, D. 2001; 'Dyspnea, Death Rattle and Cough', in BR Ferrell & N Coyle (eds.), *Textbook of Palliative Nursing*, Oxford University Press, New York.

50. Kemp, C. 1999; *Terminal Illness* (2nd ed.), Lippincott, Philadelphia.

51. Kass, RM & Ellershaw, J. 2003; 'Respiratory Tract Secretions in the Dying Patient: A Retrospective Study', *Journal of Pain and Symptom Management*, 26, 897–902.

52. Wildiers, H & Menten, J. 2002; 'Death Rattle: Prevalence, Prevention and Treatment', *Journal of Pain and Symptom Management*, 23, 310–317.

53. Furst, CJ & Doyle, D. 2004; 'The Terminal Phase', in D Doyle, G Hanks, N Cherny & K Calman (eds.), *Oxford Textbook of Palliative Medicine* (3rd ed.), Oxford University Press, Oxford.

54. Berry, PH, Griffie, J & Heidrich, DE. 2002; 'The Dying Process', in KK Kuebler, PH Berry & DE Heidrich (eds.), *End of Life Care Clinical Practice Guidelines*, W.B. Saunders, Philadelphia.

55. Berry, P & Griffie, J. 2001; 'Planning for the Actual Death', in BR Ferrell & N Coyle (eds.), *Textbook of Palliative Nursing*, Oxford University Press, New York.

56. Arnold, G. 2001; 'The Pathophysiology of Death and the Dying Process', in B Poor & G Poirrer, *End of Life Nursing Care*, Jones and Bartlett & National League for Nursing, Canada.

57. Cline, S. 1995; 'Lifting the Taboo: Women, Death and Dying', Little Brown & Company, London.

Index